Inflammatory Response in Cardiovascular Surgery

Edmo Atique Gabriel • Sthefano Atique Gabriel
Editors

Inflammatory Response in Cardiovascular Surgery

Springer

Editors
Edmo Atique Gabriel
Department of Cardiovascular
Surgery University Nove de Julho
São Paulo
Brazil

Sthefano Atique Gabriel
Department of Vascular Surgery
Pontifical Catholic University of Campinas
São Paulo
Brazil

ISBN 978-1-4471-4428-1 ISBN 978-1-4471-4429-8 (eBook)
DOI 10.1007/978-1-4471-4429-8
Springer London Heidelberg New York Dordrecht

Library of Congress Control Number: 2013940098

Printed on acid-free paper

Springer is part of Springer Science+Business Media (www.springer.com)

This book is dedicated to God and to our parents Edmo Gabriel and Maria Lucia Atique Gabriel.

Edmo Atique Gabriel
Sthefano Atique Gabriel

Preface

The inflammatory response is of vital importance in any kind of cardiovascular procedure. However, for several years, this concept has been underestimated and overlooked worldwide. This textbook is intended to serve as a useful tool to provide information on the inflammatory response in cardiovascular surgery.

The scope of this textbook is of interest to various professionals, such as cardiovascular surgeons, vascular surgeons, transplantation physicians, anesthesiologists, intensive care physicians, cardiovascular and vascular fellows, basic science physicians, students, and researchers.

It is divided into sections on general topics, vascular and cardiovascular subjects of great importance for understanding the surgical inflammatory universe. Arranging topics into vascular and cardiovascular sections was difficult but key as there are many details and particularities related to vascular diseases as well as to cardiovascular or cardiothoracic diseases.

Immunologic and physiologic concepts are clarified from the early stages of the book with the aim of preparing readers for the subsequent discussions. For this purpose, topics such as the neuroendocrine response, pathogenesis of atherosclerosis, and mechanisms of inflammation are meticulously addressed. Moreover, these preliminary chapters are fundamental to a better understanding of the inflammatory response in all cardiovascular diseases.

Later chapters elucidate the inflammatory aspects of carotid, venous, arterial, and abdominal aortic aneurysm, peripheral aneurysm, trauma, and visceral pathologies. However, all were written emphasizing the surgical view of pathologic conditions.

In the section about carotid disease, we discuss in detail the inflammatory aspects present in both endarterectomy and carotid angioplasty – two important therapeutic options in the treatment of ischemic brain disease. In the section about abdominal aortic aneurysm, we emphasize its pathogenesis and associated inflammatory aspects, and we include chapters related to endovascular treatment of abdominal aortic aneurysm and endovascular treatment of ruptured abdominal aortic aneurysm.

In the section on critical limb ischemia, we address approaches to arteritis responsible for limb ischemia and include comments on a very current topic   transplantation for limb salvage. In the section on venous disease, we focus on the aspects involved in the inflammation and origin of thromboembolic complications.

Likewise, the cardiovascular or cardiothoracic sections are systematically organized in such a way that general topics as such cardiopulmonary bypass and thyroid hormones come before specific topics such as coronary artery, valve, and congenital heart diseases, thoracoabdominal aneurysm, heart/lung transplantation, ventricular assist devices, and stem cells. On these many featured topics, the authors provide a broad range of very interesting information about inflammation from surgical perspective.

In addition to the traditional topics in cardiovascular surgery, new discussions, for example on the inflammatory aspects of cardiovascular surgery for lung protection, inflammatory aspects related to heart and lung transplantation, both in children and in adults, and the role of stem cells in cardiovascular surgery are included.

We wish to thank all contributors who spent time and made untiring efforts to provide information about the inflammatory response in cardiovascular surgery by writing great chapters. Finally, we express our gratitude to the publisher, Springer, for giving us the opportunity to put together a textbook on the remarkable concept of the inflammatory response in cardiovascular surgery.

Sao Paulo, Brazil Edmo Atique Gabriel
Sao Paulo, Brazil Sthefano Atique Gabriel

Acknowledgments

We thank Springer for the diligent attention and assistance they provided us and for their efforts to make this book possible.

Edmo Atique Gabriel
Sthefano Atique Gabriel

Contents

Part IV Critical Lower Limb Ischemia

Part V Vascular Trauma

Part VI Venous Diseases

Part VII Visceral Vasculopathy

Part VIII Peripheral Aneurysms

Contributors

Fernando C. Abrão MD Department of Surgery, Faculty of Medicine, University of Sao Paulo, Hospital Sao Jose, São Paulo, Brazil

Ahmet Ruchan Akar, MD, FRCS CTh Department of Cardiovascular Surgery, Heart Center, Ankara University School of Medicine, Dikimevi, Ankara, Turkey

Department of Multi-disciplinary Stem Cell and Regenerative Medicine, Stem Cell Institute, Ankara University, Ankara, Turkey

Nasser Alkhamees, MD Divisions of Cardiac Surgery and Surgical Research, Department of Surgery, McGill University Health Center, Montreal, QC, Canada

Johane Allard, MD Department of Medicine, University Health Network (UHN), Toronto, ON, Canada

Vania Rozas Almeida Servicio Cardiovascular, National Institute of Thorax, Providencia, Santiago, Chile

George A. Antoniou, MD, PhD Department of Vascular and Endovascular Surgery, Manchester Royal Infirmary, Central Manchester University Hospitals NHS Foundation Trust, Manchester, UK

Bianca Arendt, PhD Department of Medicine, University Health Network (UHN), Toronto, ON, Canada

Manuela Aspalter, MD Department of Vascular and Endovascular Surgery, PMU Salzburg, Salzburg, Austria

Efthymios D. Avgerinos, MD, FEBVS Department of Vascular Surgery, Medical School of Athens, Attikon University Hospital, Athens, Greece

Estela Azeka, MD, PhD Pediatric Cardiology and Adult Congenital Heart Disease Unit, Heart Institute (InCor), University of Sao Paulo Medical School, Sao Paulo, Sao Paulo, Brazil

Todd L. Berland, MD Department of Surgery, New York University Medical Center, New York, NY, USA

Jean Bismuth, MD The Methodist DeBakey Heart and Vascular Center, The Methodist Hospital, Houston, TX, USA

Jonathan T. Butcher, PhD Department of Biomedical Engineering, Cornell University, Ithaca, NY, USA

Neal S. Cayne, MD Department of Surgery, New York University Medical Center, New York, NY, USA

Ricard Cervera, MD, PhD, FRCP Department of Autoimmune Diseases, Hospital Clinico, University of Barcelona, Barcelona, Spain

Chung-Wai Chow, MD Lung Transplant Program, University of Toronto, Toronto, ON, Canada

Andrea Colli, MD, PhD Department of Cardiovascular Surgery, Cardiac Surgery Unit, University of Padova, Padova, Italy

Alberto José da Silva Duarte, PhD Clinical Laboratory, Hospital do Coração, São Paulo, Brazil

Faculty of Medicine, Universidade de São Paulo, São Paulo, Brazil

Central Laboratory of the Hospital das Clínicas, Faculty of Medicine, Universidade de São Paulo, São Paulo, Brazil

Laboratory of Medical Investigation Unit 56, Faculty of Medicine, University of Sao Paulo, São Paulo, Brazil

Alan Dardik, MD, PhD VA Connecticut Healthcare System, West Haven, CT, USA

Department of Surgery and the Interdepartmental Program in Vascular Biology and Therapeutics, Yale University School of Medicine, New Haven, CT, USA

Michael Dashwood, PhD Department of Clinical Biochemistry, Royal Free and University College Medical School, London, UK

Cyro Alves de Brito, PhD Center of Immunology, Adolfo Lutz Institute, São Paulo, Brazil

Juliana Lech de Camargo Department of Medicine, University of Taubate, Sao Paulo, Brazil

Otacilio de Camargo Júnior Pontifical Catholic University of Campinas, Department of Vascular/Endovascular Surgery, Celso Pierro Maternity Hospital, Sao Paulo, Brazil

Department of Vascular Surgery, Pontifical Catholic University of Campinas, Sao Paulo, Brazil

Armando de Carvalho Lobato, PhD Department of Vascular and Endovascular surgery, Institute of Vascular and Endovascular Surgery of Sao Paulo, (ICVE-SP), Sao Paulo, Brazil

Vascular and Endovascular Surgery, Portuguese Beneficent Hospital of Sao Paulo, Sao Paulo, Brazil

Faculty of Medicine, University of Sao Paulo, Sao Paulo, Brazil

Brazilian Society of Angiology and Vascular Surgery (SBACV), Sao Paulo, Brazil

University Nove de Julho, Sao Paulo, Brazil

Ariele Milano de Oliveira University Nove de Julho, Sao Paulo, Brazil

Nikolaos A. Diakos, MD Heart Failure Program (Division of Cardiology) and Molecular Medicine Program (Eccles Institute of Human Genetics), University of Utah, Salt Lake City, UT, USA

Jose Antonio Diaz, MD Conrad Jobst Vascular Research Laboratories, Section of Vascular Surgery, Department of Surgery, School of Medicine, University of Michigan, Ann Arbor, MI, USA

Edward B. Diethrich, MD Founder and Medical Director of The Arizona Heart Foundation, Department of Cardiovascular and Endovascular Surgery, Phoenix, AZ, USA

Robert Guimarães do Nascimento Department of Vascular and Endovascular Surgery, Institute of Vascular and Endovascular Surgery of Sao Paulo, (ICVE-SP), Sao Paulo, Brazil

Brazilian Society of Angiology and Vascular Surgery (SBACV), Sao Paulo, Brazil

Stavros G. Drakos, MD Heart Failure Program (Division of Cardiology) and Molecular Medicine Program (Eccles Institute of Human Genetics), University of Utah, Salt Lake City, UT, USA

Nilo José Coêlho Duarte, MD Clinical Laboratory, Hospital do Coração, São Paulo, Brazil

Central Laboratory of Hospital das Clinicas, Faculty of Medicine, University de São Paulo, São Paulo, Brazil

Ingrid E. Dumitriu, MD, PhD, FHEA Division of Clinical Sciences, Cardiovascular Sciences Research Centre, St. George's University of London, London, UK

Cassidy Duran, MD The Methodist DeBakey Heart and Vascular Center, The Methodist Hospital, Houston, TX, USA

Serkan Durdu, MD, PhD Department of Cardiovascular Surgery, Heart Center, Ankara University School of Medicine, Dikimevi, Ankara, Turkey

Department of Multi-disciplinary Stem Cell and Regenerative Medicine, Stem Cell Institute, Ankara University, Ankara, Turkey

Maqsood M. Elahi, MD, PhD Department of Cardiothoracic Surgery, Glenfield Hospital, Leicester, UK

Gerard Espinosa, MD, PhD Department of Autoimmune Diseases, Hospital Clinico, University of Barcelona, Barcelona, Spain

Gianluca Faggioli, MD Chirurgia Vascolare, Policlinico S. Orsola, Bologna, Italy

Department of Vascular Surgery, University of Bologna, Bologna, Italy

Francesco Formica, MD Cardiac Surgery Clinic, Department of Surgical Science, University of Milano-Bicocca, San Gerardo Hospital, Milan, Italy

Antonio Freyrie, MD Department of Vascular Surgery, University of Bologna, Bologna, Italy

Ikuo Fukuda, MD, PhD Department of Thoracic and Cardiovascular Surgery, Hirosaki University Graduate School of Medicine, Hirosaki, Aomori, Japan

Wakako Fukuda, MD Department of Thoracic and Cardiovascular Surgery, Hirosaki University Graduate School of Medicine, Hirosaki, Aomori, Japan

David Fullerton, MD Division of Cardiothoracic Surgery, The University of Colorado School of Medicine, Aurora, CO, USA

Edmo Atique Gabriel, MD, PhD Department of Cardiovascular Surgery, University Nove de Julho, São Paulo, Brazil

Sthefano Atique Gabriel, MD Department of Vascular Surgery, Pontifical Catholic University of Campinas, São Paulo, Brazil

Mauro Gargiulo, MD Department of Vascular Surgery, University of Bologna, Bologna, Italy

Meinrad Gawaz, MD Department of Cardiology, University of Tübingen, Tübingen, Germany

Randolph L. Geary, MD, FACS Department of Vascular and Endovascular Surgery, Wake Forest University School of Medicine, Winston-Salem, NC, USA

Department of Pathology, Section on Comparative Medicine, Wake Forest University School of Medicine, Winston-Salem, NC, USA

Tobias Geisler, MD Department of Cardiology, University of Tübingen, Tübingen, Germany

George S. Georgiadis, MD Department of Vascular and Endovascular Surgery, University Hospital of Alexandroupolis, Democritus University of Thrace, Alexandroupolis, Greece

Ramyar Gilani, MD Division of Vascular Surgery and Endovascular Therapy of Michael E. DeBakey, Department of Surgery, Baylor College of Medicine, Houston, TX, USA

Takeshi Goto, ME Department of Thoracic and Cardiovascular Surgery, Hirosaki University Graduate School of Medicine and Hospital, Aomori, Japan

Department of Clinical Engineering, Hirosaki University School of Medicine and Hospital, Aomori, Japan

Anders Gottsäter, MD, PhD Department of Clinical Sciences, Vascular Center, Lund University, Skåne University Hospital, Malmö, Sweden

Russell A. Gould, BS Department of Biomedical Engineering, Cornell University, Ithaca, NY, USA

Tom N. Hoel, MD, PhD Department of Thoracic and Cardiovascular Surgery, University of Oslo, Rikshospitalet University Hospital, Rikshospitalet, Norway

Thomas Hölzenbein, MD, PhD Department of Vascular and Endovascular Surgery, PMU Salzburg, Salzburg, Austria

Bahadır Inan, MD Department of Cardiovascular Surgery, Heart Center, Ankara University School of Medicine, Dikimevi, Ankara, Turkey

Caroline Jadlowiec, MD Department of Surgery and the Interdepartmental Program in Vascular Biology and Therapeutics, Yale University School of Medicine, West Haven, CT, USA

VA Connecticut Healthcare System, New Haven, CT, USA

Marcelo Biscegli Jatene, MD Pediatric Cardiothoracic Surgery Unit, Heart Institute (InCor), University of Sao Paulo Medical School, Sao Paulo, Sao Paulo, Brazil

Pediatric Cardiology and Adult Congenital Heart Disease Unit, Heart Institute (InCor), University of Sao Paulo Medical School, Sao Paulo, Sao Paulo, Brazil

Li Jie-shou, MD Department of Surgery, Jinling Hospital, Medical School of Nanjing University, Nanjing, Jiangsu, China

Juan Carlos Kaski, MD, DM (Hons), DSc, FRCP, FACC, FESC Division of Clinical Sciences, Cardiovascular Sciences Research Centre, St. George's University of London, London, UK

Kaan Kaya, MD Division and Department of Cardiovascular Surgery, Ozel Ulus Hastanesi, Ankara, Turkey

Jacek Kolcz, MD, PhD, FECTS Department of Pediatric Cardiac Surgery, Polish – American Children's Hospital, Jagiellonian University, Krakow, Poland

Mario Lachat, MD Department of Vascular Surgery, University Hospital Zurich, Zurich, Switzerland

Harald Langer, MD Department of Cardiology, University of Tübingen, Tübingen, Germany

Alice Le Huu, MD, MSc Divisions of Cardiac Surgery and Surgery Research, Department of Surgery, McGill University Health Center, Montreal, QC, Canada

Christos D. Liapis, MD, FACS, FRCS Department of Vascular Surgery, Medical School of Athens, Attikon University Hospital, Athens, Greece

Harald L. Lindberg, MD, PhD Department of Thoracic and Cardiovascular Surgery, University of Oslo, Rikshospitalet University Hospital, Oslo, Norway

Klaus Linni, MD Department of Vascular and Endovascular Surgery, PMU Salzburg, Salzburg, Austria

Xue Ma, MD Department of Vascular and Endovascular Surgery, Wake Forest University School of Medicine, Winston-Salem, NC, USA

Department of Pathology, Section on Comparative Medicine, Wake Forest University School of Medicine, Winston-Salem, NC, USA

Nina Mader, MD Department of Vascular and Endovascular Surgery, PMU Salzburg, Salzburg, Austria

Janet Madill, PhD, MD Lung Transplant Program, University of Toronto, Toronto, ON, Canada

Cecilia Marcacci, MD Department of Cardiovascular Surgery, Hospital Clinico, University of Barcelona, Barcelona, Spain

Kenneth L. Mattox, MD Michael E. DeBakey Department of Surgery, Baylor College of Medicine, Houston, TX, USA

Raffaella Mauro, MD Department of Vascular Surgery, Sant'Orsola-Malpighi Hospital, Bologna, Italy

Dieter Mayer, MD Departments for Vascular Surgery and Wound Care, University Hospital Zurich, Zurich, Switzerland

Guilherme Vieira Meirelles, MD Department of Vascular Surgery, Celso Pierro Hospital and Maternity, Campinas, SP, Brazil

Xianzhong Meng, MD, PhD Division of Cardiothoracic Surgery, The University of Colorado School of Medicine, Aurora, CO, USA

Carlos A. Mestres, MD, PhD, FETCS Department of Cardiovascular Surgery, Hospital Clinico, University of Barcelona, Barcelona, Spain

Daniel D. Myers Jr., DVM, MPH, DACLAM Conrad Jobst Vascular Research Laboratories, Section of Vascular Surgery, Department of Surgery, School of Medicine, University of Michigan, Ann Arbor, MI, USA

Conrad Jobst Vascular Research Laboratories, Section of Vascular Surgery/Unit for Laboratory Animal Medicine, School of Medicine, University of Michigan, Ann Arbor, MI, USA

Toshio Nakanishi, MD Department of Pediatric Cardiology, Heart Institute, Tokyo Women's Medical University, Tokyo, Japan

Valerio Napolioni, PhD School of Biosciences and Biotechnologies, University of Camerino, Camerino, Italy

Gustavo S. Oderich, MD Division of Vascular and Endovascular Surgery, Mayo Clinic, Rochester, MN, USA

Mateus Picada-Correa, MD Division of Vascular and Endovascular Surgery, Mayo Clinic, Rochester, MN, USA

Rodolfo Pini, MD Department of Vascular Surgery, University of Bologna, Bologna, Italy

Jose L. Pomar, MD, PhD, FETCS Department of Cardiovascular Surgery, Hospital Clinico, University of Barcelona, Barcelona, Spain

Gangjian Qin, MD Department of Medicine, Cardiology, Feinberg Cardiovascular Research Institute, Northwestern University Feinberg School of Medicine, Chicago, IL, USA

Joseph D. Raffetto, MD, MS FACS, FSVM Division of Vascular and Endovascular Surgery, Brigham and Women's Hospital, Harvard Medical School, Boston, MA, USA

Department of Surgery, VA Boston Healthcare System, West Roxbury, MA, USA

Shahzad G. Raja, BSc, MBBS, MRCS, FRCS(C-Th) Department of Cardiac Surgery, Harefield Hospital, London, UK

Zoran Rancic, MD Department of Cardiovascular Surgery, University Hospital of Zurich, Zurich, Switzerland

Department of Surgery, University of Niš, Niš, Serbia

Ehrenfried Schindler Department for Pediatric Anesthesiology, German Pediatric Heart Center, Asklepios Klinik Sankt Augustin, Sankt Augustin, Germany

Dominique Shum-Tim, MD, CM, MSc, FRCSC, FACS, FAHA Divisions of Cardiac Surgery and Surgical Research, Department of Surgery, McGill University Health Center, Montreal, QC, Canada

The Montreal Children's Hospital, The Montreal General Hospital, Montreal, QC, Canada

Department of Surgery, McGill University, Montreal, QC, Canada

Christian Espinoza Silva, MD, PhD Cardiovascular and Heart Transplant Surgeon, Servicio Cardiovascular, National Institute of Thorax, Santiago, Chile

Crina Sinescu, MD, PhD, FESC Department of Cardiology, Carol Davila University of Medicine, Bucharest, Romania

Mustafa Sırlak, MD Department of Cardiovascular Surgery, Heart Center, Ankara University School of Medicine, Ankara, Turkey

Joshua Sonett, MD Lung Transplant Program, General Thoracic Surgery, Columbia University Medical Center, New York, NY, USA

Domingos S.R. Souza, MD, PhD Department of Cardiovascular Surgery and Anesthesiology, Örebro University, Örebro, Sweden

Andrea Stella, MD Department of Vascular Surgery, Sant'Orsola-Malpighi Hospital, Bologna, Italy

David Sternberg, MD Lung Transplant Program, Henry Ford Health System, Detroit, MI, USA

Anita C. Thomas, PhD Department of Cardiovascular Surgery - Bristol Heart Institute, Bristol Royal Infirmary, Bristol, UK

Sophina Trubel, MD Department of Vascular and Endovascular Surgery, PMU Salzburg, Salzburg, Austria

Peter I. Tsai, MD Cardiothoracic Surgery, Ben Taub General Hospital, Houston, TX, USA

Diego Soto Valdés Resident of General Surgery, Department of Surgery, University of Santiago of Chile, Santiago, Chile

Frank J. Veith, MD Department of Surgery, Division of Vascular Surgery, New York University Medical Center, New York, NY, USA

Department of Surgery, Division of Vascular Surgery, The Cleveland Clinic, Cleveland, OH, USA

Division of Cardiovascular Surgery, Clinic for Cardiovascular Surgery, University Hospital Zurich, Zurich, Switzerland

Matthew J. Wall Jr., MD Cardiothoracic Surgery, Trauma and Critical Care, Baylor College of Medicine, Houston, TX, USA

Ding Wei-wei, MD, PhD Department of General Surgery, Nanjing General Hospital of Nanjing Military Command, Institute of People's Liberation Army for General Surgery, The Clinical College of the Nanjing University Medical School, Nanjing, Jiangsu, China

Omar Wever-Pinzon Heart Failure Program (Division of Cardiology) and Molecular Medicine Program (Eccles Institute of Human Genetics), University of Utah, Salt Lake City, UT, USA

Shiyue Xu, MD Department of Medicine, Cardiology, Feinberg Cardiovascular Research Institute, Northwestern University Feinberg School of Medicine, Chicago, IL, USA

Riad N. Younes, MD, PhD Department of Surgery, Faculty of Medicine, University of Sao Paulo, Hospital Sao Jose, São Paulo, Brazil

Anthony S. Zannas, MD, MSc Department of Psychiatry, Duke University Medical Center, Durham, NC, USA

Kenton J. Zehr, MD Division of Cardiothoracic Surgery and Center for Aortic Disease, Scott & White Clinic, Texas A & M Health Sciences Center College of Medicine, Temple, TX, USA

Part I

General Topics

Neuroendocrine Response and Shock

1

Riad N. Younes and Fernando C. Abrão

Historical Aspects

The concept of shock has evolved throughout the centuries since the early descriptions of traumatic injury. Hippocrates (460–380 BC) recognized certain principles of wound care, such as elevating an injured limb; however, at that time the correlation between blood loss and death had not yet been identified. In the 20th century, two physiologists, Cannon and Bayliss [1], developed studies in laboratory animals, postulating that systemic responses resulting from severe muscle injury were caused by a toxin that caused motor tonus loss, venous blood sequestration, and hypotension.

Nevertheless, in 1930 Alfred Blalock [2] defined the concept of hypovolemia as a primary mechanism in the pathogenesis of traumatic shock. Blalock was able to demonstrate in experiments with dogs that the local loss of blood and plasma through injuries was sufficient to contribute to a blood pressure decrease. Currently, through advances in molecular biology, studies of shock are intended to identify and manipulate several inflammatory mediators that are activated in severe stress situations. Prevention of organ ischemia and oxygen uptake by tissues are also very exciting lines of research in the study of shock and may lead to better results than the 50 % of mortality in some specific types of shock [3].

Definition

Shock, regardless of its cause, can be defined as a syndrome that results from inadequate tissue perfusion, causing cells to not be able to meet their metabolic needs. As a consequence, metabolism alterations occur, which cause cell dysfunction, inflammatory mediator production, and cell injury. At this point, two outcomes are possible. If cell perfusion can be restored, shock is reversed. However, in cases where injury is severe and prolonged, cell perfusion is not restored before several cell mediators are released and activated, triggering a cascade of irreversible reactions and leading to irreversible shock. Thus, this syndrome can range from subclinical hypoperfusion to multiple organ dysfunction.

The key point of hypoperfusion is tissue hypoxia. Oxygen, as an essential nutrient for proper metabolism, becomes less available in relation to tissue demands. Then oxygen debt occurs, where the oxygen demand is greater than the oxygen supply. Therefore, even in conditions of adequate oxygen supply, such as sepsis, metabolism acceleration caused by systemic inflammatory response results in increased oxygen demand, which is not supplied.

Shock Mediators

As mentioned before, any severe or prolonged injury can trigger tissue hypoperfusion and shock. The way shock is triggered has been the object of many studies, and it is currently known that neuroendocrine and inflammatory mediators are closely related to the onset, maintenance, and irreversibility of shock. This occurs through several interrelated reaction cascades that constitute the concept of systemic inflammatory response. Before we discuss the neuroendocrine part of the inflammatory response, we will mention the other major groups of mediators of this inflammatory response: endotoxins, complement fragments, eicosanoids (prostaglandins), kinins, nitric oxide, cytokines (interleukins), platelet-activating factor, endogenous opioids, and oxidizing agents [4].

Signs That Trigger Trauma Response

The afferent sensory nerve fibers provide the most direct and fastest pathway for signals to reach the CNS after the stress. It has often been suggested that pain may act as an

R.N. Younes, MD, PhD (✉) • F.C. Abrão, MD
Department of Surgery, Faculty of Medicine, University of Sao Paulo, Hospital Sao Jose, São Paulo, Brazil
e-mail: rnyounes@yahoo.com

E.A. Gabriel, S.A. Gabriel (eds.), *Inflammatory Response in Cardiovascular Surgery*,
DOI 10.1007/978-1-4471-4429-8_1,

initial afferent signal after the trauma, and many studies have suggested that the afferent nerve signals from the injured area are essential to stimulate the hypothalamic-pituitary-adrenal axis [5]. The adrenocortical response to trauma was not observed in laboratory animals after sectioning of the peripheral nerves to the traumatized area, transection of the spinal cord above the injury, or sectioning through the *medulla oblongata*. A similar response pattern to denervation before the trauma has been described in humans. Growth hormone (GH) and adrenocorticotropic hormone (ACTH) levels in serum rise within 1 h after incision in patients who receive general anesthesia and are undergoing cholecystectomy or inguinal hernia repair. However, this hormone response did not occur in patients undergoing abdominal procedures when an epidural block was used together with general anesthesia [6].

Fluid loss from the vascular compartment stimulates the pressure volume receptors, initiating a series of cardiovascular adjustments measured by the CNS. The cardiac output decreases, the peripheral resistance increases, and blood is redistributed to vital organs in order to keep them working. With the progressive loss of volume in the trauma area, the resulting hypoperfusion reduces tissue oxygenation and disrupts the acid-base balance. Then, chemoreceptor stimulation acts as an additional afferent stimulus for vasomotor and respiratory centers during hypovolemia. As fluid loss after trauma is closely related to the extent of tissue injury, these specific mechanisms allow a quantitative response to occur after the trauma (i.e., the response is directly proportional to the injury extension).

The circulating substances can directly or indirectly stimulate the CNS and activate the trauma response. The release of cytokines, produced in the injured area, may signal the brain to initiate these alterations. Conversely, it has been shown that cytokines are produced within the brain and have been found in the cerebrospinal fluid of patients after head injury and meningitis.

There is an extensive nerve fiber network of interleukin 1 (IL-1) that innervates the hypothalamus, and this cytokine may be influential at the beginning and direct the metabolic response to stress. For instance, chronic brain exposure to IL-1 resulted in catabolism in the rat. Significant weight loss, negative nitrogen balance, and hyperthermia have been demonstrated in animals infused with IL-1 in the central ventricle in comparison with controls infused with saline solution. This response to stress was associated with activation of the hypothalamus-pituitary-adrenal axis [7].

The release of cytokines, as well as of prostaglandins and interleukins, may initiate homeostatic adjustments or, in case of severe injury such as sepsis, necrohemorrhagic pancreatitis, and so on, the release of these substances can cause potent stimuli that can generate a cascade effect on the metabolism, triggering poor tissue perfusion [8].

Role of the Neuroendocrine Axis in the Systemic Inflammatory Response (Shock)

Inflammation is primarily an immune response aimed at protecting the organism from the devastating effects of pathogens, chemicals, and tissue injury. It is well established that once the body sustains an insult, local inflammatory mediators, such as prostaglandins and interleukins, begin to circulate in the blood stream. These act both locally to direct inflammation and globally to indicate to the central nervous system the need for both an added nutritional substrate directed toward vital organ systems and blunted systemic inflammation. The hypothalamic-pituitary axis responds with cortisol and similar hormones, which in the short term increase circulating carbohydrates, lipids, and proteins while simultaneously leading the immunologic response [9].

Signal Integration and Effector Mechanisms

The early response to trauma/acute illness is characterized by stimulation of the hypothalamic-pituitary-adrenal (HPA) axis, increased levels of ACTH, prolactin, and growth hormone (GH), and often a reduction in thyroid hormone secretion. GH is normally released from the anterior pituitary gland in a pulsatile manner, whereas thyroid-stimulating hormone (TSH) and prolactin release is continuous, with a superimposed pulsatile component. However, in protracted critical illness, the endocrinological profile is one of suppressed anterior pituitary hormone secretion. Despite this, cortisol levels remain high, possibly because of a pathway involving endothelin [10, 11]. The pulsatile release of GH, prolactin, and TSH is markedly reduced, predominantly in amplitude, whereas the frequency of secretory pulses is maintained. The synchronous release of GH, prolactin, and TSH is also lost, but can be improved by administering growth hormone-releasing peptide (GHRP)-2, but not growth hormone-releasing hormone or thyrotropin [12]. This suggests the existence of an endogenous GHRP-like ligand, coordinating anterior pituitary hormone release.

The central nervous system, in addition to being activated by the pathway described above, has an important role in shock-related immunoregulation according to the most recent studies.

It is the catecholaminergic stimulation pathway [13]. In the acute phase of stress response, increased sympathetic outflow stimulates a surge of catecholamines, increasing the level by as much as tenfold [14, 15].

They are a well-known participant in the acute stress response and help to increase cardiac output [16], increase basal energy expenditure [17], attenuate normal anabolic activity, and increase the breakdown of skeletal muscle [18, 19] for manufacturing acute-phase proteins. Some studies

[20, 21] demonstrated that a beta blockade can interfere with the long-term catabolism of severely burned patients and decrease the heart rate [21, 22]. In addition, norepinephrine and epinephrine have been demonstrated to have immune capabilities by enhancing expression of immune mediators and exhibiting effects on T-helper cells in animal and human models [23–29].

Sympathetic activity, primarily because of its association with the stress response, has received most of the attention from researchers, but parasympathetic activity during stress has recently been discovered to attenuate the stress response as well. Afferent activity has been demonstrated to enhance cytokine for brain activation of the immune response [30–32].

Efferent activity has also been shown to decrease systemic levels of TNF-α and prevent lethal hypotension [33]. Acetylcholine, just like catecholamines, has immunoactive capabilities. It actively inhibits the release of inflammatory interleukins such as IL-6 and IL-18, but not IL-10, which is an antiinflammatory protein [33]. In addition, studies have shown that nicotine might be an effective tool in fighting inflammatory bowel disease, and there is less inflammatory activity in the bowel mucosa of smokers [34–36]. The real impact of sympathetic and parasympathetic innervation on the immune response is yet to be elucidated, but there is ample research activity trying to do so.

Even less is known about the long-term effects of autonomic stimulation during a stress response. Because of the difficulty of studying long-term critical illness in both human and animal models, it is easy to see why there is more information about the acute phase. Some have generally postulated that continued stimulation of reactionary systems by long-term stress results in an attenuated response [37, 38]. This has been demonstrated in lifetime stress and aging [38], but diminished activity of the autonomic nervous system during critical illness has yet to be shown.

Peripheral Hormonal Environment

Hypothalamic stimulation creates a range of hormonal alterations in patients after trauma: throughout all phases of trauma, there is a sharp increase in the counter-regulatory hormones glucagon, glucocorticoids, and catecholamines. In contrast, plasma concentrations of the patient's anabolic hormone, insulin, may be reduced, normal, or elevated. During the initial response phase, insulin concentrations are normal or increased. However, the effects of high concentrations of insulin on peripheral tissues (skeletal muscle and adipose tissue) are blocked. The cause of severe insulin resistance is related to decreased food intake and an altered hormonal environment, which exerts anti-insulin activity. The counter-regulatory hormones glucagon, cortisol, and catecholamines are opposed to insulin storage or anabolic functions. In the short term, they maintain blood glucose levels and prevent hypoglycemia. The more chronic hormonal development accelerates the body's catabolism [39].

Glucocorticoids are also released after stress, and steroids have potent effects on the metabolism of substrates and minerals. Cortisol is produced in response to increasing concentrations of ACTH released from the anterior pituitary. Cortisol metabolizes amino acids from skeletal muscle and increases hepatic gluconeogenesis; it also causes severe insulin resistance, and these effects cause the apparent hyperglycemia associated with acute illness [39].

The production of catecholamines – epinephrine and norepinephrine – may be the most basic of hormonal responses to stress, in addition to having an important role in the immunoregulation of shock, as described above. These hormones exert regulatory effects on cardiac output, regional circulation, blood glucose levels, and oxidative metabolism. Epinephrine stimulates glycogenolysis, which in skeletal muscle promotes lactate production and, consequently, metabolic acidosis. Furthermore, epinephrine at higher concentrations markedly inhibits insulin production, thus facilitating the mobilization of amino acids and lipids [40].

In normal subjects, the infusion of any of these catabolic hormones alone causes minimal changes in metabolism and circulation. However, when the three hormones are infused together, the effects are synergistic and sustained. A negative nitrogen balance, gluconeogenesis, and hypermetabolism, the main components in the response to trauma, are observed and associated with hydro-saline retention. Thus, it seems that the simultaneous production of the counter-regulatory hormones glucagon, cortisol, and epinephrine is in part responsible for post-trauma alterations.

We will specifically discuss the main hormones involved in the endocrine response to shock below.

Adrenal Glucocorticoids

In critical illness, plasma cortisol levels are usually increased, but exhibit loss of the normal circadian rhythm. This period of increased cortisol synthesis may result in decreased production of other adrenal steroid hormones. However, adrenal insufficiency during critical illness is being described with increasing frequency, particularly in association with systemic sepsis with shock [41], although variations in the definition of the condition have led to inconsistencies in the reported incidences. Although adrenal insufficiency in critical illness may exhibit classic manifestations such as abdominal pain, pyrexia, confusion, and hypotension (resistant to treatment), the signs are nonspecific and common in patients in the intensive care unit. The diagnosis should always be considered in patients with increasing inotropic requirements in spite of adequate antimicrobial therapy and the absence of convincing evidence of ongoing or worsening infection. Serum cortisol levels have been variably associated with mortality in critical illness, with nonsurvivors exhibiting increased, reduced, or similar cortisol levels compared with controls [42]. Thus, the appropriate cortisol levels and responses to corticotrophin in critically ill patients are controversial. Nevertheless, the importance of adequate cortisol levels in critical illness is clear. In a large group of intensive care unit trauma patients, mortality was found to have increased from the range of 19–29 to 47 % when cortisol synthesis was (unknowingly) blocked by the routine use of the sedative etomidate [43]. When the cortisol responses to corticotrophin in patients at the onset of septic shock were examined [44], a baseline serum cortisol >940 nmol/l and a maximum increase in cortisol levels <250 nmol/l in response to corticotrophin were associated with increased mortality. Three patterns of activation of the HPA axis in septic shock were identified using these parameters. The release of large amounts of nitric oxide through the action of inducible nitric oxide synthase is a feature of sepsis. Glucocorticoids inhibit the induction of this enzyme if administered before the onset of shock. However, nitric oxide induces S-nitrosylation of critical sulfhydryl groups in the glucocorticoid receptor, with subsequent reduced binding of glucocorticoids [45]. This may explain why glucocorticoids have not been previously shown to be effective when administered in patients with established sepsis.

However, studies about the treatment of adrenal insufficiency are controversial. Improvement in shock reversal and a trend toward decreased mortality were seen with supra-physiological doses of hydrocortisone (100 mg three times daily). The use of smaller doses of hydrocortisone was associated with reduced duration of vasopressor therapy and ventilation and a trend toward earlier resolution of sepsis-induced organ dysfunction [41, 42].

Growth Hormone

Growth hormone increases plasma glucose levels and facilitates protein sparing (which protects lean body mass), lipolysis, immunocompetence, and sodium and water retention. Its secretion is inhibited by long-term glucocorticoid administration and stimulated by hypoglycemia, exercise, sleep, high protein intake, and increased levels of leucine and arginine. GH is thought to act directly and also by stimulating hepatic production of insulin-like growth factor-1 (IGF-1).

During stress or illness, baseline GH is often elevated and diurnal variation reduced. However, continued stress, as typical in critical illness, may be associated with reduced GH and IGF-1 levels and therefore with an attenuation of the anabolic processes. Differences in stress responses within the immune system in experimental animals have been attributed to gender differences in the HPA axis or to an effect of sex hormones. Although total GH secretion is similar in both sexes, a greater loss of pulsatile GH secretion is seen in male compared to female patients during protracted critical illness, thus potentially conferring an outcome advantage on the female [46].

High-dose GH administration (five to ten times the standard replacement doses) has been shown to improve the nitrogen balance in patients with burns, after trauma, in early sepsis, and in postoperative surgical patients. However, high-dose GH, administered to adult patients requiring prolonged intensive care after surgery, multiple trauma, or acute respiratory failure, has been associated with increased lengths of hospital stay, longer duration of mechanical ventilation, and increased mortality. GH administration had not been previously shown to be associated with increased mortality. Patient metabolic status at the time of GH administration may be of significance in relation to effect. Another apparent anomaly is the finding that, in a porcine model of sepsis, the effects of GH and IGF-1 on carbohydrate metabolism were markedly different [47], as the GH effect takes place partly through IGF-1.

Thyroid Hormones

Laboratory measurements of thyroid function in critically ill patients are frequently "abnormal" and are always difficult to interpret. The euthyroid sick syndrome describes abnormalities in thyroid function seen in critically ill patients who do not exhibit overt thyroid disease. Such patients may or may not have problems at the cellular level [31, 48]. Biochemical features may include several of the following: reduced total triiodothyronine (T3) levels with a more modest reduction in free T3, increased reverse T3, and possible reduced total thyroxin (T4), with normal free T4 levels. TSH is usually low or within the low-normal range. The most common expression of this condition is low T3 syndrome. Patients exhibiting this condition usually have a normal total T4 level and should be considered euthyroid. Proposed mechanisms include impaired responsiveness of the thyroid to TSH, reduced serum binding of thyroid hormones, or reduced peripheral conversion of T4 to T3. Glucocorticoids inhibit 5′ monodeiodinase, which catalyzes the conversion of T4 to T3. Cytokines, however, exert no inhibitory effect on 5′-monodeiodinase activity. It has been postulated that endogenous cortisol has an inhibitory effect on TSH concentrations in patients with euthyroid sick syndrome [49]. In low T4 and T3 syndromes, those exhibiting the lowest plasma T4 levels have the highest mortality, but no outcome benefit has been shown by administering T3 or T4 to these patients [50].

Leptin

Leptin, a hormone expressed in adipocytes, is teleologically related to cytokines. Leptin stimulates energy release from fat by fatty acid oxidation and can be considered a stress-related hormone. It suppresses adrenal synthetic activity and may in part be responsible for the functional adrenocortical insufficiency that is sometimes observed in sepsis [51]. Leptin levels vary widely between individuals, are greater in female and younger subjects, and correlate with fat mass and body weight in both normal and obese patients. Leptin secretion shows diurnal variation in normal individuals, with a twofold nocturnal rise. A variety of cytokines enhance leptin production; release is also enhanced by insulin, IGF-1, thyroid hormones, somatotropin release-inhibiting factor, glucocorticoids, and beta-adrenergic agonists. Not surprisingly, leptin levels are therefore increased in acute/early sepsis (compared with controls), and there is a reversal of the diurnal cycle. Survivors among patients with sepsis exhibit higher plasma leptin levels than nonsurvivors. Indeed, leptin levels correlate more closely with outcome than serum cortisol levels [52]. However, in patients with sepsis of longer duration (≥14 days), leptin levels are not elevated, and it is unlikely that leptin is related to the hypermetabolism of sepsis [53]. In protracted critical illness, leptin does not correlate with the body mass index or levels of circulating cortisol, thyroid hormone, or insulin, and its levels do not predict outcome. GH secretagogues (growth hormone-releasing hormone and GHRP-2) increase leptin levels [54]. The ensuing increase in fatty acid oxidation may be beneficial in prolonged critical illness, in which feeding-resistant protein wasting occurs, whereas fat stores are maintained because of re-esterification and depressed fatty acid oxidation.

The neuroendocrine response is extremely complex and yet to be fully understood. However, studies on this subject are frequent and important because of the effect they may have on the treatment of shock patients, especially regarding corticosteroid replacement needs and timing.

References

1. Cannon WB, Bayliss WM. Notes on muscle injury in relation to shock: special report of the Medical Research Commission. 1919;26:19.
2. Blalock A. Experimental shock, the cause of the low blood pressure produced by muscle injury. Arch Surg. 1930;22:959.
3. Marchick MR, Kline JA, Jones AE. The significance of non-sustained hypotension in emergency department patients with sepsis. Intensive Care Med. 2009;35:1261–4.
4. Demling R, LaLonde C, Saldinger P, Knox J. Multiple-organ dysfunction in the surgical patient: pathophysiology, prevention, and treatment. Curr Probl Surg. 1993;30:345.
5. Hume DM, Egdahl RH. The importance of the brain in the endocrine response to injury. Ann Surg. 1959;150:697.
6. Kehlet H. Modification of responses to surgery and anesthesia by neural blockade. In: Cousins MJ, Bridenbaugh PO, editors. Neural blockade in clinical anesthesia and management of pain. Philadelphia: J.B. Lippincott; 1987. p. 145.
7. Jeschke MG, Mlcak RP, Herndon DN. Morphologic changes of the liver after a severe thermal injury. Shock. 2007;28(2):172–7.
8. Dellinger RP, Levy MM, Carlet JM, et al. Surviving Sepsis Campaign: international guidelines for management of severe sepsis and septic shock: 2008. Intensive Care Med. 2008;34:17–60.
9. Lavery GG, Glover P. The methabolic and nutritional response to critical illness. Curr Opin Crit Care. 2000;6:233–8.
10. Arafah BM. Hypothalamic pituitary adrenal function during critical illness: limitations of current assessment methods. J Clin Endocrinol Metab. 2006;91:3725–45.
11. Marik P. Critical illness-related corticosteroid insufficiency. Chest. 2009;135:181–93.
12. Van den Berghe G, Wouters P, Bowers CY, et al. Growth hormone-releasing peptide-2 infusion synchronizes growth hormone, thyrotropin and prolactin release in prolonged critical illness. Eur J Endocrinol. 1999;140:17–22.
13. Reichlin S. Neuroendocrine-immune inter-actions. N Engl J Med. 1993;329:1246–53.
14. Goodall MC, Stone C, Haynes Jr BW. Urinary output of adrenaline and noradrenaline in severe thermal burns. Ann Surg. 1957;145:479–87.
15. Wilmore DW, Aulick LH. Metabolic changes in burned patients. Surg Clin North Am. 1978;58:1173–87.
16. De Backer D, Biston P, Devriendt J, et al. Comparison of dopamine and norepinephrine in the treatment of shock. N Engl J Med. 2010;362:779–89.
17. Reiss W, Pearson E, Artz CP. The metabolic response to burns. J Clin Invest. 1956;35:62–77.
18. Newsome TW, Mason Jr AD, Pruitt Jr BA. Weight loss following thermal injury. Ann Surg. 1973;178:215–7.
19. Hart DW, Wolf SE, Mlcak RP, et al. Persistence of muscle catabolism after severe burn. Surgery. 2000;128:312–9.
20. Herndon D, Hart D, Wolf S, et al. Reversal of catabolism by beta-blockade after severe burns. N Engl J Med. 2001;345:1223–9.
21. Gore DC, Wolfe RR. Hemodynamic and metabolic effects of selective beta1 adrenergic blockade during sepsis. Surgery. 2006;139:686–94.
22. Baron PW, Barrow RE, Pierre EJ, et al. Prolonged use of propranolol safely decreases cardiac work in burned children. J Burn Care Rehabil. 1997;18:223–7.
23. Panina-Bordignon P, Mazzeo D, Lucia PD, et al. Beta2-agonists prevent Th1 development by selective inhibition of interleukin-12. J Clin Invest. 1997;100:1513–9.
24. Hasko G, Szabo C, Nemeth ZH, et al. Stimulation of beta-adrenoreceptors inhibits endotoxin-induced IL-12 production in normal and IL-10 deficient mice. J Neuroimmunol. 1998;88:57–61.
25. Sanders VM, Baker RA, Ramer-Quinn DS, et al. Differential expression of the beta2- adrenergic receptor by TH1 and Th2 clones: implications for cytokine production and B cell help. J Immunol. 1997;158:4200–10.
26. Borger P, Hoekstra Y, Esselink MT, et al. Beta-adrenoceptor-mediated inhibition of IFN-gamma, IL-3, and GM-CSF mRNA accumulation in activated human T lymphocytes is solely mediated by the beta2-adrenoceptor subtype. Am J Respir Cell Mol Biol. 1998;19:400–7.
27. Hasko G, Elenkov IJ, Kvetan V, et al. Differential effect of selective block of alpha 2-adrenoreceptors on plasma levels of tumor necrosisfactor – alpha, interleukin – 6 and corticosterone induced by bacterial lipopoly-saccharide in mice. J Endocrinol. 1995;144:457–62.
28. Kovacs KJ, Elenkov IJ. Differential dependence of ACTH secretion induced by various cytokines on the integrity of the paraventricular nucleus. J Neuroendocrinol. 1995;7:15–23.
29. Woiciechowsky CK, Asadullah K, Nestler D, et al. Sympathetic activation triggers systemic interleukin-10 release in immunodepression induced by brain injury. Nat Med. 1998;4:808–13.

30. Fleshner M, Goehler LE, Schwartz BA, et al. Thermogenic and corticosterone responses to intravenous cytokines are attenuated by sub diaphragmatic vagotomy. J Neuroimmunol. 1998;86:134–41.
31. Maier SF, Goehler LE, Fleshner M, et al. The role of the vagus nerve in cytokine-to-brain communication. Ann N Y Acad Sci. 1998;840:289–300.
32. Watkins LR, Goehler LE, Relton JK, et al. Blockade of interleukin-1 induced hyperthermia by sub diaphragmatic vagotomy: evidence for vagal mediation of immune-brain communication. Neurosci Lett. 1995;183:27–31.
33. Borovikova LV, Ivanova S, Zhang M, et al. Vagus nerve stimulation attenuates the systemic inflammatory response to endotoxin. Nature. 2000;405:458–62.
34. Guslandi M. Nicotine treatment for ulcerativecolitis. Br J Physiol Opt. 1998;274:L970–9.
35. Sandborn WJ. Transdermal nicotine for mildly to moderately active ulcerative colitis: a randomized, double-blind, placebo-controlled trial. Ann Intern Med. 1997;126:364–71.
36. Sher ME. The influence of cigarette smoking on cytokine levels in patients with inflammatory bowel disease. Inflamm Bowel Dis. 1999;5:73–8.
37. McEwen B. Protective and damaging effects of stress mediators. N Engl J Med. 1998;338:171–9.
38. Seeman TE, Robbins RJ. Aging and hypothalamic-pituitary-adrenal response to challenge in humans. Endocr Rev. 1994;15:233–60.
39. Bessey PQ, Watters JM, Aoki TT, Wilmore DW. Combined hormonal infusion simulates the metabolic response to injury. Ann Surg. 1984;200:264.
40. Wilmore DW. The metabolic management of the critically ill. New York: Plenum Medical; 1977.
41. Annetta MG, Maviglia R, Proietti R, Antonelli M. Use of corticosteroids in critically ill septic patients: a review of mechanisms of adrenal insufficiency in sepsis and treatment. Curr Drug Targets. 2009;10:887–94.
42. Marik P, Pastores SM, Annane D, Meduri GU, Sprung CL, Arlt W, et al. Recommendations for the diagnosis and management of corticosteroid insufficiency in critically ill adult patients: consensus statements from an international task force by the American College of Critical Care Medicine. Crit Care Med. 2008;36:1937–49.
43. Watt I, Ledingham IM. Mortality amongst multiple trauma patients admitted to an intensive therapy unit. Anaesthesia. 1984;39: 973–81.
44. Annane D, Sébille V, Troché G. A 3-level prognostic classification in septic shock based on cortisol levels and cortisol response to corticotropin. JAMA. 2000;283:1038–45. Short corticotropin test has prognostic value in predicting risk of death in sepsis.
45. Galigniana MD, Piwien-Pilipuk G, Assreuy J. Inhibition of glucocorticoid receptor binding by nitric oxide. Mol Pharm. 1999;55:317–23.
46. Wohltmann CD, Spain DA, Carrillo EH. Does gender effect outcome in trauma patients? Crit Care Med. 1999;27:A176.
47. Balteskard L, Unneberg K, Mjaaland M, et al. Treatment with growth hormone and insulin-like growth factor-1 in septicemia: effects on carbohydrate metabolism. Eur Surg Res. 1998;30:79–94.
48. Chopra IJ. Clinical review 86. Euthyroid sick syndrome: is it a misnomer? J Clin Endocrinol Metab. 1997;82:329–834.
49. Davies PH, Sheppard MC, Franklyn JA. Inflammatory cytokines and type I 5'-deiodinase expression in phi1 rat liver cells. Mol Cell Endocrinol. 1997;129:191–8.
50. Brent GA, Hershman JM. Thyroxine therapy in patients with severe nonthyroidal illnesses and low serum thyroxine concentration. J Clin Endocrinol Metab. 1986;63:1–8.
51. Aygen B, Inan M, Doganay M, Kelestimur F. Adrenal functions in patients with sepsis. Exp Clin Endocrinol Diabetes. 1997;105:182–6.
52. Bornstein SR, Licinio J, Tauchnitz R, et al. Plasma leptin levels are increased in survivors of acute sepsis: associated loss of diurnal rhythm in cortisol and leptin secretion. J Clin Endocrinol Metab. 1998;83:280–3.
53. Carlson GL, Saeed M, Little RA, Irving MH. Serum leptin concentrations and their relation to metabolic abnormalities in human sepsis. Am J Physiol. 1999;276:E658–62.
54. Van den Berghe G, Wouters P, Carlsson L, et al. Leptin levels in protracted critical illness; effects of growth hormone-secretagogues and thyrotropin-releassing hormone. J Clin Endocrinol Metab. 1998;83:3062–70.

2 The Role of Lymphocytes in the Pathogenesis of Atherosclerosis: Focus on CD4⁺ T Cell Subsets

Ingrid E. Dumitriu and Juan Carlos Kaski

Introduction

Recent advances in the mechanisms that underlie the pathogenesis of atherosclerosis suggest that chronic inflammation and the immune system actively contribute to the development and aggravation of this disease. Classical atherosclerosis was mainly attributed to the deposition of lipids [e.g., low-density lipoproteins (LDLs)] into the intima of medium-sized and large arteries, resulting in the progressive thickening of the vessel wall. However, the identification of immune cells such as macrophages and T lymphocytes in atherosclerotic plaques sparked the interest of researchers in understanding the precise roles of these cells in atherosclerosis. Several lines of research in both animal models of atherosclerosis and patients have consolidated the view that the innate and adaptive immune systems are important mediators of the inflammatory process that drives atherosclerosis [1].

The Immune Response in Atherosclerosis

One of the earliest changes implicated in the development of atherosclerotic plaques is endothelial dysfunction. From an immunological point of view, this manifests as elevated levels of adhesion molecules and an increased permeability of the endothelium, which result in recruitment of immune cells from the circulation and an influx of lipids into the intima [2]. Monocytes and T cells recruited from the circulation populate the developing atherosclerotic plaques, where monocytes differentiate into macrophages that take up lipids (LDLs) in either their native form or following modification [e.g., oxidized LDLs (oxLDLs)] [3]. Uptake of oxLDLs into macrophages triggers secretion of inflammatory cytokines such as interferon (IFN)-γ that will induce further upregulation of adhesion molecules by endothelium and facilitate the recruitment of a novel wave of monocytes and lymphocytes. Atherosclerotic lesions can evolve in time and constitute a central lipid area surrounded by infiltrates of lymphocytes, macrophages, and foam cells (macrophages loaded with lipids). A proliferation of vascular smooth muscle cells (VSMCs) in the media accompanies the intimal changes, as well as the formation of a fibrous cap, which is constituted by a layer of endothelial cells and VSMCs [4]. Further progression of atherosclerotic plaques may prevent oxygenation of the center of the lesion, which results in cell death and the formation of a necrotic core. This can also activate angiogenesis pathways that associate with generation of neovessels and intraplaque haemorrhage. The presence of high numbers of immune cells, a thin cap, and a large necrotic core has been linked to vulnerability of the atherosclerotic plaques and predisposition to rupture. One of the mechanisms that can precipitate plaque rupture is the release of extracellular matrix–degrading enzymes, matrix metalloproteinases from activated intraplaque macrophages [5]. T cells and in particular $CD4^+$ T lymphocytes have pivotal roles in regulating macrophage activation and in orchestrating the chronic immune response in atherosclerosis [6].

The Basics of T-Cell-Mediated Immune Responses

Immune responses mediated by T cells are initiated by recognition of antigens (structures derived from pathogens in the case of immune responses to infectious organisms or altered endogenous cells in cancer or autoimmune disorders) and form the basis of adaptive immunity. The antigens are recognized and processed by antigen-presenting cells

I.E. Dumitriu, MD, PhD, FHEA (✉)
J.C. Kaski, MD, DM (Hons), DSc, FRCP, FACC, FESC, FAHA
Division of Clinical Sciences,
Cardiovascular Sciences Research Centre,
St. George's University of London, Cranmer Terrace,
SW17 0RE London, UK
e-mail: i.dumitriu@sgul.ac.uk

E.A. Gabriel, S.A. Gabriel (eds.), *Inflammatory Response in Cardiovascular Surgery*,
DOI 10.1007/978-1-4471-4429-8_2, © Springer-Verlag London 2013

(APCs), primarily dendritic cells (DCs) and macrophages, which are strategically positioned in the skin, mucosa of the respiratory and intestinal tract, and tissue stroma to facilitate pathogen detection and capture [7, 8]. DCs, the most potent of the APCs, are uniquely equipped to trigger the activation of naive T cells. Following antigen uptake, DCs undergo a series of changes that enable them to migrate from peripheral tissues into the lymphoid organs and to upregulate the expression of molecules such as costimulatory ligands. Naive T cells that recirculate between blood and lymph nodes in search of antigens come in contact with DCs displaying antigen on major histocompatibility complex (MHC) molecules and scan them for the presence of cognate antigen. If antigen recognition occurs, it will provide the first signal required for T cell activation, while interaction between costimulatory receptors on T lymphocytes (e.g. CD28) and their corresponding ligands on DCs generates the second (costimulatory) signal for activation [9]. Activated T cells proliferate and differentiate into various effectors, depending on the cytokines released by the antigen-presenting DCs (signal three). Two main types of T lymphocytes have been described: the helper T (Th) cells (identified by the expression of the CD4 marker) and the cytotoxic T lymphocytes (CTL) that express CD8 and lyse cells infected by viruses or cancer cells. The main function of Th cells is to alter the function of other cells of the immune system (e.g. macrophages, B cells, T cells). Distinct subsets of $CD4^+$ T cells have been characterised subsequently, which include Th1, Th2, Th17 and regulatory T (Treg) cells. As all these cells express the marker CD4, they are usually distinguished by the cytokines they produce and the transcription factors expressed. Interestingly, different subsets of $CD4^+$ T cells vary considerably with respect to the target cells on which they act and the effects induced. Recognition of pathogens by DCs (or macrophages) induces the secretion of cytokines that guide the differentiation of naive T cells into a specific $CD4^+$ T cell subset. Differentiation into Th1 cells is mediated by interleukin-12 (IL-12), while IL-4 is instrumental in the generation of Th2 cells [10, 11]. Th17 cells differentiate from naive $CD4^+$ T cells in the presence of IL-6 and possibly transforming growth factor-β (TGF-β) [12–14]. Treg cells can differentiate either in the thymus (naturally occurring Treg) similarly to conventional T lymphocytes or in the periphery (inducible Treg) under the influence of TGF-β or IL-10 [15].

Most of the T cells present in atherosclerotic plaques belong to the $CD4^+$ subset, while $CD8^+$ T cells are scarce. Very little information is available on the precise contribution of $CD8^+$ T cells to atherosclerosis, while their $CD4^+$ counterparts have been extensively investigated and found to be crucial players in the chronic immune response that drives atherosclerosis. The next sections will focus on the main $CD4^+$ T cell subsets that have been implicated in atherogenesis.

Proatherogenic T Cell Subsets

Th1 Cells

Th1 cells are characterised by production of inflammatory cytokines, of which IFN-γ is considered the signature cytokine of this $CD4^+$ T cell lineage. These cells have important roles in cell-mediated immune responses as they provide crucial signals for optimal macrophage activation. However, many disorders associated with chronic inflammation are due to uncontrolled Th1 function (e.g. diabetes, rheumatoid arthritis). Th1 cells have been found to have mainly proatherogenic effects. Indeed, they constitute an important part of the T lymphocytes infiltrating atherosclerotic plaques in both human disease and in experimental animal models.

Deletion of IFN-γ or of the receptor for this cytokine has been found to reduce atherosclerosis in murine models of atherosclerosis (*Apoe*$^{-/-}$ and *Ldlr*$^{-/-}$ mice) [16–18]. Similarly, *Apoe*$^{-/-}$ mice treated with IFN-γ developed larger atherosclerotic plaques [19]. In line with these results, another group found that *Ldlr*$^{-/-}$ mice deficient in T-bet, a transcription factor that is essential for Th1 cell differentiation, had significantly reduced atherosclerosis compared to T-bet-expressing *Ldlr*$^{-/-}$ mice [20]. In other models, IFN-γ was found to have opposite effects on atherogenesis. *Ldlr*$^{-/-}$ mice that were lethally irradiated to wipe out their immune cells and then reconstituted with bone marrow from *Ifn-γ*$^{-/-}$ mice were surprisingly found to have enhanced atherosclerosis, suggesting that IFN-γ could protect from atherosclerosis [21]. IFN-γ has multiple effects on various cells involved in atherogenesis: (1) it stimulates the expression of MHC II on endothelial cells and VSMCs [22, 23], which could endow these cells with the ability to present antigens; (2) it enhances endothelial activation and the recruitment of T cells and macrophages into atherosclerotic lesions; (3) it triggers the activation of macrophages and DCs, which increases their ability to present plaque-derived antigens to T cells and to amplify the immune response; (4) it induces production of matrix metalloproteinases from macrophages, which could cause apoptosis of VSMCs and promote thinning of the fibrous cap and plaque rupture; (5) it inhibits the differentiation and proliferation of VSMCs and the synthesis of collagen, which could further contribute to rupture of the plaques [24].

$CD4^+CD28^{null}$ T Cells

Another proinflammatory $CD4^+$ T lymphocyte subset that expands in patients with chronic inflammatory conditions but is very low in healthy individuals is known as the $CD4^+CD28^{null}$ T cells [25]. The feature that distinguishes these cells is the absence of the costimulatory receptor CD28, which has important roles in the optimal activation of T cells following antigen recognition on APCs [9]. CD28 is expressed constitutively on naive $CD4^+$ T cells and it interacts with ligands expressed on APCs (i.e. CD80 and CD86). In the absence of co-stimulatory signals transduced by CD28, T cells become unresponsive to antigen. The frequency of $CD4^+CD28^{null}$ T cells increases significantly in patients with acute coronary syndrome (ACS) compared to patients with stable angina (SA) and healthy subjects [25]. This T cell subset has been suggested to contribute to plaque rupture as they have been isolated from unstable coronary plaques and are known to be an important source of IFN-γ [26, 27]. In addition, $CD4^+CD28^{null}$ T cells express molecules that endow them with cytotoxic function (perforin, granzyme A and B) [28]. Of note, conventional $CD4^+CD28^+$ T cells do not express perforin and granzymes, which are usually found only in cytotoxic $CD8^+$ T lymphocytes and natural killer (NK) cells. $CD4^+CD28^{null}$ T cells have been shown to kill endothelial cells and SMCs in vitro, which could further suggest a role in plaque rupture [29] for this T cell subset.

Recently, it was found that patients with high frequencies of $CD4^+CD28^{null}$ T cells are more likely to undergo recurrent acute coronary events (i.e. myocardial infarction) [30] than those with limited expansion of these cells. Diabetes mellitus, a risk factor for ACS, also associates with $CD4^+CD28^{null}$ T cell expansion [31]. Moreover, high frequencies of $CD4^+CD28^{null}$ T cells correlate with the occurrence of the first cardiovascular event and a poor ACS outcome in diabetic patients [31].

The precise mechanisms that lead to the expansion of $CD4^+CD28^{null}$ T cells in ACS are not completely known. The proinflammatory cytokine TNF-α was suggested to down-regulate the expression of CD28 [32, 33]. Previous work from our group demonstrated that 50 % of $CD4^+CD28^{null}$ T cell clones derived from ACS patients recognise the endogenous antigen human heat shock protein 60 (hHSP60) [34, 35]. We have recently demonstrated that $CD4^+CD28^{null}$ T cells from ACS patients express elevated levels of costimulatory receptors of the tumour necrosis family receptor and that these receptors regulate the production of inflammatory cytokines and expression of perforin and granzyme B by $CD4^+CD28^{null}$ T cells [36]. Targeting this subset of T cells could yield promising results for the induction of plaque stability in ACS patients.

Th17 Cells

Th17 cells secrete IL-17, a proinflammatory cytokine, and have important roles in the immune response to infectious pathogens [37]. TGF-β and IL-6 have been shown to induce the differentiation of naive $CD4^+$ T lymphocytes into Th17 cells [12, 14], while IL-23 regulates the production of IL-17 and Th17 cell expansion [38]. As Th17 cells have potent proinflammatory functions and contribute to the pathogenesis of many autoimmune diseases, they are being actively investigated in atherosclerosis. As Th17 cells have proinflammatory roles, it would be expected that they promote atherosclerosis. Indeed, IL-17A blockade in *Apoe*$^{-/-}$ mice reduced the development of atherosclerotic plaques [39]. In addition, attenuated atherosclerosis is observed in lethally irradiated *Ldlr*$^{-/-}$ mice upon reconstitution with IL-17R-deficient bone marrow cells compared to bone marrow from wild-type counterparts [40]. Other studies on Th17 in atherosclerosis have generated contradictory results. Depletion of B cells from *Apoe*$^{-/-}$ or *Ldlr*$^{-/-}$ mice resulted in atherosclerosis reduction, which surprisingly was the consequence of elevated secretion of IL-17 from T cells [41]. The contribution of Th17 cells to human atherosclerosis is not much clearer. Th17 cells were proposed to promote atherosclerosis by acting in concert with Th1 cells following evidence that T cells from human coronary arteries express IL-17 in addition to IFN-γ [42]. However, increased expression of IL-17 was found to correlate with markers of stability in plaques from carotid or coronary atherosclerosis [43]. Therefore, further research in both animal models and patients with atherosclerosis is required to clarify the roles of Th17 cells in this disease.

Anti-atherogenic T Cell Subsets

Th2 Cells

Th2 cells produce IL-4, IL-5 and IL-13 cytokines and generally have opposing effects to Th1 lymphocytes. The cytokines secreted by Th2 cells have important roles in driving the production of antibodies from B lymphocytes, which are involved in the immune response to extracellular microbes [44]. However, Th2 cells have also been implicated in disorders associated with chronic inflammation such as allergies and asthma [45]. Initially it was thought that Th2 cells protect from atherosclerosis. BALB/c *Apoe*$^{-/-}$ mice, which are known to have predominant Th2 responses, were found to have significantly less atherosclerosis than C57BL/6 *Apoe*$^{-/-}$ mice (in which the immune response is mediated preferentially by Th1 cells) [46]. Similarly, deletion of the transcription factor that regulates the generation of Th1 cells (i.e. T-bet) in *Ldlr*$^{-/-}$ mice results in immune responses mediated preferentially by Th2 cells; this associated with decreased atherosclerosis compared to wild-type *Ldlr*$^{-/-}$ mice [20]. However, animal models deficient in IL-4 have generated controversial findings. Deletion of IL-4 in *Apoe*$^{-/-}$ mice (which impairs the differentiation of naive T cells into Th2 effectors) was found to reduce atherogenesis [47]. Similar results were obtained following reconstitution of *Ldlr*$^{-/-}$ mice with IL-4-deficient bone marrow [48], suggesting that Th2 cells could promote atherogenesis. Therefore, the role of Th2 cells in atherosclerosis is not completely understood.

Regulatory CD4$^+$ T Cells

Regulatory T cells (previously known as suppressor T cells) are a subset of CD4$^+$ T lymphocytes specialised in the maintenance of immune tolerance to self and inhibition of excessive immune responses. Treg cells can develop either in the thymus or be generated in the periphery during an active immune response. The thymus-derived Tregs are known as naturally occurring (nTreg), while the ones generated in the periphery are named inducible Tregs (iTreg) [15]. The markers that distinguish Tregs from other CD4$^+$ T lymphocytes and allow identification of regulatory T cells are CD25 (the α chain of the IL-2 receptor, which is expressed at high levels on Tregs), CD127 (which is not expressed/present in low levels in Tregs) and the transcription factor Foxp3 [49]. Defects in Tregs have been implicated in the pathogenesis of autoimmune disorders [50, 51] and could also contribute to atherogenesis. In animal models Tregs were found to protect from atherosclerosis both in the initial and late stages of the disease [52]. Depletion of CD4$^+$CD25^{hi} Tregs from *Apoe*$^{-/-}$ mice by treatment with anti-CD25 monoclonal antibodies significantly enhanced atherosclerosis [53]. In addition, an increased number of inflammatory T cells and macrophages infiltrated atherosclerotic plaques in *Apoe*$^{-/-}$ mice depleted of Tregs. This was accompanied by a decrease in collagen levels in the plaques, similar to findings in vulnerable plaques from human patients [53]. In another model, lethally irradiated *Ldlr*$^{-/-}$ mice reconstituted with Treg-deficient bone marrow developed larger atherosclerotic plaques compared to mice reconstituted with wild-type bone marrow [53]. Another proof for a protective role of Tregs in atherosclerosis comes from a model in which TGF-β signalling was disrupted, which resulted in increased atherosclerosis in *Apoe*$^{-/-}$ mice [54]. TGF-β is a potent immunosuppressive cytokine that is secreted by Tregs and is believed to be one of the mechanisms responsible for the immunosuppressive effects of these cells.

In humans, the markers used for identification of Tregs are less specific than in animals, as they can also be upregulated in recently activated conventional T cells. Initial studies in humans have suggested that Tregs were altered in patients with ACS similarly to findings in autoimmune diseases. Indeed, the frequency of circulating CD4$^+$CD25^{hi} Tregs was significantly decreased in patients with ACS (STEMI) when compared to stable angina patients or healthy subjects [55]. Moreover, the suppressive function of Tregs from ACS patients was impaired compared to the suppressive ability of Tregs from healthy individuals [56]. However, these findings have been recently contradicted by a study that investigated a larger group of patients. No relationship was found between the frequency of circulating Tregs and the extent or severity of carotid or coronary atherosclerosis [57]. Surprisingly, STEMI patients showed a decrease in Tregs, NSTEMI associated with an increased frequency of this cell subset, and in stable angina there was no change in Treg frequency. Whether these contrasting results are due to inclusion of a larger number of patients or to the markers used to identify Tregs (i.e. characterised as CD4$^+$CD25^{hi}CD127^{lo} Tregs in [57], while Tregs were quantified as CD4$^+$CD25^{hi} in the previous two studies [55, 56]) is not known and remains to be addressed by future research.

Immunotherapy in Atherosclerosis: Fact or Fiction?

Further proof that the immune system has a central role in atherosclerosis and that it could be targeted therapeutically with beneficial effects is provided by some of the therapeutic agents currently in use in coronary atherosclerosis. Recent data suggest that the efficiency of these drugs is not due just to their main pharmacological targets but that they additionally alter the function of immune cells such as T lymphocytes. Statins, which are prescribed to lower LDL levels in patients with atherosclerosis, have been shown to decrease the frequency of inflammatory CD4$^+$CD28^{null} T cells significantly [58] and increase Tregs [59] in ACS patients. Selective blockade of TNF-α could represent another strategy to decrease the inflammatory immune response in atherosclerosis. Indeed, TNF-α blockade improves endothelial function in RA patients [60]. In addition, neutralising antibodies against TNF-α have been shown to restore CD28 expression by CD4$^+$CD28^{null} T cells cultured in vitro, which may suggest that TNF-α blockade could inhibit the expansion of this inflammatory lymphocyte subset in patients with atherosclerosis [61].

Another therapeutic strategy to modulate chronic inflammatory immune responses that could be applied in atherosclerosis focuses on expanding the numbers or function of Tregs in patients. This hypothesis has been tested with successful results in animal models of atherosclerosis. *Ldlr*$^{-/-}$ mice tolerised to oxLDL or HSP60 (antigens involved in atherogenesis) developed significantly smaller atherosclerotic lesions compared to *Ldlr*$^{-/-}$ animals [62, 63]. Of note, tolerised *Ldlr*$^{-/-}$ mice had higher numbers of CD4$^+$CD25$^+$Foxp3$^+$ Tregs in the spleen and mesenteric lymph nodes, suggesting that oral tolerance to oxLDL or HSP60 associated with expansion of Tregs and suppression of the immune response. In another model, adoptive transfer of Tr1 cells (a subtype of inducible Tregs that characteristically secrete the immunosuppressive cytokine IL-10) reduced atherosclerosis in *Apoe*$^{-/-}$ mice [64]. These results suggest that activation and expansion of Tregs in vivo may provide a novel strategy to modulate the immune response and decrease or prevent atherosclerosis. However, to successfully design targeted immuno-modulation protocols would require a clearer knowledge of the roles of immune cells in atherosclerosis and in particular of the alterations that are present in these cells in human patients. These preliminary studies suggest that T cell modulation is likely to yield favourable results in patients with atherosclerosis.

Acknowledgements The authors' research is supported by the British Heart Foundation (grant no. PG/10/50/28434, to IED and JCK) and St. George's Hospital Charity, London, UK.

Conflict of Interest

None.

References

1. Libby P, Ridker PM, Hansson GK. Inflammation in atherosclerosis: from pathophysiology to practice. J Am Coll Cardiol. 2009;54(23): 2129–38.
2. Libby P, Theroux P. Pathophysiology of coronary artery disease. Circulation. 2005;111(25):3481–8.
3. Weber C, Zernecke A, Libby P. The multifaceted contributions of leukocyte subsets to atherosclerosis: lessons from mouse models. Nat Rev Immunol. 2008;8(10):802–15.
4. Hansson GK, Libby P. The immune response in atherosclerosis: a double-edged sword. Nat Rev Immunol. 2006;6(7):508–19.
5. Newby AC. Metalloproteinases and vulnerable atherosclerotic plaques. Trends Cardiovasc Med. 2007;17(8):253–8.
6. Hansson GK, Hermansson A. The immune system in atherosclerosis. Nat Immunol. 2011;12(3):204–12.
7. Banchereau J, Steinman RM. Dendritic cells and the control of immunity. Nature. 1998;392(6673):245–52.
8. Steinman RM, Banchereau J. Taking dendritic cells into medicine. Nature. 2007;449(7161):419–26.
9. Acuto O, Michel F. CD28-mediated co-stimulation: a quantitative support for TCR signalling. Nat Rev Immunol. 2003;3(12): 939–51.
10. Le Gros G et al. Generation of interleukin 4 (IL-4)-producing cells in vivo and in vitro: IL-2 and IL-4 are required for in vitro generation of IL-4-producing cells. J Exp Med. 1990;172(3): 921–9.
11. Seder RA et al. Interleukin 12 acts directly on CD4+ T cells to enhance priming for interferon gamma production and diminishes interleukin 4 inhibition of such priming. Proc Natl Acad Sci USA. 1993;90(21):10188–92.
12. Bettelli E et al. Reciprocal developmental pathways for the generation of pathogenic effector TH17 and regulatory T cells. Nature. 2006;441(7090):235–8.
13. Das J et al. Transforming growth factor beta is dispensable for the molecular orchestration of Th17 cell differentiation. J Exp Med. 2009;206(11):2407–16.
14. Mangan PR et al. Transforming growth factor-beta induces development of the T(H)17 lineage. Nature. 2006;441(7090):231–4.
15. Sakaguchi S et al. Regulatory T cells and immune tolerance. Cell. 2008;133(5):775–87.
16. Buono C et al. Influence of interferon-gamma on the extent and phenotype of diet-induced atherosclerosis in the LDLR-deficient mouse. Arterioscler Thromb Vasc Biol. 2003;23(3): 454–60.
17. Gupta S et al. IFN-gamma potentiates atherosclerosis in ApoE knock-out mice. J Clin Invest. 1997;99(11):2752–61.
18. Whitman SC, Ravisankar P, Daugherty A. IFN-gamma deficiency exerts gender-specific effects on atherogenesis in apolipoprotein E–/– mice. J Interferon Cytokine Res. 2002;22(6):661–70.
19. Whitman SC et al. Exogenous interferon-gamma enhances atherosclerosis in apolipoprotein E–/– mice. Am J Pathol. 2000;157(6): 1819–24.
20. Buono C et al. T-bet deficiency reduces atherosclerosis and alters plaque antigen-specific immune responses. Proc Natl Acad Sci USA. 2005;102(5):1596–601.
21. Niwa T et al. Interferon-gamma produced by bone marrow-derived cells attenuates atherosclerotic lesion formation in LDLR-deficient mice. J Atheroscler Thromb. 2004;11(2):79–87.
22. Jonasson L, Holm J, Hansson GK. Smooth muscle cells express Ia antigens during arterial response to injury. Lab Invest. 1988;58(3): 310–5.
23. Pober JS et al. Lymphocytes recognize human vascular endothelial and dermal fibroblast Ia antigens induced by recombinant immune interferon. Nature. 1983;305(5936):726–9.
24. McLaren JE, Ramji DP. Interferon gamma: a master regulator of atherosclerosis. Cytokine Growth Factor Rev. 2009;20(2): 125–35.
25. Liuzzo G et al. Perturbation of the T-cell repertoire in patients with unstable angina. Circulation. 1999;100(21):2135–9.
26. Frostegard J et al. Cytokine expression in advanced human atherosclerotic plaques: dominance of pro-inflammatory (Th1) and macrophage-stimulating cytokines. Atherosclerosis. 1999;145(1):33–43.
27. Liuzzo G et al. Monoclonal T-cell proliferation and plaque instability in acute coronary syndromes. Circulation. 2000;101(25):2883–8.
28. Namekawa T et al. Functional subsets of CD4 T cells in rheumatoid synovitis. Arthritis Rheum. 1998;41(12):2108–16.
29. Nakajima T et al. T-cell-mediated lysis of endothelial cells in acute coronary syndromes. Circulation. 2002;105(5):570–5.
30. Liuzzo G et al. Unusual CD4+CD28null T lymphocytes and recurrence of acute coronary events. J Am Coll Cardiol. 2007;50(15): 1450–8.
31. Giubilato S. Expansion of CD4+CD28null T-lymphocytes in diabetic patients: exploring new pathogenetic mechanisms of increased cardiovascular risk in diabetes mellitus. Eur Heart J. 2011;32(10): 1214–26.
32. Bryl E et al. Modulation of CD28 expression with anti-tumor necrosis factor alpha therapy in rheumatoid arthritis. Arthritis Rheum. 2005;52(10):2996–3003.
33. Bryl E et al. Down-regulation of CD28 expression by TNF-alpha. J Immunol. 2001;167(6):3231–8.
34. Zal B, Baboonian C, Kaski JC. Autoreactive CD4+ CD28- T cells and acute coronary syndromes. Arterioscler Thromb Vasc Biol. 2007;27(3):e18; author reply e19.
35. Zal B et al. Heat-shock protein 60-reactive CD4+CD28null T cells in patients with acute coronary syndromes. Circulation. 2004; 109(10):1230–5.
36. Dumitriu IE, Baruah P, Finlayson CJ, Loftus IM, Antunes RF, Lim P, et al. High levels of co-stimulatory receptors OX40 and 4-1BB characterise CD4^{+}CD28null T cells in patients with acute coronary syndrome. Circ Res. 2012;110:857–69.
37. Ye P et al. Requirement of interleukin 17 receptor signaling for lung CXC chemokine and granulocyte colony-stimulating factor expression, neutrophil recruitment, and host defense. J Exp Med. 2001; 194(4):519–27.
38. Langrish CL et al. IL-23 drives a pathogenic T cell population that induces autoimmune inflammation. J Exp Med. 2005;201(2):233–40.

39. Smith E et al. Blockade of interleukin-17A results in reduced atherosclerosis in apolipoprotein E-deficient mice. Circulation. 2010;121(15):1746–55.
40. van Es T et al. Attenuated atherosclerosis upon IL-17R signaling disruption in LDLr deficient mice. Biochem Biophys Res Commun. 2009;388(2):261–5.
41. Ait-Oufella H et al. B cell depletion reduces the development of atherosclerosis in mice. J Exp Med. 2010;207(8):1579–87.
42. Eid RE et al. Interleukin-17 and interferon-gamma are produced concomitantly by human coronary artery-infiltrating T cells and act synergistically on vascular smooth muscle cells. Circulation. 2009;119(10):1424–32.
43. Taleb S et al. Loss of SOCS3 expression in T cells reveals a regulatory role for interleukin-17 in atherosclerosis. J Exp Med. 2009; 206(10):2067–77.
44. Wan YY. Multi-tasking of helper T cells. Immunology. 2010;130(2): 166–71.
45. Lloyd CM, Hessel EM. Functions of T cells in asthma: more than just T(H)2 cells. Nat Rev Immunol. 2010;10(12):838–48.
46. Schulte S, Sukhova GK, Libby P. Genetically programmed biases in Th1 and Th2 immune responses modulate atherogenesis. Am J Pathol. 2008;172(6):1500–8.
47. Davenport P, Tipping PG. The role of interleukin-4 and interleukin-12 in the progression of atherosclerosis in apolipoprotein E-deficient mice. Am J Pathol. 2003;163(3):1117–25.
48. King VL, Szilvassy SJ, Daugherty A. Interleukin-4 deficiency decreases atherosclerotic lesion formation in a site-specific manner in female LDL receptor–/– mice. Arterioscler Thromb Vasc Biol. 2002;22(3):456–61.
49. Vignali D. How many mechanisms do regulatory T cells need? Eur J Immunol. 2008;38(4):908–11.
50. Costantino CM, Baecher-Allan C, Hafler DA. Multiple sclerosis and regulatory T cells. J Clin Immunol. 2008;28(6):697–706.
51. Venigalla RK et al. Reduced CD4+, CD25- T cell sensitivity to the suppressive function of CD4+, CD25high, CD127 -/low regulatory T cells in patients with active systemic lupus erythematosus. Arthritis Rheum. 2008;58(7):2120–30.
52. Mallat Z, Ait-Oufella H, Tedgui A. Regulatory T-cell immunity in atherosclerosis. Trends Cardiovasc Med. 2007;17(4):113–8.
53. Ait-Oufella H et al. Natural regulatory T cells control the development of atherosclerosis in mice. Nat Med. 2006;12(2): 178–80.
54. Robertson AK et al. Disruption of TGF-beta signaling in T cells accelerates atherosclerosis. J Clin Invest. 2003;112(9):1342–50.
55. Sardella G et al. Frequency of naturally-occurring regulatory T cells is reduced in patients with ST-segment elevation myocardial infarction. Thromb Res. 2007;120(4):631–4.
56. Mor A et al. Altered status of CD4(+)CD25(+) regulatory T cells in patients with acute coronary syndromes. Eur Heart J. 2006; 27(21):2530–7.
57. Ammirati E et al. Circulating CD4+CD25hiCD127lo regulatory T-Cell levels do not reflect the extent or severity of carotid and coronary atherosclerosis. Arterioscler Thromb Vasc Biol. 2010; 30(9):1832–41.
58. Brugaletta S et al. Novel anti-inflammatory effect of statins: reduction of CD4+CD28null T lymphocyte frequency in patients with unstable angina. Heart. 2006;92(2):249–50.
59. Mausner-Fainberg K et al. The effect of HMG-CoA reductase inhibitors on naturally occurring CD4+CD25+ T cells. Atherosclerosis. 2008;197(2):829–39.
60. Hurlimann D et al. Anti-tumor necrosis factor-alpha treatment improves endothelial function in patients with rheumatoid arthritis. Circulation. 2002;106(17):2184–7.
61. Rizzello V et al. Modulation of CD4(+)CD28null T lymphocytes by tumor necrosis factor-alpha blockade in patients with unstable angina. Circulation. 2006;113(19):2272–7.
62. van Puijvelde GH et al. Induction of oral tolerance to oxidized low-density lipoprotein ameliorates atherosclerosis. Circulation. 2006; 114(18):1968–76.
63. van Puijvelde GH et al. Induction of oral tolerance to HSP60 or an HSP60-peptide activates T cell regulation and reduces atherosclerosis. Arterioscler Thromb Vasc Biol. 2007;27(12): 2677–83.
64. Mallat Z et al. Induction of a regulatory T cell type 1 response reduces the development of atherosclerosis in apolipoprotein E-knockout mice. Circulation. 2003;108(10):1232–7.

Immunological Mechanisms of Inflammation

3

Nilo José Coêlho Duarte, Cyro Alves de Brito, and Alberto José da Silva Duarte

Introduction

Cardiovascular diseases (CVDs) are the leading cause of death worldwide. The World Health Organization has estimated that around 17.3 million people died from CVDs in 2008, representing 30 % of all global deaths. Of these deaths, an estimated 7.3 million were due to coronary heart disease and 6.2 million to stroke [1].

The majority of the CVDs are induced by atherosclerosis, which is associated with a chronic inflammatory process in which the immune system has an important role. The natural evolution of this process is the formation of a thrombus that can cause a partial or complete blockage of the blood flow, inducing damage to the organ, such as the heart or brain.

Because of the blood flow blockage in a coronary artery, the ischemic environment results in myocardial infarction and the death of cardiomyocytes. The established disorder attracts substances out of the blood and retains them. These substances, such as cytokines and chemokines, are produced during the inflammatory response to ischemic injury, mediating various reactions and attracting leukocytes to the lesion.

Despite the clinical therapeutic advances for CVDs, surgery is still widely used to treat them, and it has been reported that major general surgery causes profound alterations in immunity. After an initial proinflammatory phase associated with innate immunity, an immunosuppressive response mediated mainly by cells of the adaptive immune system takes place. Therefore, surgical stress inhibits innate immunity from the time of incision until about the first postoperative day. This is a crucial period with greater susceptibility to bacterial infections. In generaly, this susceptibility may be caused by the absence of recovery of innate immunity and lead to postoperative complications. The goal of further clinical studies must be to establish the immunomodulating property of the individual, which is very important for controlling innate immunity and inflammation in each patient.

For understanding the alterations established in the postoperative period, we first describe how the inflammation, innate immunity, and adaptive immune response take place and sequentially understand which modifications are imposed by the surgery. Finally, we describe some trials attempting to modulate immunity to inhibit the immunosuppression generated by the perioperative period.

Inflammation

Inflammation is the body's reply to injury or irritation, a protective attempt to both remove the stimulant and initiate the healing process. This response involves both innate and adaptive immunity, as well as diverse molecular and cellular processes (e.g., chemotaxis, phagocytosis, mitosis, and cell differentiation) by the affected tissues.

In the past, inflammation was associated with infections and the immune system. However, recent evidence

N.J.C. Duarte, MD (✉)
Clinical Laboratory, Hospital do Coração,
São Paulo, Brazil

Central Laboratory of Hospital das Clínicas, Faculty of Medicine,
University of São Paulo,
São Paulo, Brazil
e-mail: njcduarte@gmail.com

C.A. de Brito, PhD
Center of Immunology, Adolfo Lutz Institute,
São Paulo, Brazil

A.J. da Silva Duarte, PhD
Clinical Laboratory, Hospital do Coração,
São Paulo, Brazil

Faculty of Medicine, University of São Paulo,
São Paulo, Brazil

Central Laboratory of Hospital das Clínicas, Faculty of Medicine,
University of São Paulo,
São Paulo, Brazil

Laboratory of Medical Investigation Unit 56, Faculty of Medicine,
University of São Paulo,
São Paulo, Brazil

E.A. Gabriel, S.A. Gabriel (eds.), *Inflammatory Response in Cardiovascular Surgery*,
DOI 10.1007/978-1-4471-4429-8_3, © Springer-Verlag London 2013

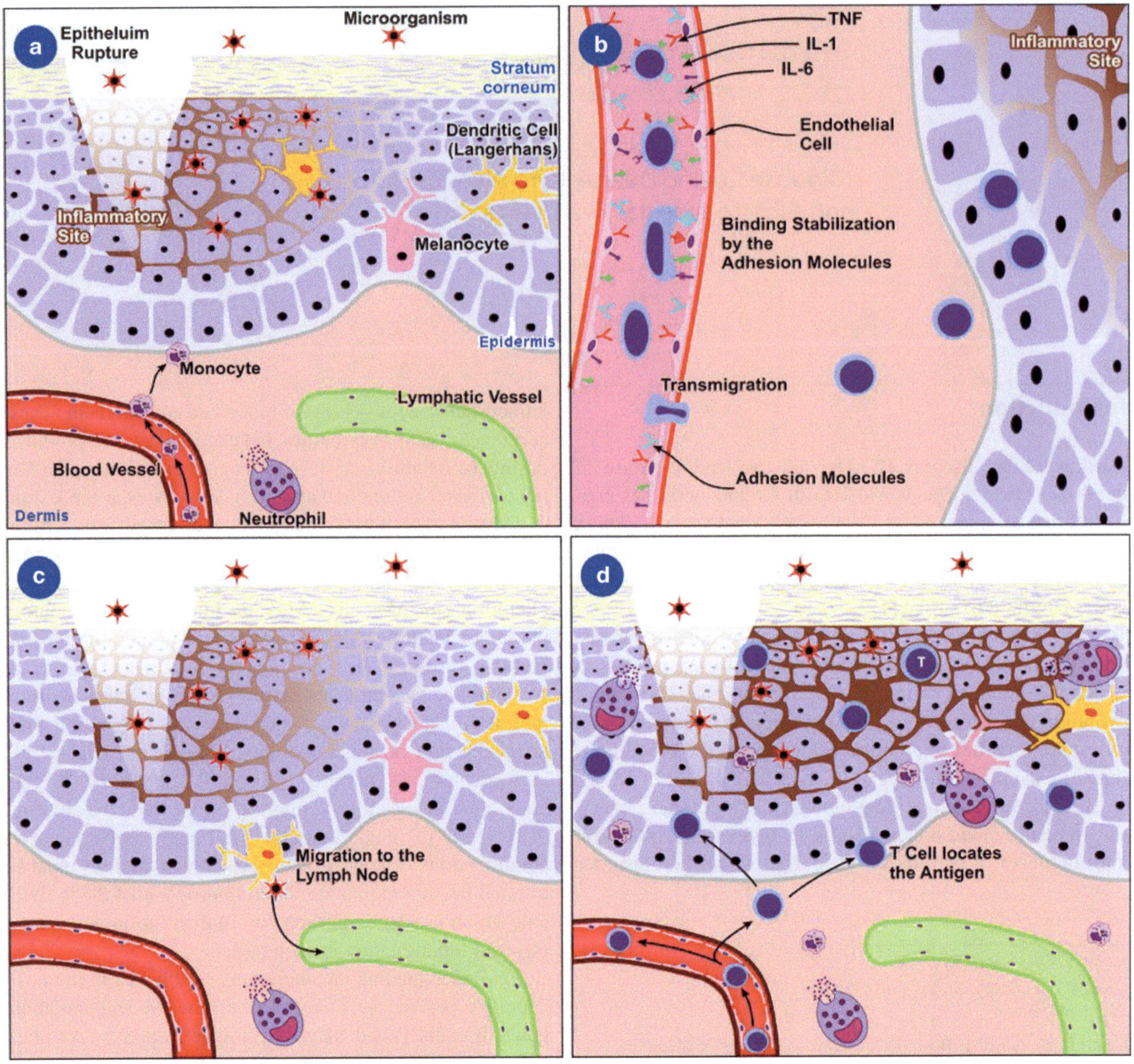

Fig. 3.1 Mechanisms involved in cell migration. (**a**) Inflammatory mediators, such as cytokines and chemokines, are produced during the inflammatory response to the pathogen or tissue proteins resulting from the cell damage. This response aims to isolate and destroy the pathogen and regenerate the injured tissue. (**b**) Expression of adhesion molecules facilitates the attachment of circulating cells to the endothelium and to tissue structures. The alteration in the blood flow allows the leukocytes in the blood to approach the endothelium, starting with a process of "rolling" by the interaction between the adhesion molecules expressed by the endothelial cells and the leukocyte molecules. At this time, the chemokines will influence the cell migration pattern. (**c**) Antigen-presenting cells migrate from the tissue to lymphoid organs where the adaptive immune response begins. (**d**) Activated lymphocytes leave the lymphatic circulation and migrate to the inflammation site

suggests that a broader range of disorders have inflammation markers. These include cancer, acute cerebrovascular stroke, Alzheimer's disease, chronic arterial and venous disease, myocardial ischemia, and systemic arterial hypertension [2].

The various forms of inflammation differ according to their location in the tissue, the organ where they occur, and the nature and severity of the tissue injury (e.g., mechanical injury, infectious agent, chemical injury, burn injury, radiation, tissue injury due to lack of organ perfusion, and oxygen supply) (Fig. 3.1a). In general, the inflammatory cascade includes several microvascular reactions, such as elevated permeability in microvessels, attachment of circulating cells to the vessels in the vicinity of the injury site, migration of several cell types, cell apoptosis, and growth of new tissue and blood vessels.

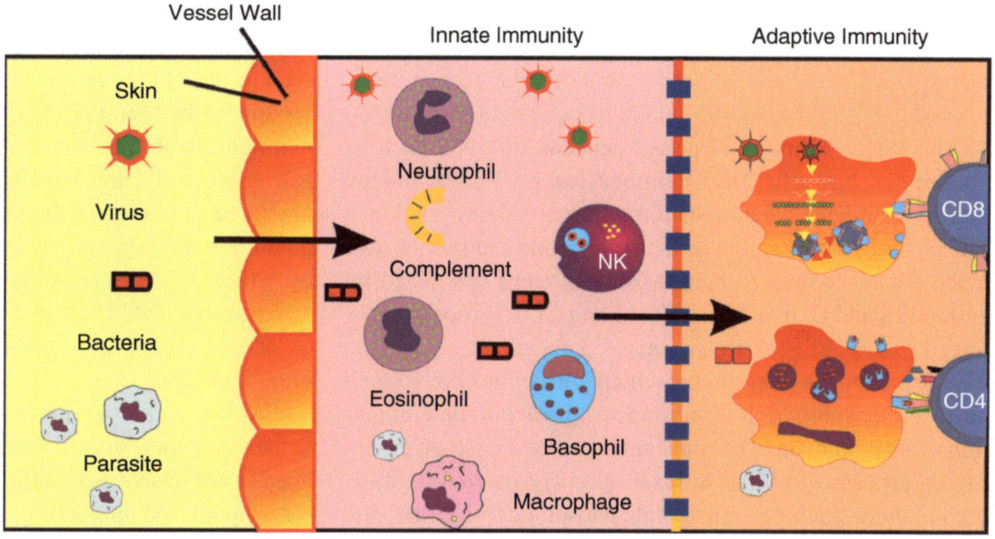

Fig. 3.2 Defense barriers against infections. The first line of defense is composed by the natural barriers, which are formed by the skin and mucosal epithelial surface, the corporal fluids, and the normal bacterial flora. The loss of integrity in any of these barriers, with or without infection, initiates the innate immunity. Next, the adaptive immune response is initiated, which is characterized by specificity and memory

An important form of cell activation in the microcirculation is the expression of membrane adhesion molecules that facilitate the attachment of circulating cells to the endothelium and to tissue structures over which they migrate. The alteration in the blood flow allows the leukocytes in the blood to approach the endothelium, starting with a process of "rolling" by the interaction between the adhesion molecules expressed by the endothelial cells (E-selectin, expressed by the activated endothelial cell, and P-selectin, which has constitutive expression) and leukocyte molecules (L-selectins) (Fig. 3.1b). After this, the action of leukotriene B4, platelet activation factor, and interleukin (IL)-8 triggers a conformational change of the integrins expressed in the leukocytes [leukocyte function-associated (LFA)-1 or CD11a/18 and Mac-1 or CD11b/18] enabling a firm interaction with the intercellular adhesion molecule (ICAM)-1 and ICAM-2 molecules expressed by the endothelial cells. The interaction of the leukocytes with platelet endothelial cell adhesion molecules allows its passage to the tissue through diapedesis and migration to the inflammatory site. At this time, the chemokines will influence the cell migration pattern, IL-8 and CXCL7 being important to neutrophil migration, CCL2, CCL3, and CCL4 to monocyte migration, and CCL11 to eosinophil migration [3, 4].

Inflammatory mediators, such as cytokines and chemokines, are produced during the inflammatory response to the pathogen or tissue proteins resulting from the cell damage. This response aims to isolate and destroy the pathogen and regenerate the injured tissue (Fig. 3.1c, d). It starts with the contraction or dilation of the arteriole muscle wall and the dilation of the venules by contraction of the actin and myosin filaments of the endothelial cells. This mechanism is due to the action of the mediators produced by local mast cells and macrophages. Some of these mediators are histamine, lipid mediators (leukotrienes- B4, C4, and D4, prostaglandins, and platelet activation factor), and neuropeptides [substance p and calcitonin gene-related peptide]. Parallel to this event, there is the activation of the blood coagulation cascade (production of chemotactic peptides), fibrinolytic system, complement activation, and kinin system (production of bradykinin) [3, 4].

The activation of the cells involved in the innate immune response induces the secretion of various cytokines, such as IL-1, IL-6, IL-8, IL-12, IL-18, and TNF-α. IL-1 acts in the vascular endothelium, increasing leukocyte adhesion, and in the bone marrow, increasing leukocyte production. In synergy with IL-18, IL-1 triggers the intracellular signalization with the activation via nuclear factor κB (NF-κB), which induces the production of many cytokines and chemokines [3, 4]. IL-1 and TNF-α bind to the thermoregulatory receptors in the hypothalamus, causing fever. TNF-α increases the vascular permeability of the endothelium, allowing the accumulation of immunoglobulins and complement proteins in the injured tissue. IL-6 is responsible for the stimulation and differentiation of the B lymphocytes and together with IL-1 and TNF-α acts in the liver, promoting the synthesis of the acute phase proteins, such as C-reactive protein (CRP). IL-8 is important in the cell migration to the damaged tissue, especially neutrophils, and IL-12, which is responsible for the activation of the natural killer cells (NK) [2].

Innate Immunity

The first line of defense of the organism against infections is composed by its natural barriers, which are formed by the skin and mucosal epithelial surface, the corporal fluids, and the normal bacterial flora (Fig. 3.2). The loss of integrity in any of these barriers, with or without infection, initiates the innate immune response. Other elements that compose the innate immunity include the complement system, inflammatory mediators, chemokines, cytokines, pathogen-associated molecular pattern recognition receptors, antimicrobial peptides, and some populations of the immune cells.

The innate immune response depends on cells such as phagocytes, NK cells, NKT lymphocytes, γ:δ T cells, and the B-1 lymphocytes capable of directly recognizing antigens. The phagocytes comprehend the neutrophils and monocytes/macrophages, which recognize the pathogens opsonized by antibodies and C3b or by the CD14 and CD204 receptors. In phagocytosis antigens are internalized, forming a membrane vesicle named the phagosome, which joins with a pre-formed vesicle (lysosome) rich in substances that act in the elimination of the pathogen. This substances are produced primarily by the process of oxidative respiration [lysosomal oxidase, nicotinamide adenine dinucleotide phosphate (NADPH), and other enzymes] where several cytotoxic products derived from oxygen are formed, such as the superoxide anion (O_2-), hydrogen peroxide (H_2O_2), free oxygen (O_2), hydroxyl radical (OH), and hypochlorous acid (HOCl). Nitrogen oxides (nitric oxide-NO), antimicrobial peptides (cationic), lysozyme, acid hydrolases, and competitors, such as lactoferrin, an iron chelator, are also produced. The macrophages are also responsible for secretion of IL-12, a cytokine important to the cellular activation.

The NK cells can potentially secrete IFN-γ, which is vital to the control of infection by intracellular pathogens, such as the Herpes virus, *Leishmania*, and *Listeria monocytogenes*, before the activation of the antigen-specific T lymphocytes. Other cytokines involved in the innate response are interferon type α and β (IFN-α and IFN-β), which have the capacity to inhibit viral replication, activate NK cells, and increase the expression of major histocompatibility complex (MHC-1) molecules in the infected cells, increasing their susceptibility to attack by cytotoxic T cells.

Innate Receptors

As a result of evolutionary progress, all multicellular organisms have developed mechanisms to recognize invading organisms by specific receptors to structures common to the majority of pathogens. These molecular patterns associated with pathogens are called pathogen-associated molecular patterns (PAMPs). They are highly conserved products associated with several microorganisms, such as the bacterial outer membrane, lipopolysaccharides (LPS), glycopeptides (PGN), lipotechoic acid (LTA), cytosine-phosphate-guanine unmethylated motifs (CpG), double-stranded RNA from RNA viruses, and mannans from fungal walls [3].

However, molecular patterns associated with tissue damage are called damage/danger-associated molecular patterns (DAMPs) [5]. In theory, every single molecule that normally resides within the cells is a potential DAMP when released after cell death. In fact, the systemic and/or local DAMPS, such as heat shock proteins (HSP), surfactant protein A, and protein of the high mobility group 1 (HMGB1), are elevated in inflammatory and autoimmune disorders, including CVDs [6]. These molecules have gained much attention in DAMP-mediated activation of the innate immune system and subsequent inflammation after cardiac ischemia. The mechanisms by which DAMPs activate and control leukocyte behavior and whether DAMPs can be used as therapeutic targets in order to modulate detrimental inflammatory responses remain unclear.

PAMPs and DAMPs activate innate immunity through some receptors, contributing to the inflammatory process even in the absence of pathogens. The molecules and receptors capable of interacting with those molecules are called pattern-recognition receptors/molecules (PRRs/PRMs). PRRs are responsible for the cell/antigen interaction in the inflammatory site, collaborating in phagocytosis, cytokines secretion, and intracellular signalization. PRMs are soluble, secreted proteins, such as surfactant protein (SP)-A, SP-D, mannose binding protein (MBL), ficolins, and CRP.

Two categories of PRRs are recognized: (1) scavenger receptors, which mediate the capture, uptake, and presentation of antigen, and (2) Toll-like receptors (TLR), which lead the activation of proinflammatory pathways.

Toll-like receptors (TLRs) constitute a family of host defense receptors, which are expressed in different cell types, especially in immune system cells, but also in keratinocytes and epithelial cells, among others (Fig. 3.3). To date, 13 TLRs have been identified in mammals, including 10 in humans and 12 in mice [7]. Among the TLR ligands are microbial compounds, such as peptideoglycan (TLR 1, 2, 3, 6), viral double-stranded RNA (TLR 3), lipopolysaccharide (TLR 4), flagellin (TLR 5), single-stranded RNA (TLR 7, 8), bacterial and viral DNA containing non-methylated cytosine-guanine dinucleotide (CpG) (TLR 9) [8], and uropathogenic *E. coli* and *T. gondii* profilin (TLR 11 in mice) [9].

The intracellular events that occur during the activation of TLR are mediated by myeloid differentiation factor 88 (MyD88), except in the activation of TLR3, which is mediated by the molecule TRIF (TIR domain-containing adapter inducing IFN-β). The activation of TLR4 is mediated by both MyD88 and TRIF [10]. MyD88-dependent pathway promotes early activation of nuclear factor kappa B (NF-κB), which leads to production of proinflammatory cytokines, particularly TNF-α. Furthermore, the MyD88-independent pathway, mediated by TRIF, promotes activation of the late phase of NF-κB and interferon regulatory factor (IRF), inducing the synthesis of IFN-β and the expression of genes induced by type 1 IFN. The activation of NF-κB is well recognized as a hallmark of innate immunity activation after cardiac ischemia. As the signaling cascade triggered by

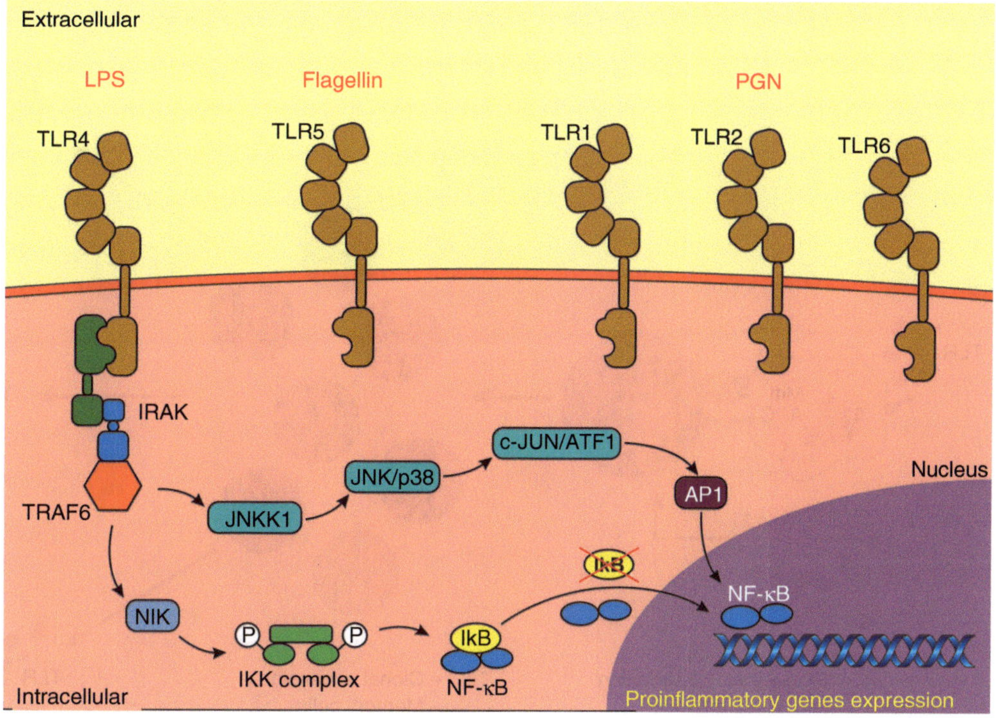

Fig. 3.3 Toll-like receptors (TLRs) constitute a family of innate immunity receptors. The intracellular events that occur during the activation of TLR are mediated by myeloid differentiation factor 88 (MyD88) or by the molecule TIR domain-containing adapter-inducing IFN-β (TRIF). TLR activation promotes activation of nuclear factor kappa B (NF-κB), which leads to production of proinflammatory cytokines

TLRs also involves NF-κB, a new paradigm of noninfectious activation of the innate immune system following cardiac ischemia can be postulated.

In an experimental model, a rapid activation of Irak-1, an important kinase in the response via TLR, has been shown after transient ischemia. This activation is caused by increased levels of HSP60 binding to TLR4 in triggering the inflammatory process in cardiac tissue [11]. It was also observed that treatment of cardiomyocytes with HSP60 leads to the activation of caspase-3 and -8, suggesting the activation of apoptotic pathways. Indeed, HSP60 induces apoptosis in rat cardiomyocytes in part by binding to TLR4 [12]. Moreover, apoptosis induced by myocardial ischemia/reperfusion injury is significantly attenuated in mice deficient in TLR4 or treated with anti-HSP60 [11].

Adaptive Immunity

The main characteristics of the adaptive immune response are specificity and memory. Unlike the innate immune responses, adaptive immune responses are not initiated in the inflammatory site, but in the peripheral lymphoid tissues. It occurs after antigen-presenting cells (APCs), such as macrophages and dendritic cells, migrate from the inflamed tissue to the nearest lymphoid tissue, carrying antigen particles that are presented to T lymphocytes (Fig. 3.4).

Unlike B cells, T lymphocytes recognize antigen only when it is associated with major histocompatibility complex (MHC) molecules expressed on the cell surface. The MHC molecules are glycoproteins encoded by highly polymorphic genes, also called HLA (human leukocyte antigen) genes in humans. There are two types of MHC molecules related to antigen presentation, the class I and class II, which differ in structure and expression pattern in different cell types. MHC-I molecules are composed of two polypeptide chains: a largest α chain, consisting of three domains, non-covalently linked to a smaller chain named β2 microglobulin. MHC-I is expressed on all nucleated cells of the body and associated with the peptides present in the cytosol, such as molecules of cytosolic pathogens, especially viruses, to present them to CD8+ T cells [3]. Class II MHC molecules, on the other hand, are expressed on antigen-presenting cells (APCs) and activated T lymphocytes. They consist of a non-covalent complex of two chains, α and β, each with two domains, which cross the membrane. These molecules bind to peptides derived from the degradation of antigens in vesicular compartments of macrophages, dendritic cells, and B lymphocytes, which will be presented to CD4+ T cells.

The binding of the complex peptide:MHC to a specific TCR is the first event necessary for activation of T lymphocytes. However, for the occurrence of an efficient activation of the immune response the involvement of accessory molecules is required. The binding of LFA-1 molecules, CD2 and ICAM-3, expressed by T lymphocytes, and ICAM-1 and 2, LFA-3, and dendritic cell-specific intercellular adhesion molecule-3-grabbing non-integrin (DC-SIGN) by APCs allows T lymphocytes to come into contact with large numbers of MHC molecules on the APC surface [4].

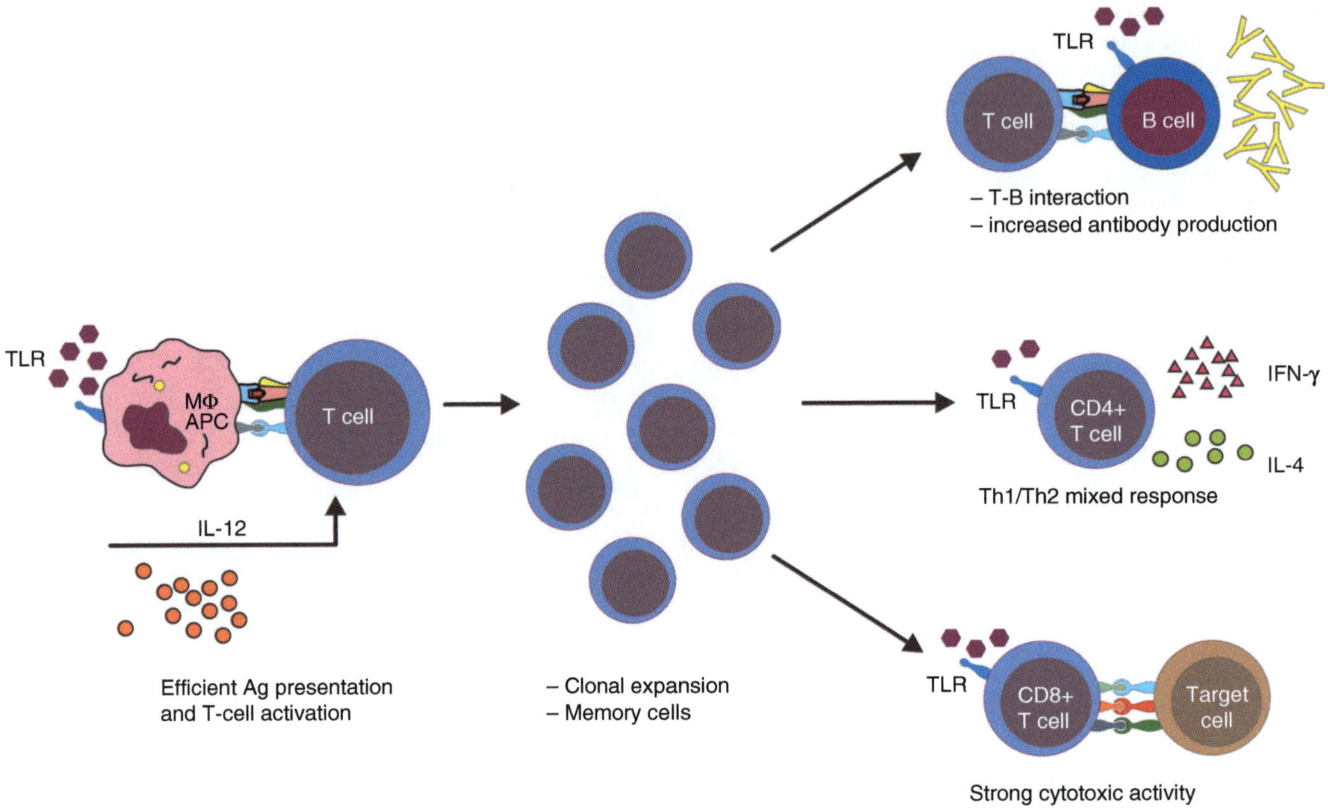

Fig. 3.4 Linking innate and adaptive immunity. Toll-like receptor agonists, such as DAMPs, increase expression of MHC and costimulatory molecules in APCs, causing proper activation of T cells, which promotes T cell clonal expansion and generation of memory cells. Immune adjuvants improve the interaction between T and B cells, secretion of Th1/Th2 cytokines, and antibody production, and they increase CTL activity in newborns (Adapted from de Brito et al. [13])

Another group of molecules involved in cell activation is the group of co-stimulatory molecules. In addition to antigen recognition via the TCR, a "second signal" or co-stimulatory signal is necessary for cell activation. The absence of co-stimulatory molecule interaction can promote T cell anergy or deletion by apoptosis [14]. The anergy is characterized by the inability of lymphocytes to produce IL-2, even after an antigenic stimulus, preventing the proliferation of specific clones and the generation of effector cells. Once activated, T cells initiate the proliferation phase, induced by autocrine production of IL-2. At this stage there is an increased expression of the α chain of the IL-2 receptor and increased receptor affinity for the cytokine. After a period of rapid growth, which can range from 3 to 7 days, T lymphocytes differentiate into effector cells that will perform specialized functions, such as helper or cytotoxic T cells [3, 4]. Effector T lymphocytes exhibit a series of phenotypic and functional changes that distinguish them from naïve T lymphocytes. The change in expression of some adhesion molecules, such as decreased CD62L and increased CD2, LFA-1, and CD44, stops the recirculation through the lymph nodes and favors the effector T cell migration to the inflammatory focus and other non-lymphoid tissues.

Cytokines secreted by cells involved in the innate response are crucial in determining a specific "T helper" (Th) response despite many factors, such as the antigen's route of entry into the body, antigen dose, and co-stimulators, and also influence the adaptive immune response. The CD4+ T cells can differentiate into different subtypes (Th1, Th2, Th3, Th17, regulatory T cells, etc.) according to the pattern of cytokine secretion. Th1 lymphocytes secrete mainly IFN-γ, IL-2, and TNF-α, whereas Th2 lymphocytes produce IL-4, IL-5, and IL-13 [15].

In general, Th1 lymphocytes stimulate a cellular immune response characterized primarily by the activation of macrophages. This process is mediated by soluble or cell surface molecules of T lymphocytes, such as IFN-γ, granulocyte-macrophage colony-stimulating factor (GM-CSF), TNF-α, CD40L, and FasL [16]. Activated macrophages produce high levels of oxygen radicals and nitric oxide (NO), antibacterial peptides, and proteases. The activation of these cells increases the expression of MHC-II molecules and B7, CD40, and TNFR receptors, enhancing antigen presentation to T lymphocytes and amplifying the immune response. Th2 lymphocytes produce cytokines that stimulate mainly the humoral immune response, i.e., the production of antibodies. IL-4 induces the switch to IgE, increases the expression of MHC-II molecules on B lymphocytes, stimulates T lymphocytes, increases the proliferation of mast cells, and inhibits macrophage activation. IL-5 stimulates the growth and differentiation of eosinophils [17].

Immune Dysfunction on Perioperative Period

In 1999, the Center for Disease Control and Prevention (CDC) in the USA presented the guideline for prevention of surgical site infection. Surgical site infections are the third most frequently reported nosocomial infection. When surgical patients with nosocomial surgical site infection died, 77 % of the deaths were reported to be related to the infection. Therefore, it is necessary be aware of the major alterations caused in the body by surgery, detectable during the perioperative days. In general, it starts by the vanishing of the skin barrier, which protects against bacterial invasion, and the inflammatory process, which is established during surgery. These alterations affect the innate immunity, the first line of host defense, as much as the adaptive response, during major general surgery [18].

In fact, it has been possible to recognize that even an elective aortic surgery utilizing synthetic graft material, as well as experiments with vascular graft materials in vitro, induce systemic reactions and inflammatory responses [19–25]. Rudensky et al. [26] have attempted to compare the systemic response following two specific cardiac surgery procedures, coronary artery bypass grafting (CABG), versus isolated valve surgery. This study concluded that valve surgery seemed to induce a stronger proinflammatory state than CABG. A significant postoperative increase was observed in both white blood cells (WBC) and monocyte counts, probably reflecting the postoperative inflammatory response invoked by the trauma.

WBCs are the key effector cells that are rapidly mobilized to heal devitalized tissue to prevent secondary microbial invasion (Fig. 3.1a–d). This mobilization is associated with the inflammatory status achieved in order to protect the organism. At this point, numerous alterations due to the damage environment are established. Analysis of the inflammatory response in endovascular stent treatment of aortic aneurysms, for example, also showed elevation of the leukocyte count, which occurred in the premature phase of follow-up, while the lymphocyte and platelet count occurred in a late phase of follow-up. The sedimentation velocity values began to increase 6 h after the surgical procedure, increasing to its peak value in 7 days. The levels of C reactive protein (CRP) increased 6 h after surgery, resulting in a peak value at 48 h. Between 48 h and 7 days, a decrease in serum values was observed, and around the second postoperative month, the CRP values were practically undetectable [27].

The inflammatory state can also be related to the kind and the complexity of the surgery. Major surgery is associated with neutrophil dysfunction, as indicated by the reduced chemotactic ability, phagocytic ability, and superoxide anion production [28, 29]. In addition, surgical injury can lead to a multifactorial perioperative response including activation of complement, coagulation, fibrinolytic, and kallikrein cascades, activation of WBCs with degranulation and protease enzyme release, production of other free radicals, synthesis of various cytokines, and their consequences [30].

In fact, a correlation between the increased level of TNF-α with subsequent significant alteration of cell surface receptors (CD11a, CD11b, CD11c, CD18 and L-selectin) at 60 min post-balloon inflation has been reported. It is necessary to remember that these molecules play an important role in diapedesis, associated with the inflammatory process established after the surgery [31].

Similarly, Schumacher et al. [32] reported an upregulation of adhesion molecules, such as ICAM-1, E-selectin, and P-selectin, and release of cytokines within 12–24 h after implantation of the endovascular device even though a short period of moderate increase of IL-6 and IL-8 has been observed. Asimakopoulis et al. [33] also observed increased CD11b (Mac-1) expression on neutrophils at 24 h post-operation extending to the third postoperative day. CD11b is the intercellular adhesion molecule-1 ligand and could reflect the modulation of this adhesion molecule during the perioperative period. In contrast, Gabriel et al. [27] identified the peak level of ICAM-1 and L-selectin in the first postoperative month and after this period of time a decrease in the levels of both markers. Others demonstrated a significant increase in neutrophil CD11b expression in samples taken 15 min after commencement of surgery, but not in subsequent samples, possibly attributable to marginalization of the activated leucocytes into tissues. In addition, these results demonstrated that the expected inflammatory response is present in both premature and late phases after cardiac surgery, such as implantation of a vascular prosthesis [27]. Together, these results suggest that during the entire inflammatory period the expression of those adhesion molecules will be raised, reflecting increased mobilization of cells between the vessels and the extracellular environment, an action necessary in all phases of the injury caused by the surgery.

Cytokines play an important role in both up- and down-regulation of inflammation, and it is involved from the beginning of the innate immune response, trying to stop all injuries and avoiding any infections [34]. In particular, cytokines have been studied as a means to demonstrate the severity of surgical tissue injury.

The response of cytokines to trauma can be divided in three phases [35]. In the first phase, there is a local production of cytokines to neutralize the trauma stimulus and initiate healing and repair. In the second phase, small amounts of the cytokines are present in the systemic circulation, which help to optimize the defense mechanism. In the third phase, the amount of circulating cytokines is higher than in the initial phases because it is required for the repair process, leading to an abnormal inflammatory response. This may result in an extensive endothelial injury by both the direct effect of the mediating agents and the WBC-endothelial interaction.

The recent discovery of naturally occurring soluble receptors for TNF-α (sTNFr1, sTNFr2), a competitive antagonist for IL-1β (IL-1ra), and true antiinflammatory cytokines, such as IL-10, IL-4, and IL-13, has led to the concept of a "cytokine balance" [36]. The antiinflammatory cytokines block the process or at least suppress the intensity of the cascade. Therefore, a "balance" between the effects of proinflammatory (IL-1β, TNF-α, IL-6) and antiinflammatory cytokines is thought to determine the outcome of disease or inflammation established by any tissue injury [37].

Especially with ruptured aneurysms, IL-1β and TNF-α proinflammatory cytokines produce fever, inflammation, tissue destruction, and in some cases shock and death. However, it has been possible to reduce the biological activities of IL-1β and TNF-α by neutralizing antibodies, soluble receptors, and receptor antagonists. In fact, blocking IL-1β and TNF-α has been successful in patients with rheumatoid arthritis or inflammatory bowel disease but has not been successful in humans with sepsis [19–25].

Several studies have tried to correlate the clinical outcome and inflammatory response. Plasma concentrations of IL-1β and TNF-α were found to be significantly higher in patients presenting a ruptured abdominal aortic aneurysm compared with those operated on electively [19, 38].

The surgical trauma *per se* also correlates well with the measurements of IL-6. The premature elevation of IL-6 levels before the first hour after the end of the procedure achieved a peak value at 24 h and began to decrease in the first postoperative month, when values similar to before the procedure were observed. Sequentially, the release of IL-6, together with other proinflammatory factors, enables WBCs to release TNF-α. However, the TNF-α levels may reflect, but do not strictly predict the clinical outcome in patients with a ruptured aneurysm.

The inflammatory curve response during the perioperative period shows elevated IL-8 values, which decline up to 24 h. In sequence, it begins to increase until 48 h, being followed by a new decrease until 3 months after the procedure. These results deserve more studies, looking for IL-8's importance as a preoperatively preexisting marker of the inflammation level and as a possible prognostic marker [27].

It is also important to stress that chemokine/cytokine production, as we have seen before, plays an important role in host defense via the TLR. In fact, recent studies conducted by Dybdahl et al. [18] have demonstrated that surgical stress influences the expression of TLRs on leukocytes in addition to the synthesis of various cytokines. The stress due to the CABG because of cardiopulmonary bypass induces immediate release of HSP70 and TLRs from myocardial cells to the circulation. The HSP70 released modulates the monocyte TLR2 and TLR4 expression, mediating the synthesis of inflammatory cytokines. In fact, human adherent monocytes responded to recombinant HSP70 with IL-6 and TNF release when tested in vitro.

These results indicate that TLR4 appears to be involved in an HSP70-mediated activation of innate immunity through cytokine synthesis [18]. Confirming these findings, it has been shown that TLR4 monoclonal antibodies inhibited the cytokine response.

What will be the consequences of these alterations over the adaptive immune response? It is known that TNF-α production can be inhibited by cortisol, whose concentration increases during surgery and can potentiate IL-10 production [39, 40]. These findings correlate with a decrease in monocyte HLA-DR expression and could reflect the participation of the adaptive immune response in the immunosuppression observed during surgical trauma.

In fact, a significant decrease in absolute lymphocyte counts is observed, especially of the T cell population, and a significant decrease in human leukocyte antigen-DR (HLA-DR) antigen expression on monocytes has also been reported [41, 42]. Expression of these antigens reflects the adaptive immune response activity.

Many others studies have found similar depression of cellular immunity parameters in cardiac surgery patients [43–49]. Several investigators have found a correlation between the degree of postoperative immunosuppression, especially the decrease in HLA-DR antigen expression, and the subsequent development of postoperative infection or complications in both general and cardiac surgery [49, 50]. Others, such as Asimakopoulis et al. [33], have reported a postoperative immunosuppressive response represented by the significant decrease in lymphocyte count and in HLA-DR antigen expression on monocytes maintained during the 2 postoperative days in valve surgery versus the CABG group. The significant drop in the absolute lymphocyte count observed by these authors must reflect a significant decrease in all types, including T cells, B cells, and NK cells. These authors also observed a decrease in CD4+ and CD8+ T cells.

The consequences of the decrease in HLA-DR expression can be very important to the outcome of the perioperative period. Several studies have reported a significant correlation between the degree of decrease in HLA-DR antigen expression and the duration of this decrease with the development of infectious and non-infectious postoperative complications [49–51]. However, Kawasaki et al. [52] could not demonstrate such a correlation in their study. The cellular immunological responses, LPS hyporesponsiveness, and suppression of monocyte mCD14 may explain the involvement of the innate immune dysfunction via the deactivation of macrophages/monocytes and neutrophils established during the perioperative period. In addition to CD14, recent studies have demonstrated that surgical stress also influences the expression of TLRs on leukocytes, which is important, as discussed before, to the outcome of the postoperative period.

Despite the feeling that the state of immune depression might contribute to the development of postoperative infection, the studies reported here did not find that any measured parameters can predict the eventual infectious state that can be established during the perioperative period.

Perioperative Immune Modulation

Detrimental inflammatory responses during surgery have been consistently observed over several decades. Despite our detailed understanding of inflammation, novel therapeutic strategies from the preclinical arena have not yet been introduced into the clinical setting. Therefore, it is necessary to describe some promising ways to control the immune reactions that take place during surgical stress.

Immunonutrition is one of the strategies for improving patient outcome during the perioperative period. In fact, immunonutrients, such as several amino acids, glutamine, omega-3 fatty acids, antioxidant vitamins and minerals, and nucleotides, are able to modulate innate immune function [53].

Mayer et al. demonstrated that omega-3 fatty acids have antiinflammatory effects, including lowering blood leukocyte counts, serum C-reactive protein (CRP) concentration, and production of inflammatory cytokines by isolated endotoxin-stimulated mononuclear cells [54]. On other hand glutamine may enhance HSP expression and reduce inflammatory cytokine release [55].

Other strategies involving different goals have been described. TLRs, for example, have been postulated as ideal candidates to bridge the gap between cardiac-related injury and circulating mediators of inflammation. Evidence exists that TLRs are indeed crucial for post-infarction healing processes, but are also mediators of reperfusion injury. They can recognize injury-related molecules released after cell stress, cell death, or both, as DAMPS [56] and be activated by them [57, 58].

Endogenous activators of TLRs are interesting as therapeutic targets, and they are likely to be safe because most of them are only released after tissue injury and might not have a systemic biological function under physiological conditions.

Current strategies concerning the clinical development of the TLR blockade include: (1) global blockade of individual TLR functions using neutralizing antibodies, soluble TLR extracellular domains (ECDs), natural antagonists, and small molecule inhibitors, (2) inhibition of signaling pathways activated downstream of TLR stimulation using small molecules to target MyD88/TRAF/IRAK complex formation, mitogen-activated protein kinases (MAPK), or IκB kinase (IKK) activity, and (3) using PAMP antagonists, such as LPS inhibitors. Some of these compounds have reached phase II clinical trials, and the results are currently awaited, while others, particularly those targeting common signaling pathways, such as MAPK, have proved to be of limited efficacy [59].

Purification of beneficial DAMPs for therapeutic applications is another attractive idea, but also very challenging. In addition, genetic variations can influence the responsiveness of the immune system to certain DAMPs and therefore be of great importance to cardiac repair mechanisms. For this reason, future studies should address the genetic determinants of processes associated with danger signaling.

The current body of knowledge about the role of DAMPs in the infarcted myocardium does not explain why the local enhancement of several candidates, as opposed to their systemic elevation, improves cardiac function. A better understanding of both spatial and temporal functions of endogenous ligands will be of utmost importance to the development of successful therapies for cardiac ischemia.

In fact, it has been suggested that TLR 4 may mediate, at least in part, myocardial ischemia/reperfusion injury. Therefore, inhibition of TLR 4 activation, for example, may be a potential therapeutic target to attenuate ischemia/reperfusion-induced tissue damage in the clinical settings [60].

Another therapeutic way to manipulate the immune system could be based on immunomodulation in which the overall immune response deviates from a Th1- to a Th2-type response, but also have side effects. In models of multiple sclerosis, tolerization with myelin antigens induces a protective Th2 response in the acute phase, but, in the long term, such a Th2 response promotes B cell differentiation and leads to a humoral attack against myelin that worsens the neurological outcome [61]. Worsening in the chronic phase has also been reported in tolerization applied to models of cerebral ischemia [62]. Therefore, the delayed effects of humoral immunity could counteract the short-term benefit of suppression of cellular immunity. Protocols involving cytokines as possible modulators of the immune response have also been designed.

The release of IL-6, possibly together with other proinflammatory factors, enables white blood cells to release TNF-α [63]. Especially in ruptured aneurysms, IL-1β and TNF-α are proinflammatory cytokines that produce fever, inflammation, tissue destruction, and in some cases shock and death [64, 65]. It is possible to reduce the biological activities of IL-1β and TNF-α by neutralizing antibodies, soluble receptors, and receptor antagonists [66–71]. In fact, blocking IL-1β and TNF-α has been successful in patients with rheumatoid arthritis or inflammatory bowel disease but has not been successful in humans with sepsis [68, 72].

Similarly, other proinflammatory cytokines besides IL-6 have been implicated in the pathogenesis of several CVDs. Interleukin 33, for example, is a new member of the IL-1 family of cytokines that promotes Th2-type immune responses by signaling through the ST2L and interleukin-1 receptor accessory protein (IL-1RAcP) dimeric receptor complex [73]. Furthermore, IL-33 is a crucial cytokine for Th2-mediated host defense. The biological effects of IL-33 are limited by a soluble decoy form of ST2 (sST2).

Recent studies have shown that IL-33 is expressed in the vasculature and, besides ST2L, appears to have multiple protective effects in atherosclerosis, obesity, and diabetes and in cardiac remodeling [73–75]. Data could be found showing the role of IL-33 and its receptor ST2L within CVD and the potential use of sST2 as a predictor of mortality in several cardiovascular disorders, acting as a cardiovascular biomarker [76–81]. Manipulation of the IL-33/ST2 pathway therefore represents a promising new therapeutic strategy for treating or preventing CVD [82].

Finally, looking for cells as targets for immunomodulation, research conducted so far has focused on leukocyte/lymphocyte and cardiomyocyte functions after altering innate immune activity. Fibroblast transdifferentiation is crucial in post infarction repair responses. TLRs could also exert their action by affecting myofibroblast function and differentiation after cardiac ischemia, although this possibility remains to be studied.

Taken together, all this information makes clear that a better understanding of the immunology of tissue damage would enable the development of targeted approaches to selectively suppress the deleterious effects of inflammation.

Conclusion

Inflammation and impaired innate immune functions are common features in surgical patients and have a direct influence on their recovery from surgery. In recent years, an increase in immune depression established during the perioperative period has been reported. Meanwhile, enormous progress has been made in learning about the mechanisms involved in these situations. However, we are still searching for more information about how to prevent these deleterious dysfunctions.

Considering all the information discussed here, we understand that it is necessary to learn about the immunity and inflammation in each patient, since a great deal of variability can be found in each case. With this objective, we believe that it will be possible to find the correct way to modulate the inflammatory and immune response in the perioperative period.

References

1. Organization, W.H. Cardiovascular diseases (CVDs) fact sheet. 2011. Available from: http://www.who.int/mediacentre/factsheets/fs317/en/index.html. Accessed Sept 2011.
2. Schmid-Schonbein GW. Analysis of inflammation. Annu Rev Biomed Eng. 2006;8:93–131.
3. Murphy K, Travers P, Walport M. Janeway's immunobiology (immunobiology: the immune system (Janeway)). New York: Garland Science; 2007.
4. Paul WE, Paul WE. Fundamental immunology. New York: Raven Press; 1984.
5. Tsan MF, Gao B. Endogenous ligands of Toll-like receptors. J Leukoc Biol. 2004;76(3):514–9.
6. Scaffidi P, Misteli T, Bianchi ME. Release of chromatin protein HMGB1 by necrotic cells triggers inflammation. Nature. 2002;418(6894):191–5.
7. Bowie AG, Haga IR. The role of Toll-like receptors in the host response to viruses. Mol Immunol. 2005;42(8):859–67.
8. Takeda K, Kaisho T, Akira S. Toll-like receptors. Annu Rev Immunol. 2003;21:335–76.
9. Lauw FN, Caffrey DR, Golenbock DT. Of mice and man: TLR11 (finally) finds profilin. Trends Immunol. 2005;26(10):509–11.
10. Akira S, Takeda K. Toll-like receptor signalling. Nat Rev Immunol. 2004;4(7):499–511.
11. Li Y et al. Myocardial ischemia activates an injurious innate immune signaling via cardiac heat shock protein 60 and Toll-like receptor 4. J Biol Chem. 2011;286(36):31308–19.
12. Kim SC et al. Extracellular heat shock protein 60, cardiac myocytes, and apoptosis. Circ Res. 2009;105(12):1186–95.
13. de Brito CA, Goldoni AL, Sato MN. Immune adjuvants in early life: targeting the innate immune system to overcome impaired adaptive response. Immunotherapy. 2009;1(5):883–95.
14. Sharpe AH, Freeman GJ. The B7-CD28 superfamily. Nat Rev Immunol. 2002;2(2):116–26.
15. Murphy KM, Reiner SL. The lineage decisions of helper T cells. Nat Rev Immunol. 2002;2(12):933–44.
16. Gordon S. Alternative activation of macrophages. Nat Rev Immunol. 2003;3(1):23–35.
17. Agnello D et al. Cytokines and transcription factors that regulate T helper cell differentiation: new players and new insights. J Clin Immunol. 2003;23(3):147–61.
18. Dybdahl B et al. Inflammatory response after open heart surgery: release of heat-shock protein 70 and signaling through Toll-like receptor-4. Circulation. 2002;105(6):685–90.
19. Roumen RM et al. Cytokine patterns in patients after major vascular surgery, hemorrhagic shock, and severe blunt trauma. Relation with subsequent adult respiratory distress syndrome and multiple organ failure. Ann Surg. 1993;218(6):769–76.
20. Baigrie RJ et al. Systemic cytokine response after major surgery. Br J Surg. 1992;79(8):757–60.
21. De Mol Van Otterloo JC. The effects of aortic reconstruction and collagen impregnation of Dacron prostheses on the complement system. J Vasc Surg. 1992;16(5):774–83.
22. Brothers TE, Graham LM, Till GO. Systemic effects of prosthetic vascular graft implantation. Surgery. 1988;104(2):375–82.
23. Swartbol P et al. Aortobifemoral surgery induces complement activation and release of interleukin-6 but not tumour necrosis factor-alpha. Cardiovasc Surg. 1996;4(4):483–91.
24. Shepard AD et al. Complement activation by synthetic vascular prostheses. J Vasc Surg. 1984;1(6):829–38.
25. Bonfield TL et al. Cytokine and growth factor production by monocytes/macrophages on protein preadsorbed polymers. J Biomed Mater Res. 1992;26(7):837–50.
26. Rudensky B et al. The cellular immunological responses of patients undergoing coronary artery bypass grafting compared with those of

patients undergoing valve replacement. Eur J Cardiothorac Surg. 2010;37(5):1056–62.
27. Gabriel EA et al. Analysis of the inflammatory response in endovascular treatment of aortic aneurysms. Eur J Cardiothorac Surg. 2007;31(3):406–12.
28. Duignan JP et al. The association of impaired neutrophil chemotaxis with postoperative surgical sepsis. Br J Surg. 1986;73(3):238–40.
29. Utoh J et al. Effect of surgery on neutrophil functions, superoxide and leukotriene production. Br J Surg. 1988;75(7):682–5.
30. Butler J, Rocker M, Westaby S. Inflammatory response to cardiopulmonary bypass. Ann Thorac Surg. 1993;55(2):552–9.
31. Swartbol P, Truedsson L, Norgren L. The inflammatory response and its consequence for the clinical outcome following aortic aneurysm repair. Eur J Vasc Endovasc Surg. 2001;21(5):393–400.
32. Schumacher H, Huber FX, Aulmann M, Kallinowski F, Allenberg JR. Effect of endovascular surgery of infrarenal aortic aneurysms on circulating endothelial adhesion molecules, cytokines and proteinase inhibitors. Langenbecks Arch Chir Suppl Kongressbd. 1997;114:15–19.
33. Asimakopoulos G et al. Leukocyte integrin expression in patients undergoing cardiopulmonary bypass. Ann Thorac Surg. 2000;69(4):1192–7.
34. Fong Y et al. The biologic characteristics of cytokines and their implication in surgical injury. Surg Gynecol Obstet. 1990;170(4):363–78.
35. Bone RC. Toward a theory regarding the pathogenesis of the systemic inflammatory response syndrome: what we do and do not know about cytokine regulation. Crit Care Med. 1996;24(1):163–72.
36. Gilliland HE et al. The choice of anesthetic maintenance technique influences the antiinflammatory cytokine response to abdominal surgery. Anesth Analg. 1997;85(6):1394–8.
37. Dinarello CA. Proinflammatory cytokines. Chest. 2000;118(2):503–8.
38. Froon AH et al. Increased concentrations of cytokines and adhesion molecules in patients after repair of abdominal aortic aneurysm. Eur J Surg. 1996;162(4):287–96.
39. van der Poll T et al. Hypercortisolemia increases plasma interleukin-10 concentrations during human endotoxemia – a clinical research center study. J Clin Endocrinol Metab. 1996;81(10):3604–6.
40. Steer JH, Vuong Q, Joyce DA. Suppression of human monocyte tumour necrosis factor-alpha release by glucocorticoid therapy: relationship to systemic monocytopaenia and cortisol suppression. Br J Clin Pharmacol. 1997;43(4):383–9.
41. Ogawa K et al. Suppression of cellular immunity by surgical stress. Surgery. 2000;127(3):329–36.
42. Ni Choileain N, Redmond HP. Cell response to surgery. Arch Surg. 2006;141(11):1132–40.
43. Rinder CS et al. Lymphocyte and monocyte subset changes during cardiopulmonary bypass: effects of aging and gender. J Lab Clin Med. 1997;129(6):592–602.
44. Franke A et al. Hyporesponsiveness of T cell subsets after cardiac surgery: a product of altered cell function or merely a result of absolute cell count changes in peripheral blood? Eur J Cardiothorac Surg. 2006;30(1):64–71.
45. Sbrana S et al. Monitoring of monocyte functional state after extracorporeal circulation: a flow cytometry study. Cytometry B Clin Cytom. 2004;58(1):17–24.
46. Akbas H et al. Effects of coronary artery bypass grafting on cellular immunity with or without cardiopulmonary bypass: changes in lymphocytes subsets. Cardiovasc Surg. 2002;10(6):586–9.
47. Wehlin L et al. Activation of complement and leukocyte receptors during on- and off pump coronary artery bypass surgery. Eur J Cardiothorac Surg. 2004;25(1):35–42.
48. Jankovicova K et al. The effect of cardiac surgery on peripheral blood lymphocyte populations. Acta Medica (Hradec Kralove). 2008;51(1):25–9.
49. Franke A et al. Delayed recovery of human leukocyte antigen-DR expression after cardiac surgery with early non-lethal postoperative complications: only an epiphenomenon? Interact Cardiovasc Thorac Surg. 2008;7(2):207–11.
50. Cheadle WG et al. HLA-DR antigen expression on peripheral blood monocytes correlates with surgical infection. Am J Surg. 1991; 161(6):639–45.
51. Strohmeyer JC et al. Standardized immune monitoring for the prediction of infections after cardiopulmonary bypass surgery in risk patients. Cytometry B Clin Cytom. 2003;53(1):54–62.
52. Kawasaki T et al. Effects of epidural anaesthesia on surgical stress-induced immunosuppression during upper abdominal surgery. Br J Anaesth. 2007;98(2):196–203.
53. Kawasaki T, Sata T. Perioperative innate immunity and its modulation. J UOEH. 2011;33(2):123–37.
54. Mayer K et al. Parenteral nutrition with fish oil modulates cytokine response in patients with sepsis. Am J Respir Crit Care Med. 2003;167(10):1321–8.
55. Ziegler TR et al. Parenteral glutamine increases serum heat shock protein 70 in critically ill patients. Intensive Care Med. 2005;31(8):1079–86.
56. Chao W. Toll-like receptor signaling: a critical modulator of cell survival and ischemic injury in the heart. Am J Physiol Heart Circ Physiol. 2009;296(1):H1–12.
57. Frantz S, Ertl G, Bauersachs J. Toll-like receptor signaling in the ischemic heart. Front Biosci. 2008;13:5772–9.
58. Arslan F et al. TLR2 and TLR4 in ischemia reperfusion injury. Mediators Inflamm. 2010;2010:704202.
59. Midwood KS, Piccinini AM, Sacre S. Targeting Toll-like receptors in autoimmunity. Curr Drug Targets. 2009;10(11):1139–55.
60. Chong AJ et al. Toll-like receptor 4 mediates ischemia/reperfusion injury of the heart. J Thorac Cardiovasc Surg. 2004;128(2):170–9.
61. Genain CP et al. Late complications of immune deviation therapy in a nonhuman primate. Science. 1996;274(5295):2054–7.
62. Gee JM et al. Long term immunologic consequences of experimental stroke and mucosal tolerance. Exp Transl Stroke Med. 2009;1:3.
63. Hall GM, Desborough JP. Interleukin-6 and the metabolic response to surgery. Br J Anaesth. 1992;69(4):337–8.
64. Swartbol P, Truedsson L, Norgren L. Adverse reactions during endovascular treatment of aortic aneurysms may be triggered by interleukin 6 release from the thrombotic content. J Vasc Surg. 1998;28(4):664–8.
65. Juvonen J et al. Elevated circulating levels of inflammatory cytokines in patients with abdominal aortic aneurysm. Arterioscler Thromb Vasc Biol. 1997;17(11):2843–7.
66. Hawkins PN, Lachmann HJ, McDermott MF. Interleukin-1-receptor antagonist in the Muckle-Wells syndrome. N Engl J Med. 2003;348(25):2583–4.
67. Joosten LA et al. IL-1 alpha beta blockade prevents cartilage and bone destruction in murine type II collagen-induced arthritis, whereas TNF-alpha blockade only ameliorates joint inflammation. J Immunol. 1999;163(9):5049–55.
68. Abramson SB, Amin A. Blocking the effects of IL-1 in rheumatoid arthritis protects bone and cartilage. Rheumatology (Oxford). 2002;41(9):972–80.
69. Mertens M, Singh JA. Anakinra for rheumatoid arthritis: a systematic review. J Rheumatol. 2009;36(6):1118–25.
70. Abbate A et al. Interleukin-1beta modulation using a genetically engineered antibody prevents adverse cardiac remodelling following acute myocardial infarction in the mouse. Eur J Heart Fail. 2010;12(4):319–22.
71. Abbate A et al. Anakinra, a recombinant human interleukin-1 receptor antagonist, inhibits apoptosis in experimental acute myocardial infarction. Circulation. 2008;117(20):2670–83.

72. Bresnihan B, Cobby M. Clinical and radiological effects of anakinra in patients with rheumatoid arthritis. Rheumatology (Oxford). 2003;42 Suppl 2:ii22–8.
73. Schmitz J et al. IL-33, an interleukin-1-like cytokine that signals via the IL-1 receptor-related protein ST2 and induces T helper type 2-associated cytokines. Immunity. 2005;23(5):479–90.
74. Moussion C, Ortega N, Girard JP. The IL-1-like cytokine IL-33 is constitutively expressed in the nucleus of endothelial cells and epithelial cells in vivo: a novel 'alarmin'? PLoS One. 2008;3(10):e3331.
75. Kuchler AM et al. Nuclear interleukin-33 is generally expressed in resting endothelium but rapidly lost upon angiogenic or proinflammatory activation. Am J Pathol. 2008;173(4):1229–42.
76. Januzzi Jr JL et al. Measurement of the interleukin family member ST2 in patients with acute dyspnea: results from the PRIDE (Pro-Brain Natriuretic Peptide Investigation of Dyspnea in the Emergency Department) study. J Am Coll Cardiol. 2007;50(7):607–13.
77. Martinez-Rumayor A et al. Soluble ST2 plasma concentrations predict 1-year mortality in acutely dyspneic emergency department patients with pulmonary disease. Am J Clin Pathol. 2008;130(4): 578–84.
78. Rehman SU et al. Independent and incremental prognostic value of multimarker testing in acute dyspnea: results from the ProBNP Investigation of Dyspnea in the Emergency Department (PRIDE) study. Clin Chim Acta. 2008;392(1–2):41–5.
79. Shah RV et al. Serum levels of the interleukin-1 receptor family member ST2, cardiac structure and function, and long-term mortality in patients with acute dyspnea. Circ Heart Fail. 2009;2(4): 311–9.
80. Dieplinger B et al. Prognostic value of established and novel biomarkers in patients with shortness of breath attending an emergency department. Clin Biochem. 2010;43(9):714–9.
81. Weinberg EO et al. Identification of serum soluble ST2 receptor as a novel heart failure biomarker. Circulation. 2003;107(5):721–6.
82. Miller AM, Liew FY. The IL-33/ST2 pathway – A new therapeutic target in cardiovascular disease. Pharmacol Ther. 2011;131(2): 179–86.

Part II

Carotid Diseases

Role of Lipoproteins in Carotid Arterial Disease

4

Efthymios D. Avgerinos and Christos D. Liapis

Introduction

Lipoproteins and their disorders are among the most substantiated risk factors for atherosclerosis and cardiovascular diseases, acting through a well-established pathway: abnormalities in lipid metabolism lead to pathologic lipid accumulation in the vessel wall, oxidative and chronic inflammatory sequelae, and the formation of atherosclerotic lesions, ultimately leading to clinical events.

Although the majority of the evidence implicating lipoproteins in atherosclerosis have traditionally emerged from the coronary vasculature, we now know that carotid artery disease (CAD), as a coronary heart disease (CHD) equivalent, shares similar links to both the pathophysiological pathways and treatment strategies. Over the past decade, however, many studies have begun to yield important information on the effect of lipoproteins' on the natural history of CAD and on the benefits of recognizing and managing these disorders.

This chapter addresses the role of lipoproteins in patients with CAD, including their physiology and metabolism, clinical evidence of their effects, and contemporary management of their disorders.

Physiology and Metabolism of Lipoproteins

Plasma lipoproteins are molecular complexes that transport and facilitate exchanges of water-insoluble lipids (cholesterol and triglycerides) from the intestine and liver through the bloodstream to the various cells of the body, where they can be stored, used for important synthetic processes, and metabolized to yield energy. They consist of a central core of triglycerides and cholesteryl esters surrounded by phospholipids, cholesterol, and constituent proteins known as apolipoproteins [1–3].

Lipoproteins are classified is based on their density (ratio of lipid to protein). They can be separated using a centrifuge into high-density lipoproteins (HDLs), low-density lipoproteins (LDLs), intermediate-density lipoproteins (IDLs), very-low-density lipoproteins (VLDLs), and the least dense particles, known as chylomicrons (Table 4.1). Apolipoproteins (apos), carried in the outer layer of lipoproteins, have functional significance that can be split into four major roles: (1) assembly and secretion of the lipoprotein (apo A-I, apo B-100, apo B-48), (2) structural integrity of the lipoprotein (apo B, apo E, apos A–I, apo A-II), (3) coactivator or inhibitor of enzymes (apos A-I, apos A-V, apo C-I, apo C-II, apo C-III), and (4) binding or docking to specific receptors and proteins for cellular uptake of the entire particle or selective uptake of a lipid component (apos A-I, apo B-100, apo E) (Table 4.2). The effects of many other apolipoproteins (apo A-IV, apo A-V, apo D, apo H, apo J, apo L, apo M) are still not completely understood [1–3].

Lipoproteins have different affinities for different lipids. In fasting serum, most of the cholesterol is carried on LDL particles, while most of the triglycerides are found in VLDL and chylomicron particles. Chylomicrons contain more than 80 % triglycerides, approximately 60 % VLDL, 10 % LDLs, and 50 % HDLs. Esterified cholesterol comprises 37 % LDLs, 10 % VLDLs, and 15 % HDLs; free cholesterol comprises approximately 10 % LDLs and VLDLs; phospholipids comprise 15 % VLDLs, 20 % LDLs, and 30 % HDLs [1–3].

The lipid metabolism follows two pathways, the exogenous (dietary, intestinal) and the endogenous (hepatic). The intestine transports lipids from digested food into the bloodstream through the lymphatic system, and the liver exports the lipids it synthesizes. Pathway defects in lipoprotein synthesis, processing, and clearance can lead to accumulation of atherogenic lipids in the plasma and endothelium.

E.D. Avgerinos, MD, FEBVS • C.D. Liapis, MD, FACS, FRCS (✉)
Department of Vascular Surgery, Medical School of Athens,
Attikon University Hospital,1 Rimini Street, Chaidari,
Athens 12462, Greece
e-mail: liapis@med.uoa.gr

E.A. Gabriel, S.A. Gabriel (eds.), *Inflammatory Response in Cardiovascular Surgery*,
DOI 10.1007/978-1-4471-4429-8_4, © Springer-Verlag London 2013

Table 4.1 Characteristics of major lipoproteins

Component	Origin	Size (nm)	Density (g/ml)	Protein (%)	Apolipoproteins
Chylomicrons	Intestine	100–1,000	<0.95	1–2	C-I, C-II, C-III, E, A-I, A-II, A-IV, B-48
VLDL	Liver, intestine	30–80	0.95–1.006	7–10	B-100, C-I, C-II, C-III
IDL	VLDL	25–50	1.006–1.019	11–18	B-100, E
LDL	VLDL	20–25	1.019–1.063	18–25	B-100
HDL	Liver, intestine VLDL, chylomicrons	5–15	1.063–1.210	32–57	A-I, A-II, A-IV C-I, C-II, C-III D, E

Table 4.2 Location and function of apolipoproteins

Apolipoprotein	Location	Function
A-I	HDL	Major component of HDL particle, ACAT activation
A-II	HDL	Major component of HDL particle
A-IV	HDL	Major component of HDL particle, absorption
A-V	VLDL, HDL	Triglyceride metabolism
B-100	VLDL, IDL, LDL, Lp(a)	LDL receptor ligand
B-48	Chylomicrons	Major component of chylomicrons
C-I	Chylomicrons	Triglyceride metabolism
C-II	Chylomicrons, VLDL, HDL	LPL activation
C-III	Chylomicrons, VLDL	LPL inhibition
D	HDL	LCAT
E	Chylomicrons, VLDL, IDL, HDL	LDL receptor ligand and apo-E receptor ligand
H	Chylomicrons, VLDL, LDL, HDL	B2 glycoprotein
J	HDL	Complement system
L 1-6	HDL	Not known
M	HDL	Not known
(a)	Lp(a)	Tissue injury

ACAT Acetyl-CoA acetyltransferase, *LPL* lipoprotein lipase, *LCAT* lecithin cholesterol acyltransferase

Exogenous (Dietary) Lipid Metabolism

Over 95 % of dietary lipids are triglycerides. The gastrointestinal tract has highly efficient fat absorption mechanisms. Dietary triglycerides are digested in the stomach and duodenum into monoglycerides and free fatty acids by gastric lipase, emulsification from vigorous stomach peristalsis, and pancreatic lipase. Dietary cholesterol esters are de-esterified into free cholesterol by these same mechanisms. Monoglycerides, free fatty acids, and free cholesterol are then solubilized in the intestine by bile acid micelles, which shuttle them to the intestinal villi for absorption. Once absorbed into the enterocyte, they are reassembled into triglycerides and packaged with cholesterol into chylomicrons, the largest lipoproteins. Chylomicrons transport dietary TGs and cholesterol from within enterocytes through the lymphatics into the circulation and finally to adipose and muscle tissue for energy use or storage. Cholesterol-rich chylomicron remnants then circulate back to the liver for degradation and reuptake of their core constituents.

Endogenous Lipid Metabolism

As dietary fat content varies, the body must ensure readily available triglyceride to meet energy demands. Hepatic secretion of VLDL particles serves this function. IDL, LDL, and HDL particles are derived following several complex VLDL de-lipidation processes and bi-directional transfer of constituents. Lipoproteins synthesized by the liver transport endogenous triglycerides and cholesterol. Lipoproteins circulate through the blood continuously until the triglycerides they contain are taken up by peripheral tissues or the lipoproteins themselves are cleared by the liver. Factors that stimulate hepatic lipoprotein synthesis generally lead to elevated plasma cholesterol and triglyceride levels.

Very-Low-Density Lipoproteins

Each VLDL particle contains apolipoproteins from the C and E family and one molecule of apo B-100 per particle. VLDL is the way the liver exports excess triglycerides derived from plasma-free fatty acids and chylomicron remnants. As triglycerides are removed from the peripheral adipose and muscle tissue, two additional atherogenic lipoprotein particles are formed, VLDL remnants and IDLs.

Intermediate-Density Lipoproteins

Intermediate-density lipoproteins are the product of VLDL and chylomicron metabolism. IDLs are cholesterol-rich VLDLs and chylomicron remnants that are either cleared by the liver or metabolized by hepatic lipase into LDL, which retains apo B.

Low-Density Lipoproteins

Low-density lipoproteins are the products of VLDL and IDL metabolism and the most cholesterol-rich and atherogenic of all lipoprotein particles. LDL binds to specific LDL receptors on the surface of each cell, and such binding facilitates transfer of the remaining cholesterol to these cells, where it can be stored for future use to make such chemical products as cell membranes, steroid hormones, and bile acids. About 70 % of these receptors are located within the liver, which clears the majority of LDL particles, while the rest are taken up by non-hepatic scavenger receptors. The number of LDL receptors is regulated by the intracellular concentration of cholesterol within each cell. When the intracellular cholesterol content of the cells is low, LDL receptor synthesis is upregulated, receptor numbers increase, and the LDL concentration of circulating plasma diminishes. On the other hand, when intracellular cholesterol is increased, LDL receptor synthesis is downregulated, receptor numbers diminish, and LDL within the circulation rises. When plasma LDL is present in excess, atherosclerosis results in proportion to the degree of circulating LDL [1–3].

There are two forms of LDL: large (buoyant) and small, dense LDL. Small, dense LDL (sdLDLD) is rich in cholesterol esters and particularly atherogenic. The increased atherogenicity of small, dense LDL derives from less efficient hepatic LDL receptor binding, leading to prolonged circulation and exposure to the endothelium and increased oxidation.

High-Density Lipoproteins

High-density lipoproteins are initially cholesterol-free lipoproteins that are synthesized in both enterocytes and the liver as lipid-poor discoid particles. HDL's overall role is to obtain cholesterol from peripheral tissues and other lipoproteins and transport it to where it is needed most, to other cells, other lipoproteins, and the liver (for clearance). This process is known as "reverse cholesterol transport" and plays an important role in the antiatherogenic properties of the HDL particle.

Pathophysiology of Atherosclerosis

Increased lipid levels can cause endothelial injury, which eventually results in endothelial dysfunction and increased permeability, allowing circulating atherogenic lipoprotein particles (VLDL, IDL, LDL) to penetrate and initiate the pathologic process of atherosclerosis. The developmental atherosclerotic process is the same for all vascular beds, including the carotids.

LDL has a leading role in the atherogenic process, predominately mediated through its oxidized fraction, as suggested by its accumulation within macrophages at all stages of plaque formation. Various reactive intermediates, derivatives of reactive oxygen and/or reactive nitrogen species, mediate the oxidative modification of LDL (oxLDL) [4–6]. OxLDL co-stimulates an inflammatory response to attract and stimulate the proliferation of both macrophages and vascular smooth muscle cells [7, 8].

Nonhepatic scavenger receptors, most notably on macrophages, take up excess circulating oxLDL not processed by hepatic receptors. Monocytes rich in oxLDL migrate into the subendothelial space and become macrophages; these macrophages then take up more oxLDL and form foam cells [9]. Groups of foam cells then accumulate underneath the endothelium and become the initial lesion of atherosclerosis, the fatty streak. As this process continues, the foam cells undergo the process of apoptosis, or cell death, which allows the lipid contained in them to spill out to from the lipid core of an atherosclerotic plaque. Some plaques continue to grow, become fibrotic, and intrude on the arterial lumen. These fibrotic plaques may be stable; however, when the lipid core enlarges and oxidizes an intense local inflammatory reaction is induced that results in the infiltration of additional macrophages and inflammatory cells. The fibrous cap thins and becomes prone to rupture and ulceration, which may lead to atherothromboembolic cerebrovascular events. This unstable plaque is also known as vulnerable plaque [1–3].

Clinical Evidence Implicating Lipoproteins to Carotid Atherosclerosis

Multiple clinical data have currently elucidated the underlying association of the major lipoproteins to atherosclerosis. Several studies have particularly focused on carotid atherosclerosis, but even more studies on the incidence of stroke related to serum lipids. While there are several possible mechanisms underlying the association of lipids and stroke, one of the most important is probably the effects of lipids on the formation of carotid artery plaque. Available clinical data relating lipids to carotid atherosclerosis and stroke are further analyzed.

Low-Density Lipoprotein

LDL cholesterol has been shown to be among the most predictive lipoprotein fractions for determining carotid atherosclerosis and stroke, being directly proportional to its concentration over a wide range of values. The majority of evidence derives from large statin trials to lower LDL cholesterol that showed reductions in carotid atherosclerosis progression, a need for carotid intervention, and cerebrovascular events, mainly the Heart Protection Study and SPARCL [10–12].

In addition, LDL fractions are intensively investigated as potentially more accurate predictors of carotid artery disease, mainly oxLDL and sdLDL. Clinical studies have shown an increase in plasma and plaque levels of oxLDL in patients with symptomatic carotid plaques compared to asymptomatic ones [13, 14]. Even more, baseline oxLDL levels may predict carotid disease progression in asymptomatic subjects, independent of other cardiovascular risk factors [15]. Regarding sdLDL, several lines of evidence suggest that it could be more atherogenic than the large (buoyant) particles of LDL and a more accurate predictor of carotid atherosclerosis compared to the traditionally measured LDL [16–21]. Many authors advocate that both plasma oxLDL and sdLDL assessments can be used as biomarkers for carotid disease progression, providing a link between lipoprotein disorders and inflammation [13–15, 18–21].

Intermediate Density Lipoprotein

Although LDL cholesterol is widely accepted as the major risk factor for the development and progression of atherosclerosis, its measurements generally include IDL. The Monitored Atherosclerosis Regression Study (MARS) provided further evidence for the role of these lipoproteins in the progression of carotid atherosclerosis and supported the suggestion that the risk of atherosclerosis attributable to LDL may be the result of the IDL included within the traditional LDL measurements [22, 23]. A later study on patients with carotid artery disease (stenosis >50 %) showed that fasting and postprandial triglyceride-rich lipoproteins (mainly VLDL and IDL) are elevated compared to controls and correlate to echo-lucent, rupture-prone carotid plaques [24].

High-Density Lipoprotein

HDL has been shown to have both direct and indirect antiinflammatory effects with potential antithrombotic results [25, 26]. However, the literature remains contradictory on the real protective effect of HDL against carotid atherosclerosis and stroke [27–29]. A recent systematic review of observational epidemiological studies concluded that although more evidence exists for an inverse association between HDL cholesterol levels and stroke or carotid atherosclerosis risk, further studies are needed [30].

Triglycerides (Very-Low-Density Lipoprotein – Chylomicron)

VLDL particles and chylomicrons represent the main triglyceride carriers in the circulation. Though clearly associated with cardiovascular disease, the exact mechanisms by which triglyceride-rich lipoproteins exert their noxious effect on the vascular wall are matters of debate. It is still unclear whether it is the number of triglyceride-rich lipoprotein particles or triglyceride-rich lipoprotein cholesterol or the associated small, dense LDL and low HDL that contribute most to atherosclerosis [31–36]. A recent systematic review and meta-regression analysis of randomized trials on lipid-modifying drugs concluded that additional studies are needed to more precisely quantify the detrimental effect of triglyceride levels on stroke risk and to establish the efficacy of triglyceride-lowering therapy in addition to LDL cholesterol reduction [37].

Lipoprotein (a)

Lipoprotein (a) consists of an LDL particle with its apolipoprotein-a. The apo-a component is characterized by five cysteine-rich regions known as "kringles." One of these regions is homologous with plasminogen and is thought to competitively inhibit fibrinolysis and thus predispose to thrombosis [38]. Lp(a) has been suggested as a direct promoter of atherosclerosis through various mechanisms, but the metabolic pathways of its production and clearance are not yet well characterized. Apoprotein-(a) fragments have been demonstrated to accumulate in unstable carotid plaques close to eroded and ulcerated areas, suggesting a strong correlation with atherosclerotic plaque destabilization [39]. A recent meta-analysis of observational studies on Lp(a) and cerebrovascular disease suggested that elevated Lp(a) is an independent risk factor for stroke [40].

Lipoprotein-Associated Phospholipase A2

Lipoprotein-associated phospholipase A2 (Lp-PLA2) is a member of the phospholipase A2 superfamily of enzymes that hydrolyze phospholipids. Lp-PLA2 binds mainly to circulating LDL, multiplying its atherogenic potential [41, 42].

Lp-PLA2 was initially attributed an atheroprotective role; however, recent evidence has highlighted its important role in the promotion of atherosclerosis [42].

Lp-PLA2 has been localized to human carotid plaques. Atherosclerotic plaques from symptomatic patients demonstrated greater levels of Lp-PLA2 than plaques obtained from asymptomatic patients [43, 44]. Additionally, blood levels of Lp-PLA2 have been shown to be an independent predictor of future stroke and transient ischemic events [45–48].

Lipoprotein Ratios

There is mounting evidence that serum lipid ratios may be better predictors of vascular risk than the traditional lipid measures. The Northern Manhattan Study on carotid atherosclerosis indicated that the relative levels of LDL and HDL may be more predictive than either LDL or HDL [49]. Very recently, a large-scale epidemiological study of healthy

Table 4.3 Lipoprotein-targeted medications

	Predominant lipoprotein effect	Clinical evidence against carotid atherosclerosis and related events
Statins		
Atorvastatin Fluvastatin Lovastatin Pravastatin Rosuvastatin Simvastatin Pitavastatin	↓↓↓ LDL ↓ VLDL ↑ HDL	Carotid plaque stabilization. Attenuates disease progression Stroke prevention Reduced rates of carotid revascularization
Niacin	↓ LDL ↓ VLDL ↑↑↑ HDL ↓ Lp(a)	Regression of carotid intima-media thickness
Ezetimibe	↓↓ LDL ↓ VLDL ↑ HDL	Regression of carotid intima-media thickness
Bile acid sequestrants		
Cholestyramine Colestipol Colsevelam	↓↓ LDL ↑ VLDL	–
Fibrates		
Bezafibrate Fenofibrate Gemfibrozil	↓↑ LDL ↓↓↓ VLDL ↑ HDL	Stroke prevention
Omega-3 fatty acids		
Eicosapentaenoic Docosahexaenoic	↓ VLDL	Regression of carotid intima-media thickness

subjects undergoing carotid intima media measurements over an 8 year follow-up confirmed these results [50].

Ample evidence also exists on the strong association between the triglyceride: HDL cholesterol ratio (TG:HDL-C) and coronary heart disease. Respectively for carotid artery disease, in a retrospective analysis of more than 1,000 patients with ischemic stroke or transient ischemic attack, an elevated level of the serum TG:HDL-C ratio, but not LDL-C, was associated with large artery atherosclerotic stroke [51]. Similar results have been demonstrated for intracranial vascular disease [52]. These findings urged some authors to introduce the term "atherogenic index" [log(TG:HDL-C)]. Pathophysiologically, this index indirectly represents sdLDL [53, 54].

Lipoproteins as Target of Carotid Artery Disease Prevention Strategies

The well-defined association of lipoproteins to cardiovascular disease and to carotid atherosclerosis and its associated events has triggered several studies and large-scale trials investigating lipid reduction strategies, both pharmacological (Table 4.3) and non-pharmacological. Their results and associated recommendations are summarized in the Third Report of the National Cholesterol Education Program (NCEP) Expert Panel on Detection, Evaluation, and Treatment of High Blood Cholesterol (HBC) in Adults (Adult Treatment Panel III) [55, 56], while vascular scientific societies have already published carotid disease-focused guidelines [57–59]. In addition, new data and novel lipoprotein targets have accumulated in literature.

Pharmacologic Therapies

Statins

Statins are hydroxymethylglutaryl-coenzyme A (HMG-CoA) reductase inhibitors preventing the formation of mevalonate during sterol synthesis, increasing LDL cholesterol clearance from plasma and decreasing liver VLDL and LDL production. In addition, they have mild elevating HDL and lowering triglyceride actions, and they seem to confer antiinflammatory, so-called "pleiotropic," effects against atherosclerosis progression. Regarding their association with carotid atherosclerosis, several large-scale studies currently evidence their effects on carotid plaque stabilization, disease progression, and stroke prevention [10–12, 60–65]. Notably, The Stroke Prevention by Aggressive Reduction in Cholesterol Levels Study (SPARCL) randomly assigned patients with TIA or stroke within 1–6 months without known coronary heart disease (CHD) and low-density lipoprotein cholesterol 100–190 mg/dl to treatment with atorvastatin 80 mg per day or placebo. The study showed that, among others, intense lipid lowering reduced the risk of stroke by 16 % [11]. A secondary analysis of the subjects with carotid stenosis not requiring revascularization at the time of randomization demonstrated that they had greater benefit when all cerebro- and cardiovascular events were combined. In the group with carotid artery stenosis, treatment with atorvastatin was associated with a 33 % reduction in the risk of any stroke and a 43 % reduction in the risk of major coronary events. Later carotid revascularization was reduced by 56 % in the group randomized to atorvastatin [12].

The current guideline can be summarized as follows: Statins are recommended in patients with ischemic stroke, TIA, asymptomatic carotid stenosis >50 %, and/or comorbid coronary artery disease, or evidence of an atherosclerotic origin. The target goal is an LDL-C of <2.6 mmol/l (100 mg/dl), and < 1.8 mmol/l (70 mg/dl) for very high-risk persons with multiple risk factors [57].

Nicotinic Acid (Niacin)

Niacin is the most effective drug for increasing HDL, but also decreases triglyceride and LDL cholesterol levels. It is also probably the only medication showing a direct lowering effect on Lp(a). Its mechanism of action is conferred by inhibiting lipoprotein synthesis and improving the clearance of triglyceride-rich lipoproteins from the circulation [1–3]. Niacin is generally used to enhance the statin lipid-lowering effect. The ARBITER 6–HALTS (Arterial Biology for the Investigation of the Treatment Effects of Reducing Cholesterol 6–HDL and LDL Treatment Strategies) trial compared the effects of two combination therapies – either niacin or ezetimibe added to long-term statin therapy – on carotid intima-media thickness over a 14-month period. This comparative effectiveness trial showed that the use of extended-release niacin causes a significant regression of carotid intima-media thickness when combined with a statin [66].

Ezetimibe

Ezetimibe is a cholesterol absorption inhibitor, blocking intestinal absorption of cholesterol and phytosterol. Ezetimibe lowers LDL cholesterol and causes small increases in HDL and a mild decrease in triglycerides. Ezetimibe can be used as a monotherapy in patients intolerant to statins or added to statins for patients who do not achieve target lipoprotein levels. Controversy currently exists on its actual clinical efficacy. While the ARBITER 6-HALTS trial showed that ezetimibe added to pravastatin or atorvastatin causes significant regression of carotid intima-media thickness, the Ezetimibe and Simvastatin in Hypercholesterolemia Enhances Atherosclerosis Regression (ENHANCE) trial failed to demonstrate similar outcomes [67].

Bile Acid Sequestrants

Bile acid sequestrants (colestipol, cholestyramine, colesevelam) block intestinal bile acid reabsorption, forcing upregulation of hepatic LDL receptors to recruit circulating cholesterol for bile synthesis, however elevating plasma triglycerides. They are currently used as adjuncts to statin therapies and have been proved to reduce cardiovascular mortality, but no particular studies on their effect on carotid atherosclerosis exist [1–3].

Fibric Acid Derivatives (Fibrates)

Fibrates (gemfibrozil and fenofibrate) predominately reduce triglycerides and, at a lower rate, increase HDL cholesterol. Their effect on LDL cholesterol is variable. They seem to stimulate fatty acid oxidation in the liver and muscle and downregulate hepatic VLDL synthesis. Although they have been shown to reduce the risk of stroke [68], no independent effect on carotid atherosclerosis has yet been demonstrated.

Omega-3 Fatty Acids (Fish Oils)

Omega-3 fatty acids (eicosapentaenoic acid, docosahexaenoic acid) in high doses can be effective in reducing triglycerides. Omega-3 fatty acids are reported to have an antiatherogenic effect, reducing carotid intima thickness and cardiovascular events [69, 70]. Currently, they are used as an adjunct to other therapies.

Miscellaneous

Given the numerous studies that demonstrate an association between Lp-PLA2 and increased coronary and carotid risk, there has been interest in pharmacologically targeting Lp-PLA2. Darapladib is a selective Lp-PLA2 inhibitor; phase I and II studies have shown a dose-dependent reduction in Lp-PLA2 activity, while phase III trial results on the its clinical effect are awaited [41].

Finally, future therapies will include peroxisome proliferator-activated receptor agonists that have thiazolidinedione-like and fibrate-like properties, LDL-receptor activators, LPL activators, and recombinant apo E to be used for LDL reduction and reconstituted mutant HDL or partially delipidated HDL for increasing HDL. Cholesterol vaccination (to induce anti-LDL antibodies and hasten LDL clearance from serum) and gene transfer are attractive therapies that are under study but years away from being available for use [71].

Nonpharmacologic Therapies

Implementation of lifestyle changes, including exercise, weight loss, and a low-fat diet, is effective as a first line strategy for plasma lipid reduction. Physical activity, eating large amounts of fruits and vegetables, legumes, and whole grains, and taking dietary supplements containing plant sterols or stanols have been shown to reduce LDL and VLDL while increasing HDL [1–3]. While no particular studies exist, their lipid-lowering effect defines their beneficial action on carotid atherosclerosis.

Conclusions

The role of lipoproteins in carotid artery disease is an enormously expanding field of research currently evidencing a strong association of the disease's natural history and related events. In addition, well-defined and targeted treatment strategies are increasingly effective in carotid risk reduction. As their physiology and metabolism are better understood, novel lipoprotein subfractions are playing a role in clinical practice, and novel conceptually appealing therapies are awaited in the years to come.

References

1. Goldberg AC. Section 8: Endocrine and metabolic disorders, Chapter 100: Lipid disorders. In: Porter RS, Kaplan JL, editors. The Merck manual of diagnosis and therapy. 19th ed. Whitehouse Station, NJ: Merck Sharp & Dohme Corp; 2011.
2. Ridker P, Libby P. Chapter 44: Risk markers for atherothrombotic disease. Genest J, Libby P. Chapter 47: Lipoprotein disorders and cardiovascular disease. In: Bonow RO, Mann D, Zipes D, Libby P,

editors. Braunwald's heart disease: a textbook of cardiovascular medicine. 9th ed. Philadelphia: Saunders; 2012.
3. Liapis CD. Chapter 25: Atherosclerosis risk factor treatment – general considerations. Walcott R, Howard J. Chapter 28: Atherosclerotic risk factors – hyperlipidemia. In: Cronenwett JL, Johnston W, editors. Rutherford's vascular surgery. 7th ed. Philadelphia: W.B. Saunders; 2010.
4. Lamon BD, Haijar DP. Inflammation at the molecular interface of atherogenesis: an anthropological journey. Am J Pathol. 2008;173: 1253–64.
5. Napoli C, De Nigris F, Palinski W. Multiple role of reactive oxygen species in the arterial wall. J Cell Biochem. 2001;82:674–82.
6. Matsunaga T. Modulation of reactive oxygen species in endothelial cells by peroxynitrite-treated lipoproteins. J Biochem. 2001;130: 285–93.
7. Parthasarathy S, Steinberg D, Witztum JL. The role of oxidized low density lipoproteins in the pathogenesis of atherosclerosis. Annu Rev Med. 1992;43:219–25.
8. Steinberg D. Low density lipoprotein oxidation and its pathobiological significance. J Biol Chem. 1997;272:20963–6.
9. Flavahan NA. Atherosclerosis or lipoprotein induced endothelial dysfunction: potential mechanisms underlying reduction in EDRF/ nitric oxide activity. Circulation. 1992;85:1927.
10. Heart Protection Study Collaborative Group. MRC/BHF Heart Protection Study of cholesterol lowering with simvastatin in 20,536 high-risk individuals: a randomised placebo-controlled trial. Lancet. 2002;360:7–22.
11. SPARCL Investigators. High-dose atorvastatin after stroke or transient ischemic attack. N Engl J Med. 2006;355:549–59.
12. Sillesen H, Amarence P, Hennerici MG. Atorvastatin reduces the risk of cardiovascular events in patients with carotid atherosclerosis. A secondary analysis of the Stroke Prevention by Aggressive Reduction in Cholesterol Levels (SPARCL) trial. Stroke. 2008;39:3297.
13. Sigala F, Kotsinas A, Savari P, et al. Oxidized LDL in human carotid plaques is related to symptomatic carotid disease and lesion instability. J Vasc Surg. 2010;52:704–13.
14. Uno M, Kitazato KT, Suzue A, Itabe H, Hao L, Nagahiro S. Contribution of an imbalance between oxidant-antioxidant systems to plaque vulnerability in patients with carotid artery stenosis. J Neurosurg. 2005;103:518–22.
15. Wallenfeldt K, Fegerberg B, Wkstrand J, et al. Oxidized low-density lipoprotein in plasma is a prognostic marker of subclinical atherosclerosis development in clinically healthy men. J Intern Med. 2004;256:413–20.
16. Mackey RH, Kuller LH, Sutton-Tyrrell K, et al. Lipoprotein subclasses and coronary artery calcium in postmenopausal women from the healthy women study. Am J Cardiol. 2002;90:71i–6.
17. Koba S, Hirano T, Kondo T, et al. Significance of small dense low-density lipoproteins and other risk factors in patients with various types of coronary heart disease. Am Heart J. 2002;144:1026–35.
18. Skoglund-Andersson C, Tang R, Bond MG, et al. LDL particle size distribution is associated with carotid intima-media thickness in healthy 50-year-old men. Arterioscler Thromb Vasc Biol. 1999;19:2422–30.
19. Liu ML, Ylitalo K, Nuotio I, et al. Association between carotid intima-media thickness and low-density lipoprotein size and susceptibility of low-density lipoprotein to oxidation in asymptomatic members of familial combined hyperlipidemia families. Stroke. 2002;33:1255–60.
20. Norata GD, Raselli S, Grigore L, Garlaschelli K, et al. Small dense LDL and VLDL predict common carotid artery IMT and elicit an inflammatory response in peripheral blood mononuclear and endothelial cells. Atherosclerosis. 2009;206:556–62.
21. Shoji T, Hatsuda S, Tsuchikura A, et al. Small dense low-density lipoprotein cholesterol concentration and carotid atherosclerosis. Atherosclerosis. 2009;202:582–8.
22. Hodis HJ, Mack WJ. Triglyceride-rich lipoproteins and the progression of coronary artery disease. Curr Opin Lipidol. 1995; 6:209–14.
23. Hodis HN, Mack WJ, Dunn M, et al. Intermediate-density lipoproteins and progression of carotid arterial wall intima-media thickness. Circulation. 1997;95:2022–6.
24. Kofoed SC, Gronholdt ML, Bismuth J, et al. Echolucent, rupture-prone carotid plaques associated with elevated triglyceride-rich lipoproteins, particularly in women. J Vasc Surg. 2002;36:783–92.
25. Mineo C, Deguchi H, Griffin JH, et al. Endothelial and antithrombotic actions of HDL. Circ Res. 2006;98:1352–64.
26. Barter PJ, Nicholls S, Raye KA, et al. Antiinflammatory properties of HDL. Circ Res. 2004;95:764–72.
27. Shahar E, Chambless LE, Rosamond WD, et al. Plasma lipid profile and incident ischemic stroke: the Atherosclerosis Risk in Communities (ARIC) study. Stroke. 2003;34:623–31.
28. Koren-Morag N, Tanne D, Graff E, et al. Low- and high density lipoprotein cholesterol and ischemic cerebrovascular disease: the bezafibrate infarction prevention registry. Arch Intern Med. 2002;162:993–9.
29. Sacco RL, Benson RT, Kargman DE, et al. High-density lipoprotein cholesterol and ischemic stroke in the elderly: the Northern Manhattan Stroke Study. JAMA. 2001;285:2729–35.
30. Amarenco P, Labreuche J, Touboul PJ. High-density lipoprotein-cholesterol and risk of stroke and carotid atherosclerosis: a systematic review. Atherosclerosis. 2008;196:489–96.
31. Liapis CD, Avgerinos ED, et al. What a vascular surgeon should know and do about atherosclerotic risk factors. J Vasc Surg. 2009;49:1348–54.
32. Stalenhoef AFH, Graaf J. Association of fasting and non fasting serum triglycerides with cardiovascular disease and the role of remnant-like lipoproteins and small dense LDL. Curr Opin Lipidol. 2008;19:355–61.
33. Stalenhoef AF, Casparie AF, Demacker PN, et al. Combined deficiency of apolipoprotein C-II and lipoprotein lipase in familial hyperchylomicronemia. Metabolism. 1981;30:919–26.
34. Frick MH, Elo O, Haapa K. Helsinki Heart Study: primary prevention trial with gemfibrozil in middle-aged men with dyslipidemia. Safety of treatment, changes in risk factors, and incidence of coronary heart disease. N Engl J Med. 1987;317:1237–45.
35. Rubins HB, Robins SJ, Collins D, Veterans Affairs High-Density Lipoprotein Cholesterol Intervention Trial Study Group. Gemfibrozil for the secondary prevention of coronary heart disease in men with low levels of high-density lipoprotein cholesterol. N Engl J Med. 1999;341:410–8.
36. Otvos JD, Collins D, Freedman DS, et al. Low-density lipoprotein and high-density lipoprotein particle subclasses predict coronary events and are favorably changed by gemfibrozil therapy in the Veterans Affairs High-Density Lipoprotein Intervention Trial. Circulation. 2006;113:1556–63.
37. Labreuche J, Deplanque D, Touboul PJ, et al. Association between change in plasma triglyceride levels and risk of stroke and carotid atherosclerosis systematic review and meta-regression analysis. Atherosclerosis. 2010;212:9–15.
38. Miles LA, Fless GM, Levin EG, et al. A potential basis for the thrombotic risks associated with lipoprotein(a). Nature. 1989; 339:301–3.
39. Fortunato JE, Bassiouny HS, Song RH, et al. Apolipoprotein(a) fragments in relation to human carotid plaque instability. J Vasc Surg. 2000;32:555–63.
40. Smolders B, Lemmens R, Thijs V. Lipoprotein (a) and stroke. Stroke. 2007;38:1959–66.
41. Epps KC, Wilensky RL. Lp-PLA2 – a novel risk factor for high-risk coronary and carotid artery disease. J Intern Med. 2011;269:94–106.
42. Stafforini DM, McIntyre TM, Carter ME. Human plasma platelet-activating factor acetylhydrolase. Association with lipoprotein

particles and role in the degradation of plateletactivating factor. J Biol Chem. 1987;262:4215–22.
43. Mannheim D, Herrmann J, Versari D, et al. Enhanced expression of Lp-PLA2 and lyso PC hosphatidylcholine in symptomatic carotid atherosclerotic plaques. Stroke. 2008;39:1448–55.
44. Vickers KC, Maguire C, Wolfert RL, et al. Relationship of lipoprotein-associated phospholipase A2 and oxidized low density lipoprotein in carotid atherosclerosis. J Lipid Res. 2009;50:1735–43.
45. Tsimikas S, Willeit J, Knoflach M, et al. Lipoprotein-associated phospholipase A2 activity, ferritin levels, metabolic syndrome, and 10-year cardiovascular and non-cardiovascular mortality: results from the Bruneck study. Eur Heart J. 2009;30:107–15.
46. Oei HH, van der Meer IM, Hofman A. Lipoprotein-associated phospholipase A2 activity is associated with risk of coronary heart disease and ischemic stroke: the Rotterdam Study. Circulation. 2005;111:570–5.
47. Persson M, Berglund G, Nelson JJ, Hedblad B. Lp-PLA2 activity and mass are associated with increased incidence of ischemic stroke: a population-based cohort study from Malmo, Sweden. Atherosclerosis. 2008;200:191–8.
48. Elkind MS, Tai W, Coates K, et al. Lipoprotein associated phospholipase A2 activity and risk of recurrent stroke. Cerebrovasc Dis. 2009;27:42–50.
49. Gardener H, Morte DD, Elkind MSV, et al. Lipids and carotid plaque in the Northern Manhattan Study (NOMAS). BMC Cardiovasc Disord. 2009;9:55.
50. Enomoto M, Adachi H, Hirai Y. LDL-C/HDL-C Ratio Predicts Carotid Intima-Media Thickness Progression Better Than HDL-C or LDL-C Alone. J Lipids. 2011. doi:10.1155/2011/549137.
51. Bang OY, Saver JL, Liebeskind DS, et al. Association of serum lipid indices with large artery atherosclerotic stroke. Neurology. 2008;70:841–7.
52. Kang K, Lee K, Chung SH. The triglyceride:high-density lipoprotein-cholesterol ratio and steno-occlusive disease in the intracranial arteries. J Thromb Thrombolysis. 2011;32:103–9.
53. Boizel R, Benhamou PY, Lardy B, et al. Ratio of triglycerides to HDL cholesterol is an indicator of LDL particle size in patients with type 2 diabetes and normal HDL cholesterol levels. Diabetes Care. 2000;23:1679–85.
54. Dobiasova M, Frohlich J. The plasma parameter log (TG/HDL-C) as an atherogenic index: correlation with lipoprotein particle size and esterification rate in apoB-lipoprotein-depleted plasma (FER(HDL)). Clin Biochem. 2001;34:583–8.
55. Expert Panel on Detection, Evaluation, and Treatment of High Blood Cholesterol in Adults. Executive Summary of The Third Report of The National Cholesterol Education Program (NCEP) Expert Panel on Detection, Evaluation, And Treatment of High Blood Cholesterol In Adults (Adult Treatment Panel III). JAMA. 2001;285:2486–97.
56. Grundy SM, Cleeman JI, Merz CN, National Heart, Lung, and Blood Institute; American College of Cardiology Foundation; American Heart Association. Implications of recent clinical trials for the National Cholesterol Education Program Adult Treatment Panel III guidelines. Circulation. 2004;110:227–39.
57. Liapis CD, Bell PR, Mikhailidis D, ESVS Guidelines Collaborators. ESVS guidelines. Section A -Prevention in patients with carotid artery stenosis. Curr Vasc Pharmacol. 2010;8:673–81.
58. Ricotta JJ, Aburahma A, Ascher E, et al. Updated Society for Vascular Surgery guidelines for management of extracranial carotid disease: executive summary. J Vasc Surg. 2011;54:832–6.
59. Brott TG, Halperin JL, Abbara S. 2011 ASA/ACCF/AHA/AANN/AANS/ACR/ASNR/CNS/SAIP/SCAI/SIR/SNIS/SVM/SVS guideline on the management of patients with extracranial carotid and vertebral artery disease. Circulation. 2011;124:e54–130.
60. Crisby M, Nordin-Fredriksson G, Shah PK. Pravastatin treatment increases collagen content and decreases lipid content, inflammation, metalloproteinases, and cell death in human carotid plaques. implications for plaque stabilization. Circulation. 2001;103:926–33.
61. Taylor AJ, Flaherty PJ. ARBITER: Arterial biology for the investigation of the treatment effects of reducing cholesterol. A randomized trial comparing the effects of atorvastatin and pravastatin on carotid intima medial thickness. Circulation. 2002;106:2055–60.
62. Avgerinos ED, Kadoglou NPE, Moulakakis K, Giannakopoulos T, Liapis C. Current role of biomarkers in carotid disease: a systematic review? Int J Stroke. 2011;6:337–45.
63. Kunte H, Amberger N, Busch MA, Rückert RI, Meiners S, Harms L. Markers of instability in high-risk carotid plaques are reduced by statins. J Vasc Surg. 2008;47:513–22.
64. Kadoglou NP, Gerasimidis T, Moumtzouoglou A, et al. Intensive lipid lowering therapy ameliorates novel calcification markers and GSM score in patients with carotid stenosis. Eur J Vasc Endovasc Surg. 2008;35:661–8.
65. Kadoglou NP, Gerasimidis T, Kapelouzou A, et al. Beneficial changes of serum calcification markers and contralateral carotid plaques echogenicity after combined carotid artery stenting plus intensive lipid lowering therapy in patients with bilateral carotid stenosis. Eur J Vasc Endovasc Surg. 2010;39:258–65.
66. Taylor AJ, Villines TC, Stanek EJ, et al. Extended-release niacin or ezetimibe and carotid intima – media thickness. N Eng J Med. 2009;361:2113–22.
67. Kastelein JJ, Akdim F, Stroes ES, et al. Simvastatin with or without ezetimibe in familial hypercholesterolemia. N Engl J Med. 2008;358:1431–43.
68. Bloomfield Rubins H, Davenport J, Babikian V, VA-HIT Study Group. Reduction in stroke with gemfibrozil in men with coronary heart disease and low HDL cholesterol: the Veterans Affairs HDL Intervention Trial (VA-HIT). Circulation. 2001;103:2828–33.
69. Balk E, Chung M, Lichtenstein A, et al. Effects of omega-3 fatty acids on cardiovascular risk factors and intermediate markers of cardiovascular disease. Evidence report/technology assessment no. 93. Rockville: Agency for Healthcare Research and Quality; 2004.
70. Lorenz MW, von Kegler S, Steinmetz H, et al. Carotid intima-media thickening indicates a higher vascular risk across a wide age range: prospective data from the carotid atherosclerosis progression study (caps). Stroke. 2006;37:87–92.
71. Florentin M, Liberopoulos EN, Mikhailidis DP, et al. Emerging options in the treatment of dyslipidemias: a bright future? Expert Opin Emerg Drugs. 2011;16:247–70.

Carotid Endarterectomy: Inflammatory Aspects

5

Sthefano Atique Gabriel and Edmo Atique Gabriel

Introduction

Carotid artery stenosis is a common disease related to the occurrence of transient ischemic attacks and strokes. Carotid endarterectomy (CEA), first performed by De Bakey in 1953, is a widely applied method to prevent recurrent neurological symptoms and stroke in patients with severe carotid artery stenosis. However, 3–7 % of CEA procedures are complicated by disabling or nondisabling strokes [1, 2].

The relation among carotid plaque characteristics, plaque embolization, and adverse clinical outcome remains poorly understood. Despite growing evidence that inflammation and its biomarkers have a key role in the development of atherosclerosis and its clinical outcomes or disease stage, the precise molecular and cellular mechanisms associated with thrombotic events are still unknown [1–3].

Several studies suggest that plaque characteristics are causally related to the development of cardiovascular events. The vulnerable, unstable plaque consists of inflammatory cells, particularly macrophages and T lymphocytes, accumulated lipid, and a thin fibrous cap and is associated with plaque rupture, thrombosis, and subsequent atherosclerotic events [1–3].

S.A. Gabriel, MD (✉)
Department of Vascular Surgery,
Pontifical Catholic University of Campinas,
São Paulo, Brazil

Department of Vascular Surgery,
Celso Pierro Hospital and Maternity, Campinas, São Paulo, Brazil
e-mail: sthefanogabriel@yahoo.com.br

E.A. Gabriel, MD, PhD
Department of Cardiovascular Surgery,
University Nove de Julho,
São Paulo, Brazil
e-mail: edag@uol.com.br

Carotid Plaque Formation and Vulnerability

Various processes involved in the progression of atherosclerotic lesions have been shown to be associated with plaque vulnerability, such as inflammation, lipid accumulation, apoptosis, proteolysis, thrombosis, and angiogenesis. Several morphological characteristics are related to plaque instability, including an atheromatous, thin fibrous cap; a large lipid core; less collagen; noncalcified ulceration; intraplaque hemorrhage; infiltration of inflammatory cells; proteolysis; and remodeling [4, 5].

Serum inflammatory biomarkers are important predictors of atherosclerotic complications. In carotid artery disease, high-sensitivity C-reactive protein correlates with morphological features of rapidly progressive carotid atherosclerosis, defined by ultrasound categorization, and could be an important risk predictor for stroke [6]. This biomarker also adds prognostic information for risk prediction of cardiovascular events and discriminates between stable and unstable coronary artery disease.

Brea et al. found that serum amyloid A increases monocyte and macrophage cytokine production and is elevated in atherosclerotic lesions. Their study concluded that elevated serum amyloid A levels can identify patients with ischemic stroke caused by atherothrombosis [7].

Blankenberg et al. observed that IL-18 promotes the Th-1 immune response and enhances the production of matrix metalloproteinase. In carotid stenosis, IL-18 expression is especially increased in unstable lesions and positively correlates with carotid intima-media thickness [8].

Kerr et al. concluded that IL-6 has pro-atherogenic properties, and in patients with acute coronary syndromes, baseline IL-6 levels are associated with a greater risk of stroke. IL-6 also amplifies the inflammatory cascade, and its expression is elevated in unstable plaque regions [9].

Schindhelm et al. have linked myeloperoxidase to atherosclerosis. This enzyme is involved in the oxidation process of

E.A. Gabriel, S.A. Gabriel (eds.), *Inflammatory Response in Cardiovascular Surgery*,
DOI 10.1007/978-1-4471-4429-8_5, © Springer-Verlag London 2013

LDL and thereby promotes foam cell formation in the vascular wall. In carotid artery stenosis, however, myeloperoxidase has not proven to be of additional value in the identification of high-risk plaques [10].

Heider et al. observed that serum pregnancy-associated plasma protein-A (PAPP-A) levels in carotid artery disease showed a positive predictive value for the presence of unstable plaques. However, their study also concluded that asymptomatic patients had significantly higher PAPP-A values compared to symptomatic patients [11].

Inflammatory Cytokines in Carotid Atherosclerosis

Inflammatory cells are responsible for secreting growth factors and cytokines that are important predictors of cardiovascular events when in high levels in the blood circulation. Profumo et al., analyzing cytokine expression in circulating T lymphocytes in patients undergoing CEA, observed elevated intracellular expression of tumor necrosis factor (TNF)-α, interferon (IFN)-γ, and interleukin (IL)-4 in circulating T lymphocytes from patients with carotid atherosclerosis, particularly from patients with complicated plaques (Table 5.1) [12]. More recently, intracellular cytokine monitoring in peripheral blood lymphocytes and monocytes was shown to be useful in the follow-up of patients after CEA to predict the onset or progression of contralateral disease [13].

When studying the presence of inflammatory cytokines in patients undergoing CEA, intracellular cytokine expression was found to be significantly higher in patients undergoing CEA who had stenosis ≥70 % (TNF-α, IFN-γ, IL-1b, IL-6, IL-4, and IL-10), with previous stroke (IFN-γ, IL-1b, IL-6, IL-8, IL-4, and IL-10), and with amaurosis fugax (IFN-γ, IL-6, IL-4, and IL-10) than in patients not undergoing CEA (Table 5.2) [14]. Proinflammatory cytokines, such as TNF-α, IFN-γ, IL-1b, IL-6, and IL-8, and antiinflammatory cytokines, such as IL-4 and IL-10, were also found in significantly higher percentages in patients undergoing CEA than in patients who were not [3].

Significantly higher levels of IL-8-positive cells were observed in patients with contralateral than in those with monolateral carotid disease, demonstrating an association of IL-8-positive cells with the onset or progression of contralateral disease after CEA [13, 14].

The higher pro- and antiinflammatory cytokine expression in patients with stenosis of ≥70 % than in those with stenosis of <70 % could indicate plaque instability and immunological mechanisms leading to atherosclerotic plaque growth. However, the question of whether inflammatory cytokine expression has a direct causal relation with carotid arterial disease or only reflects the inflammatory disease process remains unanswered.

Table 5.1 Box-plot graphs showing medians and interquartile ranges of intracellular cytokines in 67 patients undergoing carotid endarterectomy (CEA) and in 39 not undergoing CEA. Patients who underwent CEA versus patients who did not: tumor necrosis factor (TNF)-a, P = 0.02; interferon (IFN)-g, P = 0.001; interleukin (IL)-1b P = 0.04; IL-6, P = 0.0003; IL-8, P = 0.009; IL-4, P = 0.0001; IL-10, P = 0.001 by Mann-Whitney non-parametric test

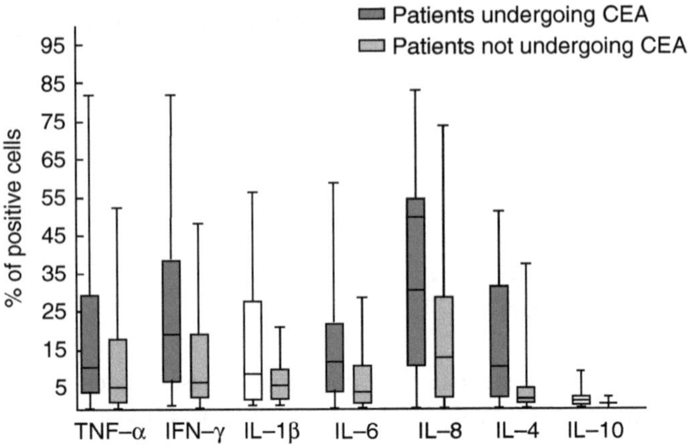

Gender Differences in Carotid Plaques

In their study on sex differences in the composition of plaques in patients undergoing CEA, Rerkasem et al. found that plaques from females had significantly less lipid and more fibrous tissue than those from males, and the perioperative stroke and death rate in females and males was 3.3 and 3.6 %, respectively [15]. This might reflect the fact that women have a more stable plaque component than men because unstable carotid plaques have a high lipid content, thin fibrous caps, a high inflammatory cell content, and increased protease activity.

Halvorsen et al. also supported the notion that women have more stable plaques with an ultrasound study on carotid arteries that showed that women had significantly fewer echolucent plaques than men [16].

Hellings et al. observed that the differences in plaque histology between men and women were paralleled by the inflammatory and protease activity in atherosclerotic plaques (Table 5.2). Women showed lower IL-8 values than men. IL-6 levels were not different between men and women. Protease activity was lower in women, with matrix metalloproteinase-8 showing significantly lower values than in men. Asymptomatic women showed lower levels of IL-8, matrix metalloproteinase-8 activity, and matrix metalloproteinase-9 activity compared with asymptomatic men [17].

Table 5.2 Box-plot graphs showing medians and interquartile ranges of intracellular cytokines in the 39 patients not undergoing carotid endarterectomy (CEA) and in the 56 patients undergoing CEA divided according to the indications for surgery [18 asymptomatic patients with stenosis ≥70 %, 14 patients with stenosis <70 % and stroke, 7 patients with stenosis <70 % and amaurosis fugax (AFX), 17 patients with stenosis <70 % and transient ischemic attack (TIA)]. Patients with stenosis of 70 % versus patients with stenosis of <70 %: tumor necrosis factor (TNF)-a and interleukin (IL)-6, $P = 0.004$; interferon (IFN)-g and IL-10, $P = 0.01$; IL-1b, $P = 0.02$; IL-4, $P = 0.006$. Patients with stroke versus asymptomatic patients: IFN-g, $P = 0.005$; IL-1b and IL-4, $P = 0.004$; IL-6, $P < 0.0001$; IL-8, $P = 0.0001$; IL-10, $P = 0.03$. Patients with AFX versus asymptomatic patients: IFN-g, $P = 0.007$; IL-6 and IL-10, $P = 0.03$; IL-4, $P = 0.003$

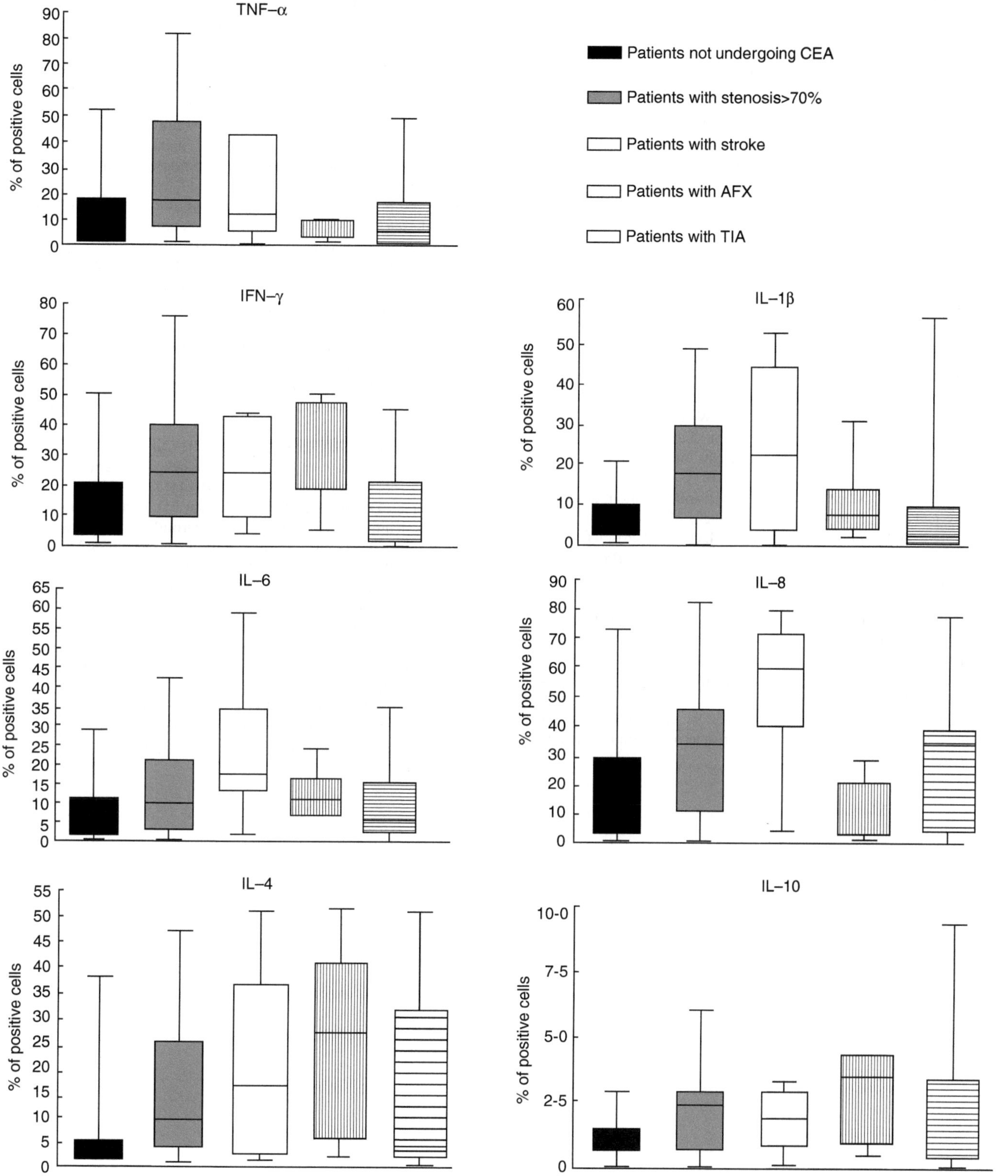

Previous studies have shown that the presence of these matrix metalloproteinases plays an important role in cell migration, degradation of the fibrous cap, expansive remodeling, and intraplaque neovessel formation. This might suggest that matrix metalloproteinase contributes to plaque instability [18, 19].

Conclusion

Investigation of inflammatory cytokine provides an insight into the inflammatory mechanisms related to carotid atherosclerosis. However, a still unanswered question is whether cytokine expression in the peripheral blood has a causal relation with carotid atherosclerosis or simply reflects the inflammatory disease process. Studies should be performed on this issue, and in the future they will lead to improved therapeutic protocols and reduced atherosclerosis-related mortality.

References

1. Ferguson GG, Eliasziw M, Barr HW, Clagett GP, Barnes RW, Wallace MC, et al. The North American Symptomatic Carotid Endarterectomy Trial: surgical results in 1415 patients. Stroke. 1999;30:1751–8.
2. Hansson GK. Mechanisms of disease: inflammation, atherosclerosis, and coronary artery disease. N Engl J Med. 2005;352:1685–95.
3. Halvorsen B, Otterdal K, Skjelland M, et al. Atherosclerotic plaque stability—what determines the fate of the plaque? Prog Cardiovasc Dis. 2008;51(3):183–94.
4. Hermus L, Lefrandt JD, Tio RA, Breek JC, Zeebregts CJ. Carotid plaque formation and serum biomarkers. Atherosclerosis. 2010;213(1):21–9.
5. Zhou W, Chai H, Ding R, Lam HY. Distribution of inflammatory mediators in carotid and femoral plaques. J Am Coll Surg. 2010; 211(1):92–8.
6. Schillinger M, Exner M, Mlekusch W, et al. Inflammation and Carotid Artery—risk for Atherosclerosis Study (ICARAS). Circulation. 2005;111(17):2203–9.
7. Brea D, Sobrino T, Blanco M, et al. Usefulness of haptoglobin and serum amyloid A proteins as biomarkers for atherothrombotic ischemic stroke diagnosis confirmation. Atherosclerosis. 2009;205(2): 561–7.
8. Blankenberg S, Luc G, Ducimetiere P, et al. PRIME Study Group Interleukin-18 and the risk of coronary heart disease in European men: the Prospective Epidemiological Study of Myocardial Infarction (PRIME). Circulation. 2003;108(20):2453–9.
9. Kerr R, Stirling D, Ludlam CA. Interleukin 6 and haemostasis. Br J Haematol. 2001;115(1):3–12.
10. Schindhelm RK, van der Zwan LP, Teerlink T, Scheffer PG. Myeloperoxidase: a useful biomarker for cardiovascular disease risk stratification? Clin Chem. 2009;55(8):1462–70.
11. Heider P, Pfäffle N, Pelisek J, et al. Is serum pregnancy-associated plasma protein a really a potential marker of atherosclerotic carotid plaque stability? Eur J Vasc Endovasc Surg. 2010;39(6): 668–75.
12. Profumo E, Siracusano A, Ortona E, et al. Cytokine expression in circulating T lymphocytes from patients undergoing carotid endarterectomy. J Cardiovasc Surg. 2003;44:237–42.
13. Profumo E, Esposito C, Buttari B, et al. Intracellular expression of cytokines in peripheral blood from patients with atherosclerosis before and after carotid endarterectomy. Atherosclerosis. 2007; 191:340–7.
14. Profumo E, Buttari B, Tosti ME, et al. Association of intracellular pro- and anti-inflammatory cytokines in peripheral blood with the clinical or ultrasound indications for carotid endarterectomy in patients with carotid atherosclerosis. Clin Exp Immunol. 2008; 152(1):120–6.
15. Rerkasem K, Gallagher PJ, Grimble RF, Calder PC, Shearman CP. Sex difference in composition of plaques of patients undergoing carotid endarterectomy. Vascular. 2010;18(2):77–81.
16. Halvorsen DS, Johnsen SH, Mathiesen EB, et al. The association between inflammatory markers and carotid atherosclerosis is sex dependent: the Tromso Study. Cerebrovasc Dis. 2009;27:392–7.
17. Hellings WE, Pasterkamp G, Verhoeven BA, et al. Gender- associated differences in plaque phenotype of patients undergoing carotid endarterectomy. J Vasc Surg. 2007;45:289–96.
18. Loftus IM, Naylor AR, Goodall S, Crowther M, Jones L, Bell PR. Increased matrix metalloproteinase-9 activity in unstable carotid plaques. A potential role in acute plaque disruption. Stroke. 2000;31:40–7.
19. Molloy KJ, Thompson MM, Jones JL, Schwalbe EC, Bell PR, Naylor AR, et al. Unstable carotid plaques exhibit raised matrix metalloproteinase-8 activity. Circulation. 2004;110:337–43.

Endovascular Treatment of Carotid Disease: Inflammatory Aspects

6

Sthefano Atique Gabriel and Edmo Atique Gabriel

Introduction

Recent studies have shown an important interest in the inflammatory aspects of carotid artery stenting; however, the pathophysiology of the vascular wall reaction after stent implantation is not yet entirely understood. Chronic vascular inflammation is associated with the development of restenosis after balloon angioplasty and stent implantation. Virmani and Farb [1] have observed that intimal and medial injury and lipid core penetration by the stent struts cause a perivascular inflammatory response. This vascular inflammatory process is also correlated with the severity of arterial injury during stent implantation [1, 2].

The inflammatory phenomenon caused by stent insertion plays an important role in vascular smooth muscle cell proliferation and late neointimal growth. It is know that vascular smooth muscle cell proliferation and subsequent hypertrophic neointima formation at the treated artery may be responsible for in-stent restenosis [1–3].

Inflammatory Biomarkers and Carotid Artery Stenting

Inflammation is currently recognized as an important factor in the development, progression, and rupture of atherosclerotic plaques. Elevated levels of circulating inflammatory markers, including high-sensitive C-reactive protein, interleukin (IL)-6, IL-18, matrix metalloproteinase (MMP), tissue inhibitor of MMP (TIMP), soluble intercellular adhesion molecule 1 (sICAM-1), and osteopontin (OPN), have an important function as predictors of future vascular events [4, 5].

In their study of the local release of inflammatory biomarkers during carotid artery stenting with plaque echogenicity and calcification, Abe et al. [6] observed that systemic IL-6 levels were associated with a recent stroke/transient ischemic attack and arteriosclerosis obliterans, and local plaque IL-6 levels were associated with a recent history of stroke/transient ischemic attack. IL-6, IL-18, and OPN levels were markedly increased at the plaque site in comparison to the systemic values. However, the local levels of TIMP-1, MMP-2, and sICAM-1 were similar to their systemic ones.

When analyzing the plaque echogenicity, the local levels of both IL-6 and OPN were significantly higher than the systemic levels in lower and higher echogenic groups. However, the level of local release of IL-6 (delta IL-6) was higher in lower echogenic lesions than in higher echogenic lesions, and the percent stenosis was not associated with the level of local release of IL-6 [6].

Considering the plaque calcification and serum inflammatory biomarkers, Abe et al. also observed that the local IL-6 levels significantly increased in both mild and severe calcification lesions. The OPN level also significantly increased in local samples of both mild and severe calcification lesions. The local level of IL-18 was slightly higher than the systemic level in both the mild and severe calcification groups [6].

These findings indicate that inflammatory markers are produced and stored in carotid plaques in vivo. Moreover, among the inflammatory markers, IL-6 and OPN are markedly released from atheromatous carotid plaques after carotid artery stenting. In addition, local IL-6 levels dramatically increased in the lower echogenic groups, suggesting that the amount of local IL-6 is related to plaque instability. However, less release of IL-6 in the severe calcification group than in the mild calcification group may suggest that extensively

S.A. Gabriel, MD (✉)
Department of Vascular Surgery, Pontifical Catholic University of Campinas, São Paulo, Brazil

Department of Vascular Surgery, Celso Pierro Hospital and Maternity, Campinas, São Paulo, Brazil
e-mail: sthefanogabriel@yahoo.com.br

E.A. Gabriel, MD, PhD
Department of Cardiovascular Surgery, University Nove de Julho, São Paulo, Brazil
e-mail: edag@uol.com.br

E.A. Gabriel, S.A. Gabriel (eds.), *Inflammatory Response in Cardiovascular Surgery*, DOI 10.1007/978-1-4471-4429-8_6, © Springer-Verlag London 2013

calcified plaques are more stable than mildly calcified ones. Therefore, patients with extensive calcification of the carotid plaque are less likely to have symptomatic disease [7].

Inflammation and In-Stent Restenosis

Wasser et al., analyzing the effect of periinterventional serum inflammation markers and procedure-related technical factors during carotid artery stenting on the development of an in-stent restenosis during long-term follow-up, concluded that a post-procedurally elevated leukocyte count as an inflammatory serum marker is an independent predictor for subsequent in-stent restenosis. Moreover, the occurrence of in-stent restenosis is markedly regulated by stent dimensions; therefore, the thinner and longer the deployed stent, the more frequently a restenosis could be detected [8].

In their study, Wasser et al. observed a statistically significantly higher median C-reactive protein value in the group of patients with an in-stent restenosis than in the group of patients without an in-stent restenosis during follow-up. The post-interventional leukocyte count showed a significant increase in patients with the occurrence of an in-stent restenosis during follow-up. The stent cell design did not differ between the groups with and without in-stent restenosis during follow-up; however, there was a significantly narrower stent width in the group with the occurrence of an in-stent restenosis, as well as a trend toward in-stent restenosis formation during follow-up in those patients with a longer stent length (Table 6.1) [8].

The role of vascular inflammation in the development of in-stent restenosis is mostly triggered by an endothelial disruption and abrasion caused by balloon inflation and stent placement. This vascular injury initiates the release of several mediators leading to adhesion of thrombocytes, neutrophils, and monocytes. These cells, for their part, release vasoactive, thrombogenic, lymphocytic, and mitogenic substances, which lead to vasoconstriction, vascular remodeling, neointimal proliferation, thrombosis, and inflammation, finally resulting in in-stent restenosis [9, 10].

In their study on the mechanisms of carotid artery stent restenosis by intravascular ultrasound study, Clark et al. considered that procedural factors during carotid artery stenting could play an important role in the development of in-stent restenosis. They concluded that the wider the stent was, the less likely the occurrence of in-stent restenosis during follow-up because a stent with a larger diameter results in a reduced flow velocity, fewer turbulences, and thus less frequent in-stent restenosis [11].

Schillinger et al., analyzing the importance of periinterventional serum levels of acute-phase reactants in 6-month restenosis after stent implantation in the carotid artery, observed that within the first 48 h after intervention, a significant increase of C-reactive protein and serum amyloid A levels was found in patients with and without restenosis. However, patients with 6-month restenosis had significantly higher postintervention serum levels of acute-phase reactants compared with the levels in patients without restenosis, and they had a significantly higher relative increase of C-reactive protein and serum amyloid A levels during the first 48 h after intervention (Table 6.2) [12, 13].

Table 6.1 Periprocedural variables

Variable	No restenosis ($n = 198$)	In-stent restenosis ($n = 12$)	p value
Serum parameters			
Leucocyte$_{pre}$ count/µl (mean, SD)	7,626 (±2,040)	8,300 (±3,013)	0.283
CRP$_{pre}$ mg/dl (median, IQR)	2 (0–6.6)	10.4 (1.45–23.7)	0.022[a]
Leucocyte$_{post}$ count/µl (mean, SD)	8,526 (±2,525)	10,433 (±4,177)	0.035[a,b]
CRP$_{post}$ mg/dl (median, IQR)	10.1 (4.5–24.9)	9 (3.0–11.2)	0.314
Cholesterol mg/dl (mean, SD)	195 (±49)	192 (±58)	0.885
Triglycerides mg/dl (mean, SD)	148 (±72)	123 (± 61)	0.439
LDL mg/dl (mean SD)	133 (± 40)	123 (± 50)	0.587
HDL mg/dl (mean, SD)	47.8 (± 13)	44.8 (± 13)	0.620
Interventional parameters			
Predilatation	21 (10.9 %)	3 (25.0 %)	0.153
Postdilatation	189 (95.5 %)	10 (83.3 %)	0.125
Multiple stents used	10 (5.1 %)	1 (8.3 %)	0.485
Stent length (mean, SD)	37.6 (±5.5)	40.7 (±7.0)	0.068[a,b]
Stent width (mean, SD)	7.4 (±1.0)	6.9 (±1.1)	0.019[a,b]
Closed cell stent design	165 (83.3 %)	11 (91.7 %)	0.695

doi:10.1371/journal.pone.0022683.t002
pre preprocedural (within 24 h before CAS), *post* postprocedural (within 24 h after CAS), *CRP* C-reactive protein
[a]Factors included in multiple regression analysis
[b]Factors remained significant after multiple regression analysis

Table 6.2 Periprocedural complications within 30 days after CAS according to preprocedural CRP levels

	Normal CRP (n=94)	Elevated CRP (n=36)	P value*
Minor stroke	2 (2.1 %)	5 (13.9 %)	0.0174
Major stroke	1 (1.1 %)	1 (2.8 %)	0.4787
Death	0 (0 %)	2 (5.6 %)	0.0751
Any stroke or death	3 (3.2 %)	8 (22.2 %)	0.0015

Note CRP indicates C-reactive protein
*P values are from χ^2 analysis

Conclusion

Inflammation is directly associated with the development, progression, and rupture of atherosclerotic plaques and with the in-stent restenosis. Serum inflammatory biomarkers, for instance, IL-6, OPN, C-reactive protein, and serum amyloid A, play an important role in the genesis of carotid artery stenosis and in the progression of atherosclerotic phenomena after carotid artery angioplasty. However, following the development of medical treatment and the increasing number of studies in the medical area, more studies should be conducted with the aim to explore the inflammatory aspects of carotid artery stenting. This effort may contribute to clarifying our understanding of the pathophysiology of inflammation in carotid artery angioplasty and improving or even preventing in-stent restenosis.

References

1. Virmani R, Farb A. Pathology of in-stent re-stenosis. Curr Opin Lipidol. 1999;10:499–506.
2. Kornowski R, Hong MK, Tio FO, et al. In-stent restenosis: contributions of inflammatory responses and arterial injury to neointimal hyperplasia. J Am Coll Cardiol. 1998;31:224–30.
3. Yutani C, Ishibashi-Ueda H, Suzuki T, et al. Histologic evidence of foreign body granulation tissue and de novo lesions in patients with coronary stent stenosis. Cardiology. 1999;92:171–7.
4. Libby P, Ridker PM, Maseri A. Inflammation and atherosclerosis. Circulation. 2002;105:1135–43.
5. Koenig W, Khuseyinova N. Biomarkers of atherosclerotic plaque instability and rupture. Arterioscler Thromb Vasc Biol. 2007;27:15–26.
6. Abe Y, Sakaguchi M, Furukado S, Okazaki S, Fujinaka T, Sakoda S, et al. Associations of local release of inflammatory biomarkers during carotid artery stenting with plaque echogenicity and calcification. Cerebrovasc Dis. 2010;30:402–9.
7. Uwatoko T, Toyoda K, Inoue T, Yasumori K, Hirai Y, Makihara N, et al. Carotid artery calcification on multislice detector-row computed tomography. Cerebrovasc Dis. 2007;24:20–6.
8. Wasser K, Schnaudigel S, Wohlfahrt J, Psychogios M-N, Knauth M, et al. Inflammation and in-stent restenosis: the role of serum markers and stent characteristics in carotid artery stenting. PLoS One. 2011;6(7):e22683. doi:10.1371/journal.pone.0022683.
9. Weintraub WS. The pathophysiology and burden of restenosis. Am J Cardiol. 2007;100(5A):3K–99.
10. Kornowski R, Hong MK, Tio FO, Bramwell O, Wu H, et al. In-stent restenosis: contributions of inflammatory responses and arterial injury to neointimal hyperplasia. J Am Coll Cardiol. 1998;31(1):224–30.
11. Clark DJ, Lessio S, O'Donoghue M, Tsalamandris C, Schainfeld R, et al. Mechanisms and predictors of carotid artery stent restenosis: a serial intravascular ultrasound study. J Am Coll Cardiol. 2006;47(12):2390–6.
12. Schillinger M, Exner M, Mlekusch W, Rumpold H, Ahmadi R, et al. Acute-phase response after stent implantation in the carotid artery: association with 6-month in-stent restenosis. Radiology. 2003;227(2):516–21.
13. Gröschel K, Ernemann U, Larsen J, Knauth M, Schmidt F, Artschwager J, et al. Preprocedural C-reactive protein levels predict stroke and death in patients undergoing carotid stenting. AJNR Am J Neuroradiol. 2007;28(9):1743–6.

Part III

Abdominal Aortic Aneurysm

Role of Matrix Metalloproteinases and Aortic Wall Degradation in Abdominal Aortic Aneurysms

7

George A. Antoniou and George S. Georgiadis

Introduction

Abdominal aortic aneurysm (AAA) is the most common type of true aneurysm. Aneurysm is defined as local dilatation of at least 1.5 times the expected normal arterial diameter. In clinical practice, a practical definition for AAA of a transverse diameter of greater than 3 cm is used. It is present in 5–10 % of men aged between 65 and 79 years [1]. Its major complication is rupture, which presents as a surgical emergency. The mortality associated with rupture is high: approximately 80 % of those who reach the hospital and 50 % of those undergoing emergency surgery for ruptured AAA will die [2]. In the United States, ruptured AAA is the 15th leading cause of death overall [3]. Elective aneurysm repair is associated with a 30-day mortality of 2–6 % [4]. These mortality figures have not changed in the past decades, despite improvements in operative techniques and perioperative management. Furthermore, the incidence of AAA seems to be increasing, which cannot be explained only by improvements in detection [5].

The aortic aneurysm constitutes a significant health problem, which creates substantial social and financial burdens for health and surgical services in several countries. The natural course is well defined and is characterized by ongoing progression and development of acute, potentially life-threatening complications. The pathogenesis of aneurysmal disease of the aorta is complex and multifactorial. Several underlying pathophysiological processes have been described to explain the mechanisms of degeneration of the aortic wall tissues resulting in aneurysm. Current concepts converge on the fact that a dysregulation in connective tissue metabolism instigating and/or resulting from local inflammatory responses under the influence of different environmental triggering events is responsible for the clinical manifestation of aneurysm [6, 7]. Delineation of underlying pathogenic mechanisms may give further insight into the biological processes of disease development and have implications in clinical practice and a pharmacotherapeutic potential.

G.A. Antoniou, MD, PhD (✉)
Department of Vascular and Endovascular Surgery, Manchester Royal Infirmary, Central Manchester University Hospitals NHS Foundation Trust, Manchester, UK
email: antoniou.ga@hotmail.com

G.S. Georgiadis, MD
Department of Vascular and Endovascular Surgery, University Hospital of Alexandroupolis, Democritus University of Thrace, Alexandroupolis, Greece

Pathogenesis and Biology of Abdominal Aortic Aneurysm

Aneurysms result from a chronic degenerative process that evolves over a long period of time. The National Heart, Lung, and Blood Institute established a consensus on current research needs to maximize the overall impact of the aneurysm research program and defined current areas of research focusing on proteolytic degradation of the aortic wall connective tissue as well as inflammatory and immunological responses as the main culprits in the pathogenic mechanisms of abdominal aortic aneurysm formation [6, 7]. Important structural elements of the aortic wall are elastin and collagen, which are found in the arterial media and adventitia and provide passive strength to the wall, whereas medial smooth muscle cells define its active properties. Elastin is the main component of the media, and it provides and distributes tensile strength along the arterial wall. It is synthesized during the early stages of aortic wall development and has an estimated half-life of 60 years. A study examining the ultrastructure of elastin elements found that there was an 81.6 % reduction in elastin lamella in the aortic wall of patients with abdominal aortic aneurysm, concluding that elastolysis is a primary event in aneurysm formation [8]. Solid evidence exists supporting that elastin degradation occurs in the early stages of the pathogenic process of aneurysm development [8–10]. On the other hand, collagen is the primary structural

E.A. Gabriel, S.A. Gabriel (eds.), *Inflammatory Response in Cardiovascular Surgery*, DOI 10.1007/978-1-4471-4429-8_7,

Table 7.1 Role of MMPs in the pathogenesis of aortic aneurysm

Matrix metalloproteinase	Enzyme	Genetic location	Main ECM substrates	Role in aortic aneurysm
MMP-1	Collagenase 1	11q22-q23	Collagens (I, II, III, VII, VIII, X), gelatin, fibronectin, vitronectin, laminin, aggrecan	Collagenolysis, associated with risk of rupture
MMP-2	Gelatinase A	16q13	Collagens (I, II, III, IV, V, VII, X, XI), gelatin, elastin, fibronectin, vitronectin, laminin	Elastolysis, dominant role in early stages of aneurysm formation
MMP-3	Stromelysin 1	11q23	Collagens (III, IV, V, VII, IX, X, XI), gelatin, elastin, fibronectin, vitronectin, laminin	Elastin and collagen degradation, activates other pro-MMPs, angiogenesis
MMP-8	Collagenase 2	11q21-q22	Collagens (I, II, III), aggrecan	Collagen degradation, aneurysm rupture
MMP-9	Gelatinase B	20q11.2-q13.1	Collagens (IV, V, XI, XIV), gelatin, elastin, vitronectin, laminin, aggrecan	Elastolysis, collagenolysis, dominant role in later stages of aneurysm formation and rupture
MMP-12	Macrophage elastase	11q22.2-q22.3	Collagens (I, IV, V), gelatin, elastin, fibronectin, vitronectin, laminin	Elastolytic activity
MMP-13	Collagenase 3	11q22.3	Collagens (I, II, III, IV, VI, IX, X, XIV), gelatin, fibronectin, aggrecan	Collagenolysis, associated with risk of rupture
MMP-14	MT1-MMP	14q11-q12	Collagens (I, II, III), gelatin, fibronectin, tenascin, vitronectin, laminin	Activates pro-MMP-2

element of the adventitia, is composed of three polypeptide chains forming a triple-helical structure, and, unlike elastin, is under a continuous process of synthesis and degradation throughout life. It provides stiffness to the arterial wall. A report found increased collagen and a prominent inflammatory cell infiltration in the aneurysm wall compared with non-aneurysmal aortas [11]. Increased collagenolytic activity in the aneurysmal aorta being correlated with aneurysm size was demonstrated in another report [12]. It seems that collagen synthesis increases during the early stage of aneurysm formation, however at later stages degradation exceeds synthesis, resulting in continuing aneurysm expansion and ultimately rupture [11–13]. The aortic wall extracellular matrix, apart from the structural elements of elastin and collagen, contains embedded inflammatory cells, smooth muscle cells, cytokines, growth factors, proteinases, and proteinase inhibitors. It is a complex structure that, apart from its scaffold properties to the aortic wall, exerts a number of biological activities and regulates elastin and collagen synthesis and degradation, smooth muscle cell apoptosis, chemotaxis and cell migration, inflammation and immune responses, and angiogenesis.

There is ample evidence that matrix degradation by a variety of proteolytic enzymes, mainly MMPs, is integral to aneurysm development and that an imbalance between MMPs and their inhibitors (TIMPs) impairs normal physiologic aortic wall remodeling [14, 15]. Elastolysis is an early event in aneurysm formation. Freestone et al. demonstrated that MMP-2 was the dominant gelatinase in small aneurysms, suggesting that it is the inciting enzyme in aneurysm genesis [16]. As opposed to MMP-2, McMillan et al. found higher MMP-9 mRNA expression in moderate-diameter (5–6.9 cm) than small-diameter (<4 cm) aneurysms [17]. Evidence suggests that MMP-9 is the dominant proteolytic enzyme promoting continued expansion and rupture [17, 18]. Peterson et al. demonstrated that levels of MMP-9 were increased in ruptured aneurysms compared to large intact aneurysms [19]. Several other MMPs have been demonstrated to play a role in the aneurysm degrading and inflammatory process (Table 7.1). Regulation of MMP activity is achieved at different levels, with TIMPs having been suggested as an important regulator of extracellular matrix degradation. The balance of aortic wall remodeling between MMPs and their inhibitors favors collagen and elastin degradation. However, the initiating events and the mechanisms for propagating these proteolytic enzymes in the aortic wall remain to be identified.

Investigations have also demonstrated a significant immunological contribution to the pathogenesis of the disease. Lymphocytes represent the main cell population found in inflammatory infiltrates in aortic aneurysms. Schonbeck et al. identified that the majority of the lymphocytes were T-helper (Th)-2-restricted CD3+ T lymphocytes, as determined by Western blot and immunohistochemical analysis, with increased Th-2-associated expression of interleukin (IL)-4, IL-5, and IL-10 [20]. It seems that exogenous and/or endogenous factors disrupting the intima/adventitia and exposing elastin and interstitial collagen instigate an immune response resulting in a cascade of inflammatory events [21, 22]. Immune cells, including macrophages and lymphocytes, along with smooth muscle cells and fibroblasts promote a strong inflammatory reaction, which activates proteolytic enzymes and extracellular matrix degradation. Elastin and collagen degradation products in turn propagate a sequestered inflammatory reaction, leading to further degeneration of the aortic wall, aneurysm expansion, and rupture. Oxidative stress significantly contributes to the pathophysiology of inflammation. Zhang et al. demonstrated increased expression of inducible nitric oxide synthase in the aneurysm wall tissues as compared with normal aorta [23]. An integral part of the whole process is a reduction in medial smooth muscle cells (apoptosis), which are the principal cell type producing extracellular matrix components [24, 25]. It seems however, that during life, as oxidative stress increases and assaults increasingly occur at the endothelial and smooth muscle levels, there is a natural biological antiinflammatory process that counteracts the tendency toward inflammatory degradation. Th-2-associated cytokines suppress macrophage expression of MMP-9, which suggests that Th-2 immune responses might restrain aneurysmal degeneration [26].

Understanding of the significance of MMPs in biology and pathology has led to the development of numerous potent synthetic inhibitors of matrix metalloproteinases. Such agents may be of great therapeutic value, and some of them are in clinical trials for the treatment of cancer and inflammatory conditions [27]. Tetracyclines non-selectively inhibit MMPs via mechanisms similar to those of endogenous inhibitors and have been shown to effectively prevent elastin and collagen destruction as well as aneurysmal dilatation [28–30].

Genetics of Aortic Aneurysm

Although the etiology of aortic aneurysm is assumed to be multifactorial, genetic influences appear to be independently associated with both disease states. A genetic predisposition to abdominal aortic aneurysm development is demonstrated by clustering of aneurysms in families and has been documented by both familial and segregation observational studies [31–33]. Baird et al. found an aneurysm prevalence of 19 % in siblings of patients with abdominal aortic aneurysm as compared to 8 % in controls using ultrasound examination, and the risk of aneurysm was demonstrated to begin earlier and increase more rapidly for siblings of affected individuals compared with controls [32]. Several investigators have also followed a candidate gene approach to further characterize the genetic component in aneurysm pathogenesis. Thompson et al. have undertaken a meta-analysis of all aneurysm candidate gene analysis studies and identified three polymorphisms associated with a significant risk of aneurysm [ACE RR 1.33 (95 % CI 1.20–1.48), MTHFR RR 1.14 (1.08–1.21), and MMP-9 RR 1.09 (1.01–1.18)] [34]. Genes encoding the components of the extracellular matrix as well as those involved in mechanisms of connective tissue metabolism and inflammatory response have been extensively investigated. In particular, polymorphic sites and gene mutations of proteins of the structural components of the connective tissue (elastin, collagen), extracellular matrix-degrading enzymes and their inhibitors (MMPs, TIMPs), and inflammation promotion agents (interleukins, platelet-activating factor, nitric oxide synthase, inflammatory receptors) have been investigated separately in gene association observational studies. Nevertheless, no single gene has yet been isolated as the key factor interpreting the genetic basis of aortic aneurysm. A small number of families have a genetically determined type III collagen defect (COL3A1), in which cases the abdominal aortic aneurysm is considered to be a manifestation of Ehlers-Danlos syndrome [35]. Furthermore, mutations in the fibrilin-1 gene (15q21.1), resulting in abnormal fibrilin-1 synthesis, secretion, or use, are responsible for Marfan syndrome, which is a hereditary connective tissue disorder associated with thoraco-abdominal aortic aneurysms and dissections [36].

Future Perspectives

Pharmacotherapeutic approaches to prevent or slow down the development and progression of the disease constitute a virgin field in medical research. Targeted approaches with the design of specific inhibitors of key players in the connective tissue degeneration process might provide novel pharmacological methods to decelerate aneurysm progression. Further knowledge about mechanisms of regulation of MMP gene expression may direct therapeutic strategies toward tissue-targeted gene therapies with agents that selectively inhibit specific MMPs.

References

1. Vardulaki KA, Prevost TC, Walker NM, Day NE, Wilmink AB, Quick CR, et al. Incidence among men of asymptomatic abdominal aortic aneurysms: estimates from 500 screen detected cases. J Med Screen. 1999;6(1):50–4.
2. Basnyat PS, Biffin AH, Moseley LG, Hedges AR, Lewis MH. Mortality from ruptured abdominal aortic aneurysm in Wales. Br J Surg. 1999;86(6):765–70.
3. Silverberg E, Boring CC, Squires TS. Cancer statistics, 1990. CA Cancer J Clin. 1990;40(1):9–26.
4. Huber TS, Wang JG, Derrow AE, Dame DA, Ozaki CK, Zelenock GB, et al. Experience in the United States with intact abdominal aortic aneurysm repair. J Vasc Surg. 2001;33(2):304–10, discussion 310–1.
5. Sakalihasan N, Limet R, Defawe OD. Abdominal aortic aneurysm. Lancet. 2005;365(9470):1577–89.
6. Ailawadi G, Eliason JL, Upchurch Jr GR. Current concepts in the pathogenesis of abdominal aortic aneurysm. J Vasc Surg. 2003;38(3):584–8.
7. Wassef M, Baxter BT, Chisholm RL, Dalman RL, Fillinger MF, Heinecke J, et al. Pathogenesis of abdominal aortic aneurysms: a

multidisciplinary research program supported by the National Heart, Lung, and Blood Institute. J Vasc Surg. 2001;34(4):730–8.
8. White JV, Haas K, Phillips S, Comerota AJ. Adventitial elastolysis is a primary event in aneurysm formation. J Vasc Surg. 1993;17(2): 371–80.
9. Krettek A, Sukhova GK, Libby P. Elastogenesis in human arterial disease: a role for macrophages in disordered elastin synthesis. Arterioscler Thromb Vasc Biol. 2003;23(4):582–7.
10. Rucker RB, Tinker D. Structure and metabolism of arterial elastin. Int Rev Exp Pathol. 1977;17:1–47.
11. Rizzo RJ, McCarthy WJ, Dixit SN, Lilly MP, Shively VP, Flinn WR, et al. Collagen types and matrix protein content in human abdominal aortic aneurysms. J Vasc Surg. 1989;10(4):365–73.
12. Busuttil RW, Abou-Zamzam AM, Machleder HI. Collagenase activity of the human aorta. A comparison of patients with and without abdominal aortic aneurysms. Arch Surg. 1980;115(11):1373–8.
13. Campa JS, Greenhalgh RM, Powell JT. Elastin degradation in abdominal aortic aneurysms. Atherosclerosis. 1987;65(1–2):13–21.
14. Keeling WB, Armstrong PA, Stone PA, Bandyk DF, Shames ML. An overview of matrix metalloproteinases in the pathogenesis and treatment of abdominal aortic aneurysms. Vasc Endovascular Surg. 2005;39(6):457–64.
15. Pearce WH, Shively VP. Abdominal aortic aneurysm as a complex multifactorial disease: interactions of polymorphisms of inflammatory genes, features of autoimmunity, and current status of MMPs. Ann N Y Acad Sci. 2006;1085:117–32.
16. Freestone T, Turner RJ, Coady A, Higman DJ, Greenhalgh RM, Powell JT. Inflammation and matrix metalloproteinases in the enlarging abdominal aortic aneurysm. Arterioscler Thromb Vasc Biol. 1995;15(8):1145–51.
17. McMillan WD, Tamarina NA, Cipollone M, Johnson DA, Parker MA, Pearce WH. Size matters: the relationship between MMP-9 expression and aortic diameter. Circulation. 1997;96(7):2228–32.
18. Thompson M, Cockerill G. Matrix metalloproteinase-2: the forgotten enzyme in aneurysm pathogenesis. Ann N Y Acad Sci. 2006; 1085:170–4.
19. Petersen E, Gineitis A, Wågberg F, Angquist KA. Activity of matrix metalloproteinase-2 and –9 in abdominal aortic aneurysms. Relation to size and rupture. Eur J Vasc Endovasc Surg. 2000;20(5):457–61.
20. Schönbeck U, Sukhova GK, Gerdes N, Libby P. T(H)2 predominant immune responses prevail in human abdominal aortic aneurysm. Am J Pathol. 2002;161(2):499–506.
21. Lindholt JS, Shi GP. Chronic inflammation, immune response, and infection in abdominal aortic aneurysms. Eur J Vasc Endovasc Surg. 2006;31(5):453–63.
22. Shimizu K, Mitchell RN, Libby P. Inflammation and cellular immune responses in abdominal aortic aneurysms. Arterioscler Thromb Vasc Biol. 2006;26(5):987–94.
23. Zhang J, Schmidt J, Ryschich E, Mueller-Schilling M, Schumacher H, Allenberg JR. Inducible nitric oxide synthase is present in human abdominal aortic aneurysm and promotes oxidative vascular injury. J Vasc Surg. 2003;38(2):360–7.
24. McCormick ML, Gavrila D, Weintraub NL. Role of oxidative stress in the pathogenesis of abdominal aortic aneurysms. Arterioscler Thromb Vasc Biol. 2007;27(3):461–9.
25. Curci JA. Digging in the "soil" of the aorta to understand the growth of abdominal aortic aneurysms. Vascular. 2009;17 Suppl 1:S21–9.
26. Curci JA, Thompson RW. Adaptive cellular immunity in aortic aneurysms: cause, consequence, or context? J Clin Invest. 2004; 114(2):168–71.
27. Zucker S, Cao J, Chen WT. Critical appraisal of the use of matrix metalloproteinase inhibitors in cancer treatment. Oncogene. 2000;19(56):6642–50.
28. Hanemaaijer R, Visser H, Koolwijk P, Sorsa T, Salo T, Golub LM, et al. Inhibition of MMP synthesis by doxycycline and chemically modified tetracyclines (CMTs) in human endothelial cells. Adv Dent Res. 1998;12(2):114–8.
29. Baxter BT, Pearce WH, Waltke EA, Littooy FN, Hallett Jr JW, Kent KC, et al. Prolonged administration of doxycycline in patients with small asymptomatic abdominal aortic aneurysms: report of a prospective (Phase II) multicenter study. J Vasc Surg. 2002;36(1): 1–12.
30. Aziz F, Kuivaniemi H. Role of matrix metalloproteinase inhibitors in preventing abdominal aortic aneurysm. Ann Vasc Surg. 2007; 21(3):392–401.
31. Salo JA, Soisalon-Soininen S, Bondestam S, Mattila PS. Familial occurrence of abdominal aortic aneurysm. Ann Intern Med. 1999;130(8):637–42.
32. Baird PA, Sadovnick AD, Yee IM, Cole CW, Cole L. Sibling risks of abdominal aortic aneurysm. Lancet. 1995;346(8975):601–4.
33. Sandford RM, Bown MJ, London NJ, Sayers RD. The genetic basis of abdominal aortic aneurysms: a review. Eur J Vasc Endovasc Surg. 2007;33(4):381–90.
34. Thompson AR, Drenos F, Hafez H, Humphries SE. Candidate gene association studies in abdominal aortic aneurysm disease: a review and meta-analysis. Eur J Vasc Endovasc Surg. 2008;35(1): 19–30.
35. Kontusaari S, Tromp G, Kuivaniemi H, Ladda RL, Prockop DJ. Inheritance of an RNA splicing mutation (G+1 IVS20) in the type III procollagen gene (COL3A1) in a family having aortic aneurysms and easy bruisability: phenotypic overlap between familial arterial aneurysms and Ehlers-Danlos syndrome type IV. Am J Hum Genet. 1990;47(1):112–20.
36. Gott VL, Laschinger JC, Cameron DE, Dietz HC, Greene PS, Gillinov AM, et al. The Marfan syndrome and the cardiovascular surgeon. Eur J Cardiothorac Surg. 1996;10(3):149–58.

Role of Haptoglobin in Abdominal Aortic Aneurysm

8

Valerio Napolioni

Haptoglobin, an Anti-inflammatory Plasma Protein

Haptoglobin (Hp) is a plasmatic protein encoded by the *HP* gene (OMIM*140100, gene map locus 16q22.1). Its main function in blood plasma is binding free hemoglobin (Hb) released from erythrocytes with high affinity and thereby inhibiting its oxidative activity. The Hp-Hb complex is then removed by the reticuloendothelial system (mostly the spleen). Hp is widely used in clinical settings where the Hp assay is implemented to screen for and monitor intravascular hemolytic anemia [1]. In intravascular hemolytic anemia, free Hb is released into the circulation, and hence Hp binds the Hb. This causes a decline in Hp levels. Conversely, in extravascular hemolysis, the reticuloendothelial system, especially splenic monocytes, phagocytoses the erythrocytes, and Hb is not released into the circulation; hence, the Hp levels are normal. Thus, Hp is a potent antioxidant playing a scavenging role for the toxic free Hb that accumulates during acute-phase inflammatory reactions [1].

However, importantly, Hp also exerts a direct angiogenic, antiinflammatory, and immunomodulatory function in extravascular tissues and body fluids. In fact, in response to various stimuli, Hp is able to migrate through vessel walls and is expressed in different tissues [2]. Furthermore, Hp can be released from neutrophil granulocytes at sites of injury or inflammation and locally dampens tissue damage [3]. Hp receptors include CD163 expressed on the monocyte-macrophage system and CD11b (CR3) found on granulocytes, natural killer cells, and in small lymphocyte subpopulations [4, 5]. Hp has also been shown to bind to the majority of $CD4^+$ and $CD8^+$ T cells, directly inhibiting their proliferation and modifying the balance of T helper (Th) 1 and 2 [6]. Notably, Hp inhibits the capacity of epidermal Langerhans cells to activate naive T cells, and abundant Hp has been detected in cytoplasmic compartments of Langerhans cells and in neutrophils [7, 8]. Also, Hp binds to mast cells through another yet unidentified receptor, possibly modulating their function [9]. Last, high density lipoprotein (HDL) particles can become proinflammatory through direct interactions of Hp-Hb complexes with apolipoprotein A1 [10].

V. Napolioni, PhD
School of Biosciences and Biotechnologies, University of Camerino, Camerino, Italy
e-mail: valerio.napolioni@unicam.it, napvale@gmail.com

Haptoglobin Protein Structure and Its Polymorphism

Hp is an α2-sialoglycoprotein endowed with Hb-binding capacity and is characterized by molecular heterogeneity; this is due to the existence of three major genotypes, i.e., *HP**1/*1, *HP**2/*1, and *HP**2/*2 [1]. The main difference between the alleles *HP**1 and *HP**2 is the presence of a duplicated ~1.7 Kb DNA segment in *HP**2, but not *HP**1 (Fig. 8.1) [11]. Of note, *HP**1 has two variants, *HP**1F (fast) and *HP**1S (slow), which are correlated with the presence of amino acids Asp-Lys (version F) or Asn-Glu (version S) at amino acid positions 52 and 53 in the α1 chain. The *HP**2 allele is supposed to originate from a breakage and reunion event at non-homologous positions within the fourth and the second introns (unequal crossing over) in an individual who was heterozygous for *HP**1F and *HP**1S [12]. Having exons 3 and 4 in duplicate, the *HP**2 monomer is bivalent and can associate with two different Hp monomers. Thus, homozygous *HP**1/*1 individuals express Hp protein as a single α1β homodimer of 86 kDa. Homozygous *HP**2/*2 individuals express cyclic Hp oligomers containing three or more α2β subunits (170–900 kDa). The Hp synthesized by *HP**2/*1 heterozygous subjects is assembled into linear homodimers and multimers of variable numbers of α2β subunits flanked at each terminus by 1α1β subunits (86–300 kDa). Thus, the *HP**2/*1 phenotype is distinctly different from the phenotypes of the *HP**2 or *HP**1 homozygotes (Fig. 8.1). Since functional differences in the antioxidant, scavenging, and immune-regulatory properties of Hp occur

E.A. Gabriel, S.A. Gabriel (eds.), *Inflammatory Response in Cardiovascular Surgery*,
DOI 10.1007/978-1-4471-4429-8_8, © Springer-Verlag London 2013

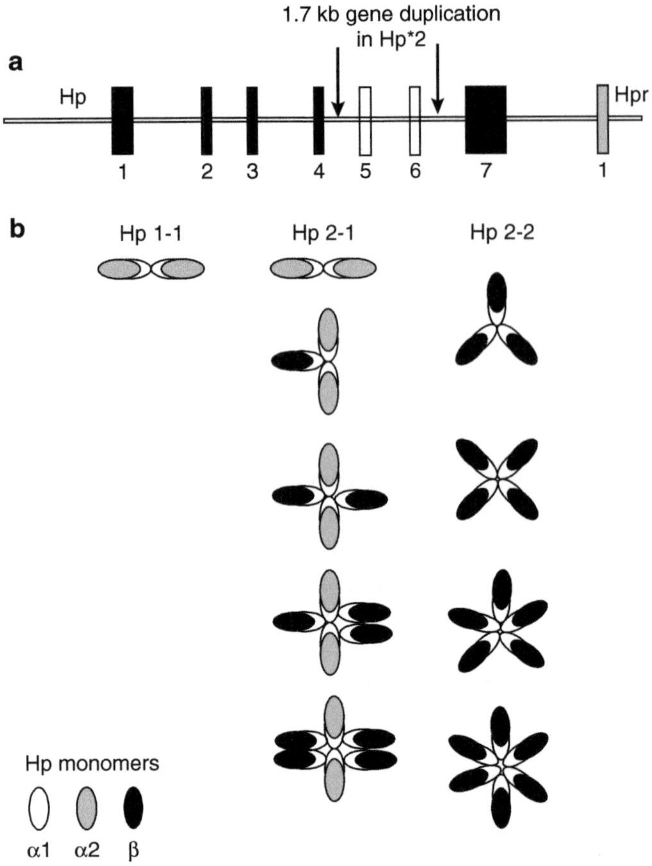

Fig. 8.1 *HP* locus genetic structure and structural differences with subunit arrangement of Hp phenotypes. (**a**) The physical map of the *HP* locus. *HP* exons are indicated by *black* boxes. The gene duplication responsible for *HP* polymorphism is indicated by two vertical *arrows*. (**b**) The three *HP* genotypes express entirely different molecular structures at the protein level

as a function of its polymorphism, the genetics of *HP* has been associated with predisposition to infections and with autoimmune, cardiovascular, and other diseases and disorders [1]. In Caucasians, the phenotype frequencies are approximately 16 % (*HP**1/*1), 48 % (*HP**2/*1), and 36 % (*HP**2/*2), but marked geographical differences exist, with Asians showing high *HP**2/*2 frequencies (up to 55 %) [1].

Haptoglobin Polymorphism and Its Role in Inflammation and Atherosclerosis

Beyond the conventional view of Hp as a marker of hemolysis, several findings point toward an immunomodulatory effect of Hp in B-cell mediated progression of atherosclerosis [13]. It has been demonstrated that the *HP**2/*2 phenotype is associated with markedly higher peripheral B-cell counts than *HP**1/*1 [14]. In contrast, B-cell percentages in bone marrow are lowest in *HP**2/*2 subjects [14]. A negative correlation between serum Hp 1–1 concentration and peripheral B-cell counts was also observed [14]. The number of free CD22 binding sites on circulating B cells was estimated to be higher in *HP**2/*2 individuals, who display lower serum Hp levels than those with *HP**1/*1. Furthermore, the concentrations of large, multimeric proteins such as IgM and Hp 2–2 are considerably lower in extravascular fluids than in plasma, because diffusion of these macromolecules into the interstitial compartment is limited. Thus, it is conceivable that some interactions of B cells that are inhibited in the blood stream are enabled within atherosclerotic plaque of *HP**2/*2 subjects.

However, it is not known whether and how the different Hp phenotypes can influence the B-T cell dialogue and T cell activation by interfering with CD22 function. Notably, higher peripheral T helper lymphocyte counts are observed in *HP**2/*2 subjects [14]. However, Hp plays a direct effect on T cells through a dose-dependent suppression of induced T-cell proliferation [6]. Hp exhibits a strong inhibitory effect on T_h2 cytokine release, thus promoting a dominant T_h1 activation over T_h2 activation and playing a modulating role on the T_h1/T_h2 balance [6]. The majority of the T cells in atherosclerotic lesions produce $T_h1$cytokines, such as IL-2, IL-12, interferon-γ, TNF-α, and TNF-β, supporting cell-mediated responses [15]. In contrast, human atheromas contain only modest quantities of the T_h2 cytokines IL-4, IL-5, and IL-10, which can promote humoral responses [15]. Whether and how the different polymorphic Hp forms can attenuate or enhance atherogenesis by direct modulation of Th1/Th2 balance requires further investigation. Some pro-atherogenic properties related to Hb binding of Hp 2–2 can have indirect effects on B- and T-cell responses as well as antibody production against oxidized LDL. First, Hp 2–2 polymers are less efficient in the clearance of free Hb after intraplaque hemorrhage, causing higher susceptibility of LDL to Hb-driven oxidation [16]. Oxidatively modified LDL epitopes are highly immunogenic and stimulate B- and T-cell responses that can promote humoral as well as cellular immunity [17]. Second, Hb/Hp 2–2 complexes display higher affinity for CD163 on monocyte-macrophages, leading to intracellular accumulation of Hb-derived iron [18]. Such iron-loaded macrophages may, in the arterial intima, expose LDL to reactive oxygen species and thus generate an inflammatory stimulus [19]. Finally, via CD163 binding, the Hb–Hp 1–1 complex stimulates the macrophage to secrete the antiinflammatory cytokine IL-10 and heme oxygenase-1 to a markedly greater degree than the Hb–Hp 2–2 complex [19]. Release of IL-10 has been suggested to reduce inflammatory cell infiltration and macrophage accumulation in atherosclerotic plaques of Hp 1–1 mice [19]. IL-10 inhibits the T_h1 response in atheroma. In contrast, macrophages activated by Hb–Hp 2–2 binding to CD163 shift the T helper response towards T_h1 cytokines [20].

Haptoglobin and Its Role in Abdominal Aortic Aneurysm

Inflammation with infiltrates of macrophages and lymphocytes is an important feature of abdominal aortic aneurysms (AAA) [21, 22]. Elevated levels of various plasma markers of inflammation have been reported in patients with AAA as compared with healthy controls or patients with cardiovascular disease [23–25]. Positive correlations between inflammatory markers and the degree of aortic dilatation have been reported in cross-sectional studies [26–29].

In this context, Hp may play a crucial role in modulation the inflammatory response characterizing AAA, both as a susceptibility factor (by its genetic polymorphism) and as a prognostic marker.

The first study on Hp's role in AAA was performed in early 1980, when Norrgärd and co-workers found that there was an increased frequency of the *HP**2/*1 phenotype in Northern Swedish individuals with AAA [30]. Following this first report, Powell et al. [31] investigated whether the different Hp phenotypes influence the degradation of aortic connective tissue. The *HP**1 allele frequency was significantly increased in patients with aneurysms compared to control subjects (0.51 vs. 0.35, $P<0.05$). However, *HP**2/*2 patients had the highest mean age at aneurysm resection. Moreover, they found that Hps containing an α1-chain accelerated the degradation of aortic elastin by elastases two- to four-fold in vitro.

This preliminary evidence led Adamson et al. [32] to test for the usefulness of the *HP* polymorphism as a family-based informative genetic marker of AAA, without significant results. After this study, the role of Hp in AAA was almost ignored until 2001, when Wiernicki et al. [33] analyzed the influence of Hp phenotypes on serum elastase activity, neutrophil count, and elastin concentration in the aorta of Polish AAA ($N=52$) and aortoiliac atherosclerotic occlusive disease (AOD; $N=37$) patients. *HP* phenotype distribution did not differ between the two groups and the third control group of 37 subjects without atherosclerosis. Nevertheless, significant increases in serum elastase activity and neutrophil count were measured in the *HP**2/*1 phenotype of AAA patients, thus supporting the association of AAA susceptibility with the *HP**2/*1 phenotype as postulated by Norrg rd et al. [30]. Nearly 10 years later, the same research group provided further evidence for the association of the *HP**2/*1 genotype with AAA [34]. They found that *HP**2/*1 patients had a significantly higher growth rate [3.69 (2.40) mm/year] of AAA compared with patients with *HP**2/*2 [1.24 (0.79), $P<0.00001$] and *HP**1/*1 [1.45 (0.68), $P=0.00004$]. Elevated elastase serum activity was also evident in AAA patients with *HP**2/*1 [0.119 (0.084) arbitrary units] in contrast to *HP**2/*2 [0.064 (0.041), $P<0.00001$] and *HP**1/*1 [0.071 (0.040), $P = 0.0006$] patients. CRP serum levels (mg/l) were significantly higher in patients with *HP**2/*1 (7.2 [7.1]) than with *HP**2/*2 [3.4 (3.1), $P=0.0058$] and *HP**1/*1 [2.8 (4.1), $P = 0.044$]. In 2011, Pan et al. [35] conducted another study aiming to assess the association of the *HP* polymorphism with AAA in the Taiwanese population. Forty-five patients with AAA and 49 non-AAA subjects were included. They found that plasma Hp concentrations were significantly higher in AAA patients compared with non-AAA subjects (254 ± 158 vs. 186 ± 108 ng/ml; $P=0.017$), in particular for *HP**2/*2 carriers compared with corresponding non-AAA subjects (238 ± 144 vs. 163 ± 86 ng/ml; $P=0.024$).

Beside studies based on the *HP* genetic polymorphism, three reports have been conducted only at the protein level. The first was performed on a large Swedish cohort, the "Malmö Preventive Study," including 6,075 men with information on 5 inflammation-sensitive plasma proteins (ISPs; fibrinogen, orosomucoid, α1-antitrypsin, haptoglobin, and ceruloplasmin) [36]. A total of 63 men had AAA (0.49 per 1,000 person/years). Fifty were non-fatal cases whose aneurysm was repaired in an open vascular or endovascular surgical procedure, and 13 of those 50 (26 %) were ruptured. The remaining 13 cases were fatal. The mean time from the baseline examination to aneurysm repair or death from AAA was 18.8 ± 4.9 years (range 1.3–26.6). Age at the time of the AAA was 67.1 ± 5.3 years (range: 55–80 years). The Hp level (g/l) was significantly higher in men who subsequently had AAA as compared with the controls (1.69 ± 0.79 vs. 1.38 ± 0.68, $p<0.001$). Moreover, a higher Hp level conferred an increased risk of fatal AAA compared with repaired AAA (O.R = 2.500, $p<0.010$). Another study examined the Hp level after postoperative surgery in elective repair of infrarenal aortic aneurysm patients [37]; AAA patients had a significant postoperative rise in IL-10 levels and a significant decrease in plasma Hp levels. Lastly, very recently, Gamberi et al. [38] performed a comprehensive plasma proteomic profiling on eight patients scheduled for AAA repair through elective aortic reconstructive surgery, identifying a significant Hp increase in plasma from AAA patients.

Overall, the emerging picture from these studies is a striking involvement of Hp in the pathophysiology of AAA. First, the *HP**2/*1 genotype seems to be an important predisposing factor of AAA liability, also influencing the prognosis. On the other side, the higher Hp level found in AAA patients is a clear demonstration of the proinflammatory nature of the AAA phenomenon. Indeed, given the antiinflammatory properties of Hp, it is conceivable that the rising of Hp level is a counteracting response to the increased inflammation due to the presence of AAA. Concerning the role of the *HP**2/*1 genotype in AAA liability, the molecular and genetic complexity of the *HP* polymorphism needs to be taken into account. Most of the authors failed to explain why the *HP**2/*1 heterozygous phenotype was different from both homozygous phenotypes and speculated that the *HP**2/*1 phenotype might cumulate harmful features associated with allele *HP**1 (stimulation of the elastin hydrolysis) and allele *HP**2 (increased risk of atherosclerosis) to yield a combination that is particularly efficient in promoting AAA growth. The reason underlying the association of the *HP**2/*1 phenotype with AAA resides in the phenomenon of molecular heterosis at the *HP* 1/2 polymorphism [39, 40] reported by several genetic association studies [40, 41] and further confirmed by the molecular structure of the haptoglobin protein (Fig. 8.1) [1]. Molecular heterosis occurs when subjects heterozygous for a specific genetic polymorphism show a significantly greater effect (positive heterosis) or lesser effect (negative heterosis) for a quantitative or dichotomous trait than subjects homozygous for either allele. Comings and MacMurray estimated that molecular heterosis may occur in up to 50 % of gene associations [40]. In this context, the *HP* 1/2 polymorphism is characterized by the production of three distinct biochemical phenotypes, each one possessing different molecular configurations (Fig. 8.1) and functions [1]. The disease-modifying effect of Hp 2–1 proteins can be related to their scarce distribution in the extravascular environment in that, being more highly polymeric proteins than Hp 1–1 dimers and displaying asymmetric structure compared with cyclic polymers produced by Hp 2–2, they are limited by their molecular mass and stereo configuration. Therefore, they have lower efficacy in both preventing oxidative tissue damage and downregulating the inflammatory processes in general. Moreover, we suggest that Hp 2–1 molecules would have lower binding to CD163 receptors and thus lower scavenging activity and angiogenic activity than Hp 2–2 molecules. They would have lower binding to hemoglobin than Hp 1–1 molecules and thus would confer a higher risk of AAA than both Hp 2–2 and Hp 1–1 molecules. Unfortunately, most of the functional studies compared Hp 1–1 with Hp 2–2, and only a few studies were applied to purified Hp 2–1 [6]. Thus, little is known about real behavior of Hp 2–1. New functional studies are clearly needed to further clarify the role of Hp 2–1 in AAA and in the inflammatory process in general.

It is also noteworthy that Hp interacts with other determinants of AAA, such as APOB [42, 43], APOE [43], and HMOX1 [44]; therefore, it is conceivable that study of epistatic relationships between polymorphism of these genes may further clarify the role of Hp in AAA.

AAA is a complex disease, and its etiology comes from the interaction of genetics and environmental factors. In the last years, the worldwide scientific community has paid much attention to the discovery of genetic determinants of common complex diseases. A more detailed understanding of genetic effects will pave the way to predictive and personalized medicine, further improving the health care of the entire community.

References

1. Langlois MR, Delanghe JR. Biological and clinical significance of haptoglobin polymorphism in humans. Clin Chem. 1996;42:1589–600.
2. Yang F, Friedrichs WE, Navarijo-Ashbaugh AL, de Graffenried LA, Bowman BH, Coalson JJ. Cell type-specific and inflammatory-induced expression of haptoglobin gene in lung. Lab Invest. 1995;73:433–40.
3. Theilgaard-Monch K, Jacobsen LC, Nielsen MJ, et al. Haptoglobin is synthesized during granulocyte differentiation, stored in specific granules, and released by neutrophils in response to activation. Blood. 2006;108:353–61.
4. Kristiansen M, Graversen JH, Jacobsen C, et al. Identification of the haemoglobin scavenger receptor. Nature. 2001;409:198–201.
5. El Ghmati SM, Van Hoeyveld EM, Van Strijp JAG, Ceuppens JL, Stevens EAM. Identification of haptoglobin as an alternative ligand for CD11b/CD18. J Immunol. 1996;156:2542–52.
6. Arredouani M, Matthijs P, Van Hoeyveld E, et al. Haptoglobin directly affects T cells and suppresses T helper cell type 2 cytokine release. Immunology. 2003;108:144–51.
7. Xie Y, Li Y, Zhang Q, Stiller MJ, Albert Wang C-L, Wayne Streilein J. Haptoglobin is a natural regulator of Langerhans cell function in the skin. J Dermatol Sci. 2000;24:25–73.
8. Wagner L, Gessl A, Parzer SB, Base W, Waldhäusl W, Pasternack MS. Haptoglobin phenotyping by newly developed monoclonal antibodies. Demonstration of haptoglobin uptake into peripheral blood neutrophils and monocytes. J Immunol. 1996;156:1989–96.
9. El Ghmati SM, Arredouani M, Van Hoeyveld EM, Ceuppens JL, Stevens EA. Haptoglobin interacts with the human mast cell line HMC-1 and inhibits its spontaneous proliferation. Scand J Immunol. 2002;55:352–8.
10. Watanabe J, Grijalva V, Hama S, et al. Hemoglobin and its scavenger protein haptoglobin associate with apoA-1-containing particles and influence the inflammatory properties and function of high density lipoprotein. J Biol Chem. 2009;284:18292–301.
11. Maeda N, Yang F, Barnett DR, Bowman BH, Smithies O. Duplication within the haptoglobin Hp2 gene. Nature. 1984;309:131–5.
12. Asakawa J, Kodaira M, Nakamura N, Satoh C, Fujita M. Chimerism in humans after intragenic recombination at the haptoglobin locus during early embryogenesis. Proc Natl Acad Sci USA. 1999;96:10314–9.
13. Delanghe JR, Langlois MR, De Buyzere ML. Haptoglobin polymorphism: a key factor in the proatherogenic role of B cells? Atherosclerosis. 2011;217(1):80–2.
14. Langlois M, Delanghe J, Philippé J. Distribution of lymphocyte subsets in bone marrow and peripheral blood is associated with haptoglobin type. Binding of haptoglobin to the B-cell lectin CD22. Eur J Clin Chem Clin Biochem. 1997;35:199–205.
15. Robertson AK, Hansson GK. T cells in atherosclerosis. For better or for worse? Arterioscler Thromb Vasc Biol. 2006;26:2421–32.
16. Brouwers A, Langlois M, Delanghe J, et al. Oxidized low-density lipoprotein, iron stores, and haptoglobin polymorphism. Atherosclerosis. 2004;176:189–95.
17. Libby P, Ridker PM, Hansson GK. Inflammation in atherosclerosis: from pathophysiology to practice. J Am Coll Cardiol. 2009;54:2129–38.
18. Langlois MR, Martin M-E, Boelaert JR, et al. The haptoglobin 2–2 phenotype affects serum markers of iron status in healthy males. Clin Chem. 2000;46:1619–25.
19. Levy AP, Levy JE, Kalet-Litman S, et al. Haptoglobin genotype is a determinant of iron, lipid peroxidation, and macrophage accumulation in the atherosclerotic plaque. Arterioscler Thromb Vasc Biol. 2007;27:134–40.
20. Guetta J, Strauss M, Levy NS, Fahoum L, Levy AP. Haptoglobin genotype modulates the balance of Th1/Th2 cytokines produced by

macrophages exposed to free hemoglobin. Atherosclerosis. 2007;191:48–53.
21. Grange JJ, Davis V, Baxter BT. Pathogenesis of abdominal aortic aneurysm: an update and look toward the future. Cardiovasc Surg. 1997;5:256–65.
22. Wassef M, Baxter BT, Chisholm RL, Dalman RL, Fillinger MF, Heinecke J, et al. Pathogenesis of abdominal aortic aneurysms: a multidisciplinary research program supported by the National Heart, Lung, and Blood Institute. J Vasc Surg. 2001;34:730–8.
23. Powell JT, Muller BR, Greenhalgh RM. Acute phase proteins in patients with abdominal aortic aneurysms. J Cardiovasc Surg (Torino). 1987;28:528–30.
24. Juvonen J, Surcel HM, Satta J, Teppo AM, Bloigu A, Syrjala H, et al. Elevated circulating levels of inflammatory cytokines in patients with abdominal aortic aneurysm. Arterioscler Thromb Vasc Biol. 1997;17:2843–7.
25. Lee AJ, Fowkes FG, Lowe GD, Rumley A. Haemostatic factors, atherosclerosis and risk of abdominal aortic aneurysm. Blood Coagul Fibrinolysis. 1996;7:695–701.
26. Domanovits H, Schillinger M, Mullner M, Holzenbein T, Janata K, Bayegan K, et al. Acute phase reactants in patients with abdominal aortic aneurysm. Atherosclerosis. 2002;163:297–302.
27. Singh K, Bonaa KH, Jacobsen BK, Bjork L, Solberg S. Prevalence of and risk factors for abdominal aortic aneurysms in a population-based study: the Tromso Study. Am J Epidemiol. 2001;154:236–44.
28. Rohde LE, Arroyo LH, Rifai N, Creager MA, Libby P, Ridker PM, et al. Plasma concentrations of interleukin-6 and abdominal aortic diameter among subjects without aortic dilatation. Arterioscler Thromb Vasc Biol. 1999;19:1695–9.
29. Vainas T, Lubbers T, Stassen FR, Herngreen SB, van Dieijen-Visser MP, Bruggeman CA, et al. Serum C-reactive protein level is associated with abdominal aortic aneurysm size and may be produced by aneurysmal tissue. Circulation. 2003;107:1103–5.
30. Norrgård O, Fröhlander N, Beckman G, Angqvist KA. Association between haptoglobin groups and aortic abdominal aneurysms. Hum Hered. 1984;34:166–9.
31. Powell JT, Bashir A, Dawson S, Vine N, Henney AM, Humphries SE, et al. Genetic variation on chromosome 16 is associated with abdominal aortic aneurysm. Clin Sci (Lond). 1990;78:13–6.
32. Adamson J, Powell JT, Greenhalgh RM. Selection for screening for familial aortic aneurysms. Br J Surg. 1992;79:897–8.
33. Wiernicki I, Gutowski P, Ciechanowski K, Millo B, Wieczorek P, Cnotliwy M, et al. Abdominal aortic aneurysm: association between haptoglobin phenotypes, elastase activity, and neutrophil count in the peripheral blood. Vasc Surg. 2001;35:345–50.
34. Wiernicki I, Safranow K, Baranowska-Bosiacka I, Piatek J, Gutowski P. Haptoglobin 2–1 phenotype predicts rapid growth of abdominal aortic aneurysms. J Vasc Surg. 2010;52:691–6.
35. Pan JP, Cheng TM, Shih CC, Chiang SC, Chou SC, Mao SJ, et al. Haptoglobin phenotypes and plasma haptoglobin levels in patients with abdominal aortic aneurysm. J Vasc Surg. 2011;53: 1189–94.
36. Engström G, Börner G, Lindblad B, Janzon L, Lindgärde F. Incidence of fatal or repaired abdominal aortic aneurysm in relation to inflammation-sensitive plasma proteins. Arterioscler Thromb Vasc Biol. 2004;24:337–41.
37. Oldenburg HS, Siroen MP, Boelens PG, Sluijter BJ, Pruitt JH, Naseri AH, et al. Aortic aneurysm repair is associated with a lower inflammatory response compared with surgery for inflammatory bowel disease. Eur Surg Res. 2004;36:266–73.
38. Gamberi T, Puglia M, Guidi F, Magherini F, Bini L, Marzocchini R, et al. A proteomic approach to identify plasma proteins in patients with abdominal aortic aneurysm. Mol Biosyst. 2011;7:2855–62.
39. Napolioni V. Regarding "haptoglobin 2–1 phenotype predicts rapid growth of abdominal aortic aneurysms". J Vasc Surg. 2011;53: 266–7.
40. Comings DE, MacMurray JP. Molecular heterosis: a review. Mol Genet Metab. 2000;71:19–31.
41. Papp M, Foldi I, Nemes E, Udvardy M, Harsfalvi J, Altorjay I, et al. Haptoglobin polymorphism: a novel genetic risk factor for celiac disease development and its clinical manifestations. Clin Chem. 2008;54(4):697–704.
42. Braeckman L, De Bacquer D, Delanghe J, Claeys L, De Backer G. Associations between haptoglobin polymorphism, lipids, lipoproteins and inflammatory variables. Atherosclerosis. 1999;143:383–8.
43. Cigliano L, Pugliese CR, Spagnuolo MS, Palumbo R, Abrescia P. Haptoglobin binds the antiatherogenic protein apolipoprotein E – impairment of apolipoprotein E stimulation of both lecithin: cholesterol acyltransferase activity and cholesterol uptake by hepatocytes. FEBS J. 2009;276:6158–71.
44. Philippidis P, Mason JC, Evans BJ, Nadra I, Taylor KM, Haskard DO, et al. Hemoglobin scavenger receptor CD163 mediates interleukin-10 release and heme oxygenase-1 synthesis: antiinflammatory monocyte-macrophage responses in vitro, in resolving skin blisters in vivo, and after cardiopulmonary bypass surgery. Circ Res. 2004; 94:119–26.

Inflammatory Aortic Aneurysm

9

Guilherme Vieira Meirelles

Introduction

The severity of aneurysmatic disease and its evolution were described long ago. Since that time, therapeutic strategies have been based on surgical procedures, which have been modified according to scientific and technical developments in the medical fields. The Papyrus of Erbes, written in approximately 2,000 B.C., described peripheral aneurysms and suggested surgical treatment with a glowing iron: "treat with the knife and burn with fire …" [1,2].

The term inflammatory abdominal aortic aneurysm (AAA) was created in 1972 by Walker et al. [5] to describe an AAA with an unusually thick wall surrounded by extensive fibrous adhesions involving adjoining tissues and structures and treated as a different clinical entity from degenerative aneurysms. This characteristic was found in 2.5–15 % of all AAAs with a 20:1 predominance in males and occurred in patients an average of 10 years younger than those with noninflammatory AAAs [3–5].

The inflammatory AAA, once believed to have a different etiology and pathogenesis, now seems to be the final result of the inflammatory process found in degenerative aneurysms. The etiology of the aortic aneurysm, attributed long ago to atherosclerosis, has not yet been fully defined.

Aneurysmatic degeneration is the end result of a multifactorial process that leads to the destruction of the connective tissues of the arterial wall. Evidence indicates that the most important structural elements of the aorta wall, the interstitial collagen and elastin, are associated with the degradation of the extracellular matrix in AAA. Many of these findings are related to matrix metalloproteinases (MMPs). Among these are 72-kDa gelatinase (MMP-2), 92-kDa gelatinase (MMP-9), matrilysn (MMP-7), and macrophage elastase (MMP-12), which are capable of degrading elastic fibers. Others, such as proteinase, plasminogen activator serum elastase, and cathepsin, also contribute to aneurysmatic degeneration [6].

Atherosclerosis is still being investigated as a participatory factor in degenerative aneurysmatic processes of the aorta. Experimental studies including atherogenic diets for extended periods produced areas of lateral inclination of the middle arterial layer, with aneurysm formation in primates (13 % in cynomolgus monkeys and 1 % in rhesus monkeys) [7].

Atherosclerotic plaques are usually more plentiful, pronounced, calcified, and complicated in the abdominal aorta compared with those in the thoracic segment. These changes are related to local differences in blood flow conditions, wall stress mechanisms, and the composition and nutrition of the structures of the arterial layers.

In humans, the abdominal aorta expands with the progression of atherosclerotic plaque. This is associated with the narrowing and loss of structural architecture of the middle layer, being particularly pronounced at its midpoint and at the fork of the iliac arteries [8].

Preliminary studies suggest cathepsin S and K as potent elastases, and the genes of this enzyme are expressed in human atheroma plaque. Atheromas also have high activity in destroying elastin, which is sensitive to the cysteine protease inhibitors. Levels of cysteine C, the most abundant of the cathepsin inhibitors, decreased in atherosclerosis arteries and in the walls of abdominal aortic aneurysms [6].

Evaluating the causal factors, elastin and collagen are the most important components of the arterial wall and are associated with smooth muscle cells and the middle layer of the abdominal aorta [9].

Elastin is the arterial wall component responsible for elasticity of the artery, allowing physiological swelling and shrinkage, determined by the heartbeat. Much evidence exists concerning the participation of aortic dilatation in elastin lesions.

The presence of swelling occurs most often in the abdominal aorta, where there are fewer elastic layers. Elastin is not synthesized in the aorta of adult individuals, and the elastic

G.V. Meirelles, MD
Department of Vascular Surgery,
Celso Pierro Hospital and Maternity,
Campinas, SP, Brazil

E.A. Gabriel, S.A. Gabriel (eds.), *Inflammatory Response in Cardiovascular Surgery*,
DOI 10.1007/978-1-4471-4429-8_9, © Springer-Verlag London 2013

capacity of the average 70 year old (period when AAAs appear most frequently) is three times less than that of a 20 year old. The use of elastase in the arterial walls in animal experiments produces dilatation, but without a relation to the proportions of the elastin lesion and the final diameter of the aorta [10]. Elastin is responsible for 35 % of the weight of the middle layer of normal aortas and is reduced up to 8 % in aneurysmatic arteries. Comparing the quantity of elastin in 81 fragments of the AAA wall surgically removed from corpses 82 with normal aortas, a reduction of approximately 90 % was found and a total reduction of 50 % in amino 84 acid aneurysms [11–13].

An additional finding was the elevated levels of elastase in these walls, suggesting an important participation of elastin in the genesis of aortic dilation in humans [14].

Collagen types I and III are the main forms of this component of the aortic wall, which is characterized by tensile strength and low distensibility in order to allow the increase in arterial diameter. Different from elastin, collagen is produced throughout life (absorbed and reconstituted) and has 20 times the tensile strength of elastin. The collagen is laid in such a way that, supported by elastin, it allows an increase in diameter (heartbeat) and upon reaching a particular stretching point is used as a protective barrier containing the arterial increase. Its concentration increases in the AAA walls. A deficiency in type III collagen (the most frequent in the aortic wall) has been associated with the rupture of cerebral aneurysms and identified as an abnormality in Ehlers-Danlos syndrome type IV (arterial weakness with formation of aneurysms) [13]. At the same time, the collagenolytic activity is increased in individuals with AAA ruptures [15]. Contrarily, metalloproteinase inhibitor (which decreases the activity of protease enzymes, such as elastase, collagenase, and gelatinase) is found in decreased concentrations in the walls of dilated arteries [6,14].

RNA messenger expression of 92-kDa gelatinase (MMP-9) on the wall of the aorta has been correlated with the presence and size of the aneurysm, being also associated with high levels of MMP-9 in the serum of these individuals. These surveys suggest there is a change in the ability to repair the arterial wall in case of an exaggerated expression of MMP-9, which results in the destruction of the arrangement [6].

The enzyme 72-kDa gelatinase (MMP-2) appears at high levels in AAA walls, in its active form, next to the extracellular matrix, suggesting a protease action. High-level membrane type I MMP (MMP-14), which constitutes the primary activator Pro-MMP-2, was also found. Doxycycline inhibits MMP-2, and this is an important factor in aneurysm formation [38].

A model of aortic wall lesion induction in rats, with administration of elastase, demonstrated the presence of transmural infiltrated mononuclear phagocytes, increased production of MMP, and progressive destruction of the protein matrix from the wall. The deletion of the degenerative process *in vivo* using nonselective antiinflammatory inhibitors of MMP (doxycycline) was also investigated. MMP-9 deficiency induced resistance to aneurysm formation, but with a bone marrow transplant to correct this deficiency, mice recovered the potential to develop aneurysms. The administration of doxycycline resulted in a fivefold decrease in the expression of MMP-9 in the aortic wall of patients undergoing elective treatment of AAA. *In vitro*, it suppressed expression of MMP-9 stimulated by forbol in mononuclear THP1 phagocytes [6].

In intermediate situations, increasing the process of reconstitution of collagen (types I and III) can maintain stable levels, but with the continuous increase of degradation, this can provide an unfavorable balance with rapid expansion and rupture of the aneurysm. Collagenase-3 (MMP-13) is most frequently found on the AAA wall [6].

In vitro studies suggest that reactive oxygen forms mediate activation of MMP-9 and MMP-8. Recent studies have shown that activated phagocytes produce oxygen, which then forms hydrogen peroxide and myeloperoxidase in the process of phagocytosis; the latter enables MMP-9 and MMP-8, creating the oxidative theory of aneurysm formation [6].

An inflammatory infiltrate composed of T cells, monocytes/macrophages, B-lymphocytes, and plasma cells associated with the presence of HLA-DR+and antigenic markers on the wall of AAAs suggests an inflammatory component. This also indicates that purified immunoglobulin G in a segment of the AAA wall in contact with the normal aorta wall will produce an immunoreaction [6,16].

Surveys on the presence of *Chlamydia pneumoniae* in aneurysmatic wall biopsies of the abdominal aorta proved to be positive in 77 % of the cases, which highlights the relationship between infection and AAA [17]. The use of plasma markers, such as IgA and IgG using ELISA or immunofluorescence, showed the presence of *Chlamydia pneumoniae* in 36 % of aneurysms. A review showed their sensitivity and specificity for the need for surgery (expansion) for AAAs to be 80 % and 66 %, respectively [17,18].

Among the mechanisms that cause weakening of the aortic wall, some are particularly crucial: genetics; smoking; factors that increase the size of the artery, such as hypertension, inflammatory, processes, and atherosclerosis.

Family history is one of the background factors related to the prevalence of aneurysm and has special characteristics, such as being most likely to be present in women or in individuals under the age of 65 years [19]. Although conditions such as mutations in type III collagen, changes in MZ alpha-1-antitrypsin, and metalloproteinase inhibitors indicate a genetic basis for AAAs, a genetic origin for the formation of the aneurysm has not yet been established. Surveys suggest that 12–19 % of people with AAA features are related to one or more first-degree relatives with this disease [20,21]. The relative risk for relatives of people with AAA is 18 times higher than for individuals without a family relationship [6]. When searching for deficiency of type III collagen in 56 people with AAA, 16 (28.6 %) had a family history and 6 (10.7 %) a deficiency in type III collagen [21].

Smoking is strongly associated with weakening of the arterial wall. The products of combustion of tobacco inactivate alpha 1-antitrypsin, oxidizing methionine, increasing wall degradation, and contributing to the genesis of AAAs and an increase in their size, which entail an increased risk of rupture [22,23]. The rupture rate in a study of small aneurysms in the UK (UK Small Aneurysm Trial) reached 1.9 % per year in patients with high serum levels of nicotine compared to 0.5 % in those with only trace amounts (AAAs of 4–5.5 cm diameter) [24].

It is still uncertain whether hypertension plays a role in the formation of AAAs or exacerbates an already existing situation. The fact is that hypertension is related to the presence of AAAs and contributes to the increase in arterial diameter [22] in the elderly (individuals aged 60 years or more, according to the World Health Organization). As described earlier, age above 60 years is related to the presence of AAAs not only in association with atherosclerotic disease, but also with changes in the elastin and collagen recruitment engine [25].

Atherosclerosis is invariably associated with AAAs in spite of different risk factors. Hyperlipidemia and diabetes are not related to AAAs, with great frequency observed in atherosclerotic disease [26].

Local factors such as composition, biomechanical strength, and nutrition are different in the abdominal and thoracic aorta [6]. There is a decrease in the vasa vasorum in the human abdominal aorta when compared with other arterial segments considering the thickness of the wall. Thus, the complement of this blood perfusion deficit is provided by direct absorption through the aortic lumen. It is believed that the presence of atherosclerotic plaques in the aorta or in the nurturing artery (vasa vasorum) helps to create layers of wall ischemia that can be related to the genesis of dilation.

The difference is basically the intense inflammatory process involving fibroses and dense adhesions to the adjacent abdominal viscera.

This condition was believed to be due to a retroperitoneal leakage of blood from tiny subclinical perforations of the non-inflammatory wall. This theory was excluded because of the absence of hemosiderin-laden macrophages in the peri-aneurysmal tissue [5,27,28].

Negative cultures for bacteria and syphilis show no relation between infectious and inflammatory AAA [3,5,27,28].

A gradual progression of inflammation from degenerative to inflammatory AAA has been described [29,30].

It is now accepted that AAAs are characterized by chronic aortic wall inflammation, destructive remodeling of the extracellular matrix, and depletion of vascular smooth muscle cells, and the difference between inflammatory and degenerative aneurysms is only the intensity of the inflammatory reaction.

The herpes simplex virus and cytomegalovirus were more frequently present in aneurysmal walls than in normal aortic walls. These viruses were more prevalent in inflammatory than in noninflammatory AAAs [31].

Risk factors that are associated with the development of inflammatory AAAs include cigarette smoking and a genetic predisposition.

Clinical Features

Different from degenerative AAAs, the exacerbations of the inflammatory process with fibrosis involving others structures are typically symptomatic (65–90 % compared to 8–18 % in the noninflammatory form), with 80 % diagnosed based on clinical symptom investigations. Abdominal or back pain, weight loss, and an elevated erythrocyte sedimentation rate (raised in 70 % of cases) in AAA patients are very probably of the inflammatory variant. Chronic renal failure is associated in 10–20 % of patients, so serum electrolyte and creatinine levels must be investigated. These AAAs are larger than the atherosclerotic type, and an intensive inflammatory process is frequently observed with duodenum entrapment (100 %) and ureteral involvement (53 % with obstructive uropathy in 21 % of patients) in the retroperitoneal fibrotic process [4,32–34].

Diagnosis

Despite a pulsatile abdominal mass (present in 15–30 %) and the associated clinical features, a computer tomography (CT) must be done to confirm the presence of a thickened aortic wall surrounded by low-attenuation soft tissue enhancement with iodine contrast creating a surrounding halo image. Other information, such as the diameter, proximal and distal colon, and involvement of the ureter or duodenum, is shown in this exam and widely used in treatment planning. Ultrasound is correct in establishing the diagnosis in 60 % compared to 90 % for CT

Surgical Management

Inflammatory aneurysms' natural history is one of enlargement and rupture, but they are less frequent than the non-inflammatory type.

Table 9.1 Surgical mortality in elective abdominal aortic aneurysmectomy

	Year	Period	Operations (n)	Mortality (%)
Revisions				
	1992	1985–1991	3.130	3.5
	2001	1985–1997	54.048	5.0
Multicenter studies				
Canadian Aneurysm Study	1989	1986	666	4.8
Veterans Administration	1996	1991–1993	3.419	4.9
United Kingdom Small Aneurysm Trial	1998	1991–1993	563	5.8
State surveys				
Michigan	1994	1980–1990	8.185	7.5
Maryland	1999	1990–1995	2.335	3.5
National Hospital Database (USA)				
	1999	1984–1994	32.389	8.4
	2000	1979–1997	358.521	5.6
	2001	1994–1996	16.450	4.2
Service survey				
	1984	1951–1980	94	7.4
	2002	1989–1998	1.135	1.2

Clinical treatment using oral corticosteroids in an effort to attenuate the inflammatory response has no scientific support. Actually, steroid therapy may increase the risk of AAA rupture by a reduction of the protective fibrosis.

Surgery remains the treatment of choice for inflammatory AAAs. The open surgical modality achieves mortality rates of 3–4 %, matching those of noninflammatory aneurysms (Table 9.1).

Due to the dissemination of the inflammatory process and retroperitoneal fibroses, there is a characteristic white, glistening cover on the aneurysmal surface, invariably incorporating portions of the duodenum and inferior vena cava.

Left renal, adrenal, and gonadal veins, the small bowel or its mesentery, the colon, and the pancreas may also be involved.

During inflammatory AAA repair, urological treatment may be necessary. Over half of CT scanning demonstrates ureteric involvement, but ureterolysis should be performed for those exhibiting signs or symptoms of obstruction or proven incipient uropathy [35].

Von Fritschen et al. found persistent fibrosis in 73 % of open-repair IAAAs after a mean follow-up of 38 months, with no significant change in periaortic fibroses in half of these patients. Bitsch et al. found complete fibrotic regression in less than a third of patients. The difference between these responses suggests that the use of Dacron prosthetic arterial grafts could initiate a pronounced inflammatory process [36].

A meta-analysis showed that the endovascular approach was associated with a primary technical success rate of 95.6 % (44/46) and a 30-day clinical success rate of 93.4 % (43/46). Of 43 patients with periaortic fibroses prior to the intervention, 22 (51.2 %) showed complete regression, 18 (41.8 %) remained unchanged, and 3 (7.0 %) showed progression after EVAR. Renal impairment disappeared in 11 (45.8 %) of 24 patients. Eight patients needed reinterventions. These results are comparable to those for open surgery and show that endovascular treatment is an option for this disease [37].

References

1. Brito JC. História da cirurgia dos aneurismas da aorta abdominal. In: Bonamigo TP, von Ristow A, editors. Aneurismas. Rio de Janeiro: Di livros; 2000. p. 23–30.
2. Kruppski WC. Arterial aneurysms. In: Rutherford RB, editor. Vascular surgery, vol. 2. 4th ed. Philadelphia: Saunders Company; 1995. p. 1025–32.
3. Rubini P, Bonati L, Parolani A, Spirito R. Inflammatory abdominal aortic aneurysms. Minerva Chir. 2001;56(3):287–98.
4. Stella A, Garinlo M, Faggioli GF. Postoperative course of inflammatory abdominal aortic aneurysms. Ann Vasc Surg. 1993;7: 229–38.
5. Walker DI, Bloor K, Williams G. Inflammatory aneurysms of the abdominal aorta. Br J Surg. 1972;59:609–14.
6. Wassef M, Baxter BT, Chisholm RL, Dalman RL, Fillinger MF, Heinecke J. Pathogenesis of abdominal aortic aneurysms: a multidisciplinary research program supported by the National Heart, Lung, and Blood Institute. J Vasc Surg. 2001;34:730–8.
7. Zarins CK, Glagov S, Vesselinovitch DE, Wissler RW. Aneurysm formation in experimental atherosclerosis: relationship to plaque evolution. J Vasc Surg. 1990;12(3):246–56.
8. Xu C, Zarins CK, Glagov S. Aneurysmal and occlusive atherosclerosis of the human abdominal aorta. J Vasc Surg. 2001;33(1):91–6.
9. Tilson MD, Gandhi RH. Arterial aneurysms: etiologic considerations. In: Rutherford RB, editor. Vascular surgery, vol. 1. 4th ed. Philadelphia: WB Saunders Company; 1995. p. 253–64.
10. Wite JV, Haas K, Phillips S, Comerota AJ. Adventitial elastolysis is a primary event in aneurysm formation. J Vasc Surg. 1993;17(2): 371–81.

11. Carmo ML, Colombo AB, Corsi FRM, Roncoroni L, Cuttin MS, Radice F. Alteration of elastin, collagen and their cross-links in abdominal aortic aneurysms. Eur J Vasc Endovasc Surg. 2002;23(6):543–9.
12. He CM, Roach MR. The composition and mechanical properties of abdominal aortic aneurysms. J Vasc Surg. 1994;20(1):6–13.
13. Hollier LH, Wisselink W. Abdominal aortic aneurysms. In: Haimovici H, editor. Vascular surgery, principles and techniques. 4th ed. Cambridge: Blackwell science; 1996. p. 797–827.
14. Cohen JR, Mandell C, Chang JB, Wise L. Elastin metabolism of the infrarenal aorta. J Vasc Surg. 1988;7(2):210–4.
15. Menashi S, Campa JS, Greenhalgh RM, Powell JT. Collagen in abdominal aortic aneurysm: typing, content, and degradation. J Vasc Surg. 1987;6:578–82.
16. Satta J, Laurila A, Pääkkö P, Haukipuro K, Parkkila RS, Uvonen TJ. Chronic inflammation and elastin degradation in abdominal aortic aneurysm disease: an immunohistochemical and electron microscopic study. Eur J Vasc Endovasc Surg. 1998;15(4):313–9.
17. Karlsson L, Gnarpe J, Nääs J, Olsson G, Lindholm J, Steen B. Chlamydia pneumoniae in abdominal aortic aneurysms. Eur J Vasc Endovasc Surg. 2000;19(6):630–5.
18. Vammen S, Lindholt JS, Andersen PL, Henneberg EW, Ostergaard L. Antibodies against chlamydia pneumoniae predict the need for elective surgical intervention on small abdominal aortic aneurysms. Eur J Vasc Endovasc Surg. 2001;22(2):165–8.
19. Darling III RC, Brewster DC, Darling RC, Lamuraglia GM, Moncure AC, Cambria RP. Are familial abdominal aortic aneurysms different? J Vasc Surg. 1989;10(1):39–43.
20. van Keulen CJ, van de Akker E, Pals G, Rauwerda JA. The role of type III collagen in the development of familial abdominal aortic aneurysms. Eur J Vasc Endovasc Surg. 1999;18(1):65–70.
21. van Vlijmen-van Keulen CJ, Pals G, Rauwerda JA. Familial abdominal aortic aneurysm: a systematic review of a genetic background. Eur J Vasc Endovasc Surg. 2002;24(2):105–16.
22. Franks PJ, Edwards RJ, Greenhalgh RM, Powell JT. Risk factors for abdominal aortic aneurysms in smokers. Eur J Vasc Endovasc Surg. 1996;11(4):487–92.
23. Rasmussen TE, Hallett JW, Tazelaar HD, Miller VM, Schulte S, O'Fallon WM. Human leukocyte antigen class II immune response genes, female gender, and cigarette smoking as risk and modulating factors in abdominal aortic aneurysms. J Vasc Surg. 2002;35(5):988–93.
24. UK SMALL Aneurism Trial. Smoking, lung function and the prognosis of abdominal aortic aneurysm. Eur J Vasc Endovasc Surg. 2000;19(6):636–42.
25. World Health Organization. Health of elderly. Genebra: WHO; 1989. p. 7–9 (World health organization technical report series 779).
26. Shteinberg D, Halak M, Shapiro S, Kinarty A, Sobol E, Lahat N. Abdominal aortic aneurysm and aortic occlusive disease: a comparison of risk factors and inflammatory response. Eur J Vasc Endovasc Surg. 2000;20(5):462–5.
27. Baskerville PA, Blakaney CJ, Joung AE. The diagnosis and treatment of periaortic fibrosis ("inflammatory" aneurysms). Br J Surg. 1983;70:381–5.
28. Crawford JL, Stowe CL, Safi HJ, Hallman CH. Inflammatory aneurysms of the aorta. J Vasc Surg. 1985;2:113–24.
29. Latifi HR, Heiken JP. CT of inflammatory abdominal aortic aneurysm: development from an uncomplicated atherosclerotic aneurysm. J Comput Assist Tomogr. 1992;16:484–6.
30. Sterpetti AV, Hunter WJ, Feldhaus RJ, et al. Inflammatory aneurysm of the abdominal aorta: incidence, pathogenesis and etiologic considerations. J Vasc Surg. 1989;9:643–9.
31. Tanaka S, Komori K, Okadome K, et al. Detection of active cytomegalovirus infection in inflammatory aortic aneurysms with RNA polymerase chain reaction. J Vasc Surg. 1994;20:235–43.
32. Cellarier J, Thonard H, Laurent P, et al. Inflammatory abdominal aortic aneurysm. J Mal Vasc. 2000;25(2):132–4.
33. Plate J, Forsty N, Stigsson L, Sällström J, Thörne J. Management of inflammatory abdominal aortic aneurysm. Acta Chir Scand. 1988;154:19–24. sources. Conn Tissue Res 1994;30:265–70.
34. Ramire AA, Riles TS, Imparato AM. CT scans of inflammatory aneurysms: a new technique for preoperative diagnosis. Surgery. 1982;91:390–3.
35. Witz M, Korzets Z. Inflammatory abdominal aortic aneurysms. Isr Med Assoc J. 2005;7:385–7.
36. Hinchliffe RJ, Macierewicz JA, Hopkinson BR. Endovascular repair of inflammatory abdominal aortic aneurysms. J Endovasc Ther. 2002;9:277–81.
37. Puchner S, Bucek RA, Rand T, Schoder M, Hölzenbein T, Kretschmer G, et al. Endovascular therapy of inflammatory aortic aneurysms: a meta-analysis. J Endovasc Ther. 2005;12:560–7.
38. Newman KM, Malon AM, Skin RD. Matrix metalloproteinases in abdominal aortic aneurysms: characterization, purification and their possible sources. Connect Tissue Res. 1994;30:265–70.

Endovascular Treatment of Abdominal Aortic Aneurysms: Current Approaches and New Devices

10

Armando de Carvalho Lobato, Robert Guimarães do Nascimento, and Ariele Milano de Oliveira

Introduction

Abdominal aortic aneurysm (AAA) is a relatively common disease among the elderly, often reaching a rate of up to 36.2 cases per 100,000 inhabitants, and it may be present in up to 5.9 % of the population aged more than 80 years. AAAs of more than 5 cm in diameter are more prone to rupture and have a mortality of up to 63 % [1].

Conventional surgical repair of AAA in patients with low or acceptable surgical risk is very effective, with morbidity and mortality rates ranging from 0 to 8 %. However, mortality in the population with moderate to high surgical risk ranges from 8 to 60 %. In view of the morbidity and mortality of conventional surgical repair of AAAs, especially in the high-risk population, the development of a less invasive and potentially safer technique is urgently needed. Stents have been developed in an attempt to avoid conventional surgical repair of AAAs [1].

The endovascular technique has gained wide acceptance for the treatment of patients with AAA. Short-term results of endovascular repair of AAAs are excellent, and the need for conversions is less than 5 %, the cumulative risk of aneurysm rupture is approximately 1 % per year, and the incidence of occlusion of the contralateral arm is less than 2.8 % in the follow-up period [2].

This chapter discusses the technical aspects of the main stents available on the market for endovascular treatment of AAAs, enabling the reader to determine the best device for each patient, and describes the "sandwich technique."

Important Aspects of Stents

Commercially available stent systems are designed with predetermined arterial diameters for implantation; therefore, the applicability of these devices is limited. In these situations, familiarity with the various devices and their correct application is important. The major anatomical determinants of endovascular treatment are the diameter and tortuosity of the arteries, the length and angulation of the proximal neck, and the presence of mural thrombus in the proximal neck [3].

Desired characteristics of stents for AAA are having a low profile; having adequate flexibility, resistance to torsion, longitudinal force; being easy to deploy; having an accurate system for determining safe and low stent permeability; and having modularity for length customization. Obviously, no ideal device is available at this time, not only because it is difficult to find all of these features in one device, but also because most of the different features are protected by specific patents that are owned by different companies [1].

Stents Available in Brazil

Up to December 2011, the NASV (National Agency for Sanitary Vigilance) listed 13 endoprostheses for the endovascular treatment of AAA: Anaconda®, Aorfix®, Apollo®, Braile®, Ella®, Endofit®, Endurant®, E-Evita®, Excluder®, Hercules®, Powerlink®, Talent®, and Zenith®.

A. de Carvalho Lobato, PhD (✉)
Department of Vascular and Endovascular Surgery, Institute of Vascular and Endovascular Surgery of Sao Paulo (ICVE-SP), Sao Paulo, Brazil

Vascular and Endovascular Surgery, Portuguese Beneficent Hospital of Sao Paulo, Sao Paulo, Brazil

Faculty of Medicine, University of Sao Paulo, Sao Paulo, Brazil

Brazilian Society of Angiology and Vascular Surgery (SBACV), Sao Paulo, Brazil

University Nove de Julho,Sao Paulo, Brazil
email: aclobato@icve.com.br

R.G. do Nascimento, MD
Department of Vascular and Endovascular Surgery, Institute of Vascular and Endovascular Surgery of Sao Paulo (ICVE-SP), Sao Paulo, Brazil

Brazilian Society of Angiology and Vascular Surgery (SBACV), Sao Paulo, Brazil

A.M. de Oliveira
University Nove de Julho, Sao Paulo, Brazil

E.A. Gabriel, S.A. Gabriel (eds.), *Inflammatory Response in Cardiovascular Surgery*,
DOI 10.1007/978-1-4471-4429-8_10, © Springer-Verlag London 2013

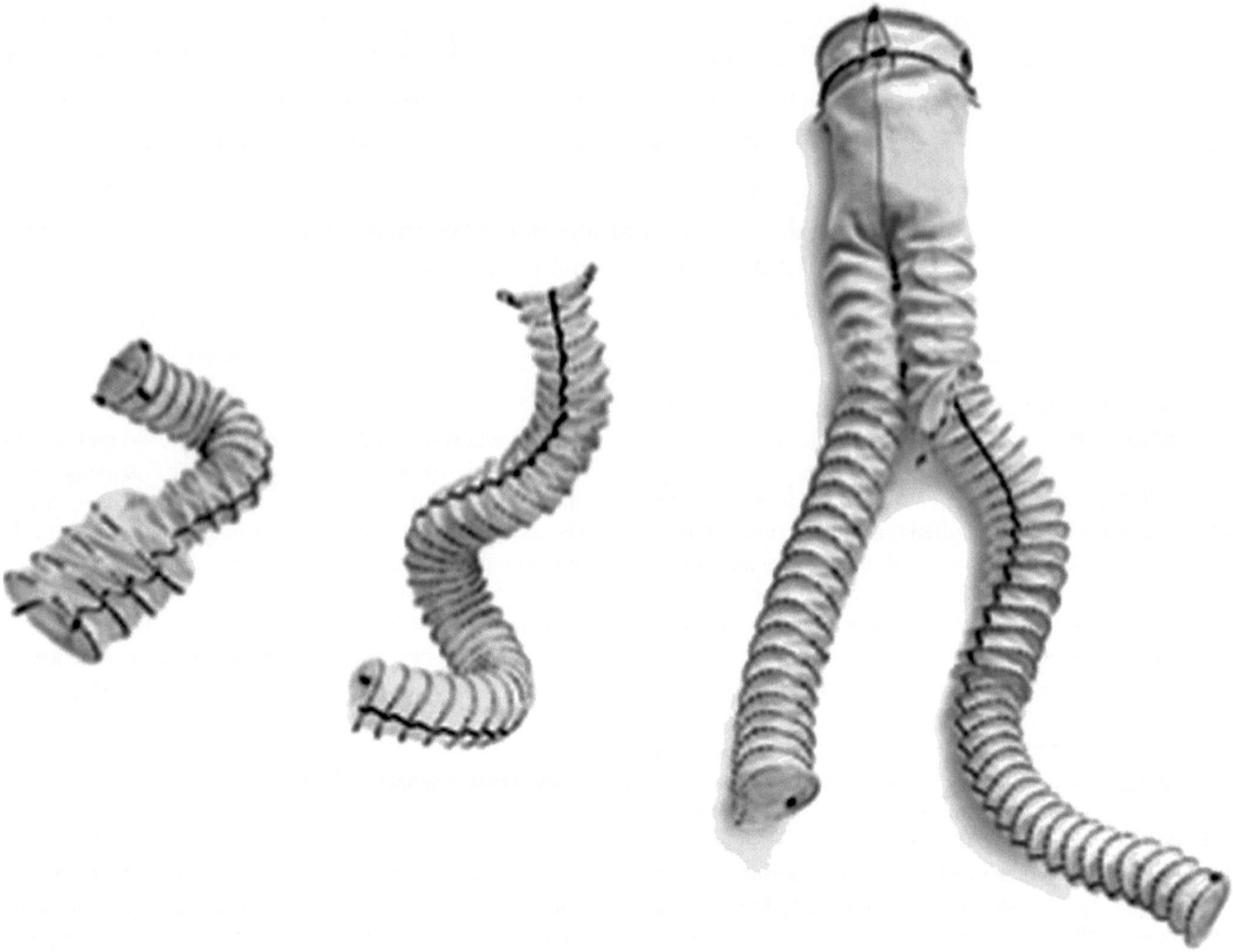

Fig. 10.1 Anaconda® stent

The Anaconda® Stent

The new Anaconda AAA™ stent, manufactured by Vascutek, a Terumo Company, was developed to correct aneurysms of the infrarenal abdominal aorta. It represents a new generation of AAA stent with a super-hydrophilic coating on the introducer; it is called "Blu Glide" and provides greater support and flexibility. It has a proximal double ring generating excellent sealing and four pairs of hooks that provide better security against fixation and migration of the endoprosthesis. The introducer has a low profile, which helps to introduce the system, and the sheath has a radiopaque tip, allowing the accurate implantation of the device. The main body has an intrinsic magnetic wire system that allows easy cannulation of the contralateral limb [8].

The main body has a diameter ranging from 19.5 to 34 mm with an area of 35 and 40 mm. The diameter of the conic iliac branch ranges from 12–15 to 17–23 mm and the length from 80 to 130 mm. The diameter of the right iliac branch ranges from 10 to 18 mm and the length from 60–140 mm.

Importantly, the Anaconda® stent allows full redeployment after the first deployment, ensuring greater accuracy, especially in tortuous anatomies (Fig. 10.1).

Endoprótese Aorfix®

AORFIX™ has the most advanced stent technology on the market [9]. It is manufactured by Lombard Medical and marketed in Europe and other countries [1].

Because of its shape and high flexibility, it fits the anatomy of the patients perfectly [12], optimizing operation performance, also in the postoperative period. Its "fish mouth" design allows optimal positioning in the proximal neck, with the lower portions lateralized, allowing flow to the renal arteries while keeping the highest parts oriented to the anterior and posterior portions of the aorta, ensuring suprarenal

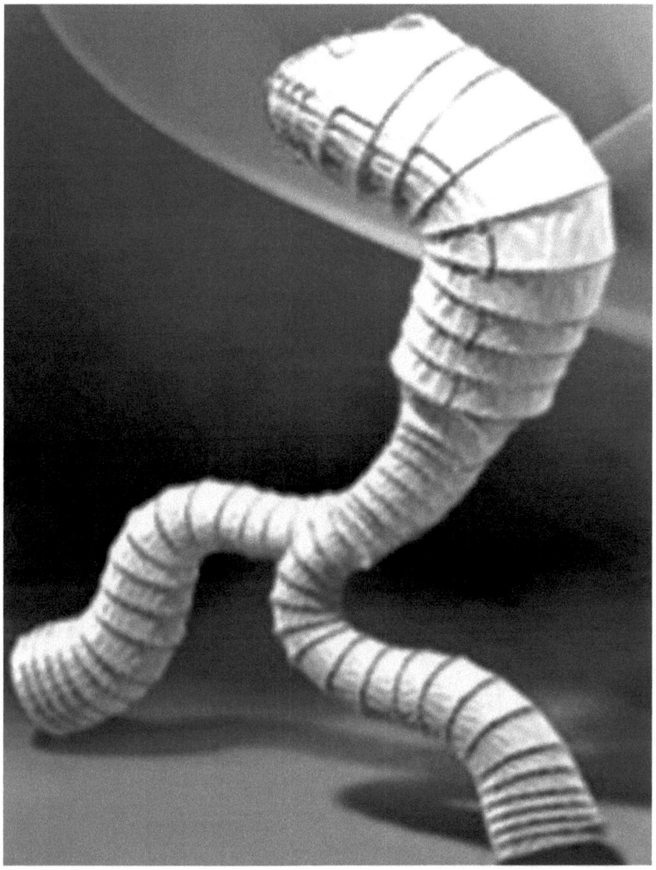

Fig. 10.2 Endoprótese Aorfix®

fixation. It is made of nitinol, which has a circular framework covered with polyester fabric, ensuring perfect adaptation of the graft, even after surgery. Radiopaque markers ensure correct positioning during the procedure, and fixing hooks ensure safer fixation [9].

For aneurysms with significant angulation of the proximal neck (60–90°) and tortuous iliac arteries, the use of this stent has proved to be extremely effective, resulting in low rates of type I endoleaks and iliac branch occlusion. Angles greater than 60° are a contraindication for the implantation of other available devices. Therefore, the development of Aorfix ® has enabled the extension of endovascular treatment to aneurysms with complex anatomies [13].

This device is available with proximal diameters of 24–31 mm, with a range of 1 mm. The length of the main body, provided by the manufacturer, is the aortal portion and has a size range of 86, 96, 111, 126, and 142 mm. The diameter of the distal ipsilateral branch can vary from 10 to 20 mm, increasing each 2 mm, and has lengths of 63, 80, and 97 mm. The contralateral branch has a proximal diameter of 12 mm, and the distal one, with the same variety of diameters as the distal ipsilateral branch, has lengths of 56, 64, 73, 81, 90, 98, and 105 mm [10] (Fig. 10.2).

Endoprótese Apolo®

This is produced by Nano Endoluminal, a Florianópolis-Santa Catarina company. It was the first Brazilian stent and has been produced since 1998. It is available in monoiliac and bifurcate formats, both with a woven metal structure formed by a single nitinol wire and coated with high-strength PTFE [14].

It is a modular, auto-expandable endoprosthesis designed for vascular reconstruction of infrarenal abdominal aneurysms. It presents a free proximal stent and barbs that ensure excellent fixation and reduce the possibility of device migration. It features gold radiopaque markers, which help in the visualization and accurate positioning of the stent [15].

The main body of the bifurcated Apollo® has diameters of 25, 28, 31, and 34 mm, and the length of the covered portion ranges from 130 to 180 mm. The monoiliac Apollo® has the same diameters as the bifurcated one, but the length ranges from 130 to 175 mm. Both have distal diameters of 12, 14, 16, and 18 mm. The straight distal iliac branches have diameters from 12 to 18 mm and lengths ranging from 60 to 115 mm. The conic iliac branches have proximal diameters of 12, 14, 16, and 18 mm and the distal ones 16, 18, 25, and 28 mm and lengths ranging from 80 to 130 mm. Proximal extensions are also offered with a length of 45 mm. Occluders have diameters of 12, 14, 16, 18, 25, and 28 mm and extension of 25 mm. Additionally, stents can be customized, with the size and design set by the physician. Thus, one can include fenestrated and branched stents [10].

Endoprótese Braile®

The new generation of stents manufactured by Braile Biomedica, a company from Sao Jose do Rio Preto-Sao Paulo, is composed of a metal frame coated with polyester. It has high flexibility and radial strength, and its release is caused by mobilization of the simple sheath. It also has proximal and distal radiopaque markers to facilitate stent placement and location [3–16]. It is indicated for the correction of abdominal aortic aneurysms (AAA) and iliac arteries.

Its main body has a proximal diameter from 24 to 36 mm and a distal one of 14 mm, with lengths of 80, 130, 155, and 170 mm. The free flow length ranges from 20 to 25 mm. It has a low profile that varies from 18 to 20 F [17].

There is also an aortomonoiliac stent with diameters of 24, 26, 28, 30, 32, and 34 mm, length of 110 mm, and distal diameter of 14 mm. Also, occluders are supplied with diameters ranging from 14 to 22 mm and lengths ranging from 14 to 22 mm [10] (Fig. 10.3).

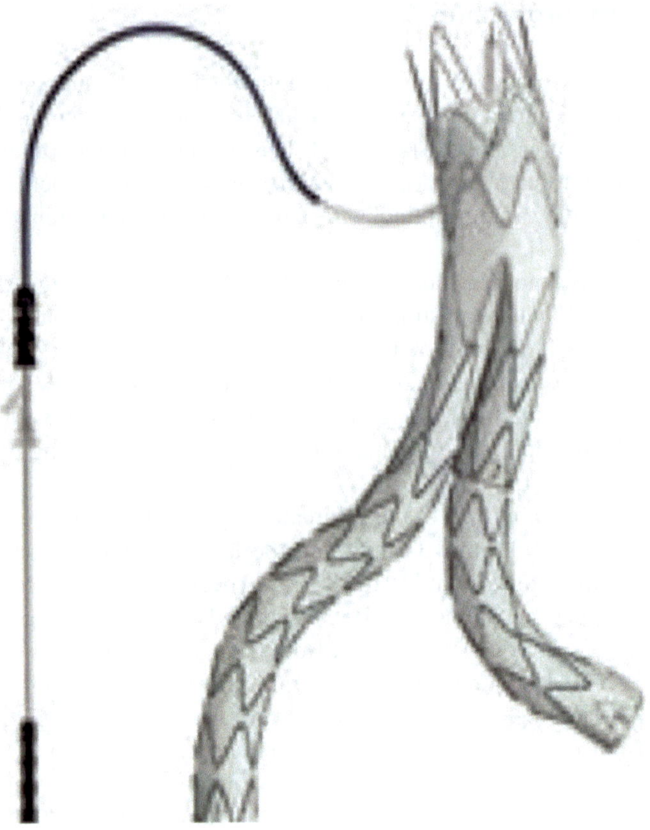

Fig. 10.3 Endoprótese Braile®

Endoprótese Ella®

Ella is manufactured by CS Ella in the Czech Republic. Treatment of AAA with this stent is effective and safe. It has been used in Brazil since 1998 with good results.

It has a resistant coating of polyester mesh attached to the stent by ultra-resistant polypropylene sutures and has two rows of barbs for stabilization and fixation to prevent migration of the stent, branches, and modular extensions that also have barbs for better fixation. It has high radial force on a continuous metal skeleton, radiopaque markers indicating the ends of the stent and the beginning of the coated portion, and a smooth surface at any angle, without risk of pressure at any site (maximum angle of 60°) [1–10].

It is indicated for less invasive alternative treatment of aortic aneurysms (AA), anastomotic pseudoaneurysms, or aneurysms without signs of infection. It can also be used to occlude the false lumen in case of dissection of the aortal portion occurring in the descending thoracic aorta and abdominal aorta or even to occlude the aorto-cava fistulas [19].

The main body has a bifurcated proximal diameter ranging from 14 to 38 mm and a distal one from 6 to 20 mm with lengths from 110 to 220 mm. These measures also apply to the monoiliac model. The iliac branch has diameters ranging from 6 to 20 mm and lengths from 22 to 120 mm. The iliac occluder has diameters from 12 to 30 mm and lengths from 35 to 60 mm (Fig. 10.4).

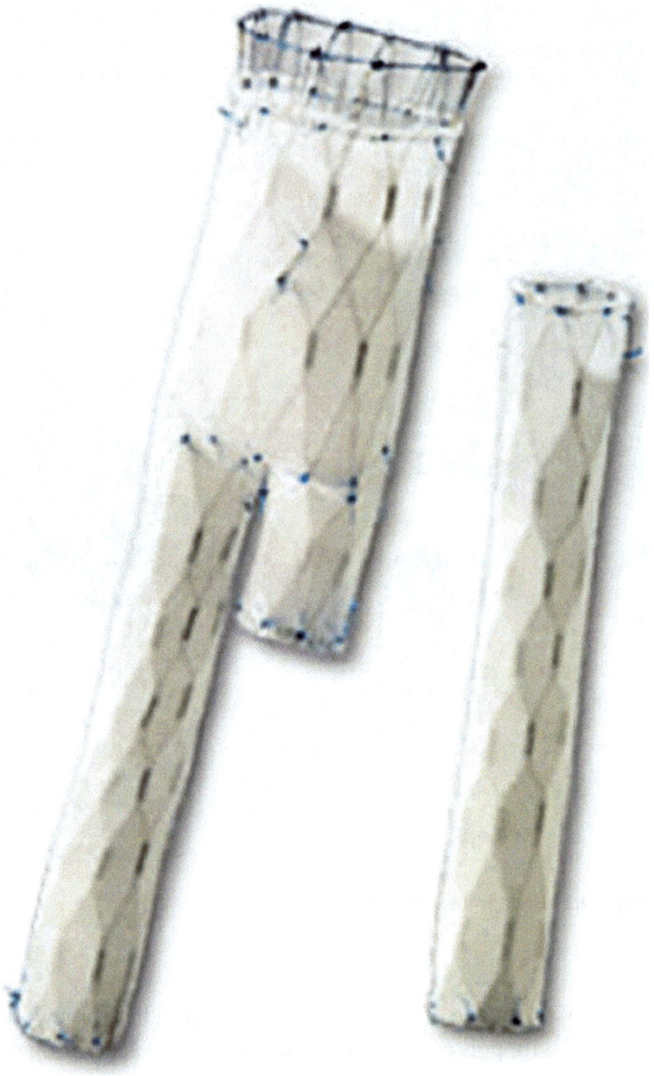

Fig. 10.4 Endoprótese Ella®

Endoprótese Endofit®

This is produced by LeMaitre Vacular, Inc. (Burlington, MA, USA), and consists of a unique, safe, and effective aorto-monoiliac device [20]. Its nitinol structure has a conical shape and layers of PTFE, without sutures. Its attachment is positioned at the suprarenal level with a free 28 mm stent, and radiopaque platinum markers indicate the initial site of the device [1–12].

Its delivery system is simple and can be positioned above the place indicated as it does not have fixation barbs. One should retract the introducer and then adjust its position [22].

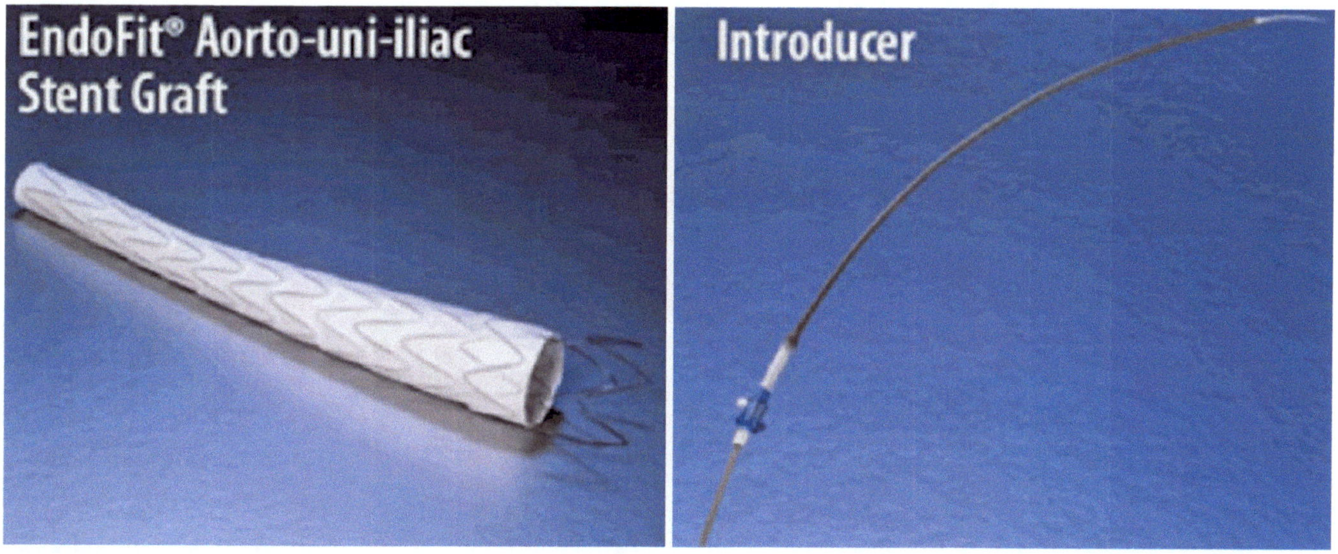

Fig. 10.5 Endoprótese Endofit®

The stent has proximal diameters of 26, 28, 30, 32, 34, or 36 mm, a distal one of 16 mm, and a length of 160 mm. There is also an 180-mm-long stent with a proximal diameter of 34 and 36 mm [22].

Distal straight tubular iliac extension has a diameter of 16 or 18 mm with a length of 80 or 100 mm. The proximal aortic extension stent is a free stent, is 50 mm long, and has the same diameter as the main body. Also the proximal extension is 38 mm long, which is compatible with the 24 F introducer. The iliac occluder has diameters of 18, 20, 23, 24, and 26 mm and is 35 mm long, being compatible with the 20 F introducer for 26 mm diameter and 18 F for other diameters [10] (Fig. 10.5).

Endoprótese Endurant®

This device is produced by Medtronic Vascular (Santa Rosa, CA). It is a last generation device designed to expand the applicability of endovascular repair of the aorta (EVAR) [24]. It was approved for use by the US Food and Drug Administration (FDA) on 16 December 2010. Its use is authorized for necks ≥ 10 mm and up to 60° angulation [24].

The endoprosthesis is made of a metallic material (nitinol) coated with polyester and fixed by polyethylene sutures. It is auto-expandable, hydrophilic, and has a low profile. It has radiopaque markers that look like the letter "e" in the proximal end, at the level of bifurcation, and in the distal end, which allow adequate positioning. The upper end has a free-flow portion composed of a single filament of nitinol. Fixing is achieved by means of a free-flow portion, which has barbs, and by the radial strength of the system [10–23].

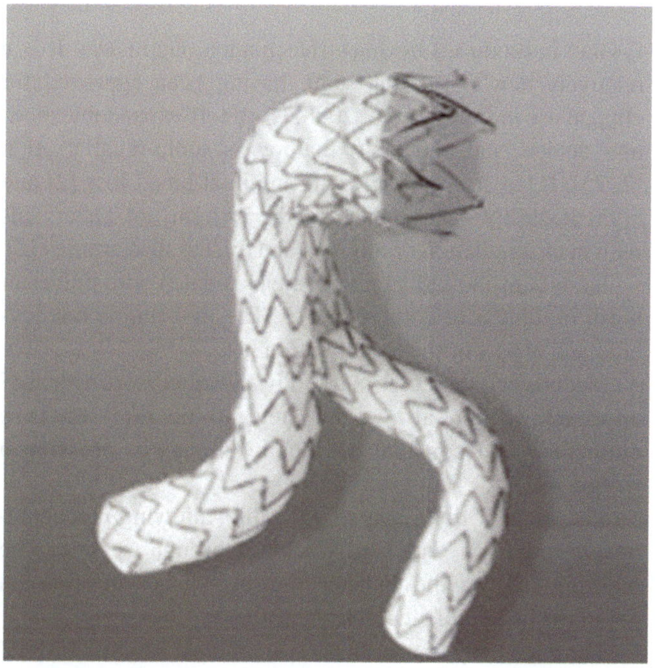

Fig. 10.6 Endoprótese Endurant®

The Endurant®device is safe and effective, with an excellent rate of successful implementation and very low leakage and reintervention rates [22].

The diameter of the main body is from 23 to 25 mm (introducer 18 F) and from 28 to 36 mm (introducer 20 F), and the length ranges from 120 to 170 mm. The iliac branches have distal diameters from 10 to 28 mm and lengths ranging from 80 to 120 mm. The iliac branches and extensions are also provided for by the "bell bottom" shape and by the distal diameter being larger than the proximal one in order to treat dilated iliac arteries. Aortouniiliac stents are available as well (Fig. 10.6).

Fig. 10.7 Endoprótese E-Evita®

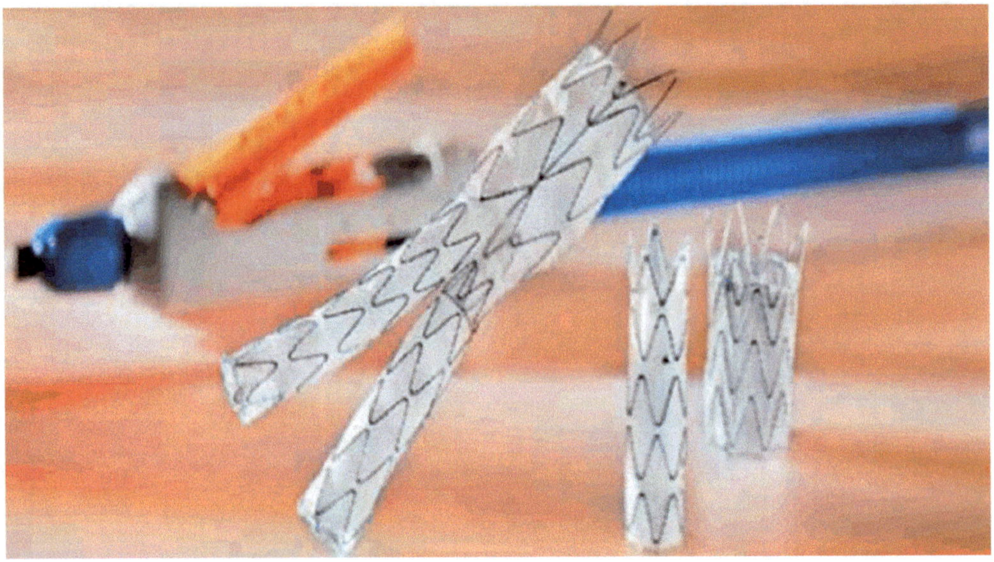

Endoprótese E-Evita®

E-vita® is produced by Jotec (Hechingen, Germany). It is a relatively new infra-renal stent, having been approved for clinical use in Europe since 2008. It is a self-expandable modular device, and one of its features is supra-renal fixation [2, 25]. It has low porosity, with minimal blood loss [2] and high flexibility, being suited to the anatomy of aneurysms with neck angulation or tortuous and dilated iliac arteries [2].

It contains individual nitinol stents, coated with polyester mesh in tubular or conical shapes. The first ring is not covered and is part of the local fixation [1].

Its delivery system is marked by a "squeeze-to-release" approach, which allows the stent to be released in a controlled and constant manner by means of pressing a trigger [2].

The catheter tip is long and flexible, allowing percutaneous introduction and easy tracking through vessels. The marking ring on the catheter sheath provides information about the degree of stent release [2].

The main body is available in two different lengths (150 and 170 mm) with trunk lengths of 50 and 70 mm, which can be combined in any manner, allowing optimization of the treatment. Its proximal diameter varies from 24 to 34 mm, and the distal one is 14 mm for the short leg and from 12 to 22 mm for the long leg. The contralateral branch presents a proximal diameter of 16 mm and distal one from 12 to 24 mm [26, 27, 28]. The length varies from 50 to 105 mm [12] (Fig. 10.7).

Endoprótese Excluder®

Excluder is a stent manufactured by W. L. Gore, approved in 2002 by the FDA for clinical use. It has a modular and self-expanding system with a spiral nitinol structure covered with PTFE and sealed by heat. Its main body has angled wire barbs located at the proximal end of the main body to provide additional anchoring support against the aortic wall [10].

The introducer system is composed of specific tube introducers for the Excluder® graft. The material is hydrophilic and has good navigability. The introducers allow safe tracking by the iliac artery, and placement is near the proximal neck. One advantage of the introducers is the possibility to check out the system's tracking on calcified or tortuous iliac arteries, preventing loss as the open stent has not gone forward [29]. Controlled proximal release is also possible through the partial opening of the proximal rings and gradual traction of the introducer sheath [30]. This technique requires training and experience of the surgical team. Remember that introducers do not have radiopaque markers, and releasing is done by pulling the sheath up to the marked site [1].

The main branch has proximal diameters of 23, 26, and 28.5 mm with an 18 F sheath and a proximal diameter of 31.5 mm with a 20 F sheath. The diameter of the iliac branch is from 12 to 14.5 mm. The length of the main trunk varies from 140 to 180 mm. The contralateral branches have diameters of 12 and 14.5 mm and a 12 F sheath, diameters of 16, 18, and 20 mm with an 18 F sheath, and lengths of 100, 120, and 140 mm [3].

In January 2011, the FDA approved the use of the new C3 device for implantation of the Excluder® graft. This device consists of a significant technological advance in the endovascular treatment of aortic aneurysms because its technology gives doctors an opportunity for a second or even third attempt to get the best possible position for stent deployment. This fourth generation delivery system has the potential to make endovascular repair easier for challenging aneurysm anatomies [3] (Fig. 10.8).

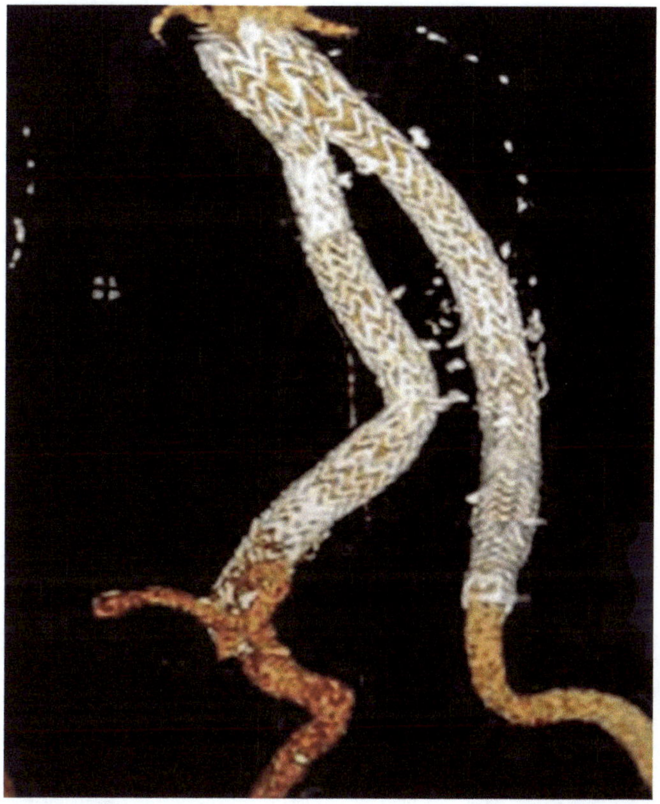

Fig. 10.8 Endoprótese Excluder®

Endoprótese Hercules®

Hercules B®, produced by the Chinese company Micro Port, is a bifurcated stent graft that has a superelastic nitinol structure that ensures radial strength and support to the polyester. It has suprarenal fixation through free stents, whose size varies from 15 to 20 mm. The initial site of the nitinol top tissue is viewed through 13 radiopaque markers that allow proper positioning of the stent.

The main body has a proximal diameter of 20, 22, 24, 26, and 28 with a 20 F profile, proximal diameters of 30, 32, and 34 with a 22 F profile, and lengths ranging from 130 to 170 mm. The ipsilateral branch has a distal diameter of 12–18 mm. The contralateral extension has a diameter 12–18 mm with an 18 F profile [32].

Endoprótese Powerlink®

This stent is made by Endologix and was approved for clinical use by the FDA on 29 October 2004. It consists of a unibody bifurcated stent graft and stents with proximal cuff extensions, and accessories are available for limbs to adapt to the specific anatomical needs of the patient [33].

It consists of a self-expandable cage of cobalt chrome alloy, with a PTFE coating of low porosity and thin walls. It is fixed proximally and distally to a metal cage with polypropylene sutures [33]. Its main body has a diameter of 28 or 25 mm and extension of 80 or 100 mm. The diameter of the iliac branches is always 16 mm, and extension is 40 or 55 mm [1].

The 19 F introducer system, IntuiTrak, is disposable, bifurcated, and integrated. The main body, branch coverings, and introducer sheath restrict the self-expandable stent in a compressed state. When the introducer sheath is retracted, the coatings of the main body and branches are exposed [33].

Complementing the main body, there are auxiliary devices for proximal extension: one model with a 20 mm free stent for suprarenal fixation and one with no stent. The models have diameters of 25 and 28 mm and lengths of 55 and 75 mm or a diameter of 34 mm with a length of 80 mm. Distal extension is available on the straight tube with 16 mm diameter and a length of 55 or 88 mm and a diameter of 20 mm with 55 mm extension. It also has a distal extension with 20 mm proximal diameter and a distal diameter of 25 mm with a length of 65 mm [1] (Fig. 10.9).

Endoprótese Talent®

This device is manufactured by Medtronic, Inc. (Santa Rosa, CA). It is bifurcated, self-expanding, and indicated for infrarenal AAA treatment [3].

It presents discontinuous stents attached to a column of nitinol. Its metal structure is composed of polyester, and the upper end has a free-flow portion. Fixation is by means of the proximal free stent and the radial strength of the system [1].

It has radiopaque markers to identify the beginning of the proximal end devoid of covering [3].

The main body has a diameter ranging from 22 to 28 mm (22 F) and from 30 to 36 mm (24 F), and total length ranging from 155 to 185 mm. It has iliac branches with proximal diameters of 10 to 22 mm and a distal one from 8 to 24 mm, with lengths ranging from 90 to 155 mm [3].

Aortic neck angulation of up to 60° has been approved, and it can be used in short necks from 10 to15 mm length, allowing aneurysm treatment for necks up to 34 mm diameter [34]. It has had excellent long-term clinical results [33].

A few points should be observed, such as the initial positioning, which must be just above the renal arteries as the system can be retracted caudally for the final release of the free-flow portion. Besides, the radiopaque marker over the stent edge must be aligned directly below the origin of the renal artery [13] (Fig. 10.10).

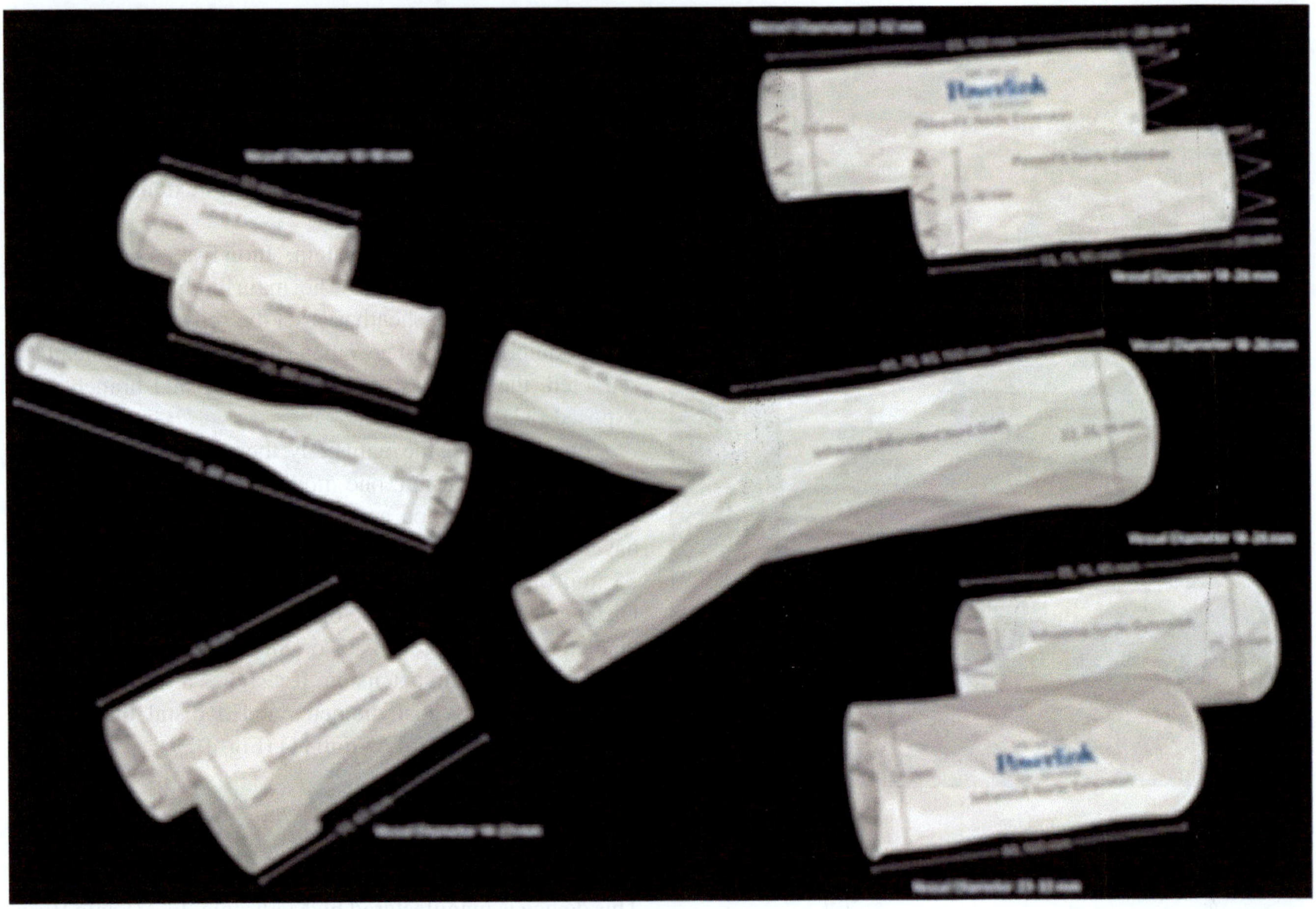

Fig. 10.9 Endoprótese Powerlink®

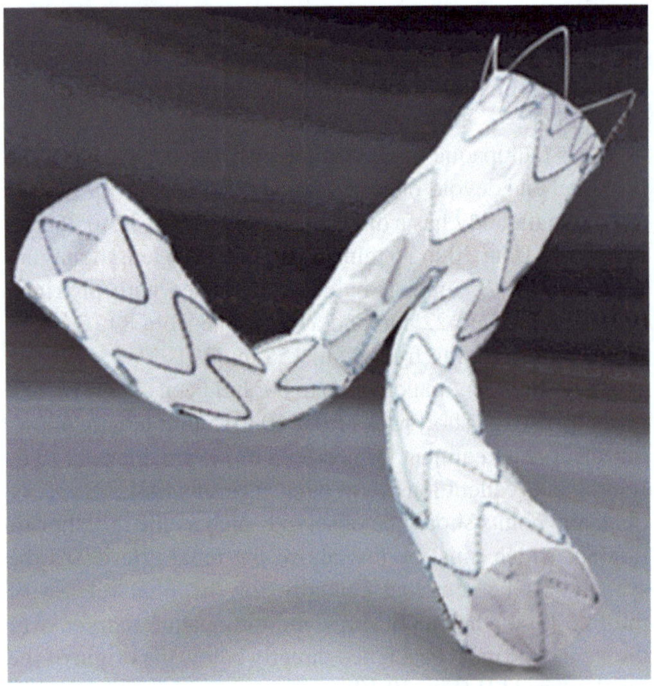

Fig. 10.10 Endoprótese Talent®

Endoprótese Zenith®

This device is produced by Cook Inc., Zenith Flex®. It is a modular system of primary and auxiliary components that are combined to form multiple configurations of the endovascular graft. Its Flexor introducer® has resistant technology and is a PTFE-coated lumen to facilitate accurate delivery.

The main body is long and designed to bifurcate just above the aortic bifurcation in order to obtain stability. It has an uncovered stent with diameters from 22 to 36 mm and a distal diameter of 12 mm. As an exception, a 22 mm prosthesis has a diameter of 11 mm. It also contains anchorage barbs for fixation with greater stability and reduced risk of leakage or migration and a hemostatic valve, New Captor®, which inhibits backflow [31].

Stent extension is identified by the contralateral short branch, and the long ipsilateral branch is over 30 mm. The branches have a diameter of 12 mm for connection to the proximal body. The distal diameters range from 8 to 24 mm and lengths from 3.7 to 12.2 mm.

It has radiopaque markers throughout the graft that promote exact placement below the renal arteries [3]. Viewing

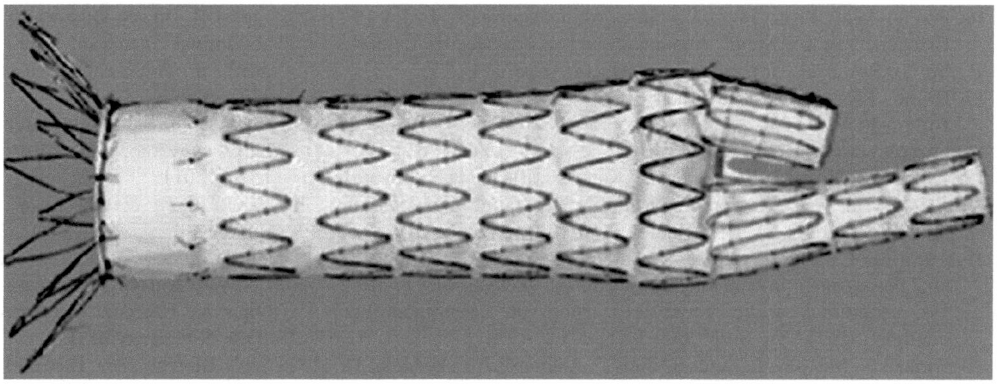

Fig. 10.11 Endoprótese Zenith®

of this distal marker indicates the position of the contralateral branch with a "J" shape anteriorly and with an inverted "J" shape posteriorly.

The Zenith Flex system is the standard for modularity. This versatility increases the number of treatment options because each Zenith Flex system can be precisely customized for each patient [3].

The stent is associated with low mortality and an acceptable rate of postoperative complications and reinterventions [3] (Fig. 10.11).

Sandwich Technique

The sandwich technique for isolated aneurysms of the common iliac artery or internal or aortoiliac aneurysms that extend to the internal iliac artery (IIA) has five steps: (1) insertion of the main body through an ipsilateral femoral approach and positioning such that the distal end of the iliac branch is placed 1 cm above the IIA origin; (2) catheterization of the ipsilateral IIA through a left arm access with a long 5 F catheter (125 cm) and a 0.035 inch, extra-stiff guidewire; (3) placing a covered stent within the IIA overlapping 6 cm in the iliac limb, followed by positioning a first iliac limb extension below the proximal end of the stent (the iliac limb extension is located first and then the covered stent); (4) modeling the iliac extension using an accommodation balloon and dilation of the covered stent with a balloon angioplasty; (5) deployment of the contralateral iliac branch [3].

This technique was developed to overcome the anatomical limitations to the use of current devices, expanding the limits of endovascular aneurysm repair in a safe, easy, and cost-effective manner. The sandwich technique is a promising tool in the armamentarium for the endovascular treatment of isolated aneurysms of the common or internal iliac artery or aortoiliac aneurysms extending to the internal iliac artery.

References

1. Uflacker R, Robison J. Endovascular treatment of abdominal aortic aneurysms. Endovascular treatment of abdominal aortic aneurysms: a review. Eur Radiol. 2001;11(5):739–53.
2. Towne JB. Endovascular treatment of abdominal aortic aneurysms. Am J Surg. 2005;189(2):140–9.
3. Brito CJ. Cirurgia vascular. Rio de Janeiro: Livraria e Editora Revinter; 2008. p. 1231–6.
4. Supporting Post-Market Clinical Data on file at Vascutek. http://www.vascutek.com/Downloads/Literature/Anaconda/BlueGlide_English.pdf. Acesso em 08 dez 2011
5. Saratzis N, Melas N, Saratzis A, Lazarides J, Ktenidis K, Sotirios T, et al. Anaconda™ aortic stent-graft: single-center experience of a new commercially available device for abdominal aortic aneurysms. J Endovasc Ther. 2008;15:33–41.
6. Stehr A, Schnitzbauer AA, Steinbauer MG, Töpel I, Pfister K, Schlitt HJ, et al. Early experience shows rapid shrinking of abdominal aortic aneurysms after endovascular treatment with anaconda™ device. Vasa. 2007;36:199–204.
7. Terumo CVS. The Vascutek AnacondaTM Stent Graft System Phase II IDE Study. 2011. http://clinicaltrials.gov/ct2/show/study/NCT00612924?term=anaconda. Acesso em 10 dez 2011.
8. Reid D. Anaconda ™: an entirely redeployable endoluminal graft with magnet-assisted limb deployment. J Endovasc Ther. 2007;14:124–5.
9. Tecmed.EndoproteseAorfix. http://www.tecmedic.com.br/linhavascular.php?codium=21&PHPSESSID=07a8fc86c962ce204c50e4e85f034d7b. Acesso em 10 dez 2011.
10. Lobato AC. Cirurgia endovascular. 2nd ed. São Paulo: Instituto de Cirurgia Vascular e Endovascular de São Paulo; 2010. p. 373–91.
11. Lombard Medical. Prospective aneurysm trial: high angle Aorfix™ bifurcated stent graft (PYTHAGORAS). 2010. http://clinicaltrials.gov/ct2/show/NCT00522535. Acesso em 12 dez 2011.
12. Weale AR, Balasubramaniam K, Hardman J, Horrocks M. Use of the AorfixTM stent graft in patients with tortuous iliac anatomy. J Cardiovasc Surg (Torino). 2010;51(4):461–6.
13. Albertini JN, Perdikides T, Soong CV, Hinchliffe RJ, Trojanowska M, Yusuf SW. Endovascular repair of abdominal aortic aneurysms in patients with severe angulation of the proximal neck using a flexible stent-graft: European Multicenter Experience. J Cardiovasc Surg (Torino). 2006;47(3):245–50.
14. Silveira PG, Galego GN, Locks L, Oliveira LG, Steckert JS, Philippi FF. Correção Endovascular dos Aneurismas de Aorta Abdominal em 143 Pacientes – Resultados Preliminares – Endoprótese Apolo®. Revista On-line da Associação Catarinense de Medicina. 2002;32(1):S42.
15. Nano. Sistema endovascular apolo. Florianópolis, SC, 2011. http://www.nano.com.br. Acesso em 14 dez 2011.

16. Pereira WM, Frota Filho JD, Sales M, Delatorre N, Leães PE, Blacher C, et al. "Stent" auto-expansível nas dissecções da aorta tipo B. Rev Bras Cir Cardiovasc. 1999;14(3):207–14.
17. Braile Biomédica. Endoprótese Auto Expansível Stent-Graft Bifurcado Percutâneo. São José do Rio Preto, São Paulo, 2011. http://www.braile.com.br/index.asp. Acesso em: 14 dez 2011
18. Köcher M, Utíkal P, Buriánková E, Koutná J, Bachleda P, Novotný J, et al. Four-year experience with an Ella Stent Graft in endovascular treatment of AAA. Cesk Radiol. 2001;55(3):159–66.
19. Lazaridis J, Melas N, Saratzis A, Saratzis N, Sarris K, Fasoulas K, et al. Reporting mid- and long-term results of endovascular grafting for abdominal aortic aneurysms using the aortomonoiliac configuration. J Vasc Surg. 2009;50(1):8–14.
20. Saratzis N, Melas N, Lazaridis J, Ginis G, Antonitsis P, Lykopoulos D, et al. Endovascular AAA repair with the aortomonoiliac EndoFit stent-graft: two years' experience. J Endovasc Ther. 2005;12(3):280–7.
21. LeMaitre Vascular Inc. Endofit AAA StentGrafts. Burlington. 2011. http://www.lemaitre.com. Acesso em: 21 dez 2011.
22. Medtronic, Inc. Endurant AAA StenGraft System. Santa Rosa. 2011. http://ww.medtronic.com. Acesso em: 14 dez 2011.
23. Böckler D, Riambau V, Fitridge R, Wolf Y, Hayes P, Silveira P, et al. Engage Investigators. Worldwide experience with the Endurant Stent graft: review of the literature. J Cardiovasc Surg (Torino). 2011;52(5):669–81. Epub 2011 Jul 28.
24. Torsello G, Troisi N, Donas KP, Austermann M. Evaluation of the Endurant stent graft under instructions for use vs off-label conditions for endovascular aortic aneurysm repair. J Vasc Surg. 2011;54(2):300–6. Epub 2011 Mar 11.
25. Moulakakis KG, Avgerinos ED, Giannakopoulos T, Papapetrou A, Brountzos EN, Liapis CD. Current knowledge on E-vita abdominal endograft. J Cardiovasc Surg (Torino). 2010;51(4):533–8.
26. Tsagakis K, Pizanis N, Baba HA, Wendt D, Wisbrun N, Altenbernd J, et al. Impermeability to blood of the E-vita open plus hybrid stent-graft: experimental and clinical evaluation. J Endovasc Ther. 2010;17(3):340–8.
27. Zipfel B, Buz S, Düsterhöft V, Hetzer R. Initial experience with abdominal aneurysm repair using the E-vita abdominal stent-graft: a single-center study. J Endovasc Ther. 2009;16(5):577–89.
28. Jotec. E-vita® abdominal stengraft system. Hechingen. 2010. 06–2. http://www.jotec.net/english/produkte-stentprot.pml. Acesso em: 15 dez 2011.
29. W. L. Gore & Associates, Inc. GORE® EXCLUDER® AAA Endoprosthesis. Flagstaff. 2002–2011. http://www.goremedical.com/excluder/. Acesso em: 17 dez 2011.
30. Lee WA, Nelson PR. Sheath-assisted controlled deployment technique for Excluder bifurcated main body. J Vasc Surg. 2006;43:1060–3. Gainesville, Fla.
31. S&G Biotech Inc., Hercules Vascular Stent. Korea. 2011. http://sngbio.en.ec21.com/Hercules_Vascular_Stent--1808153_1808585.html. Acesso em: 21 dez 2011.
32. Endologix Inc. IntuiTrak Powerlink System. Irvine. 2010. http://www.endologix.com/products/intuitrak. Acesso em: 18 dez 2011.
33. Medtronic Vascular. Talent Abdominal Stent Graft System. Santa Rosa. 2009. http://www.medtonic.com. Acesso em: 19 dez 2011.
34. Jim J, Sanchez LA, Rubin BG, Criado FJ, Fajardo A, Geraghty PJ, et al. A 5-year evaluation using the talent endovascular graft for endovascular aneurysm repair in short aortic necks. Ann Vasc Surg. 2010;24(7):851–8.
35. Cook Group. Zenith® AAA Endovascular Graft. Bloomington. 2011. www.cookmedical.com. Acesso em 20 dez 2011.
36. Mertens J, Houthoofd S, Daenens K, Fourneau I. Long-term results after endovascular abdominal aortic aneurysm repair using the Cook Zenith endograft. J Vasc Surg. 2011;54:48–57. Leuven, Belgium.
37. Lobato AC. Sandwich technique for aortoiliac aneurysms extending to the internal iliac artery or isolated common/internal iliac artery aneurysms: a new endovascular approach to preserve pelvic circulation. J Endovasc Ther. 2011;18(1):106–11.

Endovascular Treatment of Ruptured Abdominal Aortic Aneurysms

11

Frank J. Veith, Mario Lachat, Dieter Mayer, Zoran Rancic, Todd L. Berland, and Neal S. Cayne

Ruptured abdominal aortic aneurysms (RAAAs) are being treated by endovascular aneurysm repair (EVAR) and other endovascular techniques with increasing frequency. The endovascular procedures offer many potential advantages over open repair. They are less invasive, eliminate damage to periaortic and abdominal structures, decrease bleeding from surgical dissection, minimize hypothermia, and lessen the requirement for deep anesthesia.

Because of these advantages, EVAR has been used extensively to treat RAAAs by several groups who have achieved good results [1–8]. In contrast, some other groups have been unable to demonstrate superiority of EVAR over open repair in the RAAA setting [9, 10]. This chapter describes some of the strategies, techniques, and adjuncts that facilitate the endovascular treatment of RAAAs. We believe that these all contribute to improved outcomes in terms of enhanced survival in this difficult group of patients.

F.J. Veith, MD (✉)
Department of Surgery, Division of Vascular Surgery, New York University Medical Center, 4455 Douglas Avenue, Riverdale, 10471 New York, NY, USA

Department of Surgery, Division of Vascular Surgery, The Cleveland Clinic, Cleveland, OH, USA

Division of Cardiovascular Surgery, Clinic for Cardiovascular Surgery, University Hospital Zurich, Zurich, Switzerland
e-mail: fjvmd@msn.com

M. Lachat, MD
Department of Vascular Surgery, University Hospital Zurich, Zurich, Switzerland

D. Mayer, MD
Departments for Vascular Surgery and Wound Care, University Hospital Zurich, Zurich, Switzerland

Z. Rancic, MD
Department of Cardiovascular Surgery, University Hospital of Zurich, Zurich, Switzerland

Department of Surgery, University of Niš, Niš, Serbia

T.L. Berland, MD • N.S. Cayne, MD
Department of Surgery, New York University Medical Center, New York, NY, USA

Strategies, Techniques, and Adjuncts: Top Tips

Standard Approach or Protocol

These allow the most effective decision-making and treatment of these patients in what are often confusing and stressful circumstances [6, 7]. They are also important to facilitate education in and recognition of RAAAs by generalists, emergency room personnel, and others to enable early diagnosis and mobilization of the specialized caregivers best trained to optimize treatment.

Fluid Restriction (Hypotensive Hemostasis)

Fluid resuscitation should be restricted even if the patient becomes hypotensive. Experience has shown that systolic arterial pressures of 50–70 mmHg are well tolerated for short periods and limit internal bleeding and its associated loss of platelets and clotting factors [2, 3, 7, 11]. Whether or not pharmacological lowering of blood pressure is beneficial remains to be conclusively shown [3, 7].

Treatment Site

EVAR procedures are optimally performed in a site equipped for excellent fluoroscopic imaging and open surgery since some patients will require OR or open adjuncts to their EVAR.

Anesthesia and Catheter Guidewire Placement

The latter should be obtained percutaneously under local anesthesia. This permits arteriography to define aortic and arterial anatomy, facilitates large sheath and supraceliac balloon placement if needed, and prevents circulatory collapse caused by the induction of general anesthesia.

E.A. Gabriel, S.A. Gabriel (eds.), *Inflammatory Response in Cardiovascular Surgery*,
DOI 10.1007/978-1-4471-4429-8_11, © Springer-Verlag London 2013

Whether general anesthesia is used later to eliminate motion and improve fluoroscopic imaging to permit precise graft deployment remains controversial. One group has successfully used local anesthesia supplemented by sedation throughout as an alternative [1, 3, 7].

Supraceliac Aortic Sheath Placement and Balloon Control

Most experienced groups favor their use only when there is severe circulatory collapse. In such cases, deflation of the balloon before sealing of the rupture site will result in immediate recurrence of the circulatory collapse. Therefore, techniques have been developed to maintain continuous aortic control until the endograft has sealed the leak [2, 3, 7, 12, 13]. These techniques use multiple balloons to minimize renal and visceral ischemia by placing secondary balloons within the endograft as the supraceliac balloon is deflated and removed though its supporting sheath.

Endograft Type and Configuration

Both bifurcated and aortouni-iliac (or femoral) grafts can be used successfully, although some patients have unilateral iliac disease, which mandates a unilateral configuration. Modular and unibody grafts have been used successfully in both configurations. An appropriate inventory of suitable grafts and accessories must be stocked sterile in the treatment site and be available for the procedure and unexpected contingencies.

Abdominal Compartment Syndrome

This is a major cause of morbidity and mortality after EVAR for RAAA. It is advantageous to keep a high index of suspicion for this entity. Laparotomy and hematoma evacuation have alleviated the hypotension, high ventilatory compliance, and oliguria that occurs with the full blown syndrome. Monitoring bladder pressure has been helpful in the early detection of the syndrome [3, 7], and early laparotomy with open abdomen treatment (OAT) and suction/sponge (VAC) dressings may decrease mortality and allow survival in otherwise hopeless circumstances when small bowel and mesenteric edema cause loss of domain for the abdominal viscera [7, 14].

EVAR for Worst Risk Patients

It is probable that EVAR is most beneficial in augmenting survival when it is used in the worst risk patients who are unlikely to survive an OR. Patients with hemodynamic instability and profound circulatory collapse, a hostile abdomen, or those unable to receive transfusion would fall in this category. If such patients, particularly those that are hemodynamically unstable, are excluded from EVAR, it is likely that the improved survival that can accrue from this form of treatment will be diminished [8].

Discussion

It is clear that several centers, in which the physicians and surgeons are enthusiastic about EVAR treatment for RAAAs, have attempted to perform the procedure preferentially in every AAA patients with suitable anatomy [8]. This includes patients who are hypotensive and hemodynamically unstable as well as those with frank hemorrhagic shock. These centers have achieved favorable results with EVAR for RAAAs in these unstable patients and believe that it is precisely these high-risk unstable hypotensive patients in whom EVAR offers the greatest survival benefit over open repair. In these centers, between 28 and 79 % (mean 49.1 %) of all RAAA patients were treated by EVAR. In addition, the proportion of patients treated by EVAR increased with time as devices and skills improved and enthusiasm for the procedure increased, and it is likely that the proportion will increase further as new devices and techniques are introduced. All these centers that are enthusiastic about EVAR treatment of RAAAs emphasize several key factors that are important in achieving favorable outcomes in these patients. Proper use of aortic balloon control, adequate recognition and treatment of abdominal compartment syndrome, and the establishment of a structured system and protocol for the treatment of RAAA patients all contribute importantly to improved survival outcomes in patients with this diagnosis.

Although there may be other ways to deal with these and other factors and still achieve good outcomes with EVAR in the RAAA setting, the strategies, techniques, and adjuncts outlined in this chapter are one way of doing so that has proven to be effective.

References

1. Lachat ML, Pfammatter T, Witzke HJ, Bettex D, Dunzli A, Wolfensberger U, et al. Endovascular repair with bifurcated stent-grafts under local anaesthesia to improve outcome of ruptured aortoiliac aneurysms. Eur J Vasc Endovasc Surg. 2002;23(6):528–36.
2. Veith FJ, Ohki T. Endovascular approaches to ruptured infrarenal aorto-iliac aneurysms. J Cardiovasc Surg. 2002;3:369–78.
3. Hechelhammer L, Lachat ML, Wildermuth S, Bettex D, Mayer D, Pfammatter T. Midterm outcome of endovascular repair of ruptured abdominal aortic aneurysms. J Vasc Surg. 2005;41(5):752–7.
4. Mehta M, Darling III RC, Roddy SP, Fecteau S, Ozsvath KJ, Kreienberg PB, et al. Factors associated with abdominal compartment syndrome complicating endovascular repair of ruptured abdominal aortic aneurysms. J Vasc Surg. 2005;42(6):1047–51.

5. Coppi G, Silingardi R, Gennai S, Saitta G, Ciardullo AV. A single centre experience in open and endovascular treatment of hemodynamically unstable and stable patients with ruptured abdominal aortic aneurysms. J Vasc Surg. 2006;44(6):1140–7.
6. Moore R, Nutley M, Cina CS, Motamedi M, Faris P, Abuznadah W. Improved survival after introduction of an emergency endovascular therapy protocol for ruptured abdominal aortic aneurysms. J Vasc Surg. 2007;45(3):443–50.
7. Mayer D, Pfammatter T, Rancic Z, Hechelhammer L, Wilhelm M, Veith FJ, et al. 10 years of emergency endovascular aneurysm repair for ruptured abdominal aortoiliac aneurysms – lessons learned. Ann Surg. 2009;249(3):510–5.
8. Veith FJ, Lachat M, Mayer D, Malina M, Holst J, Mehta M, et al. Collected world and single center experience with endovascular treatment of ruptured abdominal aortic aneurysms. Ann Surg. 2009;250(5):818–24.
9. Peppelenbosch N, Yilmaz N, van Marrewijk C, Buth J, Cuypers P, Duijm L. Emergency treatment of acute symptomatic or ruptured abdominal aortic aneurysm. Outcome of a prospective intent-to-treat by EVAR protocol. Eur J Vasc Endovasc Surg. 2003;26(3):303–10.
10. Hinchliffe RJ, Bruijstens L, MacSweeney ST, Braithwaite BD. A randomized trial of endovascular and open surgery for ruptured abdominal aortic aneurysm – results of a pilot study and lessons learned for future studies. Eur J Vasc Endovasc Surg. 2006;32(5):506–15.
11. van der Vliet JA, van Aalst DL, Schultze Kool LJ, Wever JJ, Blankensteijn JD. Hypotensive hemostasis (permissive hypotension) for ruptured abdominal aortic aneurysm: are we really in control? Vascular. 2007;15(4):197–200.
12. Malina M, Veith F, Ivancev K, Sonesson B. Balloon occlusion of the aorta during endovascular repair of ruptured abdominal aortic aneurysm. J Endovasc Ther. 2005;12(5):556–9.
13. Larzon T, Lindgren R, Norgren L. Endovascular treatment of RAAAs: a shift of the paradigm. J Endovasc Ther. 2005;12:548–55.
14. Mayer D, Rancic Z, Meier C, Pfammater T, Veith FJ, Lachat M. Open abdominal treatment following endovascular repair of ruptured abdominal aortic aneurysms. J Vasc Surg. 2009;50:1–7.

Part IV

Critical Lower Limb Ischemia

Thromboangiitis Obliterans

12

Otacílio de Camargo Júnior
and Juliana Lech de Camargo

Introduction

Thromboangiitis obliterans (TAO) was reported in the literature for the first time in 1879 by Felix von Winiwarter [59], who described a vascular syndrome that progressed to gangrene of the lower limb, with extensive thrombosis of the arteries and small veins and preservation of the internal elastic membrane. These pathological findings were in a 57-year-old male patient presenting with foot pain that had begun 12 years earlier, turned into gangrene, and resulted in amputation. Intimal proliferation with thrombosis, fibrosis, and endarteritis different from arteriosclerosis were demonstrated in a pathological specimen.

This disease was called endarteritis obliterans until 1908 when Leo Buerger [59] published his classic study of 11 limbs that had been amputated because of ischemia with obstruction of the distal arteries and veins and preservation of entire vascular wall; he called it TAO, reinforcing what had been described by von Winiwater, presenting clinical and pathological differences regarding arteriosclerosis. For his contributions to our understanding of this disease, TAO is also known by the eponym Buerger's disease.

Arteriosclerotic inflammatory disease, characterized by the occurrence of thrombotic occlusions, often affects the medium- and small-caliber arteries and veins of the lower and upper limbs, classified histopathologically as a vasculitis, but differing from most common vasculitises in three important ways:

1. Often presents with inflammatory thrombus and preservation of the vessel wall
2. Normal levels of markers even in the acute phase
3. Normal immunoactivation markers

TAO presenting as a result of smoking, usually cigarettes, has primarily been described in males, but the number of female cases is increasing and is now already more than 20 %.

Inflammatory and Histopathological Factors

Thrombotic involvement of all layers of the arterial and venous wall characterizes the acute phase of illness. In the acute phase of the disease, the inflammatory process has polymorphonuclear leukocytes around the thrombus, often with multinucleated giant cells being the most common inflammatory thrombotic lesion in the veins. This is more characteristic of superficial thrombophlebitis and is not specific to TAO [38].

In TAO, the intensity of the periadventitial inflammatory process can be quite variable in different segments of the same vessel, showing segmental distribution, with healthy vessel segments mixed with segments of diseased vessel. In the inflammatory process, lymphohistiocytic cells, granulocytic lymphocytes, and eosinophils, can be found, though rarely in remarkable amounts [44]. In contrast, vasculitis presents very disrupted elastic laminae; in TAO, they remain intact.

The histopathology of diseased vessels is variable depending on the chronological age of the disease from which material was collected for examination. Positive histopathological findings are more likely in the acute phase; however, in the subacute phase, because of the evolution of the pathological changes, the histopathology is only suggestive. It is mostly not present in the chronic phase, when organized thrombus and fibrosis of vessels are detected (Figs. 12.1 and 12.2) [17, 39].

Which vascular damage occurs first, thrombotic or inflammatory, is undetermined, but the intense inflammatory infiltration and cell proliferation that are observed in lesions

O. de Camargo Júnior, MD (✉)
Department of Vascular/Endovascular Surgery,
Pontifical Catholic University of Campinas,
Celso Pierro Maternity Hospital,
Sao Paulo, Brazil

Department of Vascular Surgery,
Pontifical Catholic University of Campinas,
Sao Paulo, Brazil
e-mail: otacamjr@terra.com.br

J.L. de Camargo, MD.
Department of Medicine, University of Taubate,
São Paulo, Brazil

E.A. Gabriel, S.A. Gabriel (eds.), *Inflammatory Response in Cardiovascular Surgery*,
DOI 10.1007/978-1-4471-4429-8_12, © Springer-Verlag London 2013

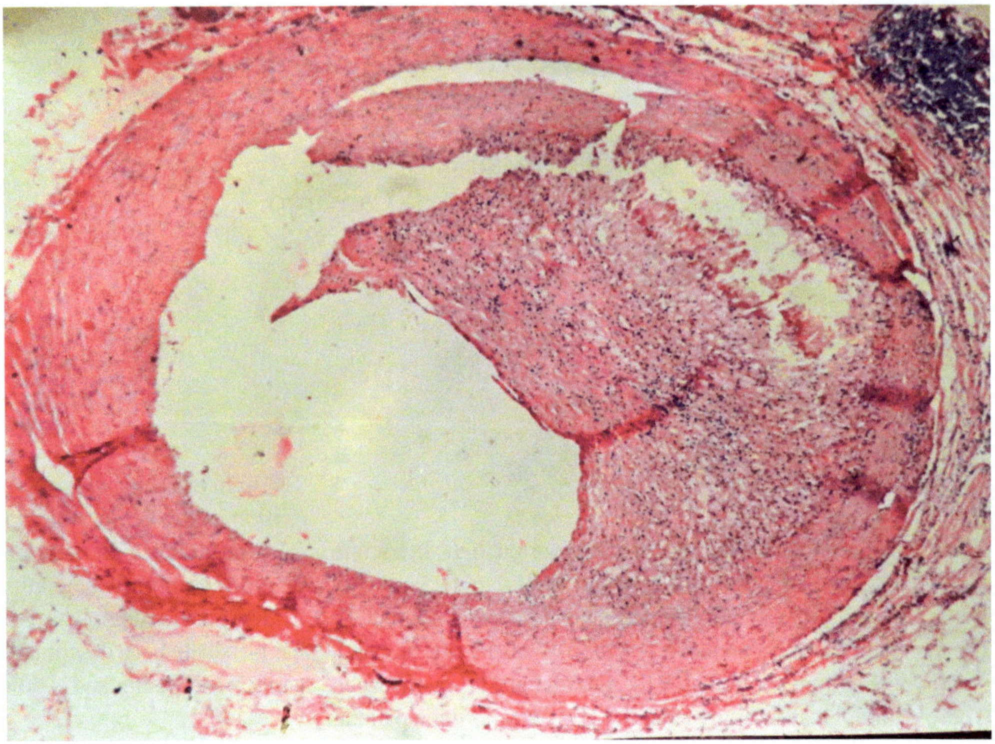

Fig. 12.1 Intimal thickening with preservation of the medial layer. Chronic inflammatory process with recanalization (Courtesy of the Study Group in Correlation Anatomy-Clinic PUCCAMP)

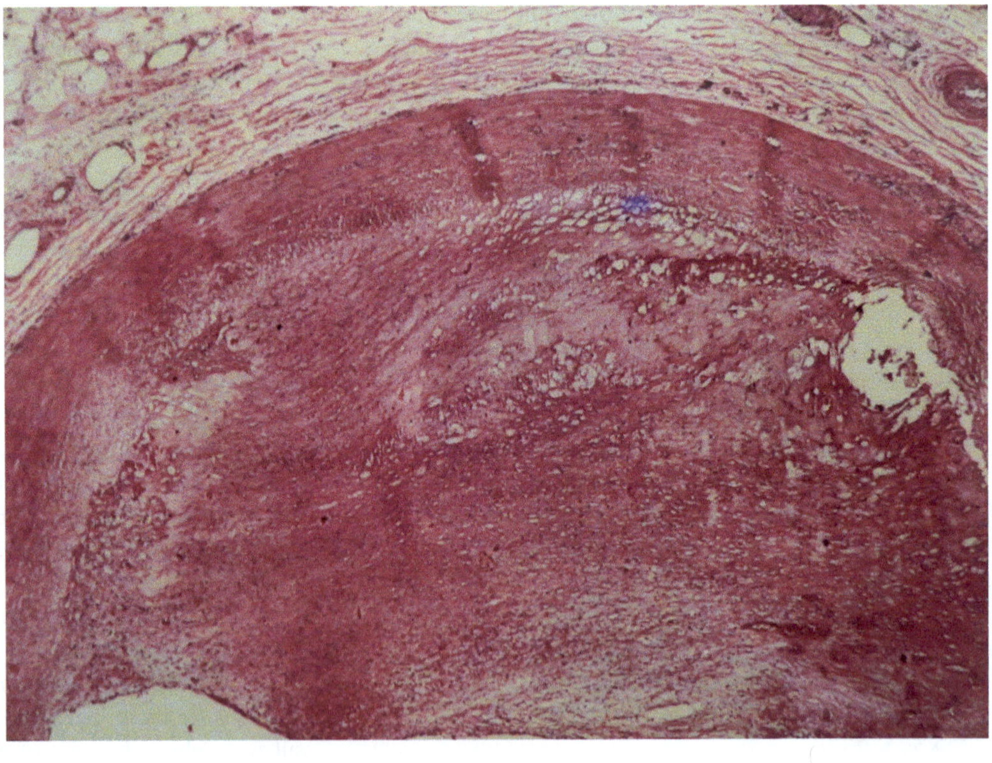

Fig. 12.2 Acute phase with thrombosis (Courtesy of the Study Group in Correlation Anatomy-Clinic PUCCAMP)

during the acute phase are different, especially when veins are affected. Various stages of lesions may occur in different segments of same vein when the biopsy is carried out in the acute phase with phlebitis and thrombophlebitis. In these stages we can find acute phlebitis without thrombosis, acute phlebitis with thrombosis, and acute phlebitis with thrombus associated with microabscesses and giant cells (Figs. 12.3 and 12.4).

The intermediate stage is characterized by progressive organization of thrombus obstruction in arteries and

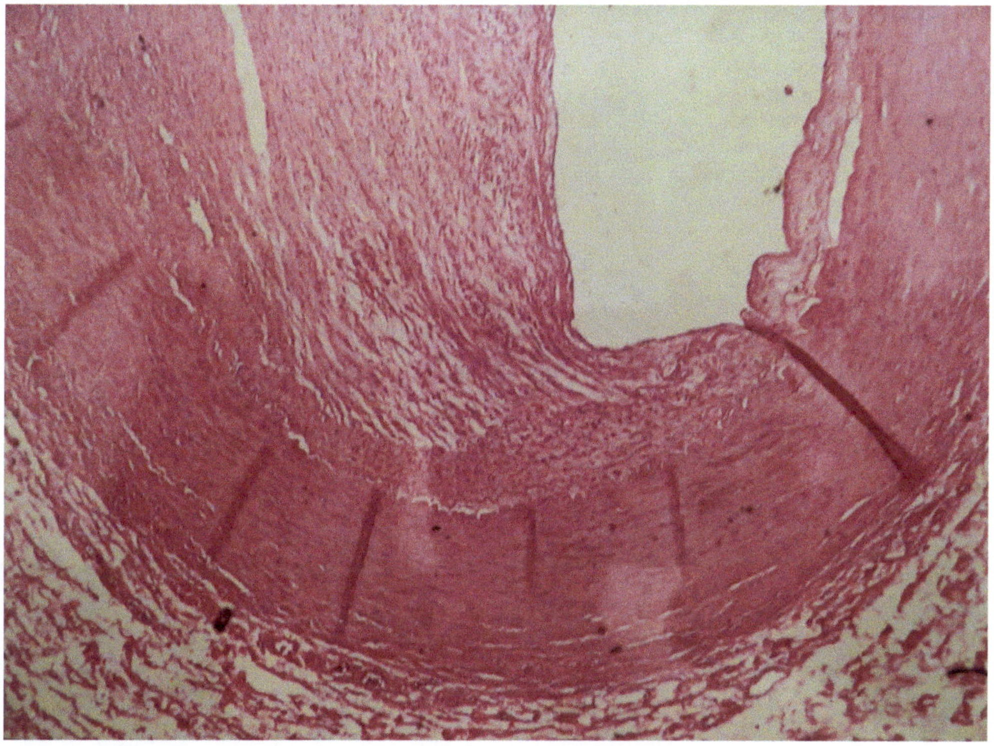

Fig. 12.3 Chronic phase with intimal and medial layer thickening (Courtesy of the Study Group in Correlation Anatomy-Clinic PUCCAMP)

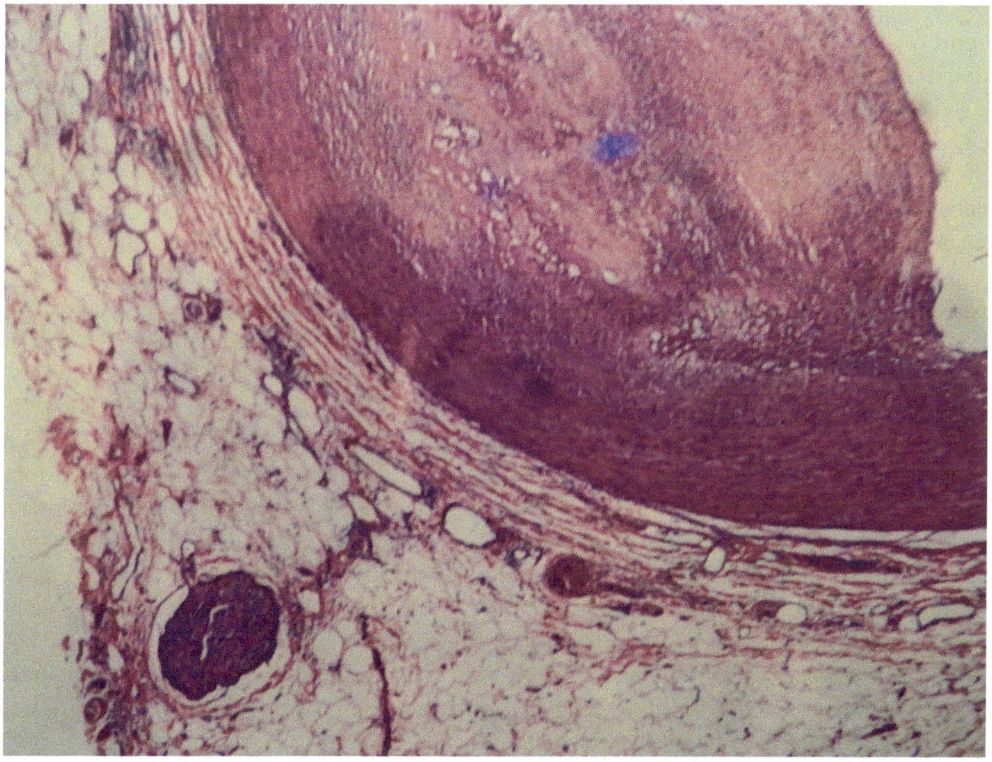

Fig. 12.4 Acute phase: intimal thickening caused by the inflammatory process. Medial layer with muscle fiber hyperplasia. Inflammatory process in the adventitia and perineural area (Courtesy of the Study Group in Correlation Anatomy-Clinic PUCCAMP)

veins, often with an inflammatory cell infiltrate within the thrombus with no expressive inflammation in the vascular wall. Obstructive thrombus organization with recanalization in various stages, prominent vascularization of the medial layer, and perivascular fibrosis of the adventitia characterize the chronic phase. These lesions are least typical.

Rupture of the internal and medial elastic laminae, which often occurs in arteriosclerosis and in systemic vasculitis, differs from TAO, in which the internal elastic lamina and

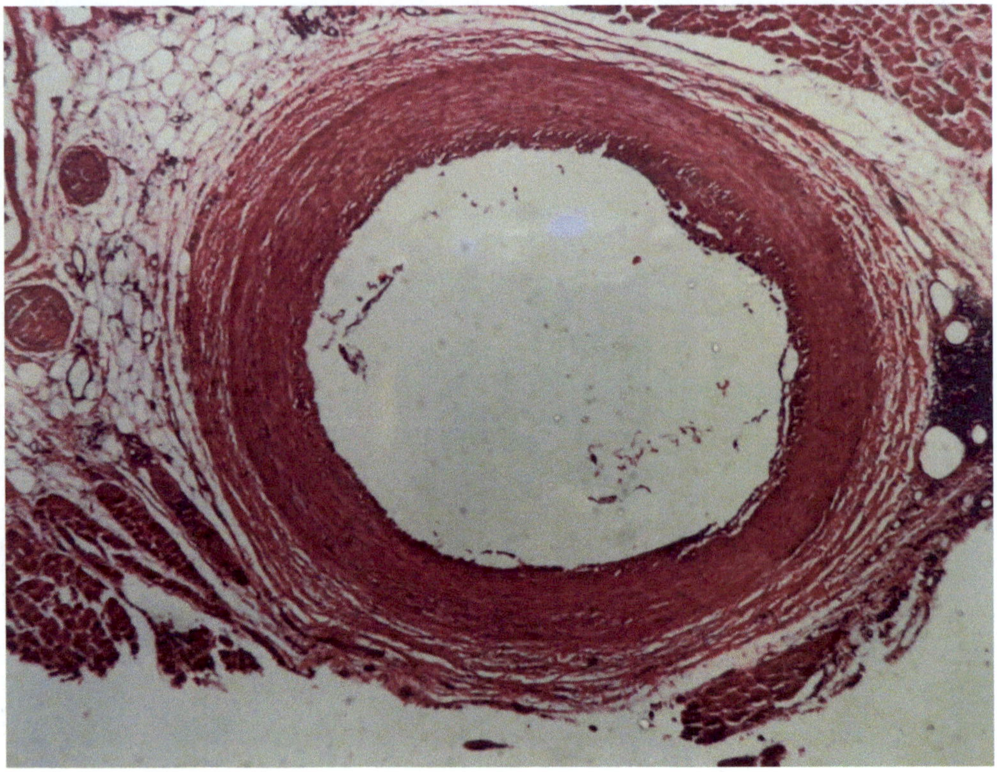

Fig. 12.5 Uniform intimal thickening. Small area of thrombosis with medial layer preservation. Inflammatory process in the adventitia and perineural area (Coronary artery courtesy of the Study Group in Correlation Anatomy-Clinic PUCCAMP)

entire vessel wall remain unchanged in the underlying location of thrombus obstruction in three stages of the disease.

There is no necrosis of the arterial wall in TAO as it presents with parietal architectural integrity, especially in the medial layer, which distinguishes it from other forms of necrotizing arteritis. Also no calcifications or atheromatous plaques are observed, distinguishing it from arteriosclerosis.

Endothelial dysfunction may also be involved in the pathogenesis of disease as high levels of antiendothelial antibodies were detected in diseased patients [22, 31].

Thromboangiitis and Arteriosclerosis

Despite histopathological differences, TAO can coexist with arteriosclerosis, especially in patients over 40 years of age, creating an additional difficulty for diagnosis. Excessive use of tobacco increases the risk of arteriosclerosis.

The histological appearance of thrombus in TAO is the same as that of arteriosclerotic thrombosis, however with an exacerbated inflammatory process, with hypercellular thrombus with intense invasion of the smooth muscle cells from the medial layer and preservation of the internal elastic lamina (Fig. 12.5).

Etiology, Pathogenesis, and Smoking

TAO is a type of vasculitis [41], but with features that differentiate it from other forms of vasculitis, presenting thrombosis with an exuberant inflammatory process, with less intense cellular activity in the vessel wall, preservation of the internal elastic lamina, and normal immunological markers.

The etiology of TAO is unknown; however, an association with the smoking habit is recognized. However, the time course of the disease can vary [13, 40, 71]. The time of onset of signs and symptoms is also associated with smoking. Manifestations are more severe in individuals who smoke all day and have less time between each cigarette; major injuries are detected in those who started smoking before the age of 20 years or have smoked for over 10 years [66].

Continued use of tobacco is closely related to disease progression, being the main factor for this progression. All researchers believe that tobacco use is a component of the TAO diagnosis. In the literature, there are no clear cases of this disease in non-tobacco-smoking patients.

Several factors have been described about how smoking affects the circulation, causing thrombosis, vasoconstriction, vascular injury produced by the altered metabolism of catecholamines, changes in the oxygen dissociation of hemoglobin in the peripheral circulation, and direct action of tobacco-derived substances in the endothelium [40, 69].

Researchers have attempted to establish an autoimmune etiology for TAO. A hypersensitivity reaction caused by tobacco in the vascular endothelium has been verified by significant amounts of active immune complexes in patients' serum, which may compromise vessels. Endothelial lesions changing the vessels' features induce the formation of anti-arterial antibodies, which react with the already exposed antigens to form circulating immune complexes, which are partially removed from the circulation. There is a consequent increase in platelet aggregation in response to the formation of immune complexes [26].

Hypotheses about an autoimmune mechanism haves been considered in studies describing the presence of antinuclear antibodies and increased specific antibodies in the arterial wall [24, 25].

Often found in patients with TAO, hyperhomocysteinemia seems to play an important role in the pathogenesis of the disease [70].

High levels of anti-endothelial antibodies, which are observed even before clinical manifestations of disease, cause endothelial dysfunction [61].

A higher occurrence of disease has been proven in countries with more significant consumption of tobacco, and an allergy or hypersensitivity to some component of tobacco is suspected. This sensitivity would lead to inflammatory obstructive disease of the small blood vessels.

Literature reports indicate that chronic anaerobic periodontal infections may also play a role in the development of TAO as almost two-thirds of patients with this disease also have severe periodontal disease. However, the prevalence of periodontal disease in smokers without TAO is also high [9, 30].

It is believed that other etiological factors with mechanisms for triggering disease onset are present because although tobacco use is predominant in the onset and progression of disease, only a small number of tobacco users worldwide develop the disease.

Epidemiology, Genetics, and Gender

Although the disease has worldwide distribution, it is most prevalent in the Mediterranean region, the Middle East, and Asia than in the West and North America. It occurs more frequently in countries where tobacco is widely used, especially where there is a habit of making cigarettes at home [23, 37, 42].

Recently, the disease has decreased in Europe and the United States because of the adoption of stricter criteria for diagnosis and also because of reducing the number of smokers.

In Japan, a study conducted in 1976 by the Committee for Buerger's Disease Research of the Ministry of Health and Welfare in analyzed 3,034 patients with the disease, 2,930 men and 104 women, finding an incidence of 5 per 100,000 people [10]. These results were similar to those of a statistical study conducted by the Committee for Research on the Epidemiology of Untreatable Diseases from the Ministry of Health and Welfare in 1986 [54].

Although to date no gene has been identified, there may be a genetic predisposition to disease onset.

Disease incidence in females younger than 70 years is low, in the range of 1–2 %, with a significant increase in the 90s, by about 20 %, probably because of the increasing number of female smokers.

Vasodilation and Coagulation

Literature data indicate reduced endothelium-dependent vasodilation in the peripheral circulation of patients with TAO. There is impaired vasodilation after infusion of the endothelium-dependent vasodilator acetylcholine [45].

In patients with TAO there is also increased platelet response to serotonin [65] and elevated plasma homocysteine [8, 60].

In the pathogenesis of TAO, prothrombotic factors play a remarkable role as mutation of prothrombin gene 20210 and the presence of anticardiolipin antibodies are associated with increased risk and severity of disease [46, 57].

Patients with high levels of antibodies and TAO are younger and at greater risk for amputations than patients with normal antibody levels [46, 57].

Immunology

Immunological factors have been the subject of several studies in patients with TAO, and several publications suggest that immune responses may be important pathogenic factors in the disease.

On one hand, more intense cellular sensitivity to collagen types I and III has been observed in patients with TAO than in healthy and arteriosclerotic patients [1, 2]. On the other hand, samples analyzed histologically for many arteries were found to have preserved the general architecture of vessel walls, irrespective of disease stage, with significant cellular infiltration in the thrombus and intima. In the acute phase, mainly macrophages and dendritic cells were identified in the intima, turning out to be TAO endarteritis caused by T-cell- and humoral-mediated cellular immunity associated with B-cell activation of macrophages or dendritic cells in the intima [34, 68].

Laboratory Aspects

There is no specific laboratory test for the diagnosis of TAO; however, all laboratory tests that contribute to the differential diagnosis should be performed, such as:

Fasting glucose
Urinalysis
Erythrocyte sedimentation rate
C-reactive protein
Antinuclear factor

Rheumatoid factor
Hemogram
Coagulation
Liver function
Renal function
Protein C
Protein S
Antithrombin III
Factor V Leiden
Prothrombin gene mutation
Toxicology: cocaine, cannabis, amphetamines

Clinical Aspects

The classic description of TAO involves a young patient, about 40 years old, a smoker, male, and often having migratory superficial thrombophlebitis and Raynaud's phenomenon in the upper and lower limbs. The usual initial involvement is obstruction of the distal arteries and veins of the hands and feet with consequent minor and asymptomatic arterial insufficiency with frequent progression to the proximal vessels, not rarely with involvement of the superficial femoral artery. This progression of arterial lesions is accompanied by worsening clinical symptoms presenting as intermittent claudication. With disease progression, symptoms appear, such as cooling of the extremities and superficial areas of ischemia that evolve into superficial ischemic ulcers on the feet, hands, and fingers. Usually, the initial trophic lesion is periungual and is often treated with excision of the nail, culminating in finger necrosis. There is infrequent involvement of the brachial artery, common iliac artery, and great vessels [4, 5, 72].

Involvement of organs is also reported in the literature. The histopathology of the vessels is the same as for the limbs, affecting the veins and arteries [27].

Although TAO affects the small and medium vessels of the extremities, the same histopathological findings have been reported in cerebral, coronary, internal mammary, renal, and mesenteric arteries [20, 36]. Involvement of multiple organs is rare [7, 49].

At least two limbs are often affected, and published reports show involvement of four limbs in 43 % of cases, three limbs in 41 % of cases, and two limbs in 16 % of cases (Figs. 12.6 and 12.7) [32, 58, 71]. In radiological tests performed in patients with disease, arteriographic changes in limb segments that have not had symptoms are frequently found.

Claudication in the legs is a common initial complaint and less frequently in the upper limbs. Plantar claudication is often an early symptom and can be confused with rheumatologic and orthopedic problems, resulting in delayed diagnosis. With disease progression, the claudication becomes more proximal, often up to the calf.

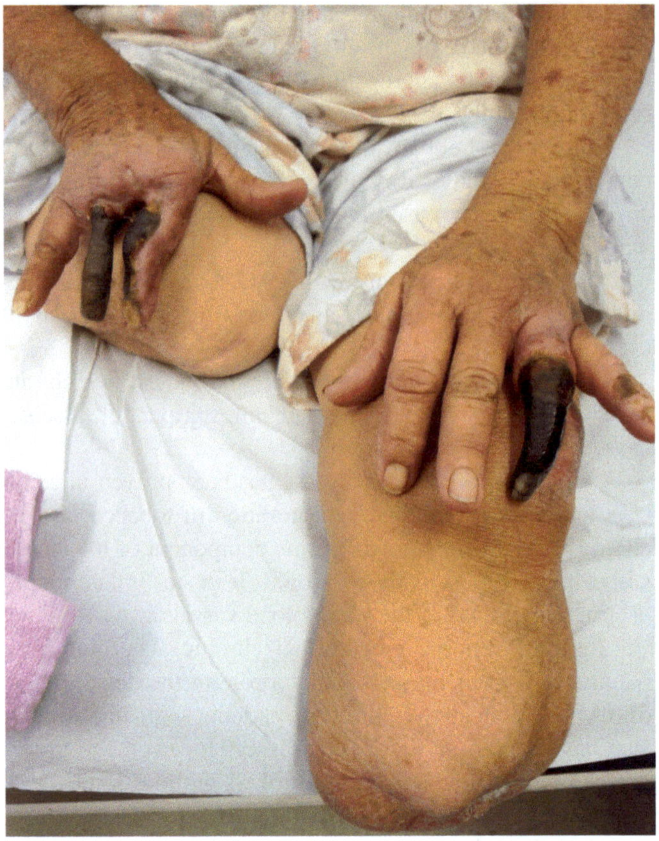

Fig. 12.6 Female patient with involvement of all four limbs

Microscopic pathological examination shows significant inflammation around the nerve fibers, which indicates ischemic neuropathy.

Rheumatological symptoms are frequent in patients with TAO, and the classic Raynaud's phenomenon is presented in approximately 50 % of patients, even asymmetrically in the limbs [21].

Recurrent arthralgia in the large joints with important local inflammatory signs may indicate prodromal signs of TAO years before the appearance of arterial occlusions [67].

Migratory thrombophlebitis can arise early, even before arterial symptoms, and can distinguish TAO from other diseases (Fig. 12.8). It may also be present in 50 % of cases and often demonstrates local disease activity; biopsies demonstrate the classic histopathological aspects of TAO [62, 64].

It may present as a first symptom of TAO in approximately 25 % of patients with recurrent episodes in 60 % of cases. Palmar or plantar hyperhidrosis may appear in up to 30 % of patients [13].

Radiological Aspects

Doppler ultrasound can be useful to measure the pressoric indices and locate the occluded artery, but duplex ultrasound mapping is a non-invasive examination that can provide the

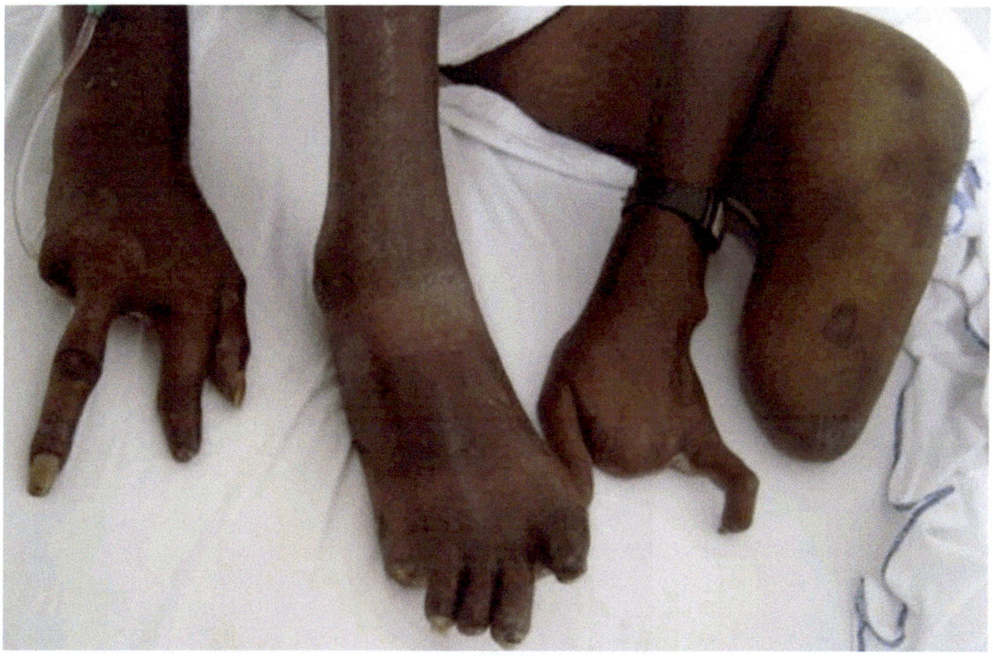

Fig. 12.7 Male patient with involvement of all four limbs

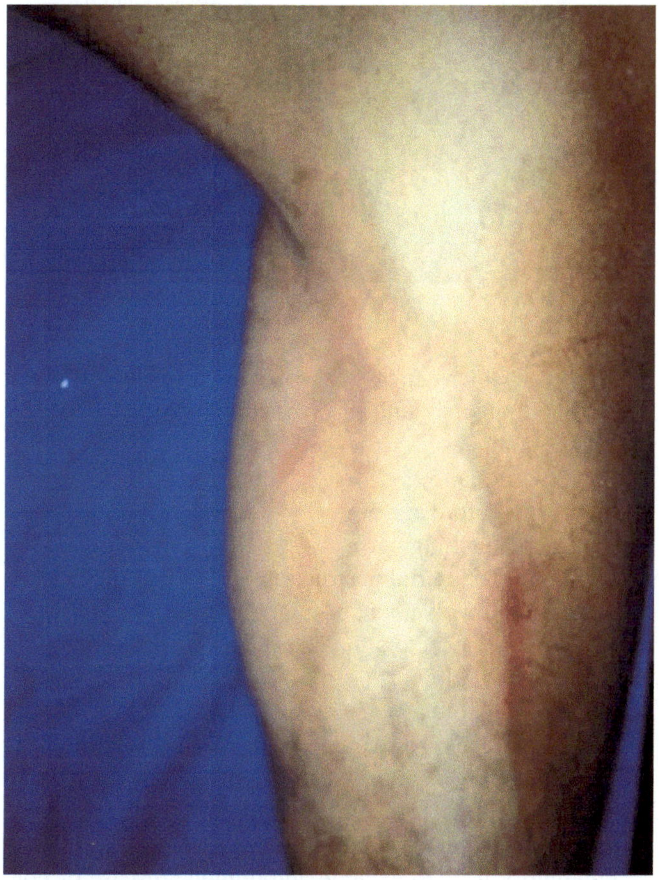

Fig. 12.8 Migratory thrombophlebitis

most data. It quantifies the distal flow of occluded arteries, even showing characteristics of the vessel wall and the location of the distal arterial occlusion.

Ultrasound can be important to rule out an embolic source and aneurysmal disease. Parietal occlusive alterations can be clearly seen on angiography and can confirm the diagnosis of TAO.

There are no pathognomonic arteriographic aspects of TAO, but aspects such as the classic sign of Martorell (corkscrew-shaped collateral vessels) do exist (Fig. 12.9).

Arteriographic aspects of TAO are:

- No signs of atherosclerosis
- Involvement of vessels of small and medium caliber: Radial, ulnar, and palmar digital arteries of the hands; tibial, peroneal, and plantar digital arteries.
- Obstructive arterial lesions and spastic segmental mixed with normal segments.
- Normal proximal circulation with intense distal involvement.
- Corkscrew-shaped collateral vessels around sites of obstruction.

Diagnosis and Differential Diagnosis

Many authors have proposed several major and minor diagnostic criteria for diagnosis, but others believe these diagnostic criteria are not useful for diagnosis and treatment of the disease. Association with other diseases should not exclude the diagnosis. Diagnostic criteria proposed are clinical, pathological, and arteriographic [50, 64].

Notable major factors are exacerbated smoking, distal ischemic symptoms before the age of 45 years, brachial and popliteal arteries without disease, arteriographic and/or histopathological signs of disease, absence of embolic sources,

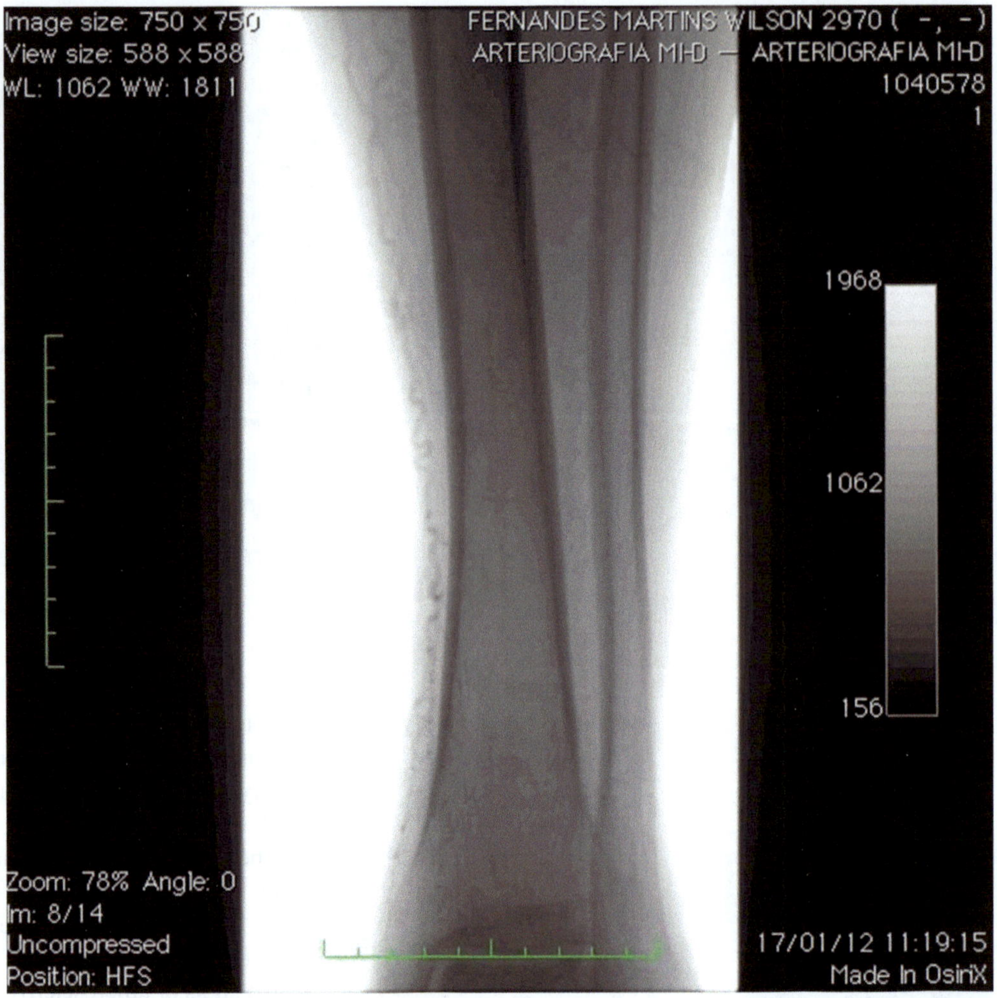

Fig. 12.9 Corkscrew-shaped collateral vessels

absence of autoimmune diseases, no change in coagulation, and no arteriosclerosis. Notable minor factors are plantar claudication, Raynaud's phenomenon, disease in the upper extremities, and migratory thrombophlebitis.

The most important diseases to consider for the differential diagnosis, with signs and symptoms similar to atherosclerosis, are embolisms and autoimmune diseases.

Other vasculitises should also be excluded, such as Takayasu's arteritis or giant cell arteritis, because of proximal arterial involvement. Ischemic symptoms are extremely similar to TAO developed because of using cocaine, amphetamines, and cannabis, with frequent reports in the literature [19, 55]. It is necessary to exclude antiphospholipid antibody syndrome, which leads to arterial and venous thrombosis, rheumatoid arthritis, mixed connective tissue disease, and scleroderma.

To rule out these diseases, serological marker tests are very important, and antiphospholipid antibody syndrome may show a positive test for lupic anticoagulant and high levels of anticardiolipin antibodies. The histopathological examination of TAO thrombus shows an intense inflammatory process that differs from those not showing an inflammatory process.

Ergotism, which can also cause ischemia of both the upper and lower limbs, should be investigated and ruled out by detailed investigation.

Shinoya's Criteria [59]

- Beginning before age 50
- History of smoking
- Infrapopliteal arterial obstruction
- Upper limb involvement or migratory phlebitis
- Absence of risk factors for atherosclerosis except smoking

Olin's Criteria [59]

- Beginning before age 45
- Current or recent smoking
- Ischemia of the distal part of the upper and/or lower limbs and claudication, rest pain, ischemic ulcers, and gangrene with documented with non-invasive tests
- Laboratory tests to exclude autoimmune disease or connective tissue disease and diabetes mellitus
- Determine the proximal source of emboli by echocardiography and angiography
- Consistent arteriographic findings in the affected limbs and in those clinically free of disease

Medical and Surgical Treatment

Several published reports show that the only appropriate treatment to stop the progression of TAO is to stop smoking or any form of tobacco and/or cannabis use. It was also shown that smoking at least one cigarette per day or chewing tobacco can cause progression of disease and serious complications [12, 32, 43, 62].

Quitting smoking by patients with TAO is known to be difficult because of the chemical dependency and psychological habit; frequently people are not able to quit smoking. To determine whether all forms of tobacco use have really been stopped, urinary levels of nicotine and cotinine can be measured [47].

Providing analgesia and anesthetic blocks, facilitating healing of ulcerations, and even preventing the patient from adopting an incorrect position of the limb, which can causes severe edema with worsening of limb perfusion, are important for patients hospitalized with ischemic rest pain and/or ulcerations. Smoking cessation at the time of admission can be beneficial; however, frequently the patient keeps smoking even when hospitalized. Keeping the patient in a proclive position can improve limb perfusion and alleviate pain.

Patients with TAO exhibit reduced glucocorticoid receptors, which may cause variable responses to corticosteroid treatment; the response varies according to the number of receptors [3, 6, 35].

Vasodilator medication, such as cilostazol capsules and intravenous or oral prostaglandin, may also improve ischemic lesions. This medication can be used alone if there is no indication for surgery [14, 15, 48]. The association of anxiolytic and antidepressant medication has proven to be beneficial in patients.

Surgical treatment can consist of minor surgery for devitalized areas, debridement, drainage of abscesses, and major amputations.

Thoracic and/or lumbar sympathectomy by an open approach or by thoracoscopy and laparoscopy can improve resting pain and healing of superficial ischemic ulcers. The results are better in more distal arterial obstructions. There is no indication for sympathectomy in cases of plantar claudication or extensive gangrene of the hand and foot (Fig. 12.10) [16, 33, 75, 76].

Surgical revascularization is still an option when good results have not been achieved by medical treatment and the patient has pain at rest and/or ulcerations. Preoperatively, angiography is the ideal examination for planning surgery. Angiography is used to find at least one accessible distal vessel, which is not a frequent disease characteristic, and its distal location. If there is an accessible distal artery, a revascularization procedure should be performed, preferably using the saphenous vein (Fig. 12.11). Despite arterial revascularization, patients with TAO have a mean patency of 20 % at 24 months, and the rate of limb salvage is considerable [18, 28, 50, 51, 53].

When the treatment options have been exhausted in case of unbearable pain at rest, carrying out neurotripsy may be advisable, which consists of crushing the nerves responsible

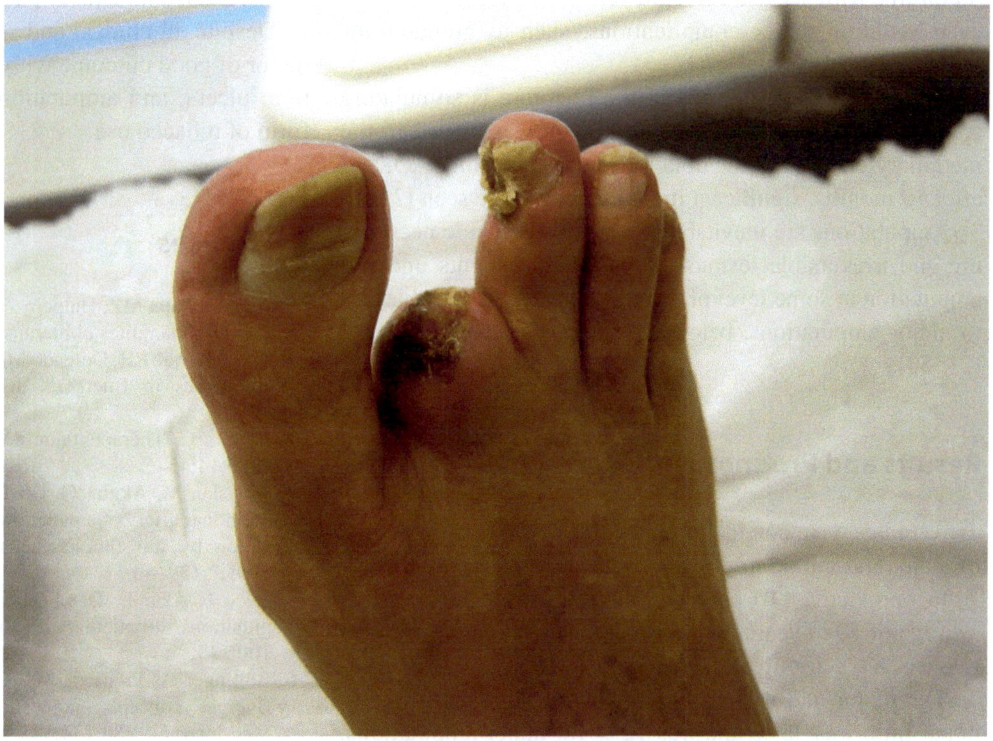

Fig. 12.10 Female patient with good healing after lumbar sympathectomy

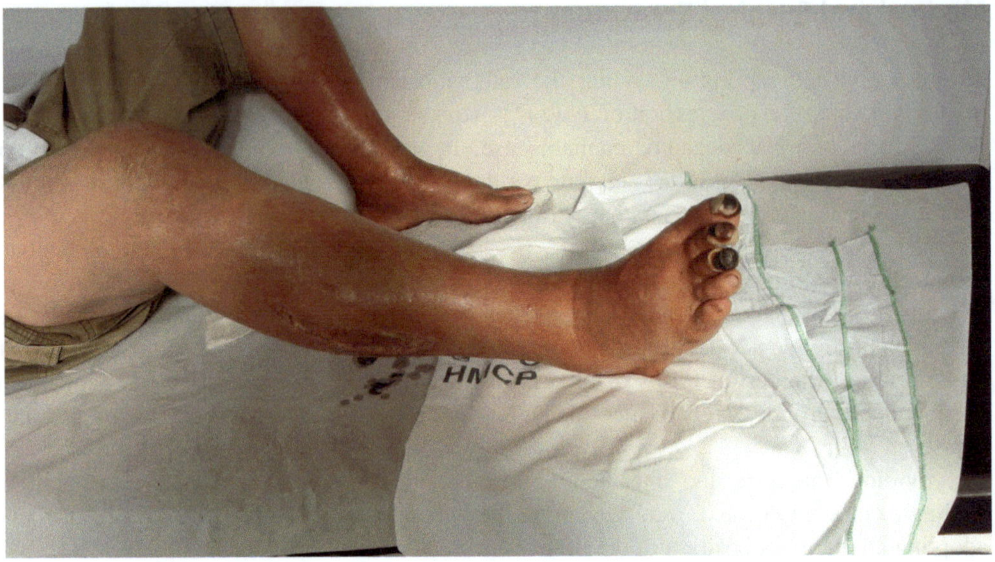

Fig. 12.11 Patient with femorofibular recanalization

for sensory innervation of the affected limb with subsequent anestesia in this segment, resulting in a better general condition and quality of life for the patient.

Neurotripsy can be performed selectively according to the injury site, although crushing of five nerves is recommended when it is performed in the foot: the tibial, superficial peroneal, deep peroneal, sural, and saphenous nerves, with the possibility of functional restoration in 6 months [52].

When medical treatment does not present clinical success and there is no possibility of surgical revascularization, implantable spinal cord stimulators can be used. There have been several successful reports concerning this in the literature, with its use for pain relief, healing ulcers, and even avoiding major complications, such as amputations [10, 63, 73, 74].

Another method reported in the literature is stimulating angiogenesis, in which a Kirschner wire was placed in the medullary channel of the tibia in six patients with TAO, and after 19 months, significant improvements were seen [29].

Amputations are inevitable in cases of ischemic necrotizing and irreversible lesions. About 20 % patients undergo amputation at some level of the foot, and 20 % are subjected to major amputations, below the knee or at the thigh level [23, 50].

Results and Prognosis

Two studies were conducted evaluating the long-term results of major and minor amputations and patient survival.

In one study, 110 patients with TAO were followed an average of 10 ½ years. In this study, the cumulative survival rate was 84 % for up to 25 years.

The major and minor amputations rate for the lower or upper limb was 43 % and was 12 % for major amputations. Patients who quit smoking did not undergo major amputations, and 19 % patients who continued smoking underwent major amputations [56].

In another study, 111 patients were followed for an average of 15 years with a major amputation rate of 11 % in 5 years, 21 % in 10 years, and 23 % in 20 years. The risk of amputation was maintained in patients who did not stop smoking, and in patients who did stop, the risk was reduced after 8 years. This study also demonstrated a decreased life expectancy in patients with TAO to a mean age of 52 years [11].

The patient profile of TAO is currently changing, with increasingly frequent involvement of the upper limbs and more female and elderly patients.

Despite all clinical and surgical treatments, the only predictor of good outcome with no symptoms, such as claudication, ulcers, and amputations, is absolute cessation of any form of tobacco use.

References

1. Adar R, Papa MZ, Halpern Z, et al. Cellular sensitivity to collagen in thromboangiites obliterans. N Engl J Med. 1983;308:1113–6.
2. Albuquerque RR, Delgado ML, Correia P, et al. Circulating immune complexes in Buerger's disease. J Cardiovasc Surg. 1989;30:821–3.
3. Allegra C. Therapeutique de la maladie de Buerger. J Mal Vasc. 1989;14:45–6.
4. Alpaslan M, Akgun G, Doven O, Oral D. Thrombus in the main pulmonar artery of a patient with thromboangiitis obliterans: observation by transthoracic echocardiography. Eur J Echocardiogr. 2001;2:139–40.
5. Avcu F, Akar E, Demirkiliç U, et al. The role of prothrombotic mutations in patients with Buerger's disease. Thromb Res. 2000;100:143.
6. Bollinger A, Piquerez MJ, Largiarder J, Scneider E. Maladie de Buerger: concepts diagnostiques et therapeutiques actueels. Ann Med Interne. 1983;134:436–40.

7. Cakmak A, Gyedu A, Akyol C, et al. Occlusion of the celiac trunk, the inferior mesenteric artery and stenosis of the superior mesenteric artery in peripheral thromboangiitis obliterans. Vasa. 2009; 38:394.
8. Caramaschi P, Biasi D, Carletto A, et al. Three cases of Buerger's disease associated with hyperhomocysteinemia. Clin Exp Rheumatol. 2000;18:264–5.
9. Chen YW, Nagasawa T, Wara-Aswapati N, et al. Association between periodontitis and anti-cardiolipin antibodies in Buerger disease. J Clin Periodontol. 2009;36:83.
10. Chierichetti F, Mambrini S, Bagliani A, Odero A. Treatment of Buerger's disease with electrical spinal cord simulations: review of three cases. Angiology. 2002;53:341–7.
11. Cooper LT, Tse TS, Mikhail MA, et al. Long-term survival and amputation risk in thromboangiitis obliterans (Buerger's disease). J Am Coll Cardiol. 2004;44:2410.
12. Corelli F. Buerger's disease: cigarette smoker disease may always be cured by medical therapy alone: uselessness of operative treatment. J Cardiovasc Surg (Torino). 1973;14:28–36.
13. Cupps TR, Fauci AS. The vasculitides. In: Lloyd H, Smith Jr MD, editors. Major problems in internal medicine, vol. XXI. Philadelphia: Saunders; 1981. p. 133–41.
14. Dean SM, Satiani B. Three cases of digital ischemia successfully treated with cilostazol. Vasc Med. 2001;6:245–8.
15. Dean SM, Vaccaro PS. Successful pharmacologic treatment of lower extremity ulcerations in 5 patients with chronic critical limb ischemia. J Am Board Fam Pract. 2002;15:55–62.
16. De Giacomo T, Rendina EA, Venuta F, et al. Thoracoscopic sympathectomy for symptomatic arterial obstruction of the upper extremities. Ann Thorac Surg. 2002;74:885–8.
17. Dible JH. The pathology of limb ischemia. Edinburgh: Oliver & Boyd; 1966.
18. Dilege S, Aksoy M, Kayabali M, et al. Vascular reconstruction in Buerger's disease: is it feasible? Surg Today. 2002;32:1042–7.
19. Disdier P, Granel B, Serratrice J, et al. Cannabis arteritis revisited: ten new case reports. Angiology. 2001;52:1–5.
20. Donatelli F, Triggiani M, Nascimbene S, et al. Thromboangiitis obliterans of coronary and internal thoracic arteries in a young woman. J Thorac Cardiovasc Surg. 1997;113:800.
21. Ehrenfeld M, Adar R. Rheumatic manifestations in patients with thromboangiitis obliterans (Buerger's disease). J Rheumatol. 2000; 27:1818–9.
22. Eichhorn J, Sima D, Lindschau C, et al. Antiendothelial cell antibodies in thromboangiitis obliterans. Am J Med Sci. 1998;315:17.
23. Grove WJ, Stansby GP. Buerger's disease and cigarette smoking in Bangladesh. Ann R Coll Surg Engl. 1992;74:115.
24. Gulati SM, Madhra K, Thusoo TK, Nair SK, Saha K. Autoantibodies in thromboangiitis obliterans (Buerger's diseas). Angiology. 1982;33:642–51.
25. Gulati SM, Saha K, Argawal V, Thusoo TK, Mehdiratta KS. Profile of non-organ specific autoantibodies in thromboangiitis obliterans. Indian J Med Res. 1984;80:228–31.
26. Gulati SM, Saha K, Kant L, Thusoo TK, Prakash A. Significance of circulatory immune complexes in thromboangiitis obliterans (Buerger's disease). Angiology. 1984;35:276–81.
27. Harten P, Muller-Huelsbeck S, Regensburger D, Loeffler H. Multiple organ manifestations in thromboangiitis obliterans (Buerger's disease): a case report. Angiology. 1996;47:419–25.
28. Inada K, Iwashima Y, Okada A, Matsumoto K. Nonatherosclerotic segmental arterial occlusion of the extremity. Arch Surg. 1974; 108:663–7.
29. Inan M, Alat I, Kutlu R, et al. Successful treatment of Buerger's disease with intramedullary K-wire: the results of the first 11 extremities. Eur J Vasc Endovasc Surg. 2005;29:277.
30. Iwai T, Inoue Y, Umeda M, et al. Oral bacteria in the occluded arteries of patients with Buerger disease. J Vasc Surg. 2005;42:107.
31. Joras M, Poredos P, Fras Z. Endothelial dysfunction in Buerger's disease and its relation to markers of inflammation. Eur J Clin Invest. 2006;36:376.
32. Joyce JW. Buerger's disease (thromboangiitis obliterans. Rheum Dis Clin North Am. 1990;16:463–70.
33. Kauffman P. Simpatectomias. In: Raia AA, Zerbini EJ, editors. Clinica Cirurgica Alipio Correa Netto, vol. 2°. 4ª ed. Sao Paulo: Sarvier; 1998. p. 84–101.
34. Kobayashi M, Ito M, Nakagawa A, et al. Immunohistochemical analysis of arterial wall cellular infiltration in Bueger's disease (endarteritis obliterans). J Vasc Surg. 1999;29:451–8.
35. Krasznai A, Krajesi P, Aranyi P, Horvath I. Glucocorticoid receptors in thromboangiitis obliterans. Int J Clin Pharmacol Ther Toxicol. 1987;25:363–5.
36. Kurata A, Nonaka T, Arimura Y, et al. Multiple ulcers with perforation of the small intestine in Buerger's disease: a case report. Gastroenterology. 2003;125:911.
37. Laohapensang K, Rerkasem K, Kattipattanapong V. Seasonal variation of Buerger's disease in Northern part of Thailand. Eur J Vasc Endovasc Surg. 2004;28:418.
38. Leu HJ, Bollinger A. Phlebitis saltans sive migrans. Vasa. 1978; 7:440–2.
39. Leu HJ. Early inflammatory changes in thromboangiitis obliterans. Pathol Microbiol (Basel). 1975;432:151–6.
40. Lie JT. Buerger's disease and inflammatory aspects of atherosclerosis. Curr Opin Rheumatol. 1990;2:76–80.
41. Lie JT. Diagnostic histopathology of major systemic and pulmonar vasculitis syndromes. Rheum Dis Clin North Am. 1990;16:269–92.
42. Lie JT. The rise and fall and resurgence of thromboangiitis obliterans (Buerger's disease). Acta Pathol Jpn. 1989;39:153.
43. Lie JT. Thromboangiitis obliterans (Buerger's disease) and smokeless tobacco. Arthritis Rheum. 1988;316:812–3.
44. Lie JT, Michet Jr CJ. Thromboangiitis obliterans with eosinophilia (Buerger's disease) of the temporal arteries. Hum Pathol. 1988;19: 598–602.
45. Makita S, Nakamura M, Murakami H, et al. Impaired endothelium-dependent vasorelaxation in peripheral vasculature of patients with thromboangiitis obliterans (Buerger's disease). Circulation. 1996;94(Suppl):II211–5.
46. Maslowski L, McBane R, Alexewicz P, Wysokinski WE. Antiphospholipid antibodies in thromboangiitis obliterans. Vasc Med. 2002;7:259–64.
47. Matsushita M, Shionoya S, Matsumoto T. Urinary cotinine measurement in patients with Buerger's disease – effects of active and passive smoking on the disease process. J Vasc Surg. 1991;14: 53–8.
48. Melian EB, Goa KL. Beraprost: a review of its pharmacology and therapeutic efficacy in the treatment of peripheral arterial disease and pulmonar arterial hypertension. Drugs. 2002;62:107–33.
49. Michail PO, Filis KA, Delladetsima JK, et al. Thromboangiitis obliterans (Buerger's disease) in visceral vessels confirmed by angiographic and histological findings. Eur J Vasc Endovasc Surg. 1998;16:445.
50. Mills JL, Porter JM. Buerger's disease: a review and update. Semin Vasc Surg. 1993;6:14–23.
51. Mills JL, Porter JM. Buerger's disease (thromboangiitis obliterans). Ann Vasc Surg. 1991;5:570–2.
52. Muraco Neto B. Neurotripsia. Tratamento da dor isquêmica de repouso nas extremidades inferiores. In: Raia AA, Zerbini EJ, editors. Clinica Cirurgica Alipio Correa Netto, vol. 2°. 4ª ed. Sao Paulo: Sarvier; 1998. p. 102–6.
53. Nishikimi N. Fate of limbs with failed vascular reconstruction in Buerger's disease patients. Int J Cardiol. 2000;75(Suppl I):S183–5.
54. Nishikimi N, Shionoya S, Mizuno S. Result of national epidemiological study of Buerger's disease. J Jpn Coll Angiol. 1987;27: 1125–30.

55. Noel B. Cocaine and arsenic induced Raynaud's phenomenon. Clin Rheumatol. 2002;21:343–4.
56. Ohta T, Ishioashi H, Hosaka M, Sugimoto I. Clinical and social consequences of Buerger disease. J Vasc Surg. 2004;39:176.
57. Olin JW. Are anticardiolipin antibodies really importante in thromboangiitis obliterans (Bueger's disease)? Vasc Med. 2002;7:257–8.
58. Olin JW. Thromboangiitis obliterans (Buerger's disease). N Engl J Med. 2000;343:864–9.
59. Olin JW. Thromboangiitis obliterans (Buerger's disease). In: Rhutherford RB, editor. Vascular surgery. 6th ed. New York: Elsevier Inc; 2007. p. 404–16.
60. Olin JW, Childs MB, Bartholomew JR, et al. Anticardiolipin antibodies and homocysteine levels in patients with thromboangiitis obliterans. Arthritis Rheum. 1996;39:S-47.
61. Olin JW, Shih A. Thromboangiitis obliterans (Buerger's disease). Curr Opin Rheumatol. 2006;18:18–24.
62. Olin JW, Young JR, Graor RA, et al. The changing clinical spectrum of thromboangiitis obliterans (Buerger's disease). Circulation. 1990;825(Suppl):IV3–8.
63. Pace AV, Saratzis N, Karokis D, et al. Spinal cord simulation in Buerger's disease. Ann Rheum Dis. 2002;61:1114.
64. Papa MZ, Adar R. A critical look at thromboangiitis obliterans (Buerger's disease). Vasc Surg. 1992;5:1–21.
65. Pietraszek MH, Choudhury NA, Koyano K, et al. Enhanced platelet response to serotonina in Buerger's disease. Thromb Res. 1990;60:241–6.
66. Puchmayer V. Smoking as a risk for the development of arterial occlusive disease. Acta Univ Carol Med Monogr (Praha). 1984;105:1.
67. Puechal X, Fiessinger JN, Kahan A, Menkes CJ. Rheumatic manifestations in patients with thromboangiitis obliterans (Buerger's disease). J Rheumatol. 1999;26:1764–8.
68. Roncon-de-Albuquerque R, Delgado L, Correia P, et al. Circulating imune complexes in Buerger's disease: endarteritis obliterans in young men. J Cardiovasc Surg (Torino). 1989;30:821–5.
69. Scarffetter K, Blasius S, Franke RP, Kohler M, Mittermayer C. Pathogenetic key position of thromboangiitis: the endotelial cell. Serum dependente proliferation studies of endotelial cells in obliteratives angiopathies. Vasa. 1986;15:34–7.
70. Stammler F, Diehm C, Hsu E, Stockinger K, Amendt K. Pravalenz der Hyperhomocysteinamic bei der Thromboangiitis obliterans. Spielt Homocystein pathogenetisch eine Rolle? Dtsch Med Wochenschr. 1996;121:1417–23.
71. Shionoya S. Buerger's disease (thromboangiitis obliterans). In: Rutherford RB, editor. Vascular surgery. 3rd ed. Philadelphia: WB Saunders; 1989. p. 207–17.
72. Shionoya S, Ban I, Nakata Y, et al. Involvement of the iliac artery in-Buerger's disease (pathogenesis and arterial reconstruction). J Cardiovasc Surg (Torino). 1978;19:69–76.
73. Swigris JJ, Olin JW, Mekhail NA. Implantable spinal cord stimulator to treat the ischemic manifestations of thromboangiitis obliterans (Buerger's disease). J Vasc Surg. 1999;29:928–35.
74. Taguchi A, Ohtani M, Soma T, et al. Therapeutic angiogenesis by autologous bone-marrow transplantation in a general hospital setting. Eur J Vasc Endovasc Surg. 2003;25:276–8.
75. Tarygin NE, Shilkina NP, Romanov VA, Lileeva MA. The morphological criteria of thromboangiitis and arteriosclerosis obliterans of the vessels of the lower extremities. Ter Arkh. 1990;62:122–6.
76. Watarida S, Shiraishi S, Fujimura M, et al. Laparoscopic lumbar sympathectomy for lower-limb disease. Surg Endosc. 2002;16:500–3.

Inflammatory Markers and Mortality in Critical Lower Limb Ischemia

13

Anders Gottsäter

Overview of Inflammatory Markers in Vascular Disease

In atherosclerotic vascular disease, endothelial dysfunction is induced by risk factors such as arterial hypertension, hypercholesterolemia, and tobacco use. Inflammatory mechanisms and inflammatory cytokines play important roles in all of these mechanisms, and the different steps in atherogenesis involve cytokines as inflammatory promoters, stimulating the expression of proatherogenic genes in endothelial cells [1, 2]. Important cytokines are, for example, tumor necrosis factor α [3], neopterin [4], and interleukin-6 [3, 5]. Expression of the immune mediator CD40 ligand is increased in atherogenesis [6, 7], and prostaglandin-like isoprostanes [8, 9] are markers of lipid peroxidation and believed to contribute to atherosclerosis and thrombosis [10].

Tumor Necrosis Factor-α

TNF-α is a multifunctional proinflammatory cytokine produced in lymphocytes, tissue macrophages, and myocardial and vascular cells [11]. TNF-α mediates proatherogenic processes, leading to altered endothelial function and enhanced expression of leukocyte adhesion molecules, which result in foam cell and fatty streak formation [3].

Interleukin-6

Interleukins are cytokines responsible for signaling between leukocytes. They mediate chemotaxis and proliferation of different cell types in the pathogenesis of atherosclerosis [3]. IL-6 is a cytokine with proinflammatory and proatherogenic activity and is secreted from activated macrophages, fibroblasts, lymphocytes, endothelial cells, and vascular smooth muscle cells [5]. Apparently healthy subjects with high IL-6 levels have increased risk of death and cerebrovascular events compared with those with low levels [12]. There is also a close relationship between concentrations of C-reactive protein (CRP), IL-6, and TNF-α and components of the insulin resistance syndrome [13].

Neopterin

Increased plasma levels of the inflammatory mediator neopterin occur in atherosclerotic patients [4], reflecting increased activity of monocytes and macrophages [4, 14]. Among patients with coronary atherosclerosis, S-neopterin and CRP are both higher in patients with acute coronary syndrome compared to those with stable angina [15]. Furthermore, statin treatment is associated with lower neopterin levels because of its antiinflammatory properties [16].

C-Reactive Protein

CRP is the major acute phase reactant in humans and is mainly synthesized by hepatocytes under control of IL-6, IL-1, and TNF-α, but extrahepatic production of CRP occurs in atherosclerotic plaques [17, 18]. CRP measured with high sensitivity assays (hs-CRP) is a strong, independent predictor of future cardiovascular events [19], such as myocardial infarction, stroke, and peripheral arterial disease (PAD) [12, 20–23].

Isoprostanes

Isoprostanes are end products of lipid peroxidation, and 8-iso-prostaglandin $F_{2\alpha}$ (8-iso-$PGF_{2\alpha}$) is an indicator of

A. Gottsäter, MD, PhD
Department of Clinical Sciences, Vascular Center,
Lund University, Skåne University Hospital,
Södra Förstadsgatan 101, SE-205 02 Malmö, Sweden
e-mail: anders.gottsater@med.lu.se

E.A. Gabriel, S.A. Gabriel (eds.), *Inflammatory Response in Cardiovascular Surgery*,
DOI 10.1007/978-1-4471-4429-8_13, © Springer-Verlag London 2013

oxidative stress [9], inducing platelet activation and smooth muscle cell proliferation and contributing to atherosclerosis and thrombosis [10]. Oxidative stress and lipid peroxidation are involved in the pathophysiology of atherosclerosis, and isoprostane levels are increased in high age, hypercholesterolemia, diabetes mellitus, and smoking [9, 10, 24].

Matrix Metalloproteinases

Matrix metalloproteinases (MMPs), enzymes degrading the extracellular matrix, are other important modulators of atherosclerosis produced by inflammatory cells. MMPs play important roles in remodeling processes, plaque formation and rupture, and aneurysm development [25].

CD40 Ligand/CD40

CD40 ligand (CD40L) is a potent immunomodulator, whereas CD40 is an integral membrane protein [26]. CD40L expressed on T lymphocytes, SMC, and macrophages triggers inflammatory responses, expression of MMPs, adhesion molecules, secretion of proinflammatory cytokines, and chemokines, playing a role in plaque rupture and acute coronary events [6, 27]. Increased levels and enhanced expression of CD40L occur in patients with acute coronary syndromes [27, 28]. Neutralization with anti-CD40L antibody inhibits these actions, and lipid-lowering therapy reduces levels and expression of CD40/CD40L [29].

Inflammatory Markers in Peripheral Arterial Disease and Critical Limb Ischemia

The importance of leukocytes and inflammatory reactions for the pathophysiology of ischemic vascular disease [1, 2] has been studied predominantly in subjects with coronary artery disease (CAD). In peripheral arterial disease (PAD) and critical limb ischemia (CLI), the role of inflammatory markers for pathophysiology is less well studied than in both coronary and precerebral atherosclerosis. Furthermore, the importance of inflammatory reactions may be especially difficult to clarify in CLI, as patients with this condition by definition [30] often have ischemic leg ulcers (Fig. 13.1) featuring inflammatory processes affecting the levels of inflammatory mediators. Circulating levels of inflammatory mediators measured in CLI patients can therefore originate partly from ulcers and gangrene of the ischemic limb and partly from the general atherosclerotic process.

Inflammatory markers have been evaluated among both asymptomatic [31–33] and symptomatic [31–34] subjects with PAD, however (Table 13.1). Furthermore, such markers have also been shown to be related to the future development of PAD and CLI already in subjects without detectable disease. For example, being in the highest quartile of hs-CRP among healthy subjects increases the risk for the development of PAD by a factor of 2.8 [22], and elevated levels of proteins such as fibrinogen, alpha 1-antitrypsin, haptoglobin, ceruloplasmin, and orosomucoid measured in 5,619 healthy men without symptoms suggestive of PAD have been associated with increased risk for the development of PAD requiring revascularization during 16 years of follow-up, even after adjustment for other relevant risk factors [35]. Multisite atherosclerotic disease is also reflected in more intensive inflammatory activity; among 234 patients undergoing coronary angiography, Brevetti and co-workers found that levels of both hs-CRP and IL-6 were higher in patients with both CAD and PAD or CAD alone or than in control subjects without either disease. Furthermore, hs-CRP was higher in patients with both diseases than in those with only CAD [34], indicating a more active inflammatory process in multisite disease.

Oxidative stress, as reflected by increased levels of 8-iso-$PGF_{2\alpha}$, has also been related to PAD. In a study of 100 patients with PAD and 100 control subjects without clinically relevant atherosclerotic disease who were all non-smokers and not taking any lipid-lowering drugs or vitamins to avoid possible effects on isoprostanes, 8-iso-$PGF_{2\alpha}$ levels were 1.5-fold higher among PAD patients than in controls [36]. Symptomatic PAD is also associated with increased levels of both IL-6 and hs-CRP compared with subjects without PAD, even after adjustment for BMI, smoking, and cholesterol [37]. In vitro culturing of whole blood and profiling of the production of several different interleukins and other cytokines confirmed this inflammatory hyperresponsiveness related to associated leukocytosis in PAD patients [38]. Matrix metalloproteinases have also been evaluated in relation to PAD, and increased plasma levels of both MMP-2 and MMP-9 were found to be correlated with development of both PAD and CLI [39]. Genetic studies have also confirmed the above-mentioned connections between inflammatory markers and CLI. Gene polymorphisms related to several markers for inflammation, both cytokines and matrix metalloproteinases, IL-6, E-selectin, ICAM-1, MCP-1, MMP-1, and MMP-3, are all independently associated with PAD, and the different risks for PAD and CLI depend on the number of high-risk genotypes concomitantly carried by the individual subject [40]. Furthermore, the IL-6 gene is upregulated in the hypoperfused musculature of CLI patients [41], corroborating the above-mentioned observation that IL-6 has been found to be increased in symptomatic peripheral artery disease [31]. It is important to note that all study results have not shown uniform results; however, in a small group of eight CLI patients including five with ischemic lesions [42] neither TNF-α nor IL-6 differed from values in healthy controls.

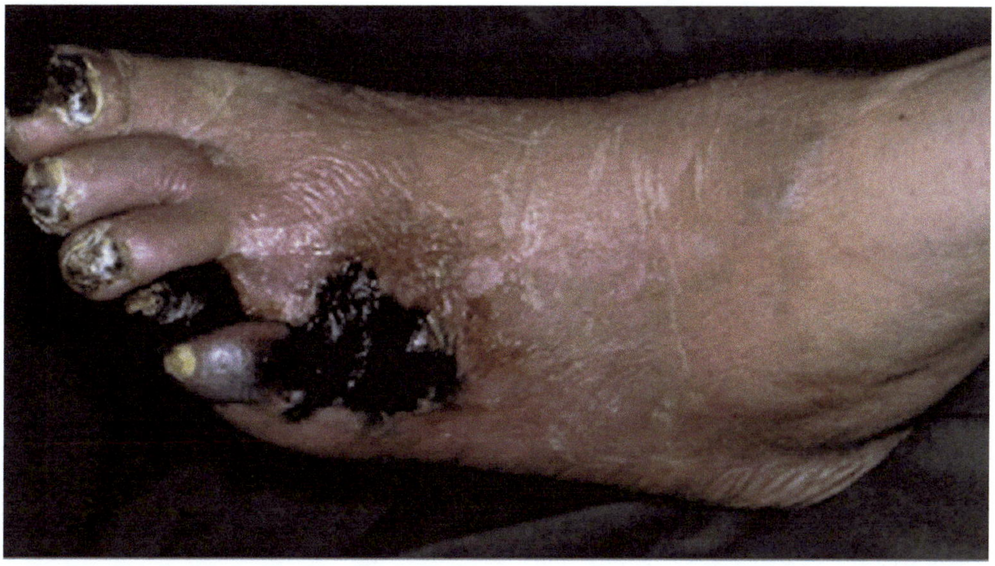

Fig. 13.1 Critical limb ischaemia with forefoot gangrene

Table 13.1 Some different markers and mediators of inflammation associated with peripheral arterial disease (PAD) and critical limb ischemia (CLI) in different studies

Variable	Feature of PAD	References
α_1-Antitrypsin	PAD development	[35]
α-Defensin	PAD severity, cardiovascular mortality in PAD	[52]
Amyloid A	Adverse prognosis after intervention for PAD	[43]
Ceruloplasmin	PAD development	[35]
Fibrinogen	PAD development, mortality in CLI	[35, 43]
Haptoglobin	PAD development	[35]
High sensitivity C-reactive protein	PAD development, occurrence, progression, and severity, adverse prognosis after intervention for PAD, cardiovascular mortality in PAD, mortality in CLI	[22, 34, 37, 43, 51–53]
Interleukin-6	PAD occurrence and progression, mortality in CLI	[31, 34, 37, 41, 51, 53]
8-Isoprostane-$PGF_{2\alpha}$	PAD occurrence	[36]
Leukocyte count	PAD occurrence, mortality in CLI	[54]
Matrix metalloproteinases 2 and 9	PAD and CLI development	[39, 40]
Neopterin	Mortality in CLI	[53]
Neutrophil/lymphocyte ratio	Mortality in CLI	[54]
Orosomucoid	PAD development	[35]
Tumor necrosis factor-α	Mortality in CLI	[53]

Inflammatory Markers During Invasive Treatment of PAD and CLI

Potential relationships between inflammatory markers and invasive treatment of PAD and CLI have also been evaluated (Table 13.1). Different markers such as high sensitivity (hs)-CRP, fibrinogen, and serum amyloid A (SAA) measured preoperatively in patients planned for lower extremity bypass all correlate with an increased risk for later adverse graft-related or cardiovascular events [43]. For hs-CRP, this relationship persisted even in multivariable analysis. In the post-treatment period after both open and endovascular repair in different vascular segments, several of the above-mentioned platelet and leukocyte mechanisms are further activated. Such post-interventional patterns have also mainly been investigated after interventions in coronary vessels, however. For example, levels of P-selectin [44] mediating platelet-leukocyte binding [45] are increased, and leukocyte-platelet interactions are increased after percutaneous coronary interventions [46]. In coronary blood, both expression of the activated platelet fibrinogen receptor [47] and release of chemoattractants affecting neutrophils [48] increase after endovascular coronary interventions. Reports on patterns of inflammatory substances during and after invasive vascular interventions for PAD are scarcer. In an observational study with repeated arterial sampling from 14 patients undergoing angiography for aortoiliac atherosclerotic disease, 9 of whom underwent PTA, we could not demonstrate any definite signs of leukocyte activation during or immediately after peripheral angiography [49]. The levels of inflammatory mediators after peripheral vascular interventions are not clinically irrelevant, however, and the occurrence of restenosis after vascular injury, such as for example an episode of invasive treatment, also has inflammatory features. A postischemic macrophage activation state evaluated in an animal model has been suggested as a new potential therapeutic approach to protect tissues from necrosis and promote tissue repair during CLI [50]. As no definite relationships have been reported between levels of inflammatory mediators and the efficacy of interventions, inflammatory mediators cannot yet be used to determine the best treatment of a certain patient.

Inflammatory Markers, Prognosis, and Mortality in Critical Lower Limb Ischemia

Even if the prognostic importance of inflammatory activation is less well established in PAD and CLI than in patients with coronary or precerebral atherosclerosis, some observations about the relevance of inflammatory activation for prognosis have been presented also in PAD patients (Table 13.1). Elevated levels of inflammatory mediators seem to be indicators of a more severe prognosis concerning both local progression of atherosclerosis in the affected limb and acute events occurring in other vascular territories. The first mechanism is exemplified by the fact that both CRP and IL-6 levels predict local progression of atherosclerosis in the lower limb during 12 year follow-up of the ankle-brachial index (ABI) [51].

A recent investigation showed that patients with CLI show significantly higher α-defensin and hs-CRP levels compared with patients with intermittent claudication (IC) [52]. Furthermore, within the IC group high concentrations of α-defensin and high hs-CRP conferred a five times higher risk for cardiovascular mortality during follow-up than in patients with either high α-defensin or high hs-CRP. The addition of α-defensin or hs-CRP to conventional risk factors thus improved risk prediction concerning cardiovascular mortality in patients with this manifestation of PAD [53].

The high 1-year mortality of around 20–25 % in patients with CLI [7, 21, 22, 52] is mainly due to cardiovascular disease. Furthermore, this already high mortality rate is increased even more in patients with features of inflammation, such as increased leukocyte count and fibrinogen level [23], or an elevated neutrophil/lymphocyte ratio and increased troponin levels [54]. The inflammatory mediators IL-6, TNFα, neopterin, and hs-CRP have also been associated with 1-year mortality in subjects with CLI [53]. For TNFα and neopterin, this association was independent of other variables, such as age, sex, gangrene, lipid-lowering therapy, leukocyte count, renal function, and HDL cholesterol. As the relationships between inflammatory mediators and mortality persisted after exclusion of patients with gangrene, these relationships may only partly be explained by the fact that patients with inflammatory processes such as gangrene of the extremities showed a high mortality [53]. Furthermore, when the patient material was later analyzed concerning 5- and 10-year mortality, the predictive value of TNFα at diagnosis persisted (Fig. 13.2). Data are partly conflicting, however, as no associations were found among α-defensin, hs-CRP, and mortality in CLI patients in the above-mentioned study by Urbonaviciene and co-workers [52].

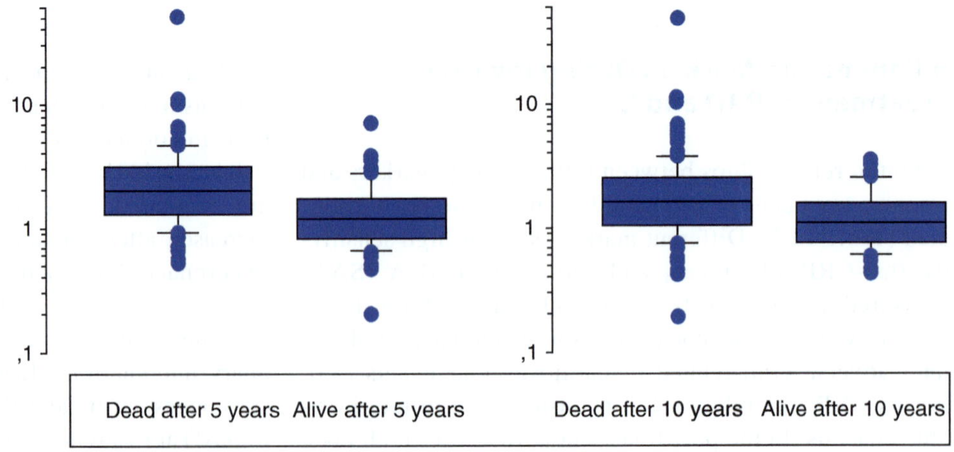

Fig. 13.2 Tumor necrosis factor-α (pg/ml, *y*-axis) at diagnosis in 259 patients [53] with critical limb ischaemia in relationship to 5- (*left panel*, $p<0.001$) and 10- (*right panel*, $p<0.001$) year survival

Conclusions

In conclusion, low-grade inflammatory activation predicts the development of PAD already in healthy subjects. The degree of such inflammatory activation is related to both the severity and progression of disease and to cardiovascular mortality in PAD patients. No definite relationships have yet been reported between levels of inflammatory mediators and the efficacy of interventions, and inflammatory mediators cannot yet be used to determine the best treatment for the individual patient.

References

1. Ross R. Atherosclerosis—an inflammatory disease. N Engl J Med. 1999;340:115–26.
2. Libby P, Ridker PM, Maseri A. Inflammation and atherosclerosis. Circulation. 2002;105:1135–43.
3. Young JL, Libby P, Schönbeck U. Cytokines in the pathogenesis of atherosclerosis. Thromb Haemost. 2002;88:554–67.
4. Tatzber F, Rabl H, Koriska K, Erhart U, Puhl H, Waeg G, et al. Elevated serum neopterin levels in atherosclerosis. Atherosclerosis. 1991;89:203–8.
5. Kishimoto T. The biology of interleukin-6. Blood. 1989;74:1–10.
6. Schönbeck U, Libby P. CD40 signaling and plaque instability. Circ Res. 2001;89:1092–103.
7. Schönbeck U, Gerdes N, Varo N, Reynolds RS, Horton DB, Bavendiek U, et al. Oxidized low-density lipoprotein augments and 3-hydroxy-methylglutaryl coenzyme A reductase inhibitors limit CD40 and CD40L expression in human vascular cells. Circulation. 2002;106:2888–93.
8. Ikeda U, Yamamoto K, Maeda Y, Shimpo M, Kanbe T, Shimada K. Endothelin-1 inhibits nitric oxide synthesis in vascular smooth muscle cells. Hypertension. 1997;29:65–9.
9. Davì G, Ciabattoni G, Consoli A, Mezzetti A, Falco A, Santarone S, et al. In vivo formation of 8-iso-prostaglandin F2α and platelet activation in diabetes mellitus; effects of improved metabolic control and vitamin E supplementation. Circulation. 1999;99:224–9.
10. Patrono C, Fitzgerald GA. Isoprostanes: potential markers of oxidant stress in atherothrombotic disease. Arterioscler Thromb Vasc Biol. 1997;17:2309–15.
11. Sack M. Tumor necrosis factor-alpha in cardiovascular biology and the potential role for anti-tumor necrosis factor-alpha therapy in heart disease. Pharmacol Ther. 2002;94:123–35.
12. Rattazzi M, Puato M, Faggin E, et al. C-reactive protein and interleukin-6 in vascular disease: culprits or passive bystanders? J Hypertens. 2003;21:1787–803.
13. Yudkin JS, Kumari M, Humphries SE, et al. Inflammation, obesity, stress and coronary heart disease: is interleukin-6 the link? Atherosclerosis. 2000;148:209–14.
14. Fuchs D, Hausen A, Reibnegger G, et al. Neopterin as a marker for cell-mediated immunity. Immunol Today. 1988;9:150–5.
15. Ilhan F, Akbulut H, Karaca I, et al. Procalcitonin, C-reactive protein and neopterin levels in patients with coronary atherosclerosis. Acta Cardiol. 2005;60:361–5.
16. Walter RB, Fuchs D, Weiss G, et al. HMG-CoA reductase inhibitors are associated with decreased serum neopterin levels in stable coronary artery disease. Clin Chem Lab Med. 2003;41:1314–9.
17. Yasojima K, Schwab C, McGeer EG, et al. Generation of C-reactive protein and complement components in atherosclerotic plaques. Am J Pathol. 2001;158:1039–51.
18. Calabro P, Willerson JT, Yeh ET. Inflammatory cytokines stimulated C-reactive protein production by human coronary artery smooth muscle cells. Circulation. 2003;108:1930–2.
19. Labarrere CA, Zaloga GP, et al. C-reactive protein: from innocent bystander to pivotal mediator of atherosclerosis. Am J Med. 2004; 117:499–507.
20. Danesh J, Whincup P, Walker M, et al. Low grade inflammation and coronary heart disease: prospective study and updated meta-analyses. BMJ. 2000;321:199–204.
21. Ridker PM, Hennekens CH, Buring JE, et al. C-reactive protein and other markers of inflammation in the prediction of cardiovascular disease in women. N Engl J Med. 2000;342:836–43.
22. Ridker PM, Stampfer MJ, Rifai N. Novel risk factors for systemic atherosclerosis: a comparison of C-reactive protein, fibrinogen, homocysteine, lipoprotein(a), and standard cholesterol screening as predictors of peripheral arterial disease. JAMA. 2001;285:2481–5.
23. Bassuk SS, Rifai N, Ridker PM. High-sensitivity C-reactive protein: clinical importance. Curr Probl Cardiol. 2004;29:439–93.
24. Gopaul NK, Änggård EE, Mallet AI, et al. Plasma 8-epi-$PGF_{2\alpha}$ levels are elevated in individuals with non-insulin dependent diabetes mellitus. FEBS Lett. 1995;368:225–9.
25. Raffetto JD, Khalil RA. Matrix metalloproteinases and their inhibitors in vascular remodeling and vascular disease. Biochem Pharmacol. 2008;75:346–59.
26. Mach F, Schönbeck U, Bonnefoy JY, et al. Activation of monocyte/macrophage functions related to acute atheroma complication by ligation of CD40: induction of collagenase, stromelysin, and tissue factor. Circulation. 1997;96:396–9.
27. Garlichs CD, Eskafi S, Raaz D, et al. Patients with acute coronary syndromes express enhanced CD40 ligand/CD154 on platelets. Heart. 2001;86:649–55.
28. Aukrust P, Muller F, Ueland T, et al. Enhanced levels of soluble and membrane-bound CD40 ligand in patients with unstable angina. Possible reflection of T lymphocyte and platelet involvement in the pathogenesis of acute coronary syndromes. Circulation. 1999;100: 614–20.
29. Anand SX, Viles-Gonzalez JF, Badimon JJ, et al. Membrane-associated CD40L and sCD40L in atherothrombotic disease. Thromb Haemost. 2003;90:377–84.
30. Norgren L, Hiatt W, Dormandy J, et al. Inter-Society Consensus for the Management of Peripheral Arterial Disease (TASC II). J Vasc Surg. 2007;45 Suppl 1:S5–67.
31. Silvestro A, Scopacasa F, Ruocco A, et al. Inflammatory status and endothelial function in asymptomatic and symptomatic peripheral arterial disease. Vasc Med. 2003;8:225–32.
32. Pradhan AD, Rifai N, Ridker PM. Soluble intercellular adhesion molecule-1, soluble vascular adhesion molecule-1, and the development of symptomatic peripheral arterial disease in men. Circulation. 2002;106:820–5.
33. McDermott MM, Green D, Greenland P, et al. Relation of levels of hemostatic factors and inflammatory markers to the ankle brachial index. Am J Cardiol. 2003;92:194–9.
34. Brevetti G, Silvestro A, Di Giacomo S, et al. Endothelial dysfunction in peripheral arterial disease is related to increase in plasma markers of inflammation and severity of peripheral circulatory impairment but not to classic risk factors and atherosclerotic burden. J Vasc Surg. 2003;38:374–9.
35. Engström G, Site-Flondell D, Lindblad B, et al. Risk of treatment of peripheral arterial disease is related to inflammation-sensitive plasma proteins: a prospective cohort study. J Vasc Surg. 2004; 40:1101–5.

36. Mueller T, Dieplinger B, Gegenhuber A, et al. Serum total 8-iso-prostaglandin F2alpha: a new and independent predictor of peripheral arterial disease. J Vasc Surg. 2004;40:768–73.
37. McDermott MM, Guralnik JM, Corsi A, et al. Patterns of inflammation associated with peripheral arterial disease: the InCHIANTI study. Am Heart J. 2005;150:276–81.
38. Chaparala RP, Orsi NM, Lindsey NJ, Girn RS, Homer-Vanniasinkam S. Inflammatory profiling of peripheral arterial disease. Ann Vasc Surg. 2009;23:172–8.
39. Busti C, Falcinelli E, Momi S, Gresele P. Matrix metalloproteinases and peripheral arterial disease. Intern Emerg Med. 2010;5:13–25.
40. Flex A, Gaetani E, Angelini F, et al. Pro-inflammatory genetic profiles in subjects with peripheral arterial occlusive disease and critical limb ischemia. J Intern Med. 2007;262:124–30.
41. Testa M, DeRuvo E, Russo A, et al. Induction of interleukin-1beta and interleukin-6 gene expression in hypoperfused skeletal muscle of patients with peripheral arterial disease. Ital Heart J. 2000;1:64–7.
42. Fiotti N, Giansante C, Ponte E, et al. Atherosclerosis and inflammation. Patterns of cytokine regulation in patients with peripheral arterial disease. Atherosclerosis. 1999;145:51–60.
43. Owens CD, Ridker PM, Belkin M. Elevated C-reactive protein levels are associated with postoperative events in patients undergoing lower extremity vein bypass surgery. J Vasc Surg. 2007;45:2–9.
44. Warzok F, Steiner M, Blann AD, et al. Immediate and late effects of coronary angiography on soluble endothelial cell markers and P-selectin in patients with and without coronary artery disease. Blood Coagul Fibrinolysis. 1999;10:381–7.
45. Furman M, Benoit S, Barnard M, et al. Increased platelet reactivity and circulating monocyte-platelet aggregates in patients with stable coronary artery disease. J Am Coll Cardiol. 1998;31:352–8.
46. Mickelson J, Lakkis N, Villarreallevy G, et al. Leukocyte activation with platelet adhesion after coronary angioplasty: a mechanism for recurrent disease? J Am Coll Cardiol. 1996;28:345–53.
47. Neumann I, Ott M, Gawaz G, et al. Neutrophil and platelet activation at baloon-injured coronary artery plaque in patients undergoing angioplasty. J Am Coll Cardiol. 1996;27:819–24.
48. Neumann F-J, Richardt G, Schneider M, et al. Cardiac release of chemoattractants after ischaemia induced by coronary baloon angioplasty. Br Heart J. 1993;70:27–34.
49. Barani J, Gottsäter A, Mattiasson I, et al. Platelet and leukocyte activation during aortoiliac angiography and angioplasty. Eur J Vasc Endovasc Surg. 2002;23:220–5.
50. Bréchot N, Gomez E, Bignon M, et al. Modulation of macrophage activation state protects tissue from necrosis during critical limb ischemia in thrombospondin-1-deficient mice. PLoS One. 2008; 3:e3950.
51. Tzoulaki I, Murray GD, Lee AJ, et al. C-reactive protein, interleukin-6, and soluble adhesion molecules as predictors of progressive peripheral atherosclerosis in the general population. Edinburgh Artery Study. Circulation. 2005;112:976–83.
52. Urbonaviciene G, Frystyk J, Flyvbjerg A, et al. Markers of inflammation in relation to long-term cardiovascular mortality in patients with lower-extremity peripheral arterial disease. Int J Cardiol. 2011;160(2):89–94.
53. Barani J, Nilsson JÅ, Mattiasson I, Lindblad B, et al. Inflammatory mediators are associated with 1-year mortality in critical limb ischemia. J Vasc Surg. 2005;42:75–80.
54. Spark JI, Sarveswaran J, Blest N, et al. An elevated neutrophil-lymphocyte ratio independently predicts mortality in chronic critical limb ischemia. J Vasc Surg. 2010;52:632–6.

Arterial Wall Remodeling and Restenosis Following Vascular Reconstruction

14

Xue Ma and Randolph L. Geary

Simply defined, restenosis is a new lumen narrowing at the site of a previous vascular reconstruction. Restenosis has been a major limitation of surgical and endovascular reconstructions since their inception, and while decades of research have yielded vastly improved results for percutaneous coronary interventions, strategies to eliminate restenosis remain elusive. Increased application of endovascular therapy to extracoronary beds has been met with sobering rates of late failures. This persistence of the problem reflects our incomplete understanding of its complex pathogenesis, and further research and novel approaches to prevention are needed before the full potential of interventions can be realized.

This chapter reviews the scope and progression of the clinical problem, the two primary structural mechanisms that contribute to restenosis, and their cellular and molecular pathogenesis.

Scope of the Problem

After the introduction of coronary angioplasty in the 1970s, widespread application was tempered by rates of restenosis as high as 60 % within 2 years (Table 14.1) [1–28]. Patients often returned with recurrent angina 3–9 months after percutaneous coronary intervention (PCI), leading to expensive and more complex repeat procedures with increased morbidity [29–31]. This prompted major investments in research to develop pharmacological inhibitors of restenosis, but drugs effective in small animal models of balloon injury failed repeatedly to reduce angioplasty restenosis in randomized clinical trials [32, 33]. In fact, the only systemic drugs that have improved PCI outcomes consistently are the antithrombotic agents (e.g., platelet IIb and IIIa antagonists and clopidogrel), largely by inhibiting thrombosis rather than restenosis per se [34].

Parallel advances in device technology also met with mixed results. The first major breakthrough came in the late 1980s with the introduction of the bare metal stent (BMS). BMSs countered elastic recoil and vasospasm that acutely decrease lumen diameter after angioplasty by 10–30 % [1, 2]. Stents were designed to hold lumen dimensions to those achieved at peak balloon inflation by providing radial strength in excess of inward radial forces exerted by the surrounding vessel wall. This strategy worked, but the greatest impact of BMSs has subsequently been recognized to be prevention of chronic arterial wall recoil, known as geometric remodeling of the healing vessel wall, as will be discussed below. Landmark PCI trials comparing BMSs to angioplasty reduced absolute and relative restenosis by 10 and 30 %, respectively [1, 2]. BMSs also improved PCI for chronic total occlusions, vein graft stenosis, and acute myocardial infarction. Nonetheless, restensosis after BMS remains unacceptably high at 15–32 % [1, 2].

Another decade passed before the next major advance, a period when exciting new approaches were embraced only to fade after disappointing results in randomized trials (e.g., atherectomy, gene therapy, and brachytherapy) [12, 13]. Drug-eluting stents (DESs) then emerged with startling results in phase I trials, reporting near 0 % restenosis with sirolimus-eluting stents [9]. Subsequent trials in less selective "real-world" populations have yielded slightly less favorable results in PCI, but after a decade of iterative refinement (e.g., new drugs and stent coatings), restenosis after DES is in the range of 5–15 %, a significant improvement over BMSs [4]. Other trials have showed that DESs are superior to angioplasty in treating the difficult problem of in-stent restenosis [35].

Restenosis in extracoronary vascular beds has received more attention in recent years, and rightly so, as the numbers of failures at these sites can be remarkably high,

X. Ma, MD • R.L. Geary, MD, FACS (✉)
Department of Vascular and Endovascular Surgery, Wake Forest University School of Medicine, Winston-Salem, NC 27104, USA

Department of Pathology, Section on Comparative Medicine, Wake Forest University School of Medicine, Winston-Salem, NC, USA
e-mail: rgeary@wakehealth.edu

E.A. Gabriel, S.A. Gabriel (eds.), *Inflammatory Response in Cardiovascular Surgery*,
DOI 10.1007/978-1-4471-4429-8_14, © Springer-Verlag London 2013

Table 14.1 Representative restenosis rates by location and intervention

Location	Procedure	Restenosis (%)	References
Coronary	PTA	21–55	[1–3]
Coronary	BMS	16–44	[1–3]
Coronary	DES	10	[4–11]
Coronary	Atherectomy	27–39	[12, 13]
Renal	PTA	26–100	[14]
Renal	BMS	17–60	[14–16]
Renal	DES	18	[16]
Iliac	PTA	22–34	[16]
Iliac	BMS	10–26	[16]
Femoral popliteal	PTA	39–62	[17–20]
Femoral popliteal	BMS	34–47	[17–20]
Femoral popliteal	DES	44	[21]
Femoral popliteal	Covered stent	37	[22]
Carotid	Endarterectomy	1.7–9.3	[23–25]
Carotid	BMS	2.7–21	[24, 25]
Mesenteric celiac	PTA	36–64	[26–28]
Mesenteric celiac	BMS	40	[25–28]

PTA percutaneous transluminal angioplasty, *BMS* bare metal stent, *DES* drug-eluting stent

particularly for atherosclerotic lesions in the extremities (Table 14.1). For example, carotid revascularization carries a relatively low (~6 %) risk of clinically significant restenosis (>70 % diameter stenosis) for both endarterectomy and stenting according to recent data from CREST (Lal et al. [36] International Stroke Conference 2012, New Orleans, LA). Much higher rates have been reported in endarterectomy trials using 50 % stenosis as the criteria for failure. Restenosis after renal angioplasty for atherosclerosis is so common that virtually all renal interventions done now employ primary stenting [14]. A meta-analysis of renal stenting by Leertouwer [14] found a mean rate of in-stent restenosis of 17 %, but late failures are probably much more common (Table 14.1). Large prospective renal stent trials have recently been completed, so the durability of BMSs will soon be characterized more accurately (e.g., ASTRAL and CORAL).

Treatment of infrainguinal peripheral artery disease is rapidly expanding as devices specifically tailored to the extremities are being developed and public awareness is increasing. However, the promise of less invasive options to replace high-risk open surgery has been slowed by rates of restenosis that often exceed 50 % at 2 years (Table 14.1). Moreover, the gains for the BMS and DES achieved in PCI have been far less consistent beyond the first few months in the lower extremities (Table 14.1) [37].

Incremental improvements from better patient and lesion selection, enhanced anticoagulation and anti-platelet agents, and improved devices and imaging have each helped reduce restenosis, but despite these advances, millions of persons are affected worldwide at an estimated cost for repeat interventions measured in the billions of healthcare dollars [38].

Structural Basis of Recurrent Lumen Narrowing

Despite the steady push to reduce the invasiveness of vascular reconstruction, virtually all methods are still mechanical in nature and cause trauma to the treated vessel wall, no matter how carefully applied. Surgery (bypass and endarterectomy) and endovascular approaches (angioplasty, atherectomy, and stenting) all injure the vessel wall, and the response to injury and subsequent healing are the common thread in the pathogenesis of restenosis.

Vessel wall trauma creates a thrombogenic lumen surface by denuding the protective endothelium, fracturing inelastic atherosclerotic plaque, and often wounding deep into the surrounding tunica media and adventitia (Fig. 14.1). This induces acute platelet and leukocyte adhesion and direct destruction of resident smooth muscle cells (SMC) and extracellular matrix (ECM), setting into motion a proliferative wound-healing response (termed "intimal hyperplasia") that is generally proportional to the extent of injury. Accumulation of new cells and ECM at sites of injury forms a "neointima" layer at the vessel lumen surface, a feature common to virtually all forms of reconstruction and one of two major factors contributing to recurrent lumen encroachment (Figs. 14.1, 14.2, and 14.3).

This observation led to an intense focus on the molecular and cellular regulation of vascular SMC growth and migration and ECM production and regrowth of a protective

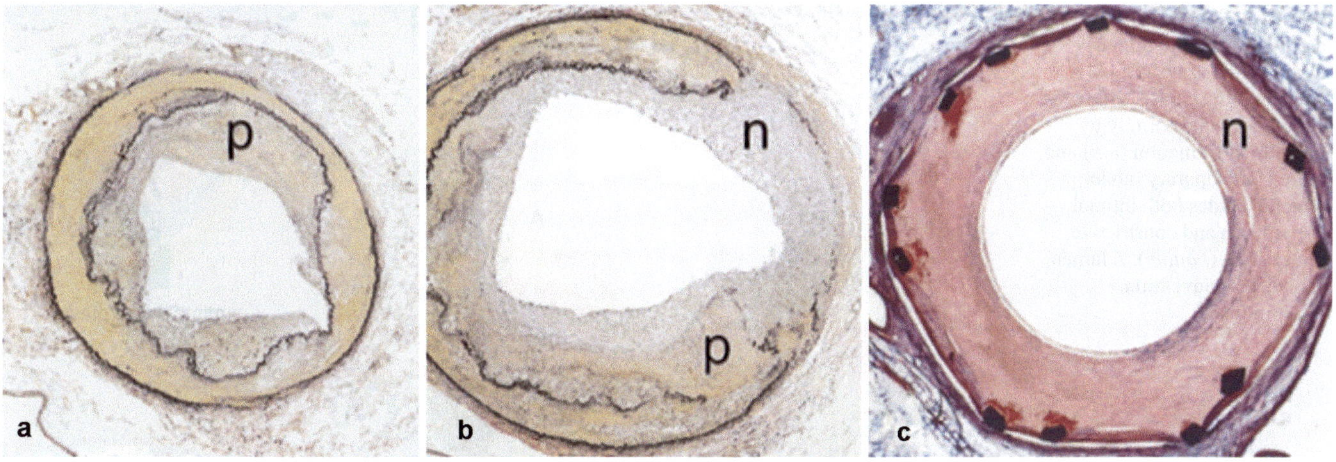

Fig. 14.1 Composite photomicrograph demonstrates a typical response 4 weeks after angioplasty and stenting in atherosclerotic primate. (**a**, **b**) Show the uninjured and injured common iliac arteries, respectively. Panel **c** shows stented iliac artery. Animals consumed an atherogenic diet for 2.5 years to create complicated plaques (*p*). (**b**) Shows fractured plaque (*p*) and overlying media that have healed with neointimal ingrowth (*n*). (**c**) Shows a stented monkey iliac artery with a typical neointimal lesion (*n*). (**a**, **b**) Verhoeff–van Gieson's stain; (**c**) trichrome stain; original magnification all panels, ×40 (Reproduced by permission of American Heart Association, Cherr et al. [73])

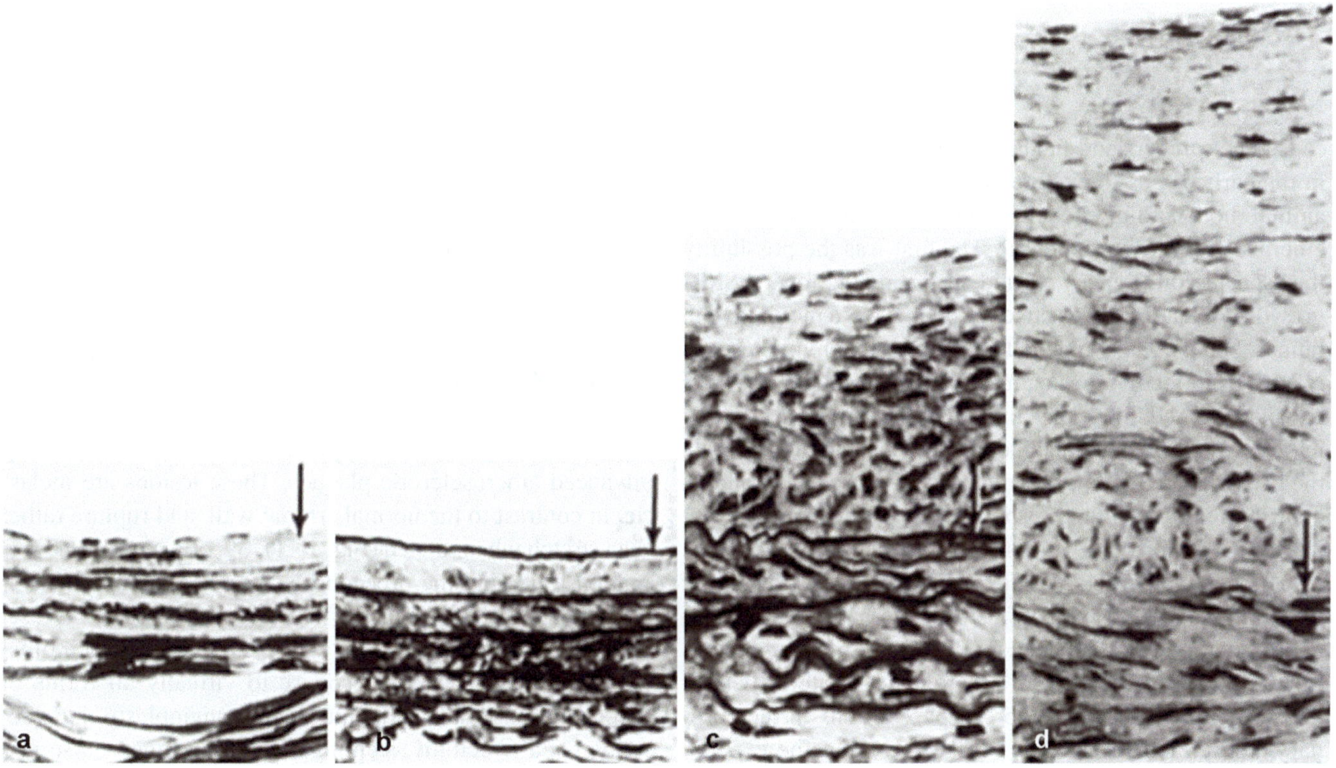

Fig. 14.2 Composite photomicrograph of the rat carotid after balloon injury. Histological cross-sections of normal rat carotid artery before injury (**a**), immediately after balloon injury (**b**), after 2 weeks (**c**), then 12 weeks (**d**). Note significant intimal hyperplasia at 2 and 12 weeks with increasing contribution from ECM. Lumen is at *top*. *Arrows* indicate IEL (Reproduced with permission from [44])

endothelial cell (EC) monolayer. Basic restenosis research initially focused on vein graft arterialization and prosthetic graft anastomotic intimal hyperplasia and then intensely on neointima formation at sites of angioplasty and within BMS. Animal models of angioplasty and bypass procedures were developed (Figs. 14.1 and 14.2) and the time course of intimal hyperplasia carefully described.

Potent inhibitors of experimental neointima formation were identified, but a series of clinical trials based on these results failed miserably with no impact on restenosis. This

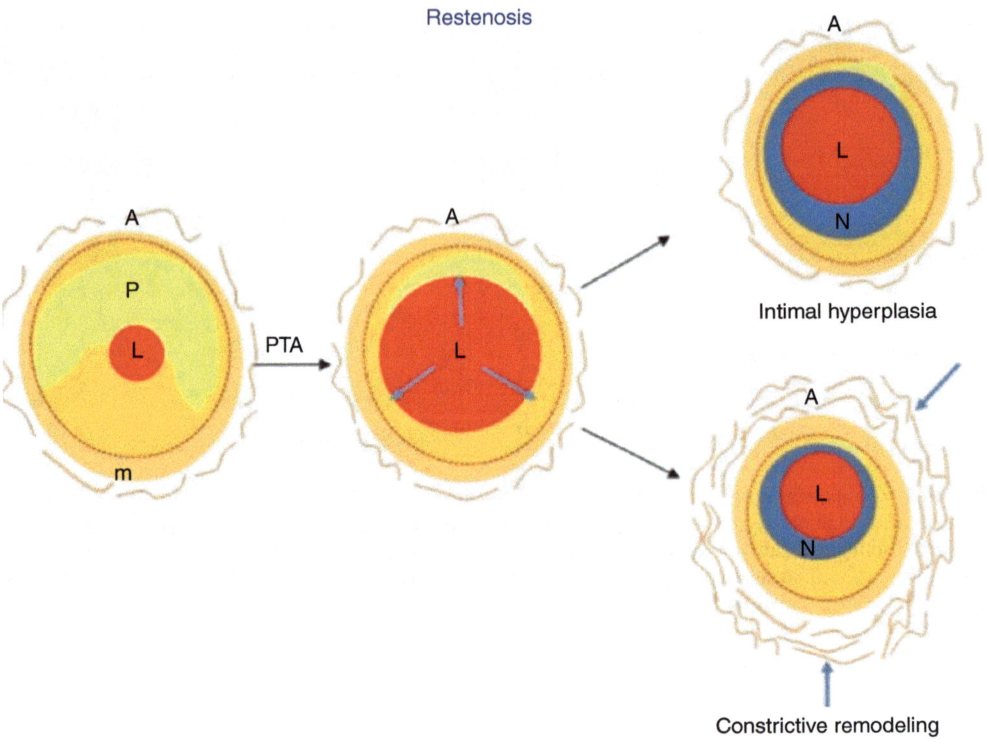

Fig. 14.3 Mechanisms of lumen narrowing after angioplasty. Diagram illustrates the early concept of restenosis following angioplasty due entirely to neointimal formation (*top*) and more contemporary model, which includes both intimal hyperplasia and constrictive remodeling (*bottom*). *L* lumen, *P* plaque, *A* adventitia, *N* neointima

caused researchers and funding agencies to take a step back in the early 1990s to explore possibilities for the failure of animal models to predict clinical benefit. Three hypotheses emerged from this reappraisal. The first was the possibility that species differences existed in the regulation of SMC growth, so that drugs effective in rodents were ineffective in human beings. Data emerged to support this hypothesis as results from studies in nonhuman primate models of restenosis mirrored those in clinical trials [39]. The second hypothesis was that animal models did not accurately depict the background of complex advanced atherosclerosis and its contribution to the injury response. Such lesions are present in the vast majority of vessels treated clinically. To this day, few models come close to developing plaques that mirror the complexity of human lesions. Perhaps the closest approximation is the monkey model of diet-induced atherosclerosis [40]. When fed an atherogenic Western diet for 2–5 years, macaques develop complex lesions in the coronary, aortic, and iliac arteries (Fig. 14.1), but the expense and time required to work in this model have severely restricted its application. The third and perhaps most important hypothesis was that factors other than neointima were contributing to lumen loss after angioplasty, and confirmatory data soon emerged from BMS and IVUS trials. The concept of geometric arterial wall remodeling after angioplasty had been largely overlooked until serial imaging of human coronary lesions with IVUS demonstrated that changes in wall diameter were even more important than new wall mass (neointima) in the loss of lumen caliber over time [41–43]. We now understand that the combination of neointima formation and inward shrinkage of the vessel wall merge to produce lumen narrowing at sites of angioplasty in the absence of a stent (Fig. 14.3). While these two processes occur together, conceptually it is easier to consider their pathogenesis separately.

Intimal Hyperplasia

In practice, angioplasty is applied to stenoses surrounded by advanced atherosclerotic plaques. These lesions are inelastic, in contrast to the normal arterial wall, and rupture rather than stretch when dilated (Fig. 14.1) [39, 40]. New tissue formation following the procedure is termed "neointima" as it accumulates at the interface between the damaged vessel wall and flowing blood (Fig. 14.1). As noted above, intimal hyperplasia is a generic response to virtually all forms of mechanical arterial wall injury (e.g., angioplasty, atherectomy, endarterectomy, stenting, etc.). The time course and regulation of intimal hyperplasia following artery injury have been extensively characterized in the rat carotid balloon injury model by Clowes and others (Fig. 14.2) [44, 45].

Balloon injury denudes the endothelium and damages the surrounding wall by stretching, which if severe can rupture the tunica media. In the rat model, a stretch injury standardized to not rupture the IEL results in the immediate death of 25–30 % of medial SMCs. The loss of an endothelial barrier promotes platelet and leukocyte adhesion forming a thin layer of mural thrombus and an acute wave of inflammation. Adherent platelets release factors that promote cell growth and migration, including PDGFs, EGF, basic FGF, and TGF-β. Dead and injured SMCs release intracellular stores of basic FGF, and the damaged ECM releases matrix-bound growth factors as well as matrix fragments that have endogenous mitogenic and inflammatory properties. A dramatic wave of replication ensues in which 30 % of medial SMCs enter S-phase within 24 h. By day 4, both quiescent and replicating SMCs can be seen migrating from the media across the IEL to form a neointima (Fig. 14.2) [44–46]. Cells arriving in the neointima continue replicating until a quiescent state is reached by 4 weeks. The neointima continues to expand for ~6 weeks from accumulation of additional ECM, and at 3 months ECM accounts for almost 80 % of the neointimal area in the rat model (Fig. 14.2d) [44].

In the rat carotid balloon injury model, the endothelium does not completely regenerate, but in other models, regrowth of an intact endothelial monolayer serves to shut down replication of the underlying SMC replication. This is due to paracrine effects of growth inhibitors secreted by the endothelium, including nitric oxide (NO) [47] and heparan sulfate proteoglycans [48]. Endothelium also serves a barrier function and excludes platelets, clotting proteins, and leukocytes from continuing to stimulate adjacent SMCs with their mitogenic, motogenic, and proinflammatory effects. These facts have formed the basis of clinical trials designed to enhance early endothelialization of prosthetic bypass grafts, BMS, and sites of angioplasty [49, 50].

As noted above, many drugs have been identified that inhibit intimal hyperplasia in the rat and other animal models of vascular injury, including heparin [48], angiotensin-converting enzyme inhibitors [51, 52], and NO donors, but when applied in human angioplasty restenosis trials, their effects have all been disappointing [32, 33]. This is due in part to the fact that intimal hyperplasia (new wall mass) is only one variable in the angioplasty restenosis equation, the other being constrictive arterial wall remodeling.

Arterial Wall Remodeling

Remodeling refers to changes in the arterial wall geometry (intima, media, and adventitia) that can occur independent of a change in the wall cross-sectional area. Normal adaptive vascular remodeling occurs when the vessel wall dilates and thickens in response to chronic increases in flow and pressure, respectively. Compensatory outward remodeling is a well-established response through which the media expands to accommodate the accumulation of atherosclerotic plaque, as described by Glagov and others. After angioplasty, the arterial wall seldom dilates to a greater caliber than was achieved when the balloon was inflated, but instead various amounts of inward wall shrinkage occur over time. As noted above, acute recoil and spasm decreases wall caliber by 10–30 % within minutes. Over the next few weeks, another constrictive process remodels the arterial wall to an even smaller caliber through a process with many parallels to wound contraction in healing cutaneous wounds.

If the reader has trouble visualizing the effects of remodeling, the data from BMS studies may be helpful. When a BMS is used, the amount of neointma that forms within the stent is generally worse, with a greater cross-sectional area than after angioplasty alone. Even so, stents reduce the frequency of restenosis compared to angioplasty alone because they completely block acute and chronic recoil/remodeling/shrinkage of the arterial wall. So the initial lumen caliber (the stent caliber) is large enough that moderate amounts of neointima have minimal impact on the lumen cross-sectional area. In contrast, an artery that constricts after angioplasty, remodeling pre-existing media and plaque area into a slightly smaller diameter, will severely narrow the lumen even if the area of the wall stays constant (i.e., no additional neointima, Fig. 14.3). These concepts have been confirmed in studies using serial imaging of arterial segments after angioplasty and after BMS. IVUS of the cross-sectional vessel area shows that after angioplasty 60–80 % of lumen loss was due to constrictive remodeling of the wall caliber, while only 20–40 % was from a change in total wall cross-sectional area (neointima) [41–43].

Changes in wall caliber are generally measured histologically by the area encompassed by the EEL [53]. The molecular mechanisms of constrictive reorganization of cells and ECM material in the injured arterial wall remain poorly understood, but attempts to explain it have drawn parallels to the process of cutaneous wound healing, wound contraction, and fibrosis [54–57]. In cutaneous wounds left to heal by secondary intent, the sequence of cellular events is similar in many ways to healing of the arterial wall after angioplasty. A platelet and fibrin plug forms in the defect, which serves as provisional matrix for the influx of leukocytes then fibroblasts from damaged wound edges as well as ingrowth of new microvessels. Wound fibroblasts dedifferentiate into myofibroblasts, which like SMCs express α-actin and are capable of contracting in response to vasoconstrictors [56]. As leukocytes remove clot and wound debris, myofibroblasts proliferate and lay down new ECM rich in glycosaminoglycans and proteoglycans to form granulation tissue [57]. Fibroblasts then reorganize and apply traction to the newly synthesized matrix, and wound contraction occurs to bring wound edges together. Subsequent ECM turnover leads to a change in matrix composition to a more collagen-rich material. This results in fibrosis and eventually a mature scar after many months [55].

Parallels occur in atherosclerotic arteries injured by angioplasty [54]. This can be modeled in nonhuman primates with complex pre-existing atherosclerosis. In this model, species differences in the regulation of SMC growth are minimized, and complex atherosclerotic lesions more closely depict the human plaque prompting reconstruction (Fig. 14.1). Angioplasty increases lumen size by fracturing the atherosclerotic plaque and stretching or tearing the surrounding media and adventitia. Thus, the arterial wall "wound" is transmural. The healing response is also transmural, and while new tissue is termed the neointima, it can develop in the media and adventitial layers if the fracture is deep.

Damage leads to acute inflammation where thrombus forms within fractures, dissections, and clefts, providing provisional scaffolding for the influx of leukocytes, initially neutrophils then monocytes after days 2–7 [40, 54]. Platelets and the fibrin plug attract leukocytes to the denuded area through a cascade of adhesion molecules including P-selectin, integrin Mac-1 and glycoprotein IIb/IIIa, and direct leukocyte attachment and migration [58, 59]. Mac-1 and platelet-mediated leukocyte adhesion plays an important role in vascular inflammation and restenosis. Following a brief but intense wave of proliferation, peaking at 4 days, SMC and other actin-positive cells (e.g., adventitial fibroblasts and circulating progenitor-derived SMCs) migrate to the lumen interface into the area of injury to form neointima starting at day 7. Inflammation then resolves, and neointima replaces the thrombus and thickens substantially from further accumulation of SMCs and ECM from days 14 to 28.

Constrictive remodeling of the arterial wall, probably from adhesive tension generated in reorganization of newly synthesized ECM, is often remarkable during this time period [53, 54]. Despite the accumulation of neointima, restenosis in this model is not caused by increased lesion size alone. Rather, the change in overall arterial wall size or remodeling with wall shrinkage is the major factor leading to lumen narrowing. Given that matrix accounts for more than 60 % of arterial wall volume, matrix reorganization is a key factor in wall remodeling and dependent on cell-matrix adhesive interactions, matrix degradation by proteases, and new matrix synthesis.

As in healing wounds, the composition of the new ECM at sites of vascular injury is distinct from that in normal arterial wall [54, 60–64]. The uninjured media is rich in types I and III collagen and elastin with lesser amounts of glycosaminoglycans and proteoglycans [61]. In contrast, ECM deposited by neointimal cells is rich in hyaluronan (HA) and versican. HA is a large hydrophilic disaccharide polymer associated with tissue remodeling in embryogenesis, wound healing, and tumor invasion. HA is important for scarless fetal wound healing and improves collagen remodeling and re-epithelialization when applied exogenously to cutaneous wound in adults [65–67]. Versican is a proteoglycan that binds to the HA backbone and changes its physical-chemical properties, increasing viscoelasticity, and together they provide hydrated space favorable for cell motility, invasion, and replication [68]. The relative ratio of HA and other stuctural matrix proteins such as collagen and elastin alters ECM reorganization in culture and within the healing arterial wall [62, 69].

HA is expressed in all arterial wall layers after angioplasty, most prominently the adventitia and neointima [54, 64]. Co-localization with type-I collagen in the healing arterial wall suggests an important interaction supported by in vitro studies of collagen remodeling. Adventitial fibroblasts and medial SMCs cultured from monkey aorta contract collagen lattices using β1 integrins. Addition of HA significantly enhances collagen reorganization and peri-cellular collagen fiber condensation [69]. This effect is mediated in part by cell surface receptors for HA, including RHAMM and CD44. Both are upregulated by arterial injury [69, 70]. Thus, these data suggest HA could alter constrictive collagen remodeling in the healing arterial wall.

Matrix metalloproteinases (MMP) are important regulators of matrix degradation that are critical in SMC migration in vitro, but their roles in constrictive remodeling are less well established. Animal studies using MMP inhibitors showed conflicting results. In rat, rabbit, and pig models of arterial injury, MMP inhibition limited the injury response [71, 72]. In contrast, a continuous infusion of a broad-spectrum MMP inhibitor after angioplasty in atherosclerotic monkeys had no effect on arterial wall remodeling or hyperplasia [73]. Not surprisingly then, clinical trials of MMP inhibitors for PCI endpoints have been negative [74].

Reactive oxygen species (ROS) have also been implicated in constrictive remodeling. ROS are transiently increased across the arterial wall after angioplasty. In rabbits undergoing iliac balloon injury, superoxide dismutase (SOD) activity, which maintains the redox balance by catalyzing the reaction of O_2- to H_2O_2, was decreased significantly as constrictive remodeling occurred [75]. Exogenous administration of SOD to the endothelium increased lumen caliber, inhibiting constrictive remodeling by 59 %. SOD also improved nitrate levels, suggesting improved remodeling was in part from increased NO production.

TGF-β and connective tissue growth factor (CTGF) are induced at sites of injury where they regulate ECM turnover and contraction during wound healing [76–78]. CTGF stimulates SMC proliferation and migration and regulates enhanced collagen remodeling by fibroblasts in vitro in response to TGF-β [76]. CTGF is significantly upregulated in monkey aortic after injury. Blocking TGF-β with neutralizing antibodies or a soluble TGF receptor used as an inhibitor has been reported to reduce lumen narrowing by inhibiting constrictive remodeling following carotid artery ligation in mice [79].

Clinical Progress in Treating Restenosis

The DES story elegantly merges therapies targeting the two major mechanisms underlying restenosis described above. DESs overcome constrictive remodeling with the stent and block intimal hyperplasia with an antiproliferative drug coating that targets high-dose inhibitors to the site of injury, avoiding systemic toxicity [6, 7]. DESs do not prevent the problem for all patients or in all vascular beds, but remarkable data from clinical studies of PCI show conclusive benefits (e.g., SIRIUS, RAVEL, TAXUS, and others) [3, 9]. New drugs combined with new coating strategies have been studied in PCI. The SPIRIT-III, SPIRIT-IV, and the COMPARE trials studied everolimus DESs and found lower restenosis than for pacitaxel DESs (2.3 % vs. 5.7 %) [10, 11].

In contrast to their efficacy in PCI, DESs in peripheral vessels, such as superficial femoral artery atherosclerotic lesions, have been less consistent in rendering advantage over the traditional BMS or angioplasty alone [17–20]. Similarly, preliminary data on DESs in renal artery atherosclerosis do not show dramatically reduced restenosis compared to BMSs. The GREAT trial showed in-stent restenosis, late lumen loss, and need for target lesion revascularization were all slightly lower with the sirolimus DES compared to the BMS, but these differences were not statistically significant [16].

In-stent restenosis tends to occur more frequently in smaller diameter vessels, which are thus more likely to benefit from DES [80, 81]. Besides artery size, a number of other factors have been associated with in-stent restenosis, including stent strut fracture, a particular problem in the superficial femoral and popliteal arteries due to major deformations that occur with bending hip and knee joints during ambulation [82]. New stent designs are being developed specifically to target this problem and the extremely high rates of primary restenosis associated with stent fractures in this location [83].

Local drug delivery with DES in large-caliber arteries is also challenging. The strut-to-lumen area ratio falls significantly in larger arteries, so the drug is more rapidly diluted using the same strategies for coating DES as used in those designed for PCI. This can lead to under-dosing in these beds. Drug resistance, hypersensitivity to coatings, lack of re-endothelialization predisposing to late thrombosis, and high cost are also potential hurdles to the success of DESs in extra-coronary applications.

DESs are also associated with increased rates of late thrombosis compared to BMSs used for PCI, likely from nonhealing or impaired reendothelialization. The scaffold remains a foreign body chronically exposed to circulating cells, and even BMSs are associated with a prolonged foreign body response around struts buried in a thick layer of neointima. Recent studies with bioabsorbable stents attempt to overcome these limitations by completely eliminating the stent after healing has occurred. The ABSORB trial concluded that a bioabsorbable everolimus-eluting stent was clinically safe, but restenosis in this preliminary study occurred in 27 %, leaving room for improvement [84].

Vascular endothelial growth factor (VEGF) has also been considered for DESs in an attempt to promote healing through affects on EC recruitment and angiogenesis [85]. VEGF gene-eluting stents promote re-endothelialization and reduce in-stent intimal hyperplasia in animal models [86]. Other strategies to induce vessel repair after PCI include the use of antibodies and peptides. The HEALING II trial employed CD34 antibody-coated stents to capture circulating CD34-positive EC progenitors to endothelialize BMSs more rapidly to inhibit neointimal formation and in-stent restenosis [50, 87, 88].

References

1. Serruys PW, de Jaegere P, Kiemeneij F, et al. A comparison of balloon-expandable-stent implantation with balloon angioplasty in patients with coronary artery disease. N Engl J Med. 1994;331:489–95.
2. Fischman DL, Leon MB, Baim DS, Schatz RA, Savage MP, Penn I, et al. A randomized comparison of coronary-stent placement and balloon angioplasty in the treatment of coronary artery disease. Stent Restenosis Study Investigators. N Engl J Med. 1994;331:496–501.
3. Mehran R, Dangas G, Abizaid A, et al. Angiographic patterns of in-stent restenosis: classification and implications for long-term outcome. Circulation. 1999;100:1872–8.
4. Brener SJ, Prasad AJ, Khan Z, Sacchi TJ. The relationship between late lumen loss and restenosis among various drug-eluting stents: a systematic review and meta-regression analysis of randomized clinical trials. Atherosclerosis. 2011;214:158–62.
5. Moses JW, Leon MB, Popma JJ, et al. Sirolimus-dluting stents versus standard stents in patients with stenosis in a native coronary artery. N Engl J Med. 2003;349:1315–23.
6. Schofer J, Schluter M, Gershlick AH, et al. Sirolimus-eluting stents for treatment of patients with long atherosclerotic lesions in small coronary arteries: double-blind, randomized controlled trial (E-SIRIUS). Lancet. 2003;362:1093–9.
7. Abizaid A, Costa MA, Blanchard D, et al. Sirolimus-eluting stents inhibit neointimal hyperplasia in diabetic patients. Insights from the RAVEL trail. Eur Heart J. 2004;25:107–12.
8. Grube E, Silber S, Hauptmann KE, et al. TAXUS I: six-and twelve-month results from a randomized, double-blind trial on a slow-release paclitaxel-eluting stent for de novo coronary lesions. Circulation. 2003;107:38–42.
9. Colombo A, Drzewiecki J, Banning A, et al. Randomized study to assess the effectiveness of slow and moderate-release polymer-based paclitaxel-eluting stents for coronary artery lesions. Circulation. 2003;108:788–94.
10. Stone GW, Midei M, Newman W, et al. Randomized comparison so everolimus-eluting and paclitaxel-eluting stents: two-year clinical follow-up from the Clinical Evaluation of the Xience V Everolimus Eluting Coronart Stent System in the Treatment of Patients with de novo Native Coronary Artery Lesions (SPIRIT) III trial. Circulation. 2009;119:680–6.
11. Kedhi E, Joesoef KS, MaFadden E, et al. Second-generation everolimus-eluting and paclitaxel-eluting stents in real life practice (COMPARE): a randomized trial. Lancet. 2010;375:201–9.
12. Stankovic G, Colombo A, Bersin R, et al. Comparison of directional coronary atherectomy and stenting versus stenting alone for the treatment of de novo and restenotic coronary artery narrowing. Am J Cardiol. 2004;93:953–8.
13. Bittl JA, Chew DP, Topol EJ, Kong DF, Califf RM. Meta-analysis of randomized trials of percutaneous transluminal coronary angioplasty versus atherectomy, cutting balloon atherotomy, or laser angioplasty. J Am Coll Cardiol. 2004;43:936–42.
14. Leertouwer TC, Gussenhoven EJ, Bosch JL, et al. Stent placement for renal arterial stenosis: where do we stand? A meta-analysis. Radiology. 2000;216:78–85.
15. Corriere MA, Edwards MS, Pearce JD, Andrews JS, Geary RL, Hansen KJ. Restenosis after renal artery angioplasty and stenting: incidence and risk factors. J Vasc Surg. 2009;50:813–9.

16. Zahringer M, Sapoval M, Pattynama PMT, et al. Sirolimus-eluting versus bare-metal low-profile stent for renal artery treatment (GREAT trial): angiographic follow-up after 6 month and clinical outcome up to 2 years. J Endovasc Ther. 2007;14:460–8.
17. Dormandy JA, Rutherford RB. Management of peripheral arterial disease (PAD). TASC Working Group. TransAtlantic Inter-Society Concensus (TASC). J Vasc Surg. 2000;31:S1–296.
18. Mwipatayi BP, Hockings A, Hofmann M, Garbowski M, Sieunarine K. Balloon angioplasty compared with stenting for treatment of femoropopliteal occlusive disease: a meta-analysis. J Vasc Surg. 2008;47:461–9.
19. Conte MS. Bypass versus Angioplasty in Severe Ischaemia of the Leg (BASIL) and the (hoped for) dawn of evidence-based treatment for advanced limb ischemia. J Vasc Surg. 2010;51(5 Suppl): 69S–75.
20. Becquemin JP, Favre JP, Marzelle J, Nemoz C, Corsin C, Liezorovicz A. Systematic versus selective stent placement after superficial femoral artery balloon angioplasty: a multicenter prospective randomized study. J Vasc Surg. 2003;37:487–94.
21. Duda SH, Bosiers M, Lammer J, Scheinert D, Zeller T, Oliva V, et al. Drug-eluting and bare nitinol stents for the treatment of atherosclerotic lesions in the superficial femoral artery: long-term results from the SIROCCO trial. J Endovasc Ther. 2006;13: 701–10.
22. McQuade K, Gable D, Hohman S, Pearl G, Theune B. Randomized comparison of ePTFE/nitinol self-expanding stent graft vs prosthetic femoral-popliteal bypass in the treatment of superficial femoral artery occlusive disease. J Vasc Surg. 2009;49:109–15.
23. Archie Jr JP. A fifteen-year experience with carotid endarterectomy after a formal operative protocol requiring highly frequent patch angioplasty. J Vasc Surg. 2000;31:724–35.
24. Mantese VA, Timaran CH, Chiu D, Begg RJ, Brott TG, CREST Investigators. The Carotid Revascularization Endarterectomy versus Stenting Trial (CREST): stenting versus carotid endarterectomy for carotid disease. Stroke. 2010;41(10 Suppl):S31–4.
25. Lal BK, Brott TG. The Carotid Revascularization Endarterectomy vs. Stenting Trial completes randomization: lessons learned and anticipated results. J Vasc Surg. 2009;50:1224–31.
26. Tallarita T, Oderich GS, Macedo TA, Gloviczki P, Misra S, Duncan AA, et al. Reinterventions for stent restenosis in patients treated for atherosclerotic mesenteric artery disease. J Vasc Surg. 2011;54: 1422–9.
27. Peck MA, Conrad MF, Kwolek CJ, LaMuraglia GM, Paruchuri V, Cambria RP. Intermediate-term outcomes of endovascular treatment for symptomatic chronic mesenteric ischemia. J Vasc Surg. 2010;51:140–7.
28. Lee RW, Bakken AM, Palchik E, Saad WE, Davies MG. Long-term outcomes of endoluminal therapy for chronic atherosclerotic occlusive mesenteric disease. Ann Vasc Surg. 2008;22:541–6.
29. Holmes DR Jr, Vilietstra RE, Smith HC, et al. Restenosis after percutaneous transluminal coronary angioplasty (PTCA): a report from the PTCA Registry of the National Heart, Lung, and Blood Institute. Am J Cardiol. 1984;53:77C–81C; Thornton MA, Gruentzig AR, Hollman J, King SB 3rd, Douglas JS. Coumadin and aspirin in prevention of recurrence after transluminal coronary angioplasty: a randomized study. Circulation. 1984;69:721–727.
30. Serruys PW, Luijen HE, Beatt KJ, et al. Incidence of restenosis after successful coronary angioplasty: a time-related phenomenon. A quantitative angiographic study in 342 consecutive patients at 1, 2, 3, and 4 months. Circulation. 1988;77:361–71.
31. Nobuyoshi M, Kimura T, Nosaka H, et al. Restenosis after successful percutaneous transluminal coronary angioplasty: serial angiographic follow-up of 229 patients. J Am Coll Cardiol. 1988;12: 616–23.
32. Faxon DP, Spiro TE, Minor S, for the ERA Investigators. Low molecular weight heparin in prevention of restenosis after angioplasty: results of enoxaparin restenosis (ERA) trial. Circulation. 1994;90:908–14.
33. MERCATOR Study Group. Does the new angiotensin converting enzyme inhibitor cilazapril prewent restenosis after percutaneous transluminal coronary angioplasty? Results of the MERCATOR study: a multicenter, randomized, double-blind placebo-controlled trial. Circulation. 1992;86:100–10.
34. Khan MM, Ellis SG, Aguirre FV, Weisman HF, Wildermann NM, Califf RM, et al. Does intracoronary thrombus influence the outcome of high risk percutaneous transluminal coronary angioplasty? Clinical and angiographic outcomes in a large multicenter trial. EPIC Investigators. Evaluation of IIb/IIIa Platelet Receptor Antagonist 7E3 in Preventing Ischemic Complications. J Am Coll Cardiol. 1998;31:31–6.
35. Kastrati A, Mehilli J, von Beckerath N, et al. Sirolimus-eluting stent or paclitaxel-eluting stents vs balloon angioplasty for prevention of recurrences in patients with coronary in-stent restenosis: a randomized controlled trial. JAMA. 2005;293:165–71.
36. Lal BK, Beach KW, Roubin GS, et al. CREST Investigators. Restenosis after carotid artery stenting and endarterectomy: a secondary analysis of CREST, a randomised controlled trial. Lancet Neurol. 2012;11(9):755–63.
37. Schillinger M, Sabeti S, Dick P, Amighi J, Mlekusch W, Schlager O, et al. Sustained benefit at 2 years of primary femoropopliteal stenting compared with balloon angioplasty with optional stenting. Circulation. 2007;115:2745–9.
38. Moliterno DJ, Topol EJ. Restenosis: epidemiology and treatment. In: Topol EJ, editor. Textbook of cardiovascular medicine. 2nd ed. Philadelphia: Lippincott-Raven; 2002. p. 1715–50.
39. Geary RL, Koyama N, Wang TW, Vergel S, Clowes AW. Failure of heparin to inhibit inrimal hyperplasia in injured baboon arteries: the role of heparin-sensitive and heparini-insensitive pathways in the stimulation of smooth muscle cell migration and proliferation. Circulation. 1995;91:2972–81.
40. Geary RL, Williams JK, Golden D, Brown DG, Benjamin ME, Adams MR. Time course of cellular proliferation, intimal hyperplasia, and remodeling following angioplasty in monkeys with established atherosclerosis: a nonhuman primate model of restenosis. Arterioscler Thromb Vasc Biol. 1996;16:34–43.
41. Mintz GS, Popma JJ, Pichard AD, et al. Arterial remodeling after coronary angioplasty. A serial intravascular ultrasound study. Circulation. 1996;94:35–43.
42. Lansky AJ, Mintz GS, Popma JJ, et al. Remodeling after directional coronary atherectomy (with and without adjuct percutaneous transluminal coronary antioplasty): a serial angiographic and intravascular ultrasound analysis from the Optimal Atherectomy Restenosis Study. J Am Coll Cardiol. 1998;32:329–37.
43. Pasterkamp G, Mali WP, Borst C. Application of intravascular ultrasound in remodeling studies. Semin Interv Cardiol. 1997;2:11–8.
44. Clowes AW, Reidy MA, Clowes MM. Kinetics of cellular proliferation after arterial injury. I. Smooth muscle growth in the absence of endothelium. Lab Invest. 1983;49:327–33.
45. Clowes AW, Reidy MA, Clowes MM. Mechanisms of stenosis after arterial injury. Lab Invest. 1983;49:208–15.
46. Clowes AW, Schwartz SM. Significance of quiescent smooth muscle migration in the injured rat carotid artery. Circ Res. 1985;56: 139–45.
47. Cooke JP, Ghebremariam YT. Dietary nitrate, nitric oxide, and restenosis. J Clin Invest. 2011;121:1258–60.
48. Majesky MW, Schwartz SM, Clowes MM, Clowes AW. Heparin regulates smooth muscle S phase entry in the injured rat carotid artery. Circ Res. 1987;61:296–300.
49. Deutsch M, Meinhart J, Zilla P, Howanietz N, Gorlitzer M, Froeschl A, et al. Long-term experience in autologous in vitro endothelialization of infrainguinal ePTFE grafts. J Vasc Surg. 2009;49: 352–62.
50. Miglionico M, Patti G, D'Ambrosio A, Di Sciascio G. Percutaneous coronary intervention utilizing a new endothelial progenitor cells antibody-coated stent: a prospective single-center registry in high-risk patients. Catheter Cardiovasc Interv. 2008;71:600–4.

51. Powell JS, Clozel JP, Muller EKM, et al. Inhibitors of angiotensin-converting enzyme prevent myointimal proliferation after vascular injury. Science. 1989;245:186–8.
52. Daemen MJAP, Lombardi DM, Bosman FT, Schwartz SM. Angiotensin II induces smooth muscle cell proliferation in the normal and injured rat arterial wall. Circ Res. 1991;68:450–6.
53. Mondy JS, Williams JK, Adams MR, Dean RH, Geary RL. Structural determinants of lumen narrowing after angioplasty in atherosclerotic nonhuman primates. J Vasc Surg. 1997;26:875–83.
54. Geary RL, Nikkari ST, Wagner WD, Williams JK, Adams MR, Dean RH. Wound healing: a paradigm for lumen narrowing following arterial reconstruction. J Vasc Surg. 1998;27:96–108.
55. Martin P. Wound healing-aiming at perfect skin regeneration. Science. 1997;276:75–81.
56. Gabbiani G, Hirshcel BJ, Ryan GB, Statkov PR, Majno G. Granulation tissue as a contractile organ. J Exp Med. 1972;135: 719–33.
57. Scott PG, Dodd CM, Tredget EE, Ghahary A, Rahemtulla F. Immunohistochemical localization of the proteoglycans decorin, biglycan and versican and transforming growth factor-β in human post-burn hypertrophic and mature scars. Histopathology. 1995;26: 423–31.
58. Inoue T, Uchida T, Yaguchi I, Sakai Y, Takayanagi K, Morooka S. Stent-induced expression and activation of the leukocyte integrin Mac-1 is associated with neointimal thickening and restenosis. Circulation. 2003;107:1757–63.
59. Biasucci LM, Liuzzo G, Buffon A, Maseri A. The variable role of inflammation in acute coronary syndromes and in restenosis. Semin Interv Cardiol. 1999;4:105–10.
60. Nikkari ST, Jarvelainen HT, Wight TN, Ferguson M, Clowes AW. Smooth muscle cell expression of extracellular matrix genes after arterial injury. Am J Pathol. 1994;144:1348–56.
61. Raines EW. The extracellular matrix can regulate vascular cell migration, proliferation, and survival: relationships to vascular disease. Int J Exp Pathol. 2000;81:173–82.
62. Wight TN, Merrilees MJ. Proteoglycans in atherosclerosis and restenosis: key roles for versican. Circ Res. 2004;94:1158–67.
63. Hedin U, Roy J, Tran PK, Lundmark K, Rahman A. Control of smooth muscle cell proliferation—the role of the basement membrane. Thromb Haemost. 1999;82 Suppl 1:23–6.
64. Riessen R, Wight TN, Pastore C, Henley C, Isner JM. Distribution of hyaluronan during extracellular matrix remodeling in human restenotic arteries and balloon-injured rat carotid arteries. Circulation. 1996;93:1141–7.
65. Fraser JRE, Laurent TC, Laurent UBG. Hyaluronan: its nature, distribution, functions and turnover. J Intern Med. 1997;242:27–33.
66. Knudson CB, Knudson W. Hyaluronan-binding proteins in development, tissue homeostasis, and disease. FASEB J. 1993;7:1233–41.
67. Price RD, Myers S, Leigh IM, Navsaria HA. The role of hyaluronic acid in wound healing: assessment of clinical evidence. Am J Clin Dermatol. 2005;6:393–402.
68. Oksalo O, Salo T, Tammi R, et al. Expression of proteoglycans and hyaluronan during wound healing. J Histochem Cytochem. 1995;43: 125–35.
69. Travis JA, Hughes MG, Wong JM, Wagner WD, Geary RL. Hyaluronan enhances contraction of collagen by smooth muscle cells and adventitial fibroblasts: role of CD44 and implications for constrictive remodeling. Circ Res. 2001;88:77–83.
70. Jain M, He Q, Lee WS, et al. Role of CD44 in the reaction of vascular smooth muscle cells to arterial wall injury. J Clin Invest. 1996;97:596–603.
71. Courtman DW, Franco CD, Meng Q, Bendeck MP. Inwark remodeling of the rabbit aorta is blocked by the matrix metalloproteinase inhibitor doxycycline. J Vasc Res. 2004;41:157–65.
72. de Smet BJ, de Kleijn D, Hanemaaijer R, et al. Metalloproteinase inhibition reduces constrictive arterial remodeling after balloon angioplasty: a study in the atherosclerotic Yucatan micropig. Circulation. 2000;101:2962–7.
73. Cherr GS, Motew SJ, Travis JA, et al. Metalloproteinase inhibition and the response to angioplasty and stenting in atherosclerotic primates. Arterioscler Thromb Vasc Biol. 2002;22:161–6.
74. Araujo CM, Rando GA, Mauro MF, Cristóvão SA, Sanchez IS, Salman AA, et al. Batimastat-eluting stent implantation for the treatment of coronary artery disease: results of the Brazilian pilot study. Arq Bras Cardiol. 2005;84:256–60.
75. Leite PF, Danilovic A, Moriel P, et al. Sustained decrease in superoxide dismutase activity underlies constrictive remodeling after balloon injury in rabbits. Arterioscler Thromb Vasc Biol. 2003;23: 2197–202.
76. Daniels JT, Schultz GS, Blalock TD, et al. Mediation of transforming growth factor-beta(1)- stimulated matrix contraction by fibroblasts: a role for connective tissue growth factor in contractile scarring. Am J Pathol. 2003;163:2043–52.
77. Geary RL, Wong JM, Rossini A, Schwartz SM, Adams LD. Expression profiling identifies 147 genes contributing to an unique primate neointimal smooth muscle cell phenotype. Arterioscler Thromb Vasc Biol. 2002;22:2010–6.
78. Kingston PA, Sinha S, Appleby CE, et al. Adenovirus-mediated gene transfer of transforming growth factor-beta3, but not transforming growth factor-beta1, inhibits constrictive remodeling and reduces luminal loss after coronary angioplasty. Circulation. 2003; 108:2819–25.
79. Ryan ST, Koteliansky VE, Gotwals PJ, Lindner V. Transforming growth factor-beta-dependent events in vascular remodeling following arterial injury. J Vasc Res. 2003;40:37–46.
80. Zeller T, Muller C, Frank U, et al. Gold coating and restenosis after primary stenting of ostial renal artery stenosis. Catheter Cardiovasc Interv. 2003;60:1–6.
81. Sacks D, Marinelli DL, Martin LG, et al. Reporting standards for clinical evaluation of new peripheral arterial revascularization devices. Technology Assessment Committee. J Vasc Interv Radiol. 1997;8:137–49.
82. Iida O, Uematsu M, Soga Y, Hirano K, Suzuki K, Yokoi H, et al. Timing of the restenosis following nitinol stenting in the superficial femoral artery and the factors associated with early and late restenoses. Catheter Cardiovasc Interv. 2011;78:611–7.
83. Lammer J, Bosiers M, Zeller T, Schillinger M, Boone E, Zaugg MJ, et al. First clinical trial of nitinol self-expanding everolimus-eluting stent implantation for peripheral arterial occlusive disease. J Vasc Surg. 2011;54:394–401.
84. Serruys PW, Ormiston JA, Onuma Y, et al. A bioabsorbable everolimus-eluting coronary stent system (ABSORB): 2-year outcomes and results from multiple imaging methods. Lancet. 2009;373: 897–910.
85. Folkman J. Angiogenesis in cancer, vascular, rheumatoid and other disease. Nat Med. 1995;1:27–31.
86. Walter DH, Cejna M, Diaz-Sandoval L, et al. Local gene transfer of phvegf-2 plasmid by gene-eluting stents: an alternative strategy for inhibition of restenosis. Circulation. 2004;110:36–45.
87. Schober A, Hoffmann R, Opree N, et al. Peripheral cd34+ cells and the risk of in-stent restenosis in patients with coronary heart disease. Am J Cardiol. 2005;96:1116–22.
88. Aoki J, Serruys PW, van Beusekom H, et al. Endothelial progenitor cell capture by stents coated with antibody against CD34: the Healing-FIM (Healthy Endothelial Accelerated Lining Inhibits Neointimal Growth-First in Man) Regestry. J Am Coll Cardiol. 2005;45:1574–9.

Shear Stress and Endothelial Cell Retention in Critical Lower Limb Ischemia

15

Caroline Jadlowiec and Alan Dardik

The Molecular-Cellular Basis for Critical Limb Ischemia

Endothelial Cell Physiology

Progressive atherosclerotic stenosis of vessels commonly leads to the development of critical limb and myocardial ischemia. When possible and appropriate, surgical revascularization is attempted, and it is here that we clinically observe the pathological processes of ischemia and reperfusion and their complex effects [1]. Understanding of the role and function of the vascular endothelium has undergone significant changes over the past several decades. In the 1960s Willms-Kretschmer and colleagues [2] and Pober [3] referred to altered endothelial cells as being activated and, in doing so, implied a functional consequence to the altered cell morphology. This dynamic view of the endothelium, however, did not ensue into the following decade when, again, it was believed that endothelial cells were nothing more than a passive barrier. It would not be until the 1980s that Bevilacqua et al [4] would reexamine the scientific principle and ultimately prove that the vascular endothelium is both dynamic and integral to vascular and systemic equilibrium. The scientific process to better understand the endothelium dates back to the 1800s when von Recklinghausen recognized that vessels were not merely inert tunnels passing through tissue, but living entities lined by cells [5]. The endothelial monolayer comprises the entirety of the vascular system, and it is now recognized that the diversity of these cells is not merely limited by cell type alone, but rather is a function of anatomic hemodynamic variation. The unique interface formed by the endothelium between blood and the surrounding vessel wall allows it to function as a primary mediator in response to shear stress alterations.

Studies have found that steady laminar shear stress is protective and, under such conditions, the endothelium is found to occupy a quiescent state where it exhibits both low proliferation and apoptosis [6]. Perhaps the most extensively investigated subject to date has been the influence of fluid shear stress applied to confluent monolayers of cultured endothelial cells [7]. Cellular morphology, under higher shear stress conditions, finds endothelial cells to have an elongated appearance and increased alignment, whereas low-flow, turbulent conditions produce rounded, nonaxially oriented endothelial cells that possess a higher cell turnover. The first in vivo documentation of flow-altered endothelial cellular morphology was conducted in the early 1970s, and the findings from this study showed that, in uniform laminar flow vessel segments, endothelial nuclei were oriented parallel to the axis of the blood vessel [8]. In contrast nonaxial, less-ordered nuclear orientation was found at vessel branch points and bifurcations where flow is recognized to be turbulent [9]. Further studies have since confirmed the morphologic observation that unidirectional laminar shear stress applied to cultured endothelial monolayers induces time- and force-dependent cytoskeletal reorganization. This restructuring produces changes in cell shape and alignment and is reversible with flow interruption [10].

Current studies identify hemodynamic shear stress as an important, if not primary, determinant of endothelial function and phenotype (Fig. 15.1). High shear stress, typically regarded as being greater than 15 dyn/cm^2, such as is found in arterial circulation, promotes endothelial cell quiescence and expression of atheroprotective genes. In contrast, low shear stress, defined as less than 4 dyn/cm^2, stimulates an activated atherogenic endothelial phenotype [11]. Nonlaminar flow correlates with endothelial cell activation and the development of atherosclerosis and neointimal hyperplasia, and, in vitro, replication of disturbed flow has shown increased endothelial cell proliferation and apoptosis. With

C. Jadlowiec, MD • A. Dardik, MD, PhD (✉)
Department of Surgery and the Interdepartmental Program in Vascular Biology and Therapeutics, Yale University School of Medicine, 10 Amistad Street, Room 437, P.O. Box 208089, New Haven, CT 06520-8089, USA

VA Connecticut Healthcare System, West Haven, CT, USA
e-mail: alan.dardik@yale.edu

E.A. Gabriel, S.A. Gabriel (eds.), *Inflammatory Response in Cardiovascular Surgery*, DOI 10.1007/978-1-4471-4429-8_15, © Springer-Verlag London 2013

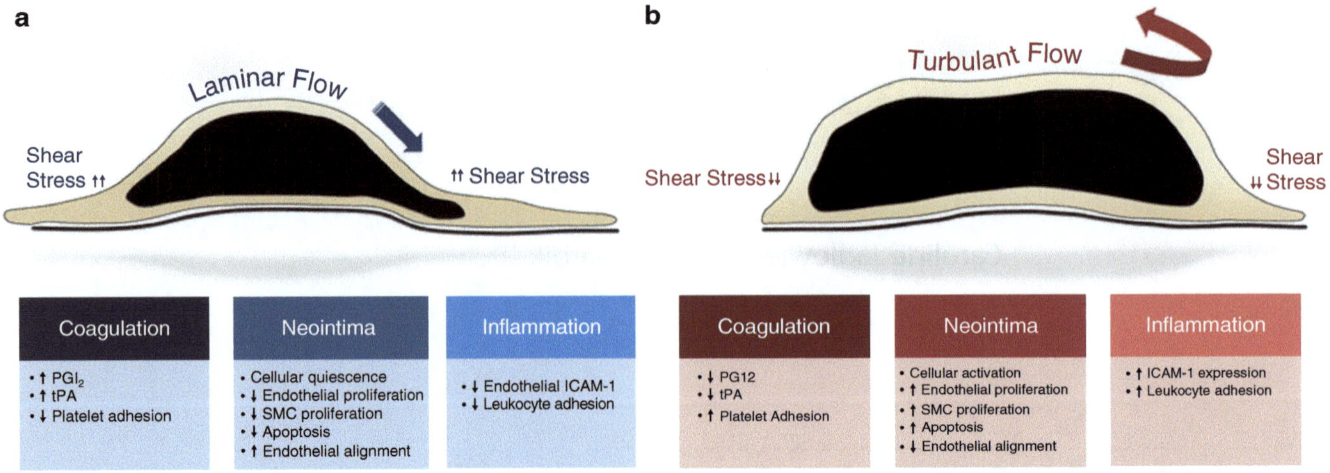

Fig. 15.1 Alterations in endothelial cell function and phenotype as determined by environmental hemodynamics. (**a**) Endothelial cell responses to high shear stress. (**b**) Endothelial cell responses to low shear stress

regard to anticoagulant properties, activated endothelium displays increased intercellular adhesion molecule expression and platelet aggregation as well as reduced production of antithrombogenic substances, such as prostacyclin (PGI_1) and tissue plasminogen activator (tPA) [7]. These qualities are in stark contrast to quiescent endothelium where leukocyte adhesion is diminished, PGI_1 and tPA production is increased, and platelet aggregation is reduced [7, 12].

Normal laminar shear stress is critical in maintaining normal physiologic vascular function including thromboresistance, barrier function, and vascular tone. In contrast, low or oscillary shear stress results in disturbed flow conditions and plays an important role in atherogenesis and bypass failure [13] (Fig. 15.1). Work done by Gimbrone and colleagues has demonstrated the relationship between decreased shear stress and atherogenesis [14]. Decreases in shear stress are accompanied by disturbances in normal endothelial cell function, and repair mechanisms within the endothelium are reduced along with the production of endothelial nitric oxide synthase (eNOS). Moreover, systemic risk factors such as hypertension and hyperlipidemia exacerbate endothelial intrinsic dysfunction. On a cellular level, this results in increased production of reactive oxygen species (ROS), altered lipoprotein permeability, leukocyte adhesion, and cellular proliferation [15].

Hypoxic Physiology

Hypoxia, depletion of the circulating oxygen content, is recognized as the driving force behind ischemic injury and, on a cellular level, endothelial cells respond to this insult by undergoing the phenotypic change now universally recognized as endothelial cell activation. This results in a series of alterations including the release of stored inflammatory mediators, changes in endothelial cell surface protein expression, and the conversion from aerobic metabolism to anaerobic alternative pathways [16]. The vascular endothelium is responsible for regulating membrane permeability, vascular tone, coagulation, and inflammation, and it does so by dynamically responding to any systemic alterations, such as hypoxia, within the vascular environment [17]. Yet, despite its wide range of adaptability, the vascular endothelium likewise remains very sensitive to hypoxic insults, inflammatory stimuli, and physical injury from surgical manipulation or hemodynamic stress, and it is this interplay between adaptation and injury that makes cardiovascular surgery a challenging paradox [16] (Fig. 15.2).

In contrast to other cell types, the vascular endothelium is comparatively resistant to decreases in oxygen content [17]. Under ischemic conditions, aerobic cellular energy depletion leads to an atypical accumulation of cytoplasmic metabolites and failure of oxygen-dependent membrane transport systems. Of most significance is the documented intracellular increase in calcium ion concentration and the upregulation of xanthine oxidase (XO) transcription and synthesis. Although restoration of blood flow after prolonged ischemia is essential for possible physiologic salvage, reperfusion itself exacerbates endothelial cell injury. XO, an endothelial cell-associated enzyme, increases under hypoxic conditions and, with the restoration of blood flow and oxygen, leads to the intracellular buildup of reactive oxygen species (ROS) [18]. Once produced, ROS cause localized and systemic cellular damage through both direct injury to membranes and proteins and indirectly through activation of proapoptotic pathways [19]. This reperfusion damage is further augmented as damaged cellular membranes are exposed to a replenished intravascular supply of calcium. Acting as a second messenger, calcium triggers activation of various enzymes crucial to the production of proinflammatory mediators [20].

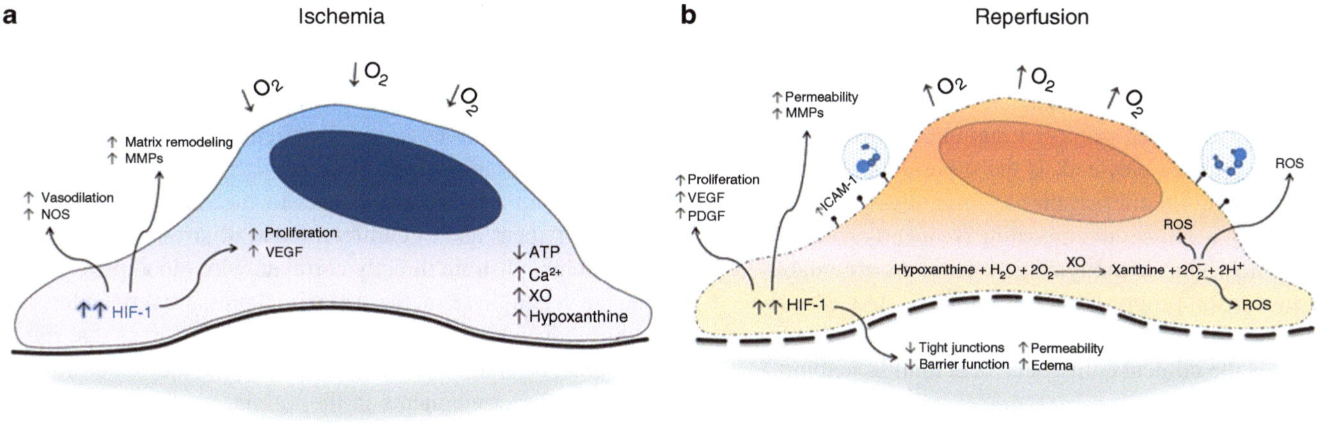

Fig. 15.2 Endothelial cell responses to ischemia. (**a**) Endothelial cell hypoxic physiology. (**b**) Endothelial cell responses to reperfusion

Under normal conditions endothelial cells form an overlapping monolayer that permits only controlled passage of molecules. This monolayer is further enhanced through the presence of tight junctions that reinforce endothelial cell barrier function. Hypoxic conditions lead to alterations in endothelial cell barrier function and vessel permeability. In response to decreased oxygen content, there is loss of tight junctions between adjacent endothelial cells leading to gap formation and increased permeability between cells. These changes are likewise accompanied by decreases in intracellular cyclic AMP, which is essential for maintenance of the actin-based cytoskeletal architecture and normal barrier function [4, 21]. This increased permeability results in what is clinically observed as ischemia reperfusion edema.

Hypoxic adaptation in endothelium leads to the transcriptional induction of a series of genes that participate in angiogenesis, metabolism, and cell proliferation, and the primary mediator of this response is hypoxia-inducible factor-1 (HIF-1), an oxygen-sensitive transcriptional activator [22]. The HIF-1 heterodimeric protein consists of two subunits, a beta subunit that is constitutively expressed (HIF-1β) and an oxygen-regulated alpha unit (HIF-1α). The stability and activity of the alpha subunit are regulated by its post-translational modifications, and, under normoxic conditions, this subunit is degraded. Conversely, in hypoxia, the beta subunit becomes stable resulting in the regulation of target gene expression [22]. Previous studies have demonstrated that HIF-1 plays a critical role in endothelial angiogenesis through both paracrine and autocrine mechanisms [23, 24]. Recent discoveries have shown that hypoxia-activated HIFs induce endothelial expression of several critical angiogenic factors, including vascular endothelial growth factor (VEGF), nitric oxide synthase (NOS), platelet-derived growth factor (PDGF), Ang2, and others [25]. HIFs have also been found to be mediators of endothelial survival pathways where hypoxic upregulation results in cellular proliferation. Clinically, this can result in a wide spectrum of remodeling, including angiogenesis and neointimal hyperplasia (Fig. 15.2).

Shear Stress and Arteriogenesis

Study of arteriogenesis, the enlargement of preexisting arterial connections into true collateral arteries, began in the 1700s with the work of Albrecht von Haller, a Swiss anatomist, who dissected human hearts and found that coronary arteries provide a system of interarterially connected vessels on the side of high arterial pressure. His findings suggested that these conduits were functional arteries, larger in size than capillaries [26]. Today, this process is recognized as arteriogenesis, and, unlike angiogenesis, which is primarily mediated by hypoxia, initiation of collateral artery growth and remodeling is dependent on alterations in hemodynamic forces. Circumferential wall stress and fluid shear stress are recognized and the two primary forces responsible for this complex process; however, uncertainties continue with regard to the specific contributions and overall importance of either toward arteriogenesis. Some uncertainty comes from the observation that fluid shear stress, with a typical range of 20–30 dyn/cm^2, is a weak force when compared with circumferential wall stress, which is 106 times greater [27].

In the early 1920s, Murray proposed that the vascular system's branching configuration exists so as to minimize the amount of mechanical and metabolic work to provide adequate blood flow. Using this model, it can be surmised that fluid shear stress remains constant throughout the vasculature and that blood flow is proportional to the cube of each individual vessel's diameter. Additionally, shear stress remains proportional to blood flow and inversely related to the cube of the radius [27, 28]. Accordingly, it is hypothesized that shear stress regulates the acute early phase of arteriogenesis where small increases in collateral artery diameter result in significant decreases in shear stress [29]. The formation of collateral circulation after an arterial occlusion correlates well with the observed increase in shear stress where increased collateral flow is caused by the pressure redistribution from pre-existent, now occluded, vessels [30]. It is also recognized that increases in collateral diameter end once shear stress normalizes.

Interestingly, despite early and abrupt normalization, cellular remodeling of collaterals persists beyond this acute period, and a shift from quiescence toward proliferation is observed in both endothelial and vascular smooth muscle cells [31]. As a result, it has been proposed that circumferential wall stress, which remains elevated, is the more dominant force in this later stage of arteriogenesis. Regardless of the dominant mediators, collateral remodeling frequently reaches a plateau, at which point hemodynamic alterations are unable to compensate for progressive atherogenesis. Indeed, when these compensatory systems fail or are overwhelmed, what follows next is the clinical entity of critical limb ischemia.

Surgical Solutions for CLI

Autologous Vein Grafts

Today, autologous vein grafting is the recognized standard for infrainguinal arterial revascularization, yet prior to the pioneering work done in the early 1900s, the predominating belief was that repair of major vasculature was beyond the capacity of surgical technique. Unconvinced that the 1894 penetrating portal venous injury of French president Carnot was not treatable, Carrel would undertake the task of refining vessel anastomosis. He would go on to establish the modern fundamentals of bypass surgery with his combined techniques of delicate vessel handling, fine suture material, and triangulation [21]. The future of bypass surgery would then be further progressed by Kunlin, who in 1948 would be the first to successfully use a reversed saphenous vein graft in the treatment of lower extremity ischemia [32]. In 1962, Sabiston would then go on to use a modification of this technique in what we recognize today as the modern coronary bypass. Interestingly, although much has changed from the pioneering days of surgical vascular research, what remains is that the conduit of choice for lower extremity bypass continues to be the greater saphenous vein.

Physiology of Vein Graft Adaptation

Venous anatomy echoes arterial, and the intima, media, and adventitia are easily identified as the major anatomic vessel wall components. It is well known that, unlike arteries, veins have a reduced medial component, which results in a thinner vessel wall and typically allows for increased compliance. From prior work, it is known that vein compliance is not a static property, but rather dependent on its environment. Although it is commonly assumed that native veins are more compliant than arteries, in actuality, this increased compliance only remains present up to pressures of 35–50 mmHg [33]. Under typical arterial pressures, vein grafts become stiff and lose compliance, while matched arteries remain moderately distensible. Accordingly, a more accurate description is that veins are more compliant than arteries at low pressures, but less compliant than arteries when subjected to arterial pressures.

Low pressure and low flow are the dominant hemodynamic entities in the normal venous environment, and, unlike the physiology observed in arterial circulation, veins are not subjected to pulsatility, high flow, or high pressures. All vessels, venous and arterial, are subject to mechanical forces in the form of shear and circumferential wall stress. Effects of circumferential strain directly correlate with blood pressure, and in the venous system, these maximal pressures are understandably reduced. The circumferential venous forces that remain go on to be counteracted by the entirety of the vessel wall, and the cellular components in the intima, media, and adventitia are uniformly affected. Conversely, shear stress, the frictional force of blood along the intima is distinctive in that it exerts its force primarily on endothelial cells. Fluid shear stress likewise displays significant variation between venous and arterial systems, and prior studies have found 1–6 dyn/cm^2 to be typical of venous shear stress. This is in large contrast to arterial vasculature where anywhere from 10 to 70 dyn/cm^2 is the prevailing norm [11]. This abrupt hemodynamic alteration has been implicated as the mechanism responsible for initial endothelial desquamation, which is observed to occur in the first week of graft placement. In such situations, graft endothelium regeneration appears to occur quickly with complete healing observed in some veins at 48 h [34]. Nonetheless, concerns regarding the long-term effects of acute arterial disruption of venous endothelium remain with respect to graft patency.

Indeed, long-term patency for autologous bypass is largely dependent on how successfully venous conduits adapt to arterialization. As first suggested by Owens et al., the process of successful vein graft adaptation appears to involve at least two distinct temporal phases: early outward remodeling of the lumen and delayed acquisition of wall stiffness [35]. In 2006, in a prospective human study, the authors showed that 72 % of venous grafts dilate during the first post-surgical month and that no appreciable changes occur beyond this time. During the first 6 months, a nearly 40 % increase in conduit stiffness was found with the greatest relative increase occurring during the initial first 3 postoperative months. Clinically, grafts that demonstrated early positive remodeling in the form of lumen dilatation appeared to have increased primary patency, and a trend toward greater wall stiffness at 1 month was noted in grafts that failed [35]. Further work done by the same authors in 2008 underscored the critical role of systemic inflammation in vein graft remodeling. In this study, there was positive correlation noted between vein graft diameter and initial shear stress. This shear-dependent response, however, was disrupted in patients with an elevated baseline high-sensitivity C-reactive protein (hsCRP). Moreover, despite similar vein diameter and shear stress at implantation, grafts in the elevated hsCRP group demonstrated less positive remodeling within the first month and likewise had a propensity to be stiffer [36]. Accordingly, although intricacies and specific mediators remain to be identified, early positive adaptation of vein grafts lends itself to successful long-term patency, and the importance of controlling systemic inflammation deserves emphasis.

Responses of Venous Endothelial Cells to Shear Stress

Hemodynamic shear stress, possibly the most influential component of vascular remodeling and pathology, is the frictional force created by the flow of blood in relation to the luminal vessel wall and endothelial surface. It is in this regard that the creation of a surgical bypass, using a venous conduit, becomes one of the most dynamic processes responsible for endothelial remodeling. Although the technicalities of performing a successful bypass are well established, much of the final outcome hinges on how successful the venous conduit will be in adapting to the high-pressure pulsatile flow arterial circulation where it is acutely placed [37]. Much remains to be learned about the underlying mechanisms responsible for both successful as well as pathologic endothelial adaptation. At present, the majority of our insight into endothelial response to hemodynamics comes from animal experiments in which shear stress is acutely or chronically altered [11].

Classically, increases in shear stress, both acute and chronic, are observed to result in upregulation of endothelial nitric oxide synthase (eNOS) mRNA and protein production [38]. Such increases in eNOS activity result in vessel lumen dilation. Studies investigating this role for nitric oxide (NO) have shown that through the use of L-NAME, a nitric oxide synthase inhibitor, flow-induced vessel dilation is inhibited [39]. In 1997, Clowes and colleagues demonstrated an important relationship between shear stress and neointimal hyperplasia. Using a primate model, the authors inserted PTFE grafts into aortoiliac circulation bilaterally. A neointima was allowed to develop for 2 months, and, at that time, half of the animals were killed. For the remaining group, graft flow was increased through the creation of a femoral arteriovenous fistula. These animals were then killed 2 months post-fistula creation. The findings from this study showed regression of the neointima in those grafts exposed to the additional 2 months of high shear stress. From prior work, using this same model, the authors were also able to show that high shear stress inhibits neointimal growth [39].

Work examining the effects of high and low flow on graft adaptation have shown increased smooth muscle cell proliferation in grafts exposed to low shear stress, and similar findings have also been observed in endothelial cells [40]. In a rat model, where unilateral ligation of the internal and external carotid arteries results in the creation of high- and low-flow arteries, increased endothelial cell proliferation is seen at 24, 48, and 72 h post-ligation in the reduced flow carotids. With this model, the achieved alteration in flow reflected true arterial and venous circulation, with a comparative shear stress of 33.4 ± 1.1 dyn/cm^2 in the high-flow carotid versus 1.4 ± 0.2 dyn/cm^2 in the ligated, low-flow complement [41]. These correlations between shear stress and neointimal remodeling provide insight into the mechanisms involved in venous bypass and likewise demonstrate the paradoxical effects that high flow and shear stress can exert on endothelial homeostasis.

Graft Characteristics and Long-Term Patency

Using the best available autologous conduit is universally accepted as the fitting approach for peripheral bypass surgery, and the conduit of choice is the ipsilateral, single-segment greater saphenous vein secondary to its documented patency in lower extremity bypass [42]. Other characteristics that define the best autologous conduit however continue to be debated, and much of the data available comes from single-institution retrospective studies that attempted to define meaningful graft characteristics in regard to long-term patency. Traditionally, three surgical configurations, reversed, nonreversed, and in situ, have been accepted for use in infrainguinal vascular bypass work, and each is believed to confer different effects on endothelial cells.

Reversed Vein Grafts

Vein excision with reversal of anatomical orientation and maintenance of intact valves is the essence of a reversed vein grafting technique. Considered to be somewhat basic, usage of reversed vein grafts is typically well adapted for most surgical bypass settings. The reversed technique eliminates the need for valve lysis and thus limits intraluminal manipulation. Concerns with regard to the altered flow dynamic in reversed vein grafts have come from studies showing intraluminal turbulence secondary to retained valves. The surgical creation of a reversed vein graft introduces valves into the arterial system and, by doing so, adds a potential source of turbulence. Such deviations from laminar flow hold the potential to initiate pathological endothelial cell activation. Despite having a reversed anatomy, venous valves do not lie flush with the graft wall, and once subjected to pulsatile arterial flow, these valves are observed to close during diastole [43]. Coupled with the cardiac cycle, valves have the potential to modify flow dynamics by becoming active and preventing the natural arterial backflow, and it has been speculated that midgraft stenotic lesions occur secondary to retained valve leaflets [44]. Other surgical concerns arise from the stasis observed within the valve cusps and the potential for them to function as a thrombogenic nidus [43].

Nonreversed Vein Grafts

In nonreversed technique, the vein is excised, its valves are subjected to mechanical lysis, and it is then oriented in its original nonreversed configuration. Observed advantages come from the preservation of a nonreversed orientation, thus improving the circumferential accord of the arterial graft anastomosis. Intraluminal valve lysis, however, is a requisite and results in endothelial cell trauma and denudation. Venous valve lysis results in significant endothelial trauma, and, from prior work, it is known that the preservation of endothelial cell integrity in venous grafts prevents subsequent morphologic changes, namely thickening of the venous intima and media in response to arterial dynamics [45]. Remarkably, despite the inherent need for more manipulation and handling with nonreversed grafts, improved hemodynamic flow is the resulting outcome following valve lysis. Studies have shown that lysis of valves increases graft flow rates anywhere from 30 to 60 % as compared to grafts with intact valves [46, 47]. Clinically, the improved bypass hemodynamics, shown through higher shear stress and flow velocity, are atheroprotective and correlate with increased long-term graft patency.

In Situ Vein Grafts

The initial concept of utilizing an autologous vein graft while minimizing surgical manipulation is attributed to the work of both Rob and Hall in the early 1960s. At that time, advanced valvulotomes had yet to be developed, and valve lysis was achieved through serial transverse venotomies and individual valve excision [48]. The modern in situ vein graft is created through limited mobilization of both the proximal and distal vein segments, thus allowing them to be used in arterial bypass but simultaneously reducing total vein manipulation and damage to the outer vessel layers, including the vasa vasorum, during harvesting. Some studies have suggested improved patency outcomes in vein bypasses harvested en-bloc with surrounding tissue where venous spasm is believed to be reduced [49]. Prior studies have also demonstrated that the disruption of the vasa vasorum results in an acute decrease in vessel distensibility as well as long-term structural changes and delayed deterioration of vessel elastic properties [50]. Based on such evidence, it has been proposed that by diminishing spasm, the need for high pressure distention, a known mediator of vein wall and endothelial damage, is reduced [49]. There is also evidence to suggest an inverse relationship between vasa vasorum preservation and neointimal hyperplasia. Findings by Gossl et al. showed that vessel areas with diminished vasa vasorum density were more susceptible to hypoxia, oxidative stress, and microinflammation, all factors known to potentiate early atherogenesis [51]. Accordingly, there is modest evidence present that the use of atraumatic techniques, which minimize damage to the adventitia and the vasa vasorum, improve bypass patency.

Although there have been many studies, mainly single center and retrospective, that have attempted to address aspects of surgical technique in relation to lower extremity bypass outcomes, the exact contribution of specific technical factors remains to be fully defined. The most comprehensive data available come from the 2006 Project of Ex-Vivo Vein Graft Engineering via Transfection III (PREVENT III) Study, which was a randomized, double-blinded, placebo-controlled trial of edifoligide for prevention of vein graft failure in patients undergoing lower extremity revascularization for critical limb ischemia. Although the primary and secondary endpoints for PREVENT III did little to modify current medical strategies for limb revascularization, the study was able to provide perhaps the most comprehensive multicenter data available to date with regard to long-debated conduit and technique characteristics, such as vessel diameter, graft type, and conduit orientation [52, 53].

Results for early 30-day graft failure identified several significant technical predictors of early loss of primary patency. Small-conduit diameter was identified as one such technical factor, and primary patency in grafts greater than 3.5 mm was observed to be 93.2 % vs. 85.7 % in grafts with diameters less than 3.0 mm. Not surprisingly, composite grafts showed worse outcomes when compared to single-segment grafts with a primary patency of 84.1 % vs. 92.2 % in non-spliced greater saphenous vein. Bypasses originating from a more distal location showed improved short-term outcomes. Grafts that originated from the popliteal artery had primary patency rates of 93.9 % as compared to those with more proximal anastomoses, such as the common or superficial femoral arteries, where rates were 91.7 % and 87.7 %, respectively. Graft length and the site of distal anastomosis were not found to be predictors of primary patency loss. Although a slight difference was observed between the early failure rates of reversed and nonreversed grafts, 91.6 % patency as compared to 93.3 %, this finding was not statistically significant [53]. At 1 year, graft patency was again found to be detrimentally affected by small conduit diameter with primary patency observed to be 68.4 % in grafts with diameters greater than 3.5 mm vs. 42.4 % for those less than 3.0 mm. Poorer outcomes were observed in bypasses composed of composite spliced vein, those greater than 60 cm in length, and more proximal bypass origination. Moreover, at 1 year, the primary patency rates for reversed (65.0 %) and nonreversed (63.3 %) orientation grafts were equivalent and not statistically significant. From these data, significant identifiable technical predictors of early and late graft failure include use of a small conduit diameter or a composite vein; however, surgical variation with the reversed and nonreversed technique does not appear to be a primary factor in bypass success [53].

Prosthetic

While the saphenous vein continues to be the superior unrivaled arterial substitute for lower extremity bypass, a significant portion of patients with critical limb ischemia does not possess an autologous vein that is usable. It is in such difficult situations that an alternative arterial conduit is frequently employed. The history regarding synthetic conduits, like much of surgical history, is long and much indebted to research pioneers. In 1952, Voorhees and Blakemore published a preliminary report describing the successful use of Vinyon "N" cloth prostheses in the infrarenal aorta of mongrel dogs [54]. Despite these limited successes, long-term durability would remain limited until the successful use of the modern polymers polytetrafluoroethylene (PTFE) and polyethylene terephthalate (Dacron).

Dacron

Within the same time period of the early 1950s, DeBakey went on to create the first Dacron tube graft for aortic reconstruction [55]. Unlike the preceding experiments using nylon, Dacron, a synthetic multifilament yarn, proved to be both a durable and suitable material for vascular reconstruction. Traditionally, Dacron grafts have either been woven or knitted, and modern grafts of both varieties continue to be manufactured and used. Woven grafts do not rely on the looping of yarn around a needle, and because of this the resulting material has a decreased porosity [56]. The more compact nature of woven grafts results in stronger fabric, but comes at the cost of decreased compliance. The stiffness of the woven graft is believed to make it more difficult to handle and suture, and the fiber orientation enhances the potential of fraying when cut in the operating room [56]. Conversely, knitted Dacron results in a softer, more compliant material that likewise is more porous. The increased porosity of these grafts makes them more susceptible to bleeding, and traditionally knitted tube grafts were subjected to preclotting where the patient's blood was passed through the graft prior to surgical interposition so as to coat the pores with fibrin and minimize operative bleeding [57]. Modern knitted grafts are now manufactured with precoated materials, such as gelatin or collagen.

PTFE

Polytetrafluoroethylene (PTFE) first came into production in the 1930s, and by the early 1970s, an expanded form, ePTFE, began to be used in animal models as an alternative to Dacron in arterial reconstruction [58]. The first successful reported clinical use followed soon after in 1976 when Campbell et al. published their experience in using ePTFE in infrainguinal bypass [59]. Today, PTFE it is predominantly processed into expanded PTFE (ePTFE), and the extrusion process results in a porous morphology that microscopically is characterized by interconnected nodes and fibrils. Unlike the woven or knitted characteristics of Dacron, ePTFE is a single seamless structure. Despite being microporous, ePTFE has a low friction coefficient making its surface smooth and hydrophobic. Although ePTFE's hydrophobic property prevents hematogenous graft permeation, plasma and platelet surface adherence is not inhibited, and the overall host response has been found to be similar to that of Dacron [60]. More recently, heparin-bonded ePTFE grafts have become available for clinical use. Early data have suggested that these grafts decrease platelet adherence and acute thrombus formation surface [61]. Animal models have also shown a reduction in anastomotic myointimal hyperplasia [62]. In 2009, The Propaten European Product Evaluation (PEPE II) study showed that heparin-bonded ePTFE grafts yield patency rates that are comparable to those obtained with other graft material in infrainguinal bypass surgery [63]. At present, however, improvements to graft patency remain to be demonstrated, and further clinical data will be required to adequately determine this. Despite such fundamental differences in material composition, prospective randomized trials have found PTFE and Dacron to be equally suitable for infrainguinal bypass. Results from a trial published in 2001 showed no differences between Dacron and PTFE with regard to primary and secondary patency or limb salvage [64]. Consequently, the surgeon's choice of PTFE versus Dacron for infrainguinal bypass in the operating room is truly based on preference and not on clinical differences in graft performance and patency.

Endothelial Cell Seeding

Early work with Dacron from the 1960s raised excitement over the finding of a complete endothelial lining present in prosthetic grafts implanted into various animal species [65]. In stark contrast to this mature endothelium found within the arterial prostheses of baboons and pigs, however, was the realization that humans grafts fail to achieve this re-endothelialization [66]. Knowledge that endothelial cells possess anti-thrombotic properties and function to limit intimal hyperplasia, both primary obstacles to graft patency, led to research investigating the potential role for endothelial cell transplantation onto synthetic vascular grafts. In 1978, Herring et al. published their work using a canine model on arterial prostheses seeded with autogenous vascular endothelium. The authors achieved this result by harvesting endothelial cells from saphenous vein using steel wool pledgets and using the admixture to preclot Dacron grafts [67]. These results were promising, and over the ensuing decade much effort would be placed into endothelial cell harvest optimization and transplant, a process that came to be referred to as cell seeding.

Further enthusiasm toward cell seeding would come from later animal studies demonstrating that ex-vivo endothelial cell incorporation into synthetic grafts enhanced patency [68]. These results only further reinforced the belief that development of mature endothelial cell surface was the missing link to maintaining long-term patency in synthetic arterial substitutes [68]. Concerns that remained to be reconciled, however, included whether any of the benefits ascribed to cell seeding in animal models actually conferred analogous human benefit [69]. In 1985, Rosenman et al. published important work relating to the kinetics of endothelial cell adhesion to synthetic graft materials. Using carotid interposition ePTFE seeded grafts with ^{111}indium oxide-labeled endothelial cells, the authors were able to examine cell retention following arterial implantation. Immediately following implantation, only 19.8 % of the originally seeded cells were found to be present, and, at 30 min, 70.2 % of these remaining cells desquamated. Cell loss continued over the next 24 h, at which time only 4.4 % of originally seeded cells remained present [70]. These results were obviously unfavorable, and for much of the next decade, experimental work would focus on methods to improve endothelial cell adhesion.

The findings of poor endothelial cell retention coupled with, at best, modest improvements in graft patency greatly diminished the surgical community's enthusiasm for cell seeding. As noted by Zilla, those who continued work with endothelial cell transplant were prepared to accept both a long and arduous route with the knowledge that their contribution would be a quiet one [71]. Not surprisingly, research using collagen or fibronectin pretreatment to synthetic grafts found that endothelial cells adhered poorly to and did not grow on untreated Dacron and PTFE, while protein-treated materials facilitated cellular retention [72]. Differences were also noted between pre-treated Dacron and PTFE. Cells seeded onto protein-treated PTFE were noted to form a confluent monolayer within 9 days, while the more irregular surface of Dacron showed inferior results [73]. The following decade would bring with it the next generation of advancement in the quest to create a biologically functional vascular prosthesis. It was observed that chronic in vitro culture of aortic endothelial cells with flow was associated with cytoskeletal reorganization and increased endocytic activity when compared to conventional static culture conditions. These data implied that, through the control of flow, differentiation of endothelial cells could be regulated [74]. It was therefore hypothesized that endothelial cell adhesion could be stimulated and enhanced by shear stress. The results of this hypothesis became apparent in 1999, when Dardik and colleagues published their work investigating the role of shear stress in endothelial cell retention. PTFE endothelial cell seeded grafts were treated with 0, 1, or 25 dyn/cm^2 shear stress in vitro and then implanted. The authors found that pretreatment with 25 dyn/cm^2 resulted in fully confluent endothelial cell retention at 24 h post in vivo implantation. Furthermore, this confluency and retention continued to be observed up to a 3-month time point. In comparison, this same observation did not hold true for low flow conditions [75].

Despite great progress in understanding the biomechanics of endothelial cell adaptation, clinical studies to date have been less successful in providing similar insight and progress. The first report of human cell seeding came from Herring et al. in 1984. Using seeded and unseeded ePTFE, the authors documented a 100 % patency for seeded femoral-popliteal bypasses at 18 months in comparison to 60 % in unseeded grafts [76]. Overall, however, results from further human clinical trials have been mixed, with many investigators finding no benefit [77]. The most promising long-term clinical cell seeding data come from work done by Zilla and colleagues. In a study published in 1999, the authors showed a notable primary 9-year patency rate of 65 % in endothelialized PTFE grafts versus 16 % in control non-seeded PTFE grafts [78]. More recently in 2009, the same authors published their long-term results using autologous in vitro endothelialization of infrainguinal ePTFE grafts. Over a span of 15 years, and inclusive of 341 infrainguinal endothelialized ePTFE grafts, the authors showed an overall femoropopliteal primary patency rate of 69 % at 5 years and 61 % at 10 years [79]. Unexpectedly, examination of retrieved ePTFE samples from this cohort revealed the presence of an endothelium on all samples after 38.9 ± 17.8 months, thus challenging prior cell seeding outcomes where long-term cell retention appeared difficult, if not impossible, to achieve [79]. The results of this group go on to suggest that in vitro long-term endothelialization of synthetic grafts is not only clinically feasible, but that it also provides a patency benefit in challenging patients without suitable autogenous vein.

References

1. Verrier ED, Boyle Jr EM. Endothelial cell injury in cardiovascular surgery. Ann Thorac Surg. 1996;62(3):915–22.
2. Willms-Kretchmer K, Flax MH, Cotran RS. The fine structure of the vascular response in haptan-specific delayed hypersensitivity and contact dermatitis. Lab Invest. 1967;17(3):334–49.
3. Pober JS. Warner-Lambert/Parke-Davis award lecture. Cytokine-mediated activation of vascular endothelium. Physiology and pathology. Am J Pathol. 1988;133(3):426–33.
4. Bevilacqua MP, Pober JS, Wheeler ME. Interleukin 1 acts on cultured human vascular endothelium to increase the adhesion of polymorphonuclear leukocytes, monocytes, and related leukocyte cell lines. J Clin Invest. 1985;76:2003–11.
5. Cines DB, Pollak ES, Buck CA, et al. Endothelial cells in physiology and in the pathophysiology of vascular disorders. Blood. 1998;91(10):3527–61.
6. Paszkowiak JJ, Dardik A. Arterial wall shear stress: observations from the bench to the bedside. Vasc Endovascular Surg. 2003;37(1):47–57.
7. Dardik A, Chen L, Frattini J, et al. Differential effects of orbital and laminar shear stress on endothelial cells. J Vasc Surg. 2005;41(5):869–80.
8. Davies PF. Flow-mediated endothelial mechanotransduction. Physiol Rev. 1995;75(3):519–60.
9. Flaherty JT, Pierce JE, Ferrans VJ, et al. Endothelial nuclear patterns in the canine arterial tree with particular reference to hemodynamic events. Circ Res. 1972;30(1):23–33.

10. Resnick N, Gimbrone MA. Hemodynamic forces are complex regulators of endothelial gene expression. FASEB J. 1995;9(10): 874–82.
11. Malek AM, Alper AL, Izumo S. Hemodynamic shear stress and its role in atherosclerosis. JAMA. 1999;282(21):2035–42.
12. Caplan BA, Schwartz CJ. Increased endothelial cell turnover in areas of in vivo Evans blue uptake in the pig aorta. Atherosclerosis. 1973;17:401–17.
13. Cunningham KS, Gotlieb AI. The role of shear stress in the pathogenesis of atherosclerosis. Lab Invest. 2005;85:9–23.
14. Gimbrone Jr MA, Nagel T, Topper JN. Biomechanical activation: an emerging paradigm in endothelial adhesion biology. J Clin Invest. 1997;99(8):1809–13.
15. Gimbrone MA, Topper JN, Nagel T, et al. Endothelial dysfunction, hemodynamic forces, and atherogenesis Atherosclerosis V: the Fifth Saratoga Conference. Ann N Y Acad Sci. 2000;902:230–40.
16. Verrier ED, Morgan EN. Endothelial response to cardiopulmonary bypass surgery. Ann Thorac Surg. 1998;66(S1):S17–9.
17. Ten VS, Pinsky DJ. Endothelial response to hypoxia: physiologic adaptation and pathologic dysfunction. Curr Opin Crit Care. 2002;8(3):242–50.
18. Ratych RE, Chuknyiska RS, Bulkley GB. The primary localization of free radical generation after anoxia/reoxygenation in isolated endothelial cells. Surgery. 1987;102(2):122–31.
19. Braunersreuther V, Jaquet V. Reactive oxygen species in myocardial reperfusion injury: from physiopathology to therapeutic approaches. Curr Pharm Biotechnol. 2012;13(1):97–114.
20. Kerrigan CL, Stotland MA. Ischemia reperfusion injury: a review. Microsurgery. 1993;14(3):165–75.
21. Cooley BC. History of vein grafting. Microsurgery. 1998;18(4): 234–6.
22. Ke Q, Costa M. Hypoxia-inducible factor-1 (HIF-1). Mol Pharmacol. 2006;70(5):1469–80.
23. Pugh CW, Ratcliffe PJ. Regulation of angiogenesis by hypoxia: role of the HIF system. Nat Med. 2003;9:677–84.
24. Manalo JD, Rowan A, Lavoie T, et al. Transcriptional regulation of vascular endothelial cell responses to hypoxia by HIF-1. Blood. 2005;105(2):659–69.
25. Carmeliet P, Jain RK. Angiogenesis in cancer and other disease. Nature. 2000;407:249–57.
26. Buschmann I, Schaper W. The pathophysiology of the collateral circulation (arteriogenesis). J Pathol. 2000;190(3):338–42.
27. Schaper W, Scholz D. Factors regulation arteriogenesis. Arterioscler Thromb Vasc Biol. 2003;23(7):1143–51.
28. Murray CD. The physiological principle of minimum work applied to the angle of branching of arteries. J Gen Physiol. 1926;9(6): 835–41.
29. Grundmann S, Piek JJ, Pasterkamp G, et al. Arteriogenesis: basic mechanisms and therapeutic stimulation. Eur J Clin Invest. 2007;37(10):755–66.
30. Pipp F, Boehm S, Cai WJ, et al. Elevated fluid shear stress enhances postocclusive collateral artery growth and gene expression in the pig hind limb. Arterioscler Thromb Vasc Biol. 2004;24(9):1664–8.
31. Heil M, Eitenmüller I, Schmitz-Rixen T. Arteriogenesis versus angiogenesis: similarities and differences. J Cell Mol Med. 2006;10(1):45–55.
32. Kunlin J. Le traitement de l'arterite obliterante par la greffe veineuse. Arch Mal Coeur. 1949;42:371–2.
33. Dobrin PB, Littooy FN, Golan J, et al. Mechanical and histologic changes in canine vein grafts. J Surg Res. 1988;44(3):259–65.
34. Krupski W, Thal ER, Gewertz BL, et al. Endothelial response to venous injury. Am Med Assoc. 1979;114(11):1240–8.
35. Owens CD, Wake N, Jacot JG, et al. Early biomechanical changes in lower extremity vein grafts–distinct temporal phases of remodeling and wall stiffness. J Vasc Surg. 2006;44(4):740–6.
36. Owens CD, Rybicki FJ, Wake N. Early remodeling of lower extremity vein grafts: inflammation influences biomechanical adaptation. J Vasc Surg. 2008;47(6):1235–42.
37. Golledge J, Turner RJ, Harley SL, et al. Circumferential deformation and shear stress induce differential responses in saphenous vein endothelium exposed to arterial flow. J Clin Invest. 1997;99(11): 2719–26.
38. Nadaud S, Philippe M, Arnal JF, et al. Sustained increase in aortic endothelial nitric oxide synthase expression in vivo in a model of chronic high blood flow. Circ Res. 1996;79:857–63.
39. Guzman RJ, Abe K, Zarins CK. Flow-induced arterial enlargement is inhibited by suppression of nitric oxide synthase activity in vivo. Surgery. 1997;122:273–80.
40. Kraiss LW, Geary RL, Mattsson EJ, et al. Acute reductions in blood flow and shear stress induce platelet-derived growth factor-A expression in baboon prosthetic grafts. Circ Res. 1996;79: 45–53.
41. Mondy JS, Lindner V, Miyashiro JK, et al. Platelet-derived growth factor ligand and receptor expression in response to altered blood flow in vivo. Circ Res. 1997;81:320–7.
42. Masser PA, Taylor LM, Moneta GL, et al. Technique of reversed vein bypass for lower extremity ischemia. Ann Vasc Surg. 1996;10(2):190–200.
43. McCaughan Jr JJ, Walsh DB, Edgcomb LP, et al. In vitro observations of greater saphenous vein valves during pulsatile and nonpulsatile flow and following lysis. J Vasc Surg. 1984;1(2):356–61.
44. Vesti BR, Primozich J, Bergelin RO, et al. Follow-up of valves in saphenous vein bypass grafts with duplex ultrasonography. J Vasc Surg. 2001;33(2):369–74.
45. Quist WC, LoGerfo FW. Prevention of smooth muscle cell phenotypic modulation in vein grafts: a hitomorphometric study. J Vasc Surg. 1992;16(2):225–31.
46. Ku DN, Klafta JM, Gewertz BL, et al. The contribution of valves to saphenous vein graft resistance. J Vasc Surg. 1987;6:274–9.
47. Chin AK, Mayer DN, Goldman RK, et al. The effect of valvulotomy on flow rate through the saphenous vein graft: clinical implications. J Vasc Surg. 1988;8(3):316–20.
48. May AG, DeWeese JA, Rob CG. Arterialization in situ saphenous vein. Arch Surg. 1965;91(5):743–50.
49. Souza SRD, Bomfim V, Skoglund H, et al. Early patency of saphenous vein graft for coronary artery bypass harvested with surrounding tissue. Ann Thorac Surg. 2001;71:797–800.
50. Stefanadis C, Vlachopoulos C, Karayannacos P, et al. Effect of vasa vasorum flow on structure and function of the aorta in experimental animals. Circulation. 1995;91:2669–78.
51. Gossl M, Versari D, Lerman LO, et al. Low vasa vasorum densities correlate with inflammation and subintimal thickening: potential role in location—determination of atherogenesis. Atherosclerosis. 2009;206:362–8.
52. Conte MS, Bandyk DK, Clowed AW, et al. Results of PREVENT III: a multicenter, randomized trial of edifoligide for the prevention of vein graft failure in lower extremity bypass surgery. J Vasc Surg. 2006;43(4):742–51.
53. Schanzer A, Hevelone N, Owens CD, et al. Technical factors affecting autogenous vein graft failure: observations from a large multicenter trial. J Vasc Surg. 2007;46(6):1180–90.
54. Voorhees AB, Jaretzki A, Blakemore AH. The use of tubes constructed from vinyon "N" cloth in bridging arterial defects: a preliminary. Ann Surg. 1952;135(3):332–3.
55. Kapadia MR, Popowich DA, Kibbe MR. Modified prosthetic vascular conduits. Circulation. 2008;117(14):1873–82.
56. Quarmby JW, Burnand KG, Lockhart SJM, et al. Prospective randomized trial of woven versus collagen¯impregnated knitted prosthetic Dacron grafts in aortoiliac surgery. Br J Surg. 1998;85(6): 775–7.

57. Guidoin R, Gosselin C, Domurado D. Dacron as arterial prosthetic material: nature, properties, brands, fate and perspectives. Biomater Med Devices Artif Organs. 1977;5(2):177–203.
58. Soyer T, Lempinen M, Cooper P, et al. A new venous prosthesis. Surgery. 1972;72(6):864–72.
59. Campbell CD, Brooks DH, Webster MW. The use of expanded microporous polytetrafluoroethylene for limb salvage: a preliminary report. Surgery. 1976;79(5):485–91.
60. Blumenberg RM, Anderson JM, Gelfand ML, et al. Histologic evaluation of Dacron® and PTFE graft material explanted from humans after 4 to 20 years in vivo. Vasc Endovascular Surg. 2000;34(6):505–12.
61. Heyligers JMM, Lisman T, Weeterings C, et al. Heparin immobilization reduces thrombogenicity on small-caliber ePTFE grafts. J Vasc Surg. 2006;43(3):587–91.
62. Lin PH, Chen C, Bush RL, et al. Small-caliber heparincoated ePTFE grafts reduce platelet deposition and neointimal hyperplasia in a baboon model. J Vasc Surg. 2004;39(6):1322–8.
63. Hugl B, Nevelsteen A, Daenens K, et al. PEPE II-a multicenter study with an end-point heparin-bonded expanded polytetrafluoroethylene vascular graft for above and below knee bypass surgery: determinants of patency. J Cardiovasc Surg. 2009;50(2):195–203.
64. Post S, Kraus T, Muller-Reinartz U, et al. Dacron vs polytetrafluoroethylene grafts for femoropopliteal bypass: a prospective randomised multicentre trial. Eur J Vasc Endovasc Surg. 2001;22(3):226–31.
65. Stump MM, Jordan GL, DeBakey ME, et al. Endothelium grown from circulating blood on isolated intravascular Dacron hub. Am J Pathol. 1963;43(3):361–7.
66. Berger K, Sauvage LR, Rao AM, et al. Healing of arterial prostheses in man: its incompleteness. Ann Surg. 1972;175(1):118–27.
67. Herring MB, Dilley R, Jersild RA. Seeding arterial prostheses with vascular endothelium. The nature of the lining. Ann Surg. 1979;190(1):84–90.
68. Stanley JC, Burkel WE, Ford JW, et al. Enhanced patency of small-diameter, externally supported Dacron iliofemoral grafts seeded with endothelial cells. Surgery. 1982;92(6):994–1005.
69. Smyth JV, Welch M, Carr HMH, et al. Fibrinolysis profiles and platelet activation after endothelial cell seeding of prosthetic vascular grafts. Ann Vasc Surg. 1995;9(6):542–6.
70. Rosenman JE, Kempczinski RF, Pearce WH, et al. Kinetics of endothelial cell seeding. J Vasc Surg. 1985;2(6):778–84.
71. Zilla P. In vitro endothelialization: its contribution towards an ideal vascular replacement. Madame Curie Bioscience Database [Internet]. Austin: Landes Bioscience; 2000.
72. Radomski JS, Jarrell BE, Williams SK, et al. Initial adherence of human capillary endothelial cells to Dacron. J Surg Res. 1987;42(2):133–40.
73. Foxall TL, Auger KR, Callow AD, et al. Adult human endothelial cell coverage of small-caliber Dacron and polytetrafluoroethylene vascular prostheses in vitro. J Surg Res. 1986;41(2):158–72.
74. Ott MJ, Ballermann BJ. Shear stress-conditioned, endothelial cell-seeded vascular grafts: improved cell adherence in response to in vitro shear stress. Surgery. 1995;117(3):334–9.
75. Dardik A, Liu A, Ballermann BJ. Chronic in vitro shear stress stimulates endothelial cell retention on prosthetic vascular grafts and reduces subsequent in vivo neointimal thickness. J Vasc Surg. 1999;29(1):157–67.
76. Herring M, Gardner A, Glover J. Seeding human arterial prostheses with mechanically derived endothelium: the detrimental effect of smoking. J Vasc Surg. 1984;1(2):279–89.
77. Herring MH, Comiton RS, Legrand DR, et al. Endothelial seeding of polytetrafluoroethylene popliteal bypasses: a preliminary report. J Vasc Surg. 1987;6(2):114–8.
78. Deutsch M, Meinhart J, Fischlein T, et al. Clinical autologous in vitro endothelialization of infrainguinal ePTFE grafts in 100 patients: a 9-year experience. Surgery. 1999;126(5):847–55.
79. Deutsch M, Meinhart J, Zilla P, et al. Long-term experience in autologous in vitro endothelialization of infrainguinal ePTFE grafts. J Vasc Surg. 2009;49(2):352–62.

Arterial Transplantation for Limb Salvage

16

Thomas Hölzenbein, Nina Mader, Manuela Aspalter, Sophina Trubel, and Klaus Linni

Introduction

Distal arterial bypass, despite being challenged by endovascular therapy, remains the cornerstone of distal revascularization for peripheral arterial disease. The autologous saphenous vein is regarded as the graft of choice for these interventions [1]. It has proven its usefulness and durability for short bypass grafts to the popliteal artery above and below the knee as well as for long distal reconstructions to tibial and pedal target arteries [2]. Although there are reports advocating prosthetic grafts for primary bypass, the saphenous vein is unrivalled with regard to its versatility, infection resistance, and long-term performance.

There are circumstances in which no saphenous vein is available because of previous vein harvesting for coronary bypass, previous leg revascularization, creation of an arteriovenous fistula for hemodialysis, or other procedures requiring vascular graft material or after removal of the vein for venous insufficiency. The vein can be of inferior quality because of inadequate size or postthrombotic changes. In these circumstances, the surgeon is forced to change the operative strategy and look for alternative graft material. The bypass surgery can be performed using alternative sources of autologous vein, such as the short saphenous vein [3], the arm veins [4, 5], or even the deep femoral vein. Currently, there is no recommendation available about the sequence in which these veins should be harvested for distal bypass, and the literature in that regard is not conclusive [5–7]. There are no prospective comparisons of the autologous alternative vein grafts available. Local policies and surgeon preference seem to be the main reasoning for decision-making [5, 6]. The bypass procedure can be altered by using only short segments of vein connecting various distal target arteries, feeding this graft with an artificial graft: the bridge graft concept [8]. Yet, although technically feasible, the results of bypass in these circumstances do not match the results using the saphenous vein. In addition, it is difficult to compare the results of alternative autologous vein to bridge graft revascularization because many of these procedures are secondary or tertiary procedures done for failed or failing distal bypass grafts. In these circumstances, the target arteries are located at more distal sites, usually at the tibial level, and the graft material is barely sufficient to reach the distal target artery sites, even with a distal origin bypass grafts [9, 10].

When no autologous graft is available, only a few options are possible. The surgeon may choose a prosthetic graft material such as expanded polytetrafluoroethylene (ePTFE) or Dacron for bypass reconstruction. However, these grafts have shown inferior long-term results with regard to infection resistance and mid-term patency in infrapopliteal reconstructions [11].

Homografts have been used since the beginning of reconstructive vascular surgery, mainly for aortic and iliac reconstruction. Initially, grafts were stored in chilled sterile saline solution without any adjuncts. These grafts often failed because of aneurysmal degeneration and secondary rupture [12]. Improvements in preservation and cryopreservation techniques have enhanced results of homograft reconstructions. However, the availability of artificial grafts and the development of the all autologous vein policy have reduced the need for homografts for distal revascularization [13, 14]. New interest in homograft revascularization, especially in distal revascularization, was driven by the need for a solution in patients requiring extension of limb salvage after several failed previous revascularizations [15, 16]. In these patients, bypass with cryopreserved arterial or venous homografts (self-prepared or commercially available) or fresh homografts ("transplantation") with or without subsequent immunosuppression can be

T. Hölzenbein, MD, PhD (✉) • N. Mader, MD
M. Aspalter, MD • S. Trubel, MD • K. Linni, MD
Department of Vascular and Endovascular Surgery, PMU Salzburg, Müllner Hauptstrasse 48, Salzburg 5020, Austria
e-mail: t.hoelzenbein@salk.at; n.mader@salk.at; m.aspalter@salk.at; s.trubel@salk.at; k.linni@salk.at

E.A. Gabriel, S.A. Gabriel (eds.), *Inflammatory Response in Cardiovascular Surgery*,
DOI 10.1007/978-1-4471-4429-8_16, © Springer-Verlag London 2013

performed [17–19]. The concept of transplantation derived from the observation that arteries in solid organ transplantation, except for cardiac grafts [20], virtually never occlude or become aneurysmal, even after long-term follow-up.

Patient Selection

In our series, only patients with extensive limb-threatening arterial disease after exhaustion of all autologous vein sources and no option for an intertibial or tibiopedal vein bridge graft as outflow for a femerodistal ePTFE graft were selected for this procedure. Usually patients require bypass to a single distal tibial or pedal artery. Patients are asked to sign a consent form in which the experimental nature of this procedure is explicitly mentioned. They have to be willing to undergo immunosuppressive therapy and a strict follow-up regimen. After informed consent has been obtained, patients undergo tissue typing, and all national transplant centers are informed to look for potential organ donors within their respective regional responsibility.

Organ Donor Selection

Younger individuals without peripheral arterial disease or major trauma to the legs may serve as donors for bypass grafts. Otherwise, the same criteria as for solid organ donors apply. These donors usually serve as multiorgan donors, and several solid organs and other tissues can be harvested. Arteries as well as veins can be harvested. Whereas the saphenous vein is relatively easy to harvest and can be taken from the groin to the ankle, the vein is often damaged because of lack of surgical experience, time constraints, or judgment, yielding only short segments of usable vein. These segments may well serve as hemodialysis grafts, but seldom as single-segment distal bypass grafts. Arteries are more difficult to harvest, requiring more advanced surgical skills, and greater care has to be taken during procurement. The probable graft length should be known before harvest, and a body height match between the donor and recipient is desirable, avoiding problems with graft length at implantation. ABO compatibility between the donor and recipient should be observed. HLA matching may be of importance for later graft rejection, but HLA mismatch or a positive crossmatch is not an exclusion criterion for fresh arterial homograft transplantation [21].

Graft Procurement

Homografts can be obtained from either heart-beating organ donors or post mortem, depending on whether one has chosen fresh or cryopreserved homografts. In both cases, the arteries are harvested under sterile conditions. In organ donor procedures, both legs are prepped down to the proximal calf. For fresh homograft preparation, the artery is used from the common iliac artery down to the tibioperoneal trunk. Although technically possible, graft harvesting becomes increasingly difficult more distally because of the depth of the arteries and tibial artery side branches. With regard to graft length, this corresponds to the saphenous vein taken from the groin down to the ankle. The hypogastric and profunda femoris arteries are also harvested together for histological purposes, viability tests, angiographic access, and possible patch plasties in the recipient. Usually the right-sided artery is harvested. The organ harvest procedure has to be slightly changed for the additional procurement of the iliac arteries. As arterial homografts are usually harvested in younger organ donors usually serving as multiorgan donors, other arterial segments will be harvested from the transplant teams. Usually both iliac bifurcations are taken for the liver and the pancreatic graft to serve as conduits. Arterial cannulation for organ perfusion, which is commonly performed through the right common iliac artery, should be carried out through either an aortic access or preferably the contralateral groin. This preserves the entire right iliofemoral arterial system for homograft procurement and allows harvest of the left femoral artery as a conduit for the liver graft. The procurement can be done either simultaneously with the transplant teams or after harvest of the solid organs, depending upon the time and availability of surgical teams.

The artery is harvested by leaving the entire artery in its bed and just ligating the side branches is situ. As most vasa vasorum of the femoral artery initiates at the origin of side branches, side branch flush ligation must be avoided, and side branches should be ligated 1 or 2 mm from the main stem in order to preserve these arteries. It is important to determine the length of the graft before excision of the artery. After systemic heparinization, the artery is removed and rinsed thoroughly with the organ perfusion solution used for the respective organ donor. We have used Eurocollins solution, HTK solution, and UW solution and found no difference with regard to graft patency or infection. The graft is then stored in a small batch of perfusate and packed in several sterile bags, similar to an organ transplant graft, and prepared for further transport on ice in an insulation bag.

Graft Description and Documentation

If the organ procurement team is different from the implantation team, it is necessary to submit a detailed description of the graft harvested. This is similar to solid organ transplantation and includes basic details of the organ donor (sex, blood group, previous medical history, basic laboratory tests, viral antibodies, location of the explantation, and exact time of excision), a vial of peripheral blood or a small piece of spleen or lymph node for crossmatching with the recipient, information on the perfusate, length of the graft before removal, description of the graft anatomy, presence of major side branches (hypogastric artery, profunda femoris artery), and areas of inferior quality or injuries.

Cold Ischemia Time

There are no reports on the limits of the cold ischemia time of these grafts. Although it is probable that arteries and veins can tolerate extended cold ischemia up to 48 h, we have never tested these limits and have implanted the grafts as soon as possible in order to assure viability of the transplanted graft.

Graft Implantation

Graft implantation follows standard surgical principles of bypass surgery. Usually sufficient graft length is available, so proximal and distal anastomotic sites can be chosen at convenient locations to avoid extremely scarred regions, such as the groin. The graft is then removed from the sterile bag, swabs are taken from the transport solution for bacteriology, and the graft is rinsed with cold heparinized saline solution. Clips are removed and exchanged for ligatures. After proper heparinization of the recipient patient and a single shot of 120 mg prednisolone-21-sodium-hydrosuccinate (Solu-Dacortine®), the proximal anastomosis is performed first with standard suturing techniques. The graft is then perfused with blood. The artery will distend considerably and lengthen back almost to its initial configuration. The graft is then tunneled as desired and placed into the tunnel with some tension. The graft is then trimmed, and the distal anastomosis is performed with standard suturing techniques. After flushing, the anastomosis is opened. The trimmed graft segment is then sent to the laboratory for viability tests and histology. A completion angiogram is then performed using the hypogastric artery or the deep femoral artery of the graft as access site. The arteries are then tied off, leaving some extra length, which may serve as a biopsy site for confirmation of rejection or an access site for later thrombectomy. In order to have easy access to the grafts routinely, we choose the subcutaneous space.

Postoperative Follow-up

Patients receive a postoperative MR angiogram before discharge. Patients are seen weekly until their wounds heal completely and every 6 weeks thereafter. Healing of the wound seems somewhat slower than expected, and this is attributed to the immunosuppressive therapy. Cyclosporin A blood levels are determined at every visit. Duplex is carried out every 6 months to look for aneurysms or signs of rejection. Antithrombotic therapy is carried out with oral anticoagulation with phenprocoumon (Marcoumar®) up to an INR of 2.5 and 100 mg of salicylic acid (ThromboASS®). This is continued until definite graft failure.

Immunosuppressive Therapy

Several of our patients are already on immunosuppressive therapy for a solid organ transplant (cardiac transplant, kidney transplant) [22]. All other patients receive a mild immunosuppressive regimen with low-dose cortisone, cyclosporin A (Sandimmun®) [23], and mycophenolate mofetil (Cellcept®) [24]. Immunosuppressive therapy is continued until definite graft failure. Cyclosporin A levels are adjusted to 80–110 ng/ml. Immunosuppressive therapy in these patients is a challenge because of their poor functional status and medical comorbidities. Many of the patients present with moderate renal insufficiency, making therapy with cyclosporin A difficult even with moderate blood levels. As most of the patients are diabetic, a cortisone-free immunosuppressive therapy would be of advantage [25].

Graft Rejection

Graft rejection is difficult to determine in these patients and can only be proven by the presence of antibodies [26] or histology of a perfused segment of artery [27]. Initially, we hoped that the long large branches of the donor profunda and donor hypogastric artery would remain patent for some time to allow for histological evaluation in case of suspected graft rejection. However, these side branches tend to thrombose within the first months of bypass function. Graft samples can be obtained, but always after graft thrombosis. There have been some signs of lymphocyte accumulation in the graft arterial wall in some cases, but clear signs of structural destruction as a sign of severe rejection have not been seen in our experience. Often reversible intimal thickening can be observed in these grafts, which could be reduced by elevating the level of cyclosporin A. Although this could possibly be a sign of graft rejection, we cannot prove this to date; The usefulness of duplex surveillance in these patients is currently under further investigation.

Late Problems

Fresh arterial homografts need intense medical attention to keep them going on a long-term basis. We have performed repeated thrombectomies and patch plasties at the site of

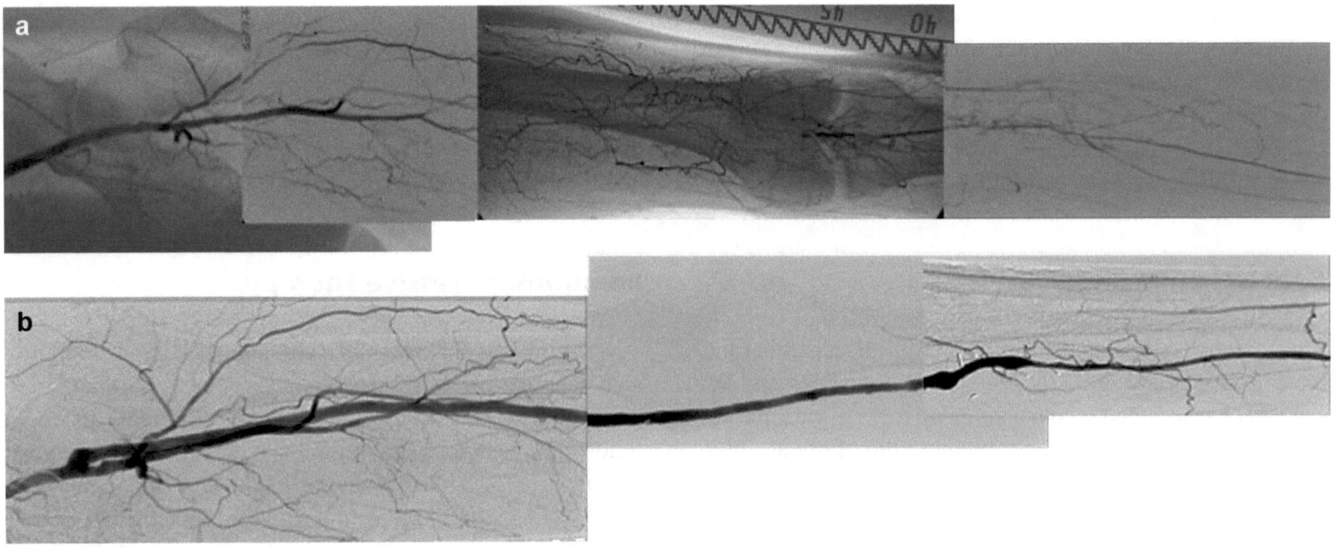

Fig. 16.1 Pre- and postoperative angiogram of a patient undergoing arterial transplantation. The patient had undergone eight pervious vascular procedures on the left leg after varicose vein surgery 35 years ago. Panel **a** shows distal runoff via the posterior tibial artery. Panel **b** shows a postoperative follow-up angiogram 2 years after the procedure with moderate aneurysmal degeneration of the graft

pseudoaneurysms. We could not determine whether these pseudoaneurysms were at the sites of side branches, sites of early donor atherosclerosis, or randomly distributed within the graft. These small patch plasties have been performed with remnants of vein, such as the lesser saphenous vein or arm vein.

Results

Our patients undergoing fresh arterial homograft transplantations usually have undergone multiple previous vascular surgeries, and all of them have been operated on for limb salvage. Under these difficult circumstances, we have achieved a 1 year limb salvage of 75 %, which otherwise would be impossible [28]. Life quality was acceptable in these patients despite several follow-up interventions because open as well as endovascular interventions [29] could be done under local anesthesia, with short hospital stays (Fig. 16.1).

Frequency

Fresh arterial homograft implantation is an infrequent procedure. We are trying hard to follow an all autologous vein bypass policy, and about 95 % of all infrainguinal bypass procedures are performed with autologous vein. The remainder of the bypass procedures comprises bridge grafts, and only 1.5 % of all infrainguinal bypass procedures are performed with arterial homografts. This is not because of a shortage of these grafts. Austria has very liberal organ donation legislation in which every patient experiencing irreversible brain death may become a potential organ donor. Despite increasing donor age, the average waiting time for a fresh arterial homograft is 2 weeks. This procedure, although not entirely experimental, is reserved for patients in whom no other option is available (Fig. 16.2) or who are under immunosuppressive therapy for a solid organ transplant.

Conclusion

Fresh arterial homograft for distal bypass with moderate immunosuppressive therapy seems to be a promising way to go in selected patients with distal arterial disease who are difficult to manage. It is unclear whether fresh or cryopreserved homografts are the way to go or if arterial or venous homografts perform better. Careful graft procurement by surgeons with vascular surgery experience is of great advantage. Patient and donor selection together with careful follow-up is a key for success in these patients and will lead to gratifying results [18, 19, 22, 28, 30].

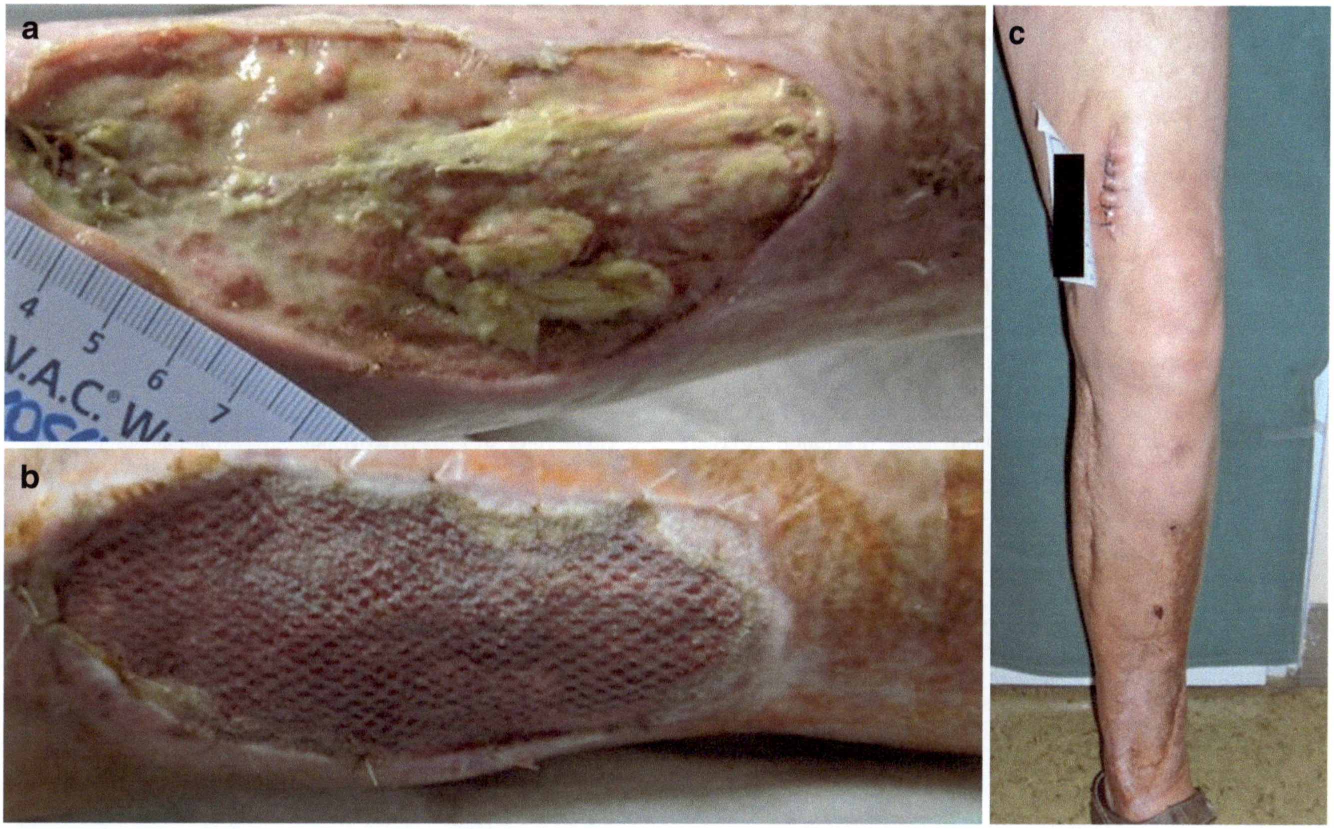

Fig. 16.2 Pre.- and postoperative view of the same patient as shown in Fig. 16.1. Panel **a**: Extensive gangrene on the anterior aspect of the calf prevented artificial graft use. Patient was MRSA positive. Panel **b**: After revascularization, debridement, and vacuum therapy, a split thickness skin graft heals nicely. Panel **c**: The lesion is completely healed 3 years after the procedure, and the patient is essentially symptom free. Nevertheless, occasional thrombectomies are necessary to maintain graft function

References

1. Albers M, Romiti M, Brochado-Neto FC, Pereira CA. Meta-analysis of alternate autologous vein bypass grafts to infrapopliteal arteries. J Vasc Surg. 2005;42:449–55.
2. Pomposelli FB, Kansal N, Hamdan AD, Belfield A, Sheahan M, Campbell DR, et al. A decade of experience with dorsalis pedis artery bypass: analysis of outcome in more than 1000 cases. J Vasc Surg. 2003;37:307–15.
3. Chang BB, Paty PS, Shah DM, Leather RP. The lesser saphenous vein: an underappreciated source of autogenous vein. J Vasc Surg. 1992;15:152–6.
4. Hölzenbein TJ, Pomposelli Jr FB, Miller A, Gibbons GW, Campbell DR, Freeman DV, et al. The upper arm basilic-cephalic loop for distal bypass grafting: technical considerations and follow-up. J Vasc Surg. 1995;21:586–92.
5. Hölzenbein TJ, Pomposelli Jr FB, Miller A, Contreras MA, Gibbons GW, Campbell DR, et al. Results of a policy with arm veins used as the first alternative to unavailable ispilateral saphenous vein for infrainguinal bypass. J Vasc Surg. 1996;23:130–40.
6. Chew DK, Owens CD, Belkin M, Donaldson MC, Whittemore AD, Mannick JA, et al. Bypass in the absence of ispilateral greater saphenous vein: safety and superiority of the contralateral saphenous vein. J Vasc Surg. 2002;35:1085–92.
7. Landry GJ, Moneta GL, Taylor LM, Edwards JM, Yeager RA, Porter JM. Choice of autogenous conduit for lower extremity vein graft revisions. J Vasc Surg. 2002;36:238–44.
8. Deutsch M, Meinhart J, Howanietz N, Fröschl A, Heine B, Moidl R, et al. The bridge graft: a new concept for infrapopliteal surgery. Eur J Vasc Endovasc Surg. 2001;21:508–612.
9. Arvela E, Söderström M, Albäck A, Aho PS, Venermo M, Lepantalo M. Arm vein conduit vs prosthetic graft in infrainguinal revascularization for critical leg ischemia. J Vasc Surg. 2010;52:616–23.
10. Kreienberg PB, Darling RC, Chang BB, Champagne BJ, Paty PS, Roddy SP, et al. Early results of a prospective randomized trial of spliced vein versus polytetrafluoroethylene graft with a distal vein cuff for limb-threatening ischemia. J Vasc Surg. 2002;35: 299–306.
11. Takagi H, Goto S, Matsui M, Manabe H, Umemoto T. A contemporary meta-analysis of Dacron versus polytetrafluoroethylene grafts for femoropopliteal bypass grafting. J Vasc Surg. 2010;52:232–6.
12. Szilagyi DE, Rodriguez FJ, Smith RF, Elliot JP. Late fate of arterial allografts. Observations 6 to 15 years after implantation. Arch Surg. 1970;101:721–33.
13. Taylor L, Edwards JM, Porter JM. Present status of reversed vein bypass grafting: five-year results of a modern series. J Vasc Surg. 1990;11:193–206.
14. Kent KC, Whittemore AD, Mannick JA. Short-term and midterm results of an all-autogenous tissue policy for infrainguinal reconstruction. J Vasc Surg. 1989;9:107–14.
15. Callow AD. Arterial homografts. Eur J Vasc Endovasc Surg. 1996;12:272–81.
16. Barner HB, DeWeese JA, Schenk EA. Fresh and frozen homologous venous grafts for arterial repair. Angiology. 1966;17: 389–401.

17. Posner MP, Makhoul RG, Altman M, Kimball P, Cohen N, Sobel M, et al. Early results of infrageniculate arterial reconstruction with using cryopreserved homograft saphenous conduit (CADVEIN) and combination low-dose systemic immunosuppression. J Am Coll Surg. 1996;183:208–16.
18. Randon C, Jacobs B, De Ryck F, Beele H, Vermassen F. Fifteen years of infrapopliteal arterial reconstructions with cryopreserved venous allografts for limb salvage. J Vasc Surg. 2010;51:869–77.
19. Albertini JN, Barral X, Brancherau A, Favre JP, Guidicelli H, Magne JL, et al. Long term results of arterial allograft below-knee bypass for limb salvage: a retrospective multicenter study. J Vasc Surg. 2000;31:426–35.
20. Rahmani M, Cruz RP, Granville DJ, McManus BM. Allograft vasculopathy versus athersosclerosis. Circ Res. 2006;99:801–15.
21. Zehr BP, Niblick CJ, Downey H, Ladowski JS. Limb salvage with CryoVein cadaver saphenous vein allografts used for peripheral bypass: role of blood compatibility. Ann Vasc Surg. 2011;25: 177–81.
22. Da Gama AD, Sarmento C, Viera T, Do Carmo GX. The use of arterial allografts for vascular reconstruction in patients receiving immunosuppression for organ transplant. J Vasc Surg. 1994;20: 271–8.
23. Vischjager M, Van Gulik TM, De Kleine RH, van Marle J, Pfaffendorf M, Klopper PJ, et al. Experimental arterial allografting under low therapeutic dosages of cyclosporin for immunosuppression. Transplantation. 1996;61:1138–42.
24. Wagner E, Roy R, Marons Y, Douville Y, Guidoin R. Fresh venous allografts in peripheral arterial reconstruction in dogs. Effects of histocompatibility and of short-term immunosuppression with cyclosporine A and mycophenolate mofetil. J Thorac Cardiovasc Surg. 1995;110:1732–44.
25. Carpenter JP, Tomaszeweli JE. Immunosuppression for human saphenous vein allograft bypass surgery: a prospective randomized trial. J Vasc Surg. 1997;26:32–42.
26. Balzer KM, Luther B, Sandmann W, Wassmuth R. Donor-specific sensitization by cadaveric venous allografts used for arterial reconstruction in peripheral arterial occlusive disease. Tissue Antigens. 2004;64:13–7.
27. Williams GM, ter Haar A, Krajewski C, Parks LC, Roth J. Rejection and repair of endothelium in major vessel transplants. Surgery. 1975;78:694–706.
28. Prager M, Hölzenbein T, Aslim E, Domenig C, Mühlbacher F, Kretschmer G. Fresh arterial homograft transplantation. A novel concept for critical limb ischemia. Eur J Vasc Endovasc Surg. 2002;24:312–21.
29. Castier Y, Alsac JM, Paraskevas N, Francis F, Coppin T, Cerceau O, et al. Endovascular treatment of aneurysmal deterioration in peripheral arterial allografts. J Endovasc Ther. 2007;14:605–8.
30. Sebesta P, Stadler P, Sedivy P, Bartik K. The seven year secondary patency of a fresh arterial allograft in the femorocrural position in a heart transplant recipient. Ann Vasc Surg. 2010;24: 953e7–10.

Part V

Vascular Trauma

17 Disseminated Intravascular Coagulation in Vascular Trauma

Ramyar Gilani, Peter I. Tsai, Matthew J. Wall Jr., and Kenneth L. Mattox

Introduction

A principal function of the vascular system is to maintain structural integrity to allow for normal physiologic activity. Insults to this delicate framework due to various forms of traumatic injury severely disrupt the dynamic homeostatic environment of the vascular and hematologic systems, resulting in physiologic derangements – not only within the local setting, but also within the global host environment. Disruption of vessel architecture often manifests as either hemorrhage or thrombosis, which leads to subsequent shock and ischemia. The resulting shift in homeostasis places physiologic stress on nearly every organ system in the body, including the system of coagulation. Corrective maneuvers employed by clinicians addressing hemorrhage and coagulopathy intend to restore normal function of coagulation and while doing so can often simultaneously lead to undesired deleterious effects. This chapter discusses the normal balance of the vascular and hematologic systems, describe the local and systemic sequelae of vascular trauma in reference to coagulation, and review the therapies utilized for treating disturbances in coagulation.

R. Gilani, MD
Division of Vascular Surgery and Endovascular Therapy of Michael E. DeBakey, Department of Surgery, Baylor College of Medicine, Houston, TX, USA

P.I. Tsai, MD
Cardiothoracic Surgery, Ben Taub General Hospital, Houston, TX, USA

M.J. Wall Jr., MD
Cardiothoracic Surgery, Trauma and Critical Care, Baylor College of Medicine, Houston, TX, USA

K.L. Mattox, MD (✉)
Michael E. DeBakey Department of Surgery, Baylor College of Medicine, Houston, TX, USA
e-mail: kmattox@aol.com; plisa@aol.com; redstart@aol.com

Coagulation and Fibrinolysis

In a normal state, a continuous equilibrium between the blood vessels and blood is maintained among endothelium, blood cells, and coagulation proteins. This balance allows for blood to remain fluid and flow while preparedness for desired hemostasis is assured. Once a source of trauma is introduced and vessel architecture is disrupted, a normal physiologic response designed to achieve hemostasis is initiated. This response seems to be advantageous for the cessation of hemorrhage; however, excessive coagulation can lead to undesired thrombosis and ischemia.

The endothelium within vessels is a critical component of the balance between fluid state and coagulation. Functionally, vascular endothelium regulates blood flow, cellular adhesion, and coagulation. Normal endothelium is a non-thrombogenic coating that is metabolically active with both antithrombotic and prothrombotic properties. The antithrombotic activity of endothelium is modulated through its structure and synthesis of anticoagulants. The continuous layer prevents circulating platelets and plasma proteins to contact the highly thrombogenic subendothelial matrix [1]. Endothelial cells produce prostacyclin, nitric oxide, and adenosine phosphatase, which are known to inhibit platelet aggregation. They also synthesize tissue plasminogen activator (t-PA), which plays a key role in fibrinolysis [2]. Further, anticoagulants depend on membrane expression of heparin-like molecules and thrombomodulin by endothelial cells for activity [3]. In addition to their antithrombotic activities, endothelial cells have synthetic functions that are prothrombotic. These cells secrete a highly thrombogenic subendothelial extracellular matrix that binds platelets [1]. Other prothrombotic synthesis products of endothelial cells include von Willebrand factor (vWF), tissue factor, and plasminogen activator inhibitors (PAIs) [4].

Circulating platelets play a key role in maintaining coagulation readiness. Normally, platelets are sequestered from contact with the extracellular matrix by the endothelium, thus preventing activation. These circulating platelets contain

E.A. Gabriel, S.A. Gabriel (eds.), *Inflammatory Response in Cardiovascular Surgery*,
DOI 10.1007/978-1-4471-4429-8_17, © Springer-Verlag London 2013

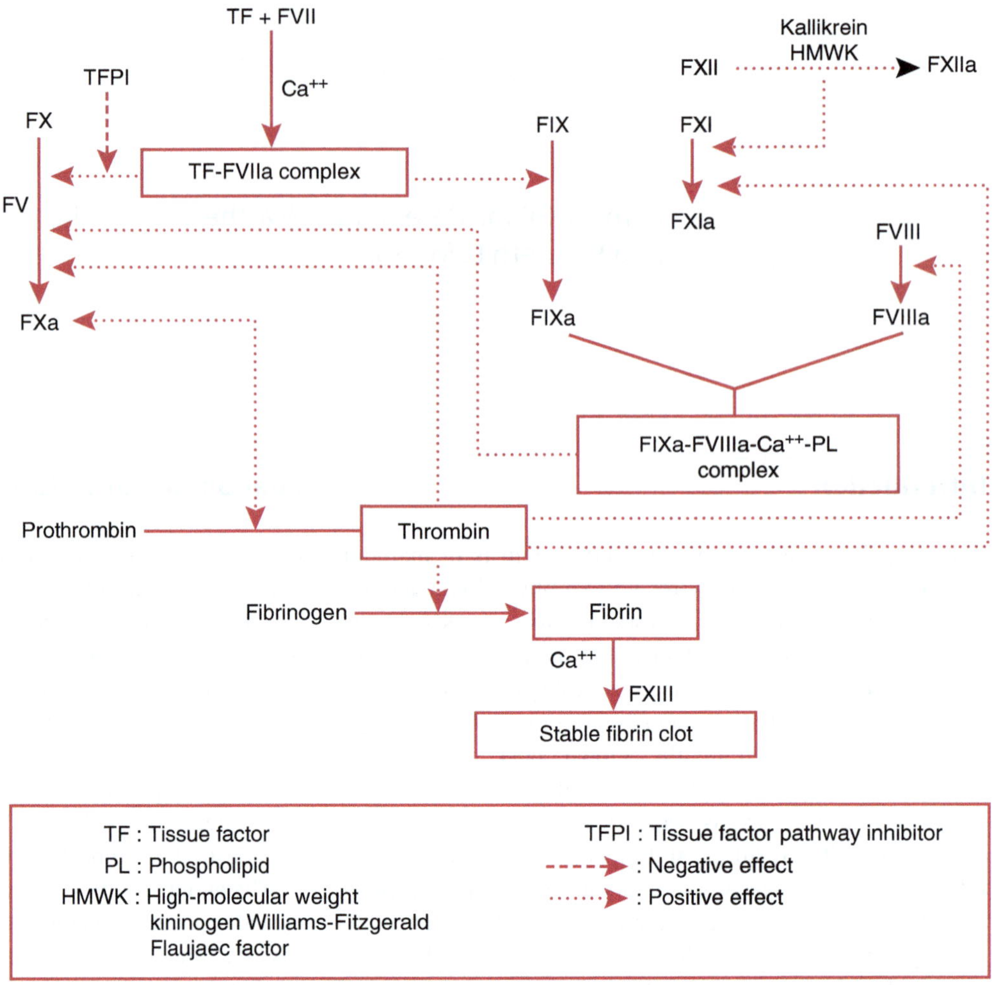

Fig. 17.1 Contemporary depiction of the blood coagulation cascade

numerous granules containing a myriad of modulating cytokines and chemokines. In the setting of vascular injury, platelets contact the extracellular matrix, which sets off a sequence of platelet-mediated activity that is essential to normal hemostasis [5]. Initially, platelets undergo adhesion to the extracellular matrix, which is dependent upon interaction between vWF and platelet surface receptors such as glycoprotein Ib [6]. After adhesion, platelet activation and subsequent secretion of secretory granules occur. This then leads to further platelet activation and aggregation, and the coagulation intrinsic pathway is prompted. The enlarging mass of aggregating platelets forms what is known as the primary hemostatic plug, the first step in achieving hemostasis. At this point, platelet aggregation is reversible; however, ongoing activation of coagulation ultimately leads to fibrin deposition within the plug, becoming irreversible and creating the more stable secondary hemostatic plug.

The final step in achieving hemostasis involves activation of the clotting cascade, ultimately resulting in the formation of stable fibrin clot. This process occurs through a sequence of enzymatic reactions leading up to the formation of fibrin (Fig. 17.1) and involving activation of coagulation factors that are normally quiescent within the circulation until a triggering mechanism is encountered. The overall schema is best represented by two activating pathways, the intrinsic and extrinsic pathways, converging into a common pathway leading to the formation of thrombin.

The intrinsic pathway does not require interaction with the injured vessel wall, but rather a negatively charged surface. In the laboratory, this surface can be glass or kaolin; however, the physiologic surface is unknown [7]. Regardless, the initiating step occurs with the activation of factor XII. It is not clear what role the intrinsic pathway plays in vivo, despite understanding that deficiencies in the pathway can lead to severe bleeding disorders, such as hemophilia.

Activation of the extrinsic pathway is initiated through the release of tissue factor from the subendothelium due to injury. The released tissue factor then comes into contact with factor VII, thus beginning the cascade. There is evidence to suggest that the tissue factor-factor VII pathway is the predominant mechanism for in vivo coagulation [8]. Both routes lead to the activation of factor X, thus initiating the common pathway leading to fibrin formation and deposition resulting in a stabilized clot and secondary hemostasis.

Also within the coagulation cascade are mechanisms exerting anti-thrombotic control. Antithrombin III (ATIII) is thought to be the principal inhibitor of coagulation factors [9]. It targets most factors, notably factors IIa and Xa, and requires heparin as a cofactor to increase efficiency. Protein C is another naturally occurring anticoagulant, the effects of which stem from its ability to inactivate factors Va and VIIIa [10]. Activity of protein C requires the presence of cofactor protein S. Low levels of both protein C and S are risk factors for thrombophilia [11].

Opposing the processes of primary and secondary hemostasis in a state of equilibrium is the system of fibrinolysis. Objectively, fibrinolysis serves to break down fibrin and provide control measures on excessive or undesired thrombosis. However, excessive or unopposed fibrinolysis can lead to coagulopathy and hemorrhage. The principle component in the fibrinolysis system is the activation of plasminogen to plasmin by t-PA. Once a vessel sustains injury, t-PA, located within the endothelium, is released at the site of injury, which then initiates the pathway resulting in plasmin degradation of fibrin into fibrin split products. This process is kept localized, partly because of the specificity of t-PA for plasminogen bound to fibrin. Also, within the circulation, alpha2-antiplasmin binds circulating plasmin, thus inhibiting it and preventing systemic fibrinolysis [12].

Further inhibition of fibrinolysis is provided by mediators known as plasminogen activator inhibitors (PAIs). PAIs are contained within platelets and endothelium, and as their name implies, they bind and inhibit t-PA. Activated platelets and an injured endothelium release PAIs in high concentration. Fibrinolysis is therefore paramount. The balance between coagulation and fibrinolysis exists in a dynamic state involving many participants to achieve the desired hemostasis and prevent unwanted thrombosis. During the maintenance phase of these processes, appropriate amounts of substrate are present with normal metabolic activity. However, the stress of vascular trauma quickly alters system requirements, resulting in shifts to the dynamic state in an attempt to maintain homeostasis. Unfortunately, demand on the system often exceeds capability, which requires external forces to reestablish the delicate balance.

Impact of Vascular Trauma

Trauma to the vascular system can cause significant disruption in the flow of blood, leading to hemorrhage and thrombosis, thus initiating a complex sequence of events designed to maintain homeostasis in the setting of injury. Injuries may be penetrating or blunt trauma, with penetrating injuries being more common. Once a vessel sustains an insult, two pathophysiologic pathways are responsible for the resulting sequelae acutely. Disruption of the vessel wall can lead to active hemorrhage of whole blood, shock, and systemic inflammatory response. Damage to the layers of the vessel wall may cause cessation of blood flow, thrombosis, and distal shock. Often times, there is overlap between both pathways, creating local and systemic responses affecting coagulation [13].

Ongoing hemorrhage begins to produce signs of hemorrhagic shock once 15 % of blood volume is lost. As hemorrhage continues, signs of hypotension, tachycardia, and malperfusion intensify. Blood volume loss beyond 40 % is immediately life-threatening [14]. With the onset of hemorrhagic shock, a variety of changes begin to take place in a cascade of closely involved events.

Shock, specifically hemorrhagic shock, is a known trigger for a systemic inflammatory response, resulting in the release of inflammatory mediators secondary to injury. One of the first mediators is tumor necrosis alpha (TNF-α), and once released, it triggers the release of other mediators, such as interleukin-1 (IL-1) and IL-6. On its own, TNF-α causes vasodilation and has procoagulant activity [15]. TNF-α, IL-1, and IL-6 all invoke endothelial cells to release tissue factor (TF) and thus trigger the coagulation cascade systemically.

As expected, normal coagulation commences locally at the site of injury. However, this may not be adequate to arrest hemorrhage, and continued bleeding ensues until surgical correction. Activated clotting at sites of injury leads to consumption of platelets and coagulation factors as well as fibrin deposition. With ongoing consumption exceeding reserves, thrombocytopenia and hypofibrinogenemia occur, leading to a consumptive coagulopathy. The balance between coagulation and fibrinolysis shifts to favor clot dissolution and also explains the late observed fibrinolysis.

Bleeding trauma patients often experience hypothermia, which has known deleterious effects on coagulation. As body temperature declines, potential energy for enzymatic activity dissipates. The reactions of coagulation require enzymatic activity and are therefore slowed with decreases in body temperature. Beyond 34 °C, impairment of coagulation becomes significant [16]. The level of derangement is not evident on routine laboratory tests as the samples are warmed to 37 °C prior to testing. Platelet function is also impacted by hypothermia. In addition to reduction in platelet enzymatic function, production of thromboxane A2 is reduced, which results in vasodilation and reduced platelet aggregation, leading to microvascular bleeding [17].

Mechanisms of DIC

Disseminated intravascular coagulation is a syndrome describing systemic observances due to derangements in activated coagulation and fibrinolysis and occurs because of some underlying etiology [18]. Trauma is a known initiator of DIC, which is found in 50–70 % of trauma patients [19]. DIC can be variable, from mild to life-threatening, and has identifiable stages indicating constant progression. Clinically, manifestations include thrombosis, coagulopathy, hemorrhage, and multiorgan system failure. Once initiated, coagulation derangements can become severe, and goal of therapy is to treat the underlying cause and restore the normal balance between coagulation and fibrinolysis.

The precipitating event in DIC is tissue factor (TF) activation of the coagulation cascade leading to fibrin deposition. Mediators, such interleukin-1 (IL-1), IL-6, and tumor necrosis factor alpha (TNF-α), play a key role in the release of TF from the subendothelium [20]. The subsequent activation of the extrinsic pathway via factor VIIa ultimately leads to generation of factor Xa and extensive thrombin formation and fibrin deposition [21]. In addition, the resulting endothelial damage results in platelet activation and aggregation, causing platelet consumption.

Normal opposing mechanisms to thrombosis are also impaired in DIC. Levels of antithrombin III are found to be low in DIC. Normal levels of protein C and S are also decreased [20]. Furthermore, fibrinolysis activity is depressed secondary to increased levels of plasminogen activator inhibitor (PAI) [22]. This systemic coagulation=exaggerated activation leads to consumption of substrate for coagulation and defines phase I of DIC [23]. Microthrombi also form within organ system vascular beds, causing thrombosis and organ ischemia, which lead to organ dysfunction.

As phase I continues, consumption ultimately exceeds available reserves, and the system of coagulation begins to decompensate, defining phase II of DIC. At this point, laboratory evaluation demonstrates increased prothrombin time (PT) and partial thromboplastin time (PTT). However, thrombin time (TT) may still be normal because of the remaining normal levels of fibrinogen. Further ongoing consumption eventually exhausts the system completely, resulting in phase III of DIC [23]. Once reaching this point, laboratory clotting times are markedly increased, platelet counts have dropped, and fibrinogen levels are now also low, as are levels of other coagulation factors. With extreme systemic coagulation insufficiency, generalized hemorrhage is an associated clinical finding with phase III DIC.

Ongoing fibrin deposition generates increasing levels of plasmin, which has a protective role in lysing the generated microthrombi and restoring the microcirculation within organs, and should not be inhibited [24]. As plasmin production continues in combination with coagulation exhaustion, secondary thrombolysis ensues. Although partly protective, this secondary thrombolysis forces the balance further toward coagulopathy and undesirable hemorrhage.

Management Strategies for DIC in Vascular Trauma

Treatment principles for managing DIC focus on first correcting the underlying cause and then attempting to reestablish homeostasis. Attempts at halting the progression of DIC, once the systemic cascade has been initiated, are ineffective until the impetus has been removed. In vascular trauma, focus should also be placed on prevention, as once DIC begins to progress, the deleterious effects can be quite devastating. Therefore, triggering mechanisms associated with vascular trauma should be avoided or mitigated through conscious efforts, recognizing the consequences of ignoring them.

Hemorrhage control is paramount in vascular trauma, not only because uncontrolled bleeding is eventually lethal, but also because it places severe stress on physiologic reserves, and corrections have additional negative effects. Therefore, without expeditious vascular control, all other maneuvers are futile. While attempting to stop hemorrhage, however, other maneuvers intended to lessen the impact of blood loss should not be ignored. A damage control strategy designed to lessen the physiologic impact of surgery should be considered even before the onset of operation. During the initial damage control strategy, there is little role for complex vascular reconstructions, and simple, expeditious, and efficacious techniques should be all that are utilized.

While ongoing hemorrhage ensues, consumption of coagulation components occurs, which can lead to exhaustion of reserves. Targeted blood component therapy should be initiated once large-volume blood loss is anticipated. Routine laboratory evaluations often offer delayed results in the analysis of the current status of coagulation and are unreliable. The thromboelastogram (TEG) has a role in trauma, as results can be generated and acted upon rapidly. However, waiting for laboratory evaluation of coagulation status should not delay blood component therapy. A transfusion strategy using a 1:1:1 ratio of packed red blood cells (pRBCs), fresh frozen plasma (FFP), and platelets (PLTs) is utilized and adjusted according to need. Effective transfusion practice is facilitated by prior arrangements of protocols for use in situations of massive transfusion.

With active ongoing hemorrhage and fluid resuscitation, hypothermia is almost inevitable. Also, with large areas of skin exposure, maintenance of body temperature and correction of hypothermia are quite difficult. Therefore, the surrounding environment must be maintained in order to maintain the core body temperature. Utilization of active warming maneuvers should be initiated early to prevent hypothermia from occurring. Keeping operative times to a minimum will also help to reduce heat loss and its consequences.

Ischemia and the resulting acidosis from shock, thrombosis, and even vascular control have a definite impact on coagulation, so attempts should be made to minimize the impact of ischemia and acidosis on coagulation. The hemodynamic status needs constant attention to optimize end organ perfusion through volume additions or inotropic support. In the setting of thrombosis, rapid restoration of blood flow helps decrease the ischemic time and subsequent acidosis. Cross-clamping for vascular control must be recognized as acidosis provoking. Furthermore, supra-celiac clamping and the resulting hepatic ischemic time in addition to other vital abdominal organs have implications of further worsening coagulopathy, and clamp times must be kept to a minimum.

Despite incorporating all possible preventable maneuvers, DIC can be unavoidable. Once surgical hemorrhage control has been achieved, treatment must focus on returning the balance of coagulation. Frequent laboratory assessment of clotting should be performed, with targeted therapy employed based on results demonstrating clotting deficiencies. Although it may be counterintuitive, anti-thrombolytic therapy should not be incorporated, as the observed fibrinolysis in DIC serves a protective purpose within the microvasculature.

Summary

Vascular trauma and its subsequent effects have a profound impact on coagulation that can ultimately lead to DIC. As a process, DIC is quite extensive, with local and systemic components resulting in significant derangements in coagulation. DIC is a secondary phenomenon, and effective treatment strategies focus on preventive strategies that are considered and incorporated early on during treatment. Once present, focused therapy intended to correct specific alterations in the coagulation profile is the best treatment strategy. However, it should be recognized that therapies can have undesired effects and must be evaluated in terms of risk versus benefit.

References

1. Wu KK, Thiagarajan P. Role of endothelium in thrombosis and hemostasis. Annu Rev Med. 1996;47:315–31.
2. Lijnen HR, Collen D. Endothelium in hemostasis and thrombosis. Prog Cardiovasc Dis. 1997;39(4):343–50.
3. Tans G, Nicolaes GA, Rosing J. Regulation of thrombin formation by activated protein C: effect of the factor V Leiden mutation. Semin Hematol. 1997;34(3):244–55.
4. Lijnen HR, Collen D. Mechanisms of physiological fibrinolysis. Baillieres Clin Haematol. 1995;8(2):277–90.
5. Packham MA. Role of platelets in thrombosis and hemostasis. Can J Physiol Pharmacol. 1994;72(3):278–84.
6. Cruz MA, Yuan H, Lee JR, Wise RJ, Handin RI. Interaction of the von Willebrand factor (vWF) with collagen. Localization of the primary collagen-binding site by analysis of recombinant vWF a domain polypeptides. J Biol Chem. 1995;270(18):10822–7.
7. Scully MF. The biochemistry of blood clotting: the digestion of a liquid to form a solid. Essays Biochem. 1992;27:17–36.
8. Broze Jr GJ. The role of tissue factor pathway inhibitor in a revised coagulation cascade. Semin Hematol. 1992;29(3):159–69.
9. Pratt CW, Church FC. Antithrombin: structure and function. Semin Hematol. 1991;28(1):3–9.
10. Esmon CT. Molecular events that control the protein C anticoagulant pathway. Thromb Haemost. 1993;70(1):29–35.
11. Dahlbäck B. The protein C anticoagulant system: inherited defects as basis for venous thrombosis. Thromb Res. 1995;77(1):1–43.
12. Müllertz S, Clemmensen I. The primary inhibitor of plasmin in human plasma. Biochem J. 1976;159(3):545–53.
13. Erickson LA, Ginsberg MH, Loskutoff DJ. Detection and partial characterization of an inhibitor of plasminogen activator in human platelets. J Clin Invest. 1984;74(4):1465–72.
14. American College of Surgeons Committee on Trauma. Advanced trauma life support coarse manual. Chicago: American College of Surgeons; 1997.
15. Akira S, Hirano T, Taga T, Kishimoto T. Biology of multifunctional cytokines: IL 6 and related molecules (IL 1 and TNF). FASEB J. 1990;4(11):2860–7.
16. Watts DD, Trask A, Soeken K, Perdue P, Dols S, Kaufmann C. Hypothermic coagulopathy in trauma: effect of varying levels of hypothermia on enzyme speed, platelet function, and fibrinolytic activity. J Trauma. 1998;44(5):846–54.
17. Valeri CR, Feingold H, Cassidy G, Ragno G, Khuri S, Altschule MD. Hypothermia-induced reversible platelet dysfunction. Ann Surg. 1987;205(2):175–81.
18. Levi M, de Jonge E, van der Poll T, ten Cate H. Disseminated intravascular coagulation. Thromb Haemost. 1999;82(2):695–705.
19. Gando S. Disseminated intravascular coagulation in trauma patients. Semin Thromb Hemost. 2001;27(6):585–92.
20. Levi M, van der Poll T, ten Cate H, van Deventer SJ. The cytokine-mediated imbalance between coagulant and anticoagulant mechanisms in sepsis and endotoxaemia. Eur J Clin Invest. 1997;27(1):3–9.
21. Baglin T. Disseminated intravascular coagulation: diagnosis and treatment. BMJ. 1996;312(7032):683–7.
22. Biemond BJ, Levi M, Ten Cate H, Van der Poll T, Büller HR, Hack CE, et al. Plasminogen activator and plasminogen activator inhibitor I release during experimental endotoxaemia in chimpanzees: effect of interventions in the cytokine and coagulation cascades. Clin Sci (Lond). 1995;88(5):587–94.
23. Müller-Berghaus G, ten Cate H, Levi M. Disseminated intravascular coagulation: clinical spectrum and established as well as new diagnostic approaches. Thromb Haemost. 1999;82(2):706–12.
24. Hesselvik JF, Blombäck M, Brodin B, Maller R. Coagulation, fibrinolysis, and kallikrein systems in sepsis: relation to outcome. Crit Care Med. 1989;17(8):724–33.

Temporary Intravascular Shunt in Complex Vascular Injury

18

Ding Wei-wei and Li Jie-shou

Despite the decline in the overall amputation rate associated with lower limb vascular injury, complex vascular injuries of the extremities accompanied by skeletal fractures or soft tissue destruction still result in a high rate of limb loss of up to 20 % [5]. The austere environment, limited instrumentation and operating room (OR) availability, large number of wounds encountered, (with many of them being relatively severe), and the front-line surgical team's paucity of experience with vascular anastomosis complicate the performance of definitive vascular repairs [6]. Ligation, balloon occlusion, or clamping of an injured blood vessel in an extremity may prevent exsanguination; however, irreversible tissue loss will occur if too much time elapses while other injuries are treated [7]. Complex repairs including end-to-end anastomosis, saphenous vein grafts, and vascular prosthesis transplantation are time-consuming, and in the cold, a coagulopathic, exsanguinating patient may develop disastrous outcomes, such as infection, amputation, thrombosis, and death. The front-line surgical team needs an easy and reliable hemostasis facility so that distal perfusion can be maintained.

The concept of temporarily bridging the vessel gap or intravascular shunting to maintain distal blood flow is not new. Silver tubes were first used in 1915 [8], and encouraging results were reported in 1922 during World War I [6]. Glass [9] and plastic [2] tubes were then used during World War I1 to maintain perfusion of the injured limb while collaterals developed. After that, shunts were abandoned because of the long evacuation times and the high incidence of shunt thrombosis. In 1971, Eger et al. [10] was the first documented author to pioneer the use of temporary intravascular shunts in the management of artêrial injuries. The shunts were irrigated with heparin to maintain patency at that time. Later, surgeons extended the use of shunts to arterial injuries associated with fractures and dislocations and supported the utility of this rational approach in selected civilian patients with complex upper and lower limb vascular injuries [7, 11–15] and recently as a component of damage control management in patients with severe multisystem trauma [16].

Temporary intravascular shunting of major vascular injuries requiring complex repair has the potential advantage of facilitating rapid control of hemorrhage and restoring flow distally while permitting deferment of definitive repair to higher echelons of care where more resources and expertise are available. Typically, these temporary intravascular shunts are used in combined orthopedic and vascular injuries or damage control surgery (DCS). Temporary shunts interrupt the warm ischemic time, providing a time window in which to carry out other tests or treatments and allowing eventual return to the vascular injury [7]. Similarly, use of these vascular shunts may reduce the risk of amputation of potentially salvageable extremities.

The evidence for the value of temporary intravascular shunts as a DCS adjunct technique mainly depends on personal experiences. This systemic review first summarize the type, configuration, duration, indications, and complications of the temporary intravascular shunts used as an adjunct to DCS in severe vascular injuries.

What Can Be Used As Temporary Intravascular Shunts?

How to choose the shunt material and configuration presumably depends on the experience and preference of the trauma surgeon. The use of commercial and self-made tubes of different diameters for intravascular shunts has been reported (listed in Table 18.1).

Commercially available shunts (i.e., Javid, Sundt, Argyle, and Pruitt-Inahara carotid shunts) are first designed to provide

D. Wei-wei, MD, PhD (✉)
Department of General Surgery, Nanjing General Hospital of Nanjing Military Command, Institute of People's Liberation Army for General Surgery, The Clinical College of the Nanjing University Medical School, Nanjing, Jiangsu, China
e-mail: dingwei_nju@hotmail.com

Li Jie-shou
Department of Surgery, Jinling Hospital, Medical School of Nanjing University, Nanjing, Jiangsu 210002, China

E.A. Gabriel, S.A. Gabriel (eds.), *Inflammatory Response in Cardiovascular Surgery*,
DOI 10.1007/978-1-4471-4429-8_18, © Springer-Verlag London 2013

Table 18.1 Cumulative review of temporary intravascular shunts used as damage control surgery adjuncts for treating complex vascular injuries

Year	Author	Type	Configuration	*N*	Duration	Patency rate	Distribution	Systemic anticoagulation
1971	Eger	PVC tube	T-shaped	36	ND	ND	ULAV	Yes
1979	Majeski	Javid	Looped	2	210 min	100 % (2/2)	ULAV	ND
1981	Nunley	Sundt	Straight	8	ND	100 % (8/8)	ULAV	ND
		Ventriculoperitoneal shunts	Straight					
1984	Eggink	ND	T-shaped	ND	ND	ND	ND	ND
1986	Khalil	Javid	Straight	5	2–6 h	100 % (5/5)	LEAV	No
		Balloon-type shunts	Straight					
		Nasogastric tube	Straight					
1986	Nichols	Javid and Sundt	Looped	13	127 min	100 % (13/13)	ULAV	No
1989	Johansen	PVC intravenous tube	Looped	1	16 h	100 % (1/1)	LEAV	No
1992	Husain	PVC Suction catheter	ND	5	3–6 h	100 % (5/5)	LEA	No
1995	Reilly	Javid	Straight	1	36 h	100 % (1/1)	SMA	No
1996	Starr	ND	ND	3	ND	100 % (3/3)	LEA	No
1999	Reber	Heyer-Schulte carotid shunt	T-shaped	7	90–390 min	100 % (7/7)	ULAV	No
2000	Granchi	Argyle	Straight	19	47–3,130 min	100 % (19/19)	ULAV	No
2002	Sriussadaporn	PVC intravenous and extension tube	Looped	7	60–180 min	100 % (7/7)	LEAV	No
2003	Parry	Argyle	Straight	18	22 h	100 % (18/18)	LEA	No
		thoracostomy tube	Straight					
		Pruitt-Inahara	T-shaped					
2003	Rozycki	Chest tube	Straight	13	24–54 h	83 % (15/18)	ULAV	No
		Angiocatheter	Straight					
		Argyle	Straight					
		Pruitt-Inahara	T-shaped					
2004	Hossny	PVC Suction catheter	Straight	7	ND	100 % (7/7)	LEAV	No
2004	Nalbandian	ND	Looped	1	24 h	100 % (1/1)	LEAV	No
2006	Rasmussen	Javid	Straight	30	2 h	86 %[a](19/22)	ULAV	No
		Argyle	Straight			12 %[b](1/8)		
2006	Chambers	Javid and Sundt	Straight	20	<6 h	78 % (21/27)	ULAV	No

Abbreviations: *ND* not determined, *SMA* superior mesenteric artery, *PVC* polyvinylchloride, *ULAV* upper and lower extremity artery and vein, *LEAV* lower extremity artery and vein, *LEA* lower extremity artery, *LEV* lower extremity venous

[a]Proximal shunt

[b]Distal shunt

temporary carotid bypasses for cerebral circulation during carotid endarterectomy procedures, and now they are widely used as an adjunct to DCS in severe vascular injuries.

The Sundt shunt (internal and external) is constructed of silicone elastomer with stainless steel spring reinforcement to minimize kinking and occlusion of the cannula lumen and to aid in the ease of insertion of the proximal and distal ends [17]. The ends of the shunt have cone-shaped bulbs to facilitate fixation of the shunt in the vessel. The bulb fits so firmly against the wall of the vessel that there is no bleeding around the distal bulb.

The Javid shunt has fusiform swellings at each end and is held in place by external clamps [18]. It is most commonly used in the superficial femoral artery and vein [19]. Argyle shunts are usually used in the tibial and brachial arteries. Both the Argyle and Javid are in-line shunts, while the few Sundt shunts are either in-line or looped. However, in the military experiences in Iraq, Rasmussen et al. [19] did not see any differences in patency rates among the Javid, Sundt, and Argyle shunts, although the patient number was small.

The Pruitt-Inahara shunt is the same length as the Javid, but is held in place by incorporated inflatable balloons at each end. They are dual-lumen devices with balloons at both the distal and proximal ends of the shunt with a T-piece. The balloons, when inflated independently, act as a stabilization mechanism to maintain the position of the shunt when it is placed within the arteries. An external safety balloon located on the inflation arm leading to the distal balloon acts as a mechanism to relieve pressure on the distal balloon in the event it inflates above maximum stated volume. The external safety balloon feature reduces the possibility of balloon overinflation and resultant vessel damage [18, 20]. The Pruitt-Inahara carotid shunt instantly verifies pulsatile flow, and an arteriogram can be performed to verify flow to the hand or foot. Its occlusion balloons eliminate the need for clamps, thereby reducing vessel trauma, using a small incision, minimal dissection, and a short arteriotomy [21].

Self-made shunts such as the endotracheal suction catheter [13, 22], nasogastric tube [15], ventriculoperitoneal shunt [23], thoracostomy tube [21, 24], and angiocatheter [24] are readily available in various sizes, inexpensive, and non-toxic. The Indian surgeon Husain et al. [13] reported the inexpensive and easily available polyvinylchloride (PVC) disposable endotracheal suction catheters, which were successfully used as temporary intravascular shunts in five popliteal artery trauma patients during the delay between the time of injury or presentation and the vascular repair. The shunts provided good outcomes with all limbs viable without complications.

Choosing the right shunt diameter size is critical. However, the surgeon selects the shunt size mostly based on clinical experience and estimation of vessel size [25]. One principle is that it is essential to never have an oversized shunt in order to minimize endothelium dysfunction. Many authors prefer to loop the shunt while securing it in vessel. However, Chambers et al. [6] suggested to avoid looping of the shunts to help minimize both the resistance to flow and likelihood of dislodgment as both complications occurred intraoperatively early in their military experience. They advocated ensuring the shunt lies straight; they needed a significant length to lie within the vessel lumen above and below the site of injury.

How Long Can the Shunt Stay Patent?

The success rate of arterial revascularization is inversely proportional to the duration of the ischemic time. According to the histological studies of Malan [26], the critical warm ischemic time for striated muscle is 6–8 h. Blood flow must be reestablished within this time to avoid irreversible muscle and nerve damage. The presence of soft tissue loss, disruption of arterial and venous collateral vessels, or hypotension may further decrease the length of this critical period. After vascular shunts have been inserted, potentially life-threatening injuries to the head, chest, or abdomen can be diagnosed and treated in a more orderly fashion. Similarly, use of these vascular shunts can prevent the need for the amputation of potentially salvageable extremities because of the prolonged ischemic time during other operative procedures. Therefore, the amount of time the intravascular shunt can maintain patency is of importance to the trauma surgeon.

The reported shunt times in the literature ranged from a couple of minutes to as long as several days. The longest shunt time of up to 10 days occurred in a civilian case (David V. Feliciano, Atlanta, GA, 2009 personal communication). But the longest dwell time recorded in the literature was reported by Granchi [25], who demonstrated that shunts could be left in place and maintained distal perfusion for up to 52 h without systemic anticoagulation in complex extremity injuries. Although Rozycki et al. [24] reported a dwell time of 54 h for a Pruitt-Inahara shunt left in the brachial artery, this shunt was occluded at reoperation, resulting amputation in the end. Intravascular shunts have been used to maintain the vascular patency of the extremities, with times ranging from 12 to 17 h in three patients undergoing air transfer to a level I trauma center for definitive care [27]. No evidence of shunt thrombosis or distal emboli was observed. However, Rasmussen et al. [19] argued that in war time maintaining the shunt patency for 2 h is sufficient because of fast evacuation patterns and relatively fewer shunt-related complications.

Experimentally, Ding compared four different shunt indwelling times in previously established superior mesenteric artery (SMA) injury models [28] and aimed to determine the safest duration in the setting of DCS. Their study suggested that TIVS can be used as an important DCS adjunct to maintain patency safely for 6 h (Fig 18.1); however, prolonged duration of an indwelling vascular shunt (over 9 h) caused endothelial injury in such SMA injuries in the

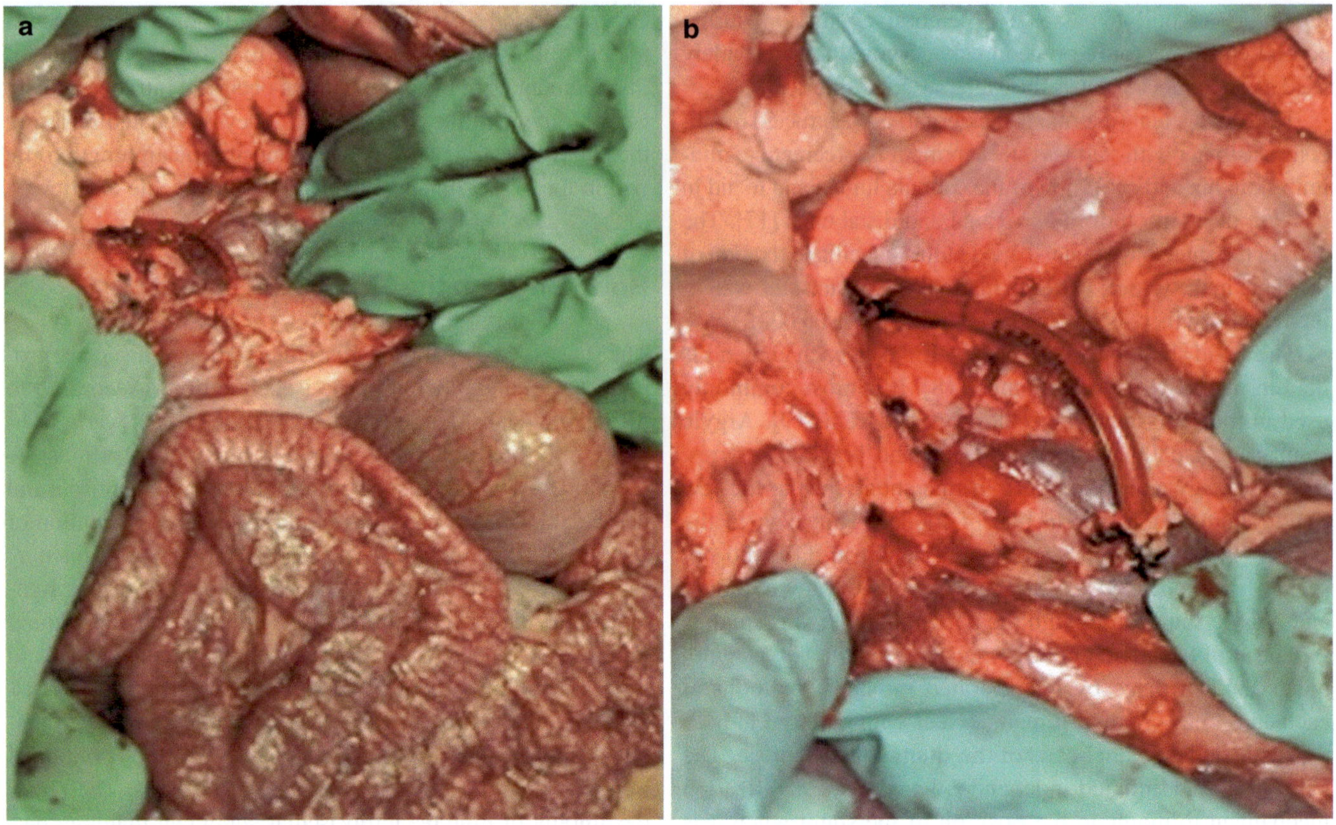

Fig 18.1 After re-establishment of intestinal circulation with a temporary intravascular shunt, the entire small bowel regained normal color and vigorous peristaltic activity (**a**). (**b**) A close view of the temporary intravascular shunt in situ, which was inserted to the proximal and distal end of transected SMA

setting of DCS [29]. Their recent study [30] showed that prolonged indwelling time of temporary vascular shunts is associated with increased endothelial injury, and, when possible, vascular reconstruction following the use of shunts should include an interposition graft after debridement of the arterial edges that interfaced with the shunt. Finally, to minimize intimal injury to the native vessel, this model suggests that the indwell times of shunts should be <9 h.

Aldridge et al. [31] found that heparin-bonded polyvinylchloride intravascular shunts remained patent in the iliac circulation for a 24-h period. They noted no distal embolization from the arterial shunts during the observation period and no increase in coagulation factor, platelet consumption, or red blood cell destruction. Dawson et al [32] demonstrated in a swine model that a temporary arterial shunt could maintain patency with adequate distal perfusion for up to 24 h without systemic anticoagulation.

Duration of patency is affected by multiple technical and physiologic factors. Several technical considerations appear to be beneficial in minimizing shunt occlusion: performance of distal fasciotomy [6], reestablishment of major venous outflow before arterial shunt in cases of concurrent arterial and venous injuries [12, 14, 32, 33], avoiding looping of the shunts [6], appropriate shunt diameter [24], avoiding external angulation of the extremity [6], and periodical distal detection using an ultrasound machine [32].

Must Systemic Anticoagulation Be Administered?

Trauma surgeons may expect the shunt to stay patent as long as possible so that they do not need to hurry when carrying out difficult and uncontrollable surgery on dying patients. Another issue is that the shunt may clot without anticoagulation therapy during the recovery period [34].

Despite administration of systemic heparin to their patients, Wagner et al. [35] reported a limb salvage rate of 85 % after blunt popliteal trauma, which is close to the salvage rate of 84 % reported by Hafez et al. [36], although they did not use systemic heparin. Daugherty et al. [37] have used systemic anticoagulation in all popliteal artery trauma patients without untoward effects; it would perhaps be more prudent to withhold systemic heparinization in such patients, particularly those with multiple injuries.

Massive transfusions with possible hypothermia and dilutional coagulopathy often complicate making the decision about anticoagulation. As shown in Table 18.1, most authors don't agree about administering systemic anticoagulation. Administering systemic anticoagulation may increase wound bleeding and thwart attempts at hemostasis [32]. Hypothetically, the patency of the shunt and perfusion of the limb might be jeopardized if anticoagulation is withheld, but the patient's life is threatened by renewed or continued bleeding if anticoagulation is given. This approach raises a variety of questions regarding shunt application in devastating vascular injury. In particular, the timing of reoperation and the need for controlled therapeutic anticoagulation once the initial coagulopathy has been corrected are unclear. Instead, according to many authors' experiences [13, 15, 19, 25, 32], local irrigation of the proximal and distal arterial segments with heparinized saline is performed to effect some local anticoagulation. They advocated avoiding systemic anticoagulation because of the risks of bleeding or worsening of existing coagulopathy. The coagulopathic state that damage control patients exhibited would lend itself to shunt patency rather than thrombosis.

With the development of heparin-bonded shunts, it seems likely that these patients may better tolerate temporary intravascular shunting while damage control part II (recovering) is being undertaken without systemic anticoagulation. Ultimately, it may improve both morbidity and mortality in this difficult patient population.

Indications

There has been debate concerning the order of management in combined skeletal and vascular trauma with proponents arguing in favor of performing arterial repair first [38, 39] and others favoring skeletal fixation as the initial mode of therapy [16, 40]. However, the crucial denominator in these injuries that heralds an adverse outcome is the relentless progression of warm ischemia and its unforgiving effect on striated muscle. Temporary intravascular shunting eliminated the dilemma.

Definitely, temporary intravascular shunting should not be used in all major limb vascular injuries, and in clean sharp amputation patients who arrive in the operating room within 2 or 3 h of injury, its use by the trauma surgeon is not recommended [23].

The use of shunts in patients with severe vascular injury can improve the overall outcome by reducing the intraoperative ischemic time and hence shortening the total ischemic time. The time that can be saved with shunting is the time needed to harvest the saphenous vein, fashion the graft, construct the anastomosis, repair other life-threatening injuries, and correct the lethal triangle (hypothermia, acidosis, and coagulopathy) before definitive vascular repair. These procedures prolong the intraoperative ischemic time, and consequently the total ischemic time, in the non-shunt patients. Shunting is more effective in minimizing the intraoperative ischemic time than in the situation in which rapid definitive arterial repair is performed as the initial step and none of the non-arterial injuries take priority.

Complex Vascular Extremity Injuries

Vascular injuries of the upper and lower extremities associated with fracture dislocation, neurovascular disruption, multiple systemic injuries, and extensive soft tissue crushing injuries are considered to be the indications for temporary intravascular shunts. Vascular injuries of the upper and lower limbs in the presence of extensive soft tissue loss, fractures, or other life-threatening injuries are associated with a high amputation rate [15]. Rapid reperfusion of the extremity via such shunts permits more comprehensive evaluation and management of the other associated injuries than would be possible in the presence of prolonged ischemia.

Several studies have demonstrated the safety and utility of temporary arterial shunts for combined arterial and orthopedic injuries. Majeski et al. [41] in 1979 recommended a standard Javid shunt for early revascularization of limbs with arterial injuries to minimize the ischemic time. According to Reber et al. [12], using an initial temporary intravascular shunt in selected patients with combined skeletal and vascular injury of the upper or lower limbs may reduce the number of complications resulting from prolonged ischemia and permits an unhurried and reasonable sequence of treatment. In 1982, Johansen et al. defined the criteria for "complex vascular injuries" and advocated the routine use of shunts in their management [27]. Hossny et al. [22] recommended routine use of shunts in patients with complete lower limb ischemia caused by blunt popliteal artery trauma in their clinical observation. They compared the benefits of routine use of a temporary intraluminal shunt in 8 shunt patients with 13 no-shunt patients with complete limb ischemia caused by blunt popliteal trauma. Insertion of a shunt succeeded in maintaining the total ischemic time within the same preoperative ischemic interval in all eight patients, whereas the total ischemic time was within the time interval after the preoperative interval in all but two patients in the non-shunt group. The shunt patients had a lower fasciotomy rate (14.3 vs. 70 %), a smaller mean number of repeat operations (0.8 vs. 1.9), shorter mean hospital stay (14.4 vs. 23 days), and an obviously lower amputation rate (0 vs. 40 %). Rasmussen et al. [19] described the largest series from the central level III echelon facility in the Iraq conflict. In this article, 30 of 53 (57 %) patients who were transferred from the front line to the central trauma center had temporary shunts in place. Chambers et al. [6] summarized their experiences from a 6-month rotation during Operation Iraqi Freedom (OIF) and supported the use of the TVS option by front-line surgical teams as an effective means of obtaining rapid control of extremity hemorrhages while simultaneously re-establishing distal flow.

Damage Control Surgery for Severe Visceral Vascular Injuries

Using damage control surgery, firstly advocated by Rotondo [16], survival rates in patients with major vascular and multiple visceral injuries can be greatly improved [42–44]. Though we cannot predict with certainty who will die after DCS, shunt placement offers a direct benefit to the surgeon who must choose between a protracted and dangerous arterial reconstruction or a precipitous amputation [45]. The temporary arterial shunt provides another option that allows the surgeon to abbreviate the operation without sacrificing the limb.

The use of an intravascular shunt in the visceral circulation is rare [21]. Reilly et al. [16] described the first and the unique clinical application of an intraluminal shunt to a patient to maintain temporary vascular continuity of the superior mesenteric artery during rewarming and correction of coagulopathy in the intensive care unit following a gunshot wound to the abdomen. The patient died because of aspiration pneumonia on day 63 after injury; however, the autopsy of the intestines showed no evidence of ischemic changes, and the SMA graft was patent.

Shunt Used During Transfer to a Higher Trauma Center

Temporary intravascular shunts can be used while transferring patients to a higher or more experienced trauma center. Johansen et al. [27] described the use of a polyethylene shunt inserted into the ends of a lacerated superficial femoral artery before a 950-mile air evacuation. Anticoagulation was not used. This shunt remained patent for over 16 h during the transfer, and arterial repair was able to be performed, although development of compartment syndrome led to later amputation. Surgeons in remote locations or practicing outside of a trauma center, especially those without significant vascular surgery experience, should consider shunt insertion as a simpler alternative to surgical reconstruction when faced with a patient with a complex limb injury.

Complications

Dislodgment, occlusion, infection, and hemorrhaging may occur when keeping a shunt in vivo. Dislodgment of a temporary shunt is rare [45] and is usually the result of inadequate fixation. The signs are those of severe hemorrhage inside the involved limb, with sudden gross swelling and severe oozing of blood between the skin sutures. If this occurs, the vessel should be occluded with finger compression or vascular clamps and another available in-house surgeon called. This surgeon, having looped the vessel proximally and distally to the injury, can replace the shunt quickly without significant blood loss or interruption of perfusion.

Shunt occlusion occurs relatively more frequent. It is usually not a problem during the first few hours postoperatively because the patient is coagulopathic. However, after the patient is rewarmed and coagulation has been restored, it is not uncommon to encounter sudden occlusion of the shunt. This usually manifests as a difference in color, temperature, or capillary filling between the two extremities and occasionally the absence of a distal Doppler signal, which has been documented previously. Consideration should then be given to the feasibility of a vascular reconstructive procedure. This would preferably occur at a second operation, but can be performed in the SICU if early shunt occlusion occurs in a patient [45]. Thrombosis may also occur because the vessels that are small at baseline are prone to significant spasm in injured patients who are cold and in shock, which limits outflow and patency [19]. Thrombectomy should be performed in this situation. Intimal disruption while inserting the shunt and securing it in the vascular lumen greatly influences the early patency of the anastomosis. Generally, the shunts should not be oversized in case of endothelial denaturation [25].

Although shunt-related complications have been noted by surgeons [12] and some refuse to use them because of the complications [46], the actual rate is low. Hossny [22] reported no technical complications in shunt insertions and no shunt-related complications such as shunt dislodgement or distal embolization in their eight shunt patients. More than 90 % of shunt patients reported in literature did not develop any complications (listed in Table 18.1).

Long-term follow-up of shunt patients seems too difficult. An attempt to contact all patients for return visits was impractical. More detailed research is needed to evaluate the long-term complications of intravascular shunts. Further experience is needed to more definitively determine the usefulness of temporary intravascular shunts in trauma patients in both military and civilian conditions. Expanded use of shunts in other unligatable arteries or veins, such as the superior mesenteric artery, portal vein, and iliac vessels, is worth considering in further research. The optimal shunt type or material, the most appropriate dwell time, the safest procedures for inserting shunts, and the right time to carry out shunting are unclear.

References

1. Fisher GW. Acute arterial injuries treated by the United States Army Medical Service in Vietnam, 1965–1966. J Trauma. 1967;7:844–55.
2. DeBakey ME, Simeone FA. Battle injuries of the arteries in World War II: an analysis of 2,471 cases. Ann Surg. 1946;123:534–79.
3. Hughes CW. Acute vascular trauma in Korean War casualties; an analysis of 180 cases. Surg Gynecol Obstet. 1954;99:91–100.
4. Rich NM, Baugh JH, Hughes CW. Acute arterial injuries in Vietnam: 1,000 cases. J Trauma. 1970;10:359–69.

5. Snyder 3rd WH. Vascular injuries near the knee: an updated series and overview of the problem. Surgery. 1982;91:502–6.
6. Chambers LW, Green DJ, Sample K, et al. Tactical surgical intervention with temporary shunting of peripheral vascular trauma sustained during Operation Iraqi Freedom: one unit's experience. J Trauma. 2006;61:824–30.
7. Nalbandian MM, Maldonado TS, Cushman J, Jacobowitz GJ, Lamparello PJ, Riles TS. Successful limb reperfusion using prolonged intravascular shunting in a case of an unstable trauma patient – a case report. Vasc Endovascular Surg. 2004;38:375–9.
8. Tuffier M. French surgery in 1915. Br J Surg. 1916;4:420–32.
9. Matheson NM, Murray G. Recent advances and experimental work in conservative vascular surgery. In: Hamilton-Bailey, editors. Surgery of modern Warfie. vol 1. Baltimore: Williams and Wilkins; 1941. p. 324–7.
10. Eger M, Golcman L, Goldstein A, Hirsch M. The use of a temporary shunt in the management of arterial vascular injuries. Surg Gynecol Obstet. 1971;132:67–70.
11. McHenry TP, Holcomb JB, Aoki N, Lindsey RW. Fractures with major vascular injuries from gunshot wounds: implications of surgical sequence. J Trauma. 2002;53:717–21.
12. Reber PU, Patel AG, Sapio NL, Ris HB, Beck M, Kniemeyer HW. Selective use of temporary intravascular shunts in coincident vascular and orthopedic upper and lower limb trauma. J Trauma. 1999;47:72–6.
13. Husain AK, Khandeparkar JM, Tendolkar AG, Magotra RA, Parulkar GB. Temporary intravascular shunts for peripheral vascular trauma. J Postgrad Med. 1992;38:68–9.
14. Barros D'Sa AA. The rationale for arterial and venous shunting in the management of limb vascular injuries. Eur J Vasc Surg. 1989;3:471–4.
15. Khalil IM, Livingston DH. Intravascular shunts in complex lower limb trauma. J Vasc Surg. 1986;4:582–7.
16. Reilly PM, Rotondo MF, Carpenter JP, Sherr SA, Schwab CW. Temporary vascular continuity during damage control: intraluminal shunting for proximal superior mesenteric artery injury. J Trauma. 1995;39:757–60.
17. Lindberg B, Norback B, Svendsen P, Synek V. Carotid endarterectomy. A review of 104 operations. J Cardiovasc Surg. 1975;16:161–70.
18. Wilkinson JM, Rochester JR, Sivaguru A, Cameron IC, Fisher R, Beard JD. Middle cerebral artery blood velocity, embolisation, and neurological outcome during carotid endarterectomy: a prospective comparison of the Javid and the Pruitt-Inahara shunts. Eur J Vasc Endovasc Surg. 1997;14:399–402.
19. Rasmussen TE, Clouse WD, Jenkins DH, Peck MA, Eliason JL, Smith DL. The use of temporary vascular shunts as a damage control adjunct in the management of wartime vascular injury. J Trauma. 2006;61:8–15.
20. Hayes PD, Vainas T, Hartley S, et al. The Pruitt-Inahara shunt maintains mean middle cerebral artery velocities within 10 % of preoperative values during carotid endarterectomy. J Vasc Surg. 2000;32:299–306.
21. Parry NG, Feliciano DV, Burke RM, et al. Management and short-term patency of lower extremity venous injuries with various repairs. Am J Surg. 2003;186:631–5.
22. Hossny A. Blunt popliteal artery injury with complete lower limb ischemia: is routine use of temporary intraluminal arterial shunt justified? J Vasc Surg. 2004;40:61–6.
23. Nunley JA, Koman LA, Urbaniak JR. Arterial shunting as an adjunct to major limb revascularization. Ann Surg. 1981;193:271–3.
24. Rozycki GS, Tremblay LN, Feliciano DV, McClelland WB. Blunt vascular trauma in the extremity: diagnosis, management, and outcome. J Trauma. 2003;55:814–24.
25. Granchi T, Schmittling Z, Vasquez J, Schreiber M, Wall M. Prolonged use of intraluminal arterial shunts without systemic anticoagulation. Am J Surg. 2000;180:493–6; discussion 6–7.
26. Malan E, Tattoni G. Physio- and anatomo-pathology of acute ischemia of the extremities. J Cardiovasc Surg. 1963;4:212–25.
27. Johansen K, Hedges G. Successful limb reperfusion by temporary arterial shunt during a 950-mile air transfer: case report. J Trauma. 1989;29:1289–91.
28. Ding W, Wu X, Gong G, Meng Q, Ni L, Li J. Establishment of an acute superior mesenteric artery injury model for damage control surgery. J Surg Res. 2009;152:249–57.
29. Ding W, Wu X, Meng Q, et al. Time course study on the use of temporary intravascular shunts as a damage control adjunct in a superior mesenteric artery injury model. J Trauma. 2010;68:409–14.
30. Ding W, Ji W, Wu X, Li N, Li J. Prolonged indwelling time of temporary vascular shunts is associated with increased endothelial injury in the porcine mesenteric artery. J Trauma. 2011;70:1464–70.
31. Aldridge SD, Badellino MM, Malaspina PJ, et al. Extended intravascular shunting in an experimental model of vascular injury. J Cardiovasc Surg (Torino). 1997;38:183–6.
32. Dawson DL, Putnam AT, Light JT, et al. Temporary arterial shunts to maintain limb perfusion after arterial injury: an animal study. J Trauma. 1999;47:64–71.
33. Harkin DW, D'Sa AA, Yassin MM, et al. Reperfusion injury is greater with delayed restoration of venous outflow in concurrent arterial and venous limb injury. Br J Surg. 2000;87:734–41.
34. Sagraves SG, Toschlog EA, Rotondo MF. Damage control surgery – the intensivist's role. J Intensive Care Med. 2006;21:5–16.
35. Wagner WH, Calkins ER, Weaver FA, Goodwin JA, Myles RA, Yellin AE. Blunt popliteal artery trauma: one hundred consecutive injuries. J Vasc Surg. 1988;7:736–43.
36. Hafez HM, Woolgar J, Robbs JV. Lower extremity arterial injury: results of 550 cases and review of risk factors associated with limb loss. J Vasc Surg. 2001;33:1212–9.
37. Daugherty ME, Sachatello CR, Ernst CB. Improved treatment of popliteal arterial injuries using anticoagulation and extra-anatomic reconstruction. Arch Surg. 1978;113:1317–21.
38. Hardy JD, Raju S, Neely WA, Berry DW. Aortic and other arterial injuries. Ann Surg. 1975;181:640–53.
39. O'Donnell Jr TF, Brewster DC, Darling RC, Veen H, Waltman AA. Arterial injuries associated with fractures and/or dislocations of the knee. J Trauma. 1977;17:775–84.
40. Freischlag JA, Sise M, Quinones-Baldrich WJ, Hye RJ, Sedwitz MM. Vascular complications associated with orthopedic procedures. Surg Gynecol Obstet. 1989;169:147–52.
41. Majeski JA, Gauto A. Management of peripheral arterial vascular injuries with a Javid shunt. Am J Surg. 1979;138:324–5.
42. Stone HH, Strom PR, Mullins RJ. Management of the major coagulopathy with onset during laparotomy. Ann Surg. 1983;197:532–5.
43. Burch JM, Ortiz VB, Richardson RJ, Martin RR, Mattox KL, Jordan Jr GL. Abbreviated laparotomy and planned reoperation for critically injured patients. Ann Surg. 1992;215:476–83; discussion 83–4.
44. Morris Jr JA, Eddy VA, Blinman TA, Rutherford EJ, Sharp KW. The staged celiotomy for trauma. Issues in unpacking and reconstruction. Ann Surg. 1993;217:576–84; discussion 84–6.
45. Aucar JA, Hirshberg A. Damage control for vascular injuries. Surg Clin North Am. 1997;77:853–62.
46. Huynh TT, Pham M, Griffin LW, et al. Management of distal femoral and popliteal arterial injuries: an update. Am J Surg. 2006;192:773–8.

Part VI

Venous Diseases

19 Metalloproteinases in Acute Venous Occlusion

Anita C. Thomas

Abbreviations

AP	Antiplasmin
AT	Antithrombin
col	Collagen
DVT	Deep vein thrombosis
ECM	Extracellular matrix
F	Factor
GF	Growth factor
IFN	Interferon
IL	Interleukin
LDL	Low density lipoprotein
LPS	Lipopolysaccharide
LRP	Low density lipoprotein receptor-related protein
MG	Macroglobulin
MMP	Matrix metalloproteinase
PAI	Plasminogen activator inhibitor
PDGF	Platelet-derived growth factor
ROS	Reactive oxygen species
TF	Tissue factor
TFPI	Tissue factor pathway inhibitor
TGF	Transforming growth factor
TIMP	Tissue inhibitor of metalloproteinase
TLR	Toll-like receptor
TM	Thrombomodulin
TNF	Tissue necrosis factor
tPA	Tissue plasminogen activator
uPA	Urokinase plasminogen activator
vWF	von Willebrand factor

A.C. Thomas, PhD
Department of Cardiovascular Surgery - Bristol Heart Institute, 7th Floor, Queens Building, Bristol Royal Infirmary, Bristol BS2 8HW, UK
e-mail: a.thomas@bristol.ac.uk

Introduction

Acute venous thrombosis is a life-threatening event proceeding from altered blood flow, abnormalities in the vessel wall, and changes in blood components (Virchow's triad). Aberrations in the coagulatory and fibrinolytic pathways contribute to the altered blood components, but other blood proteases also have roles to play [1].

Matrix Metalloproteinases

Matrix metalloproteinases (MMPs, matrixins) are a family of highly conserved, neutral, zinc-dependent peptidases, of which at least 14 are to be found in the vasculature [2, 3]. They are known to play major roles in embryology, morphogenesis, reproduction, disease, and wound repair [4, 5] as the major regulators of extracellular matrix (ECM), but their activity is not restricted to matrix turnover. They are also involved in cell communication and the activation and release of growth factors (GFs) and other bioactive molecules from the matrix; they also have nonmatrix substrates [2–7]. There are many interactions between the thrombotic, fibrinolytic, and MMP pathways. For example, MMPs are known to prevent the activity of two of the important anticoagulant pathway regulators, tissue factor pathway inhibitor (TFPI) and antithrombin (AT), and to be activated by a third pathway regulator, protein C; smooth muscle cell migration (which requires matrix remodelling) is facilitated by urokinase and tissue plasminogen activators (uPAs and tPAs, respectively); several MMPs are capable of degrading plasminogen; the plasma proteases plasmin, thrombin, uPA, and activated factor Xa may activate pro-MMP-1, -2, -3, -7, -9, -10, and -13 [2, 5–13]. The use of MMP-10 as a thrombolytic treatment has also been the subject of a patent (US application 20110091436). The particular focus of this chapter is the strong links between venous thrombosis and MMP production and activation, with MMP activity a requirement for thrombus resolution [2, 12, 14, 15]. Figure 19.1 outlines

E.A. Gabriel, S.A. Gabriel (eds.), *Inflammatory Response in Cardiovascular Surgery*,
DOI 10.1007/978-1-4471-4429-8_19, © Springer-Verlag London 2013

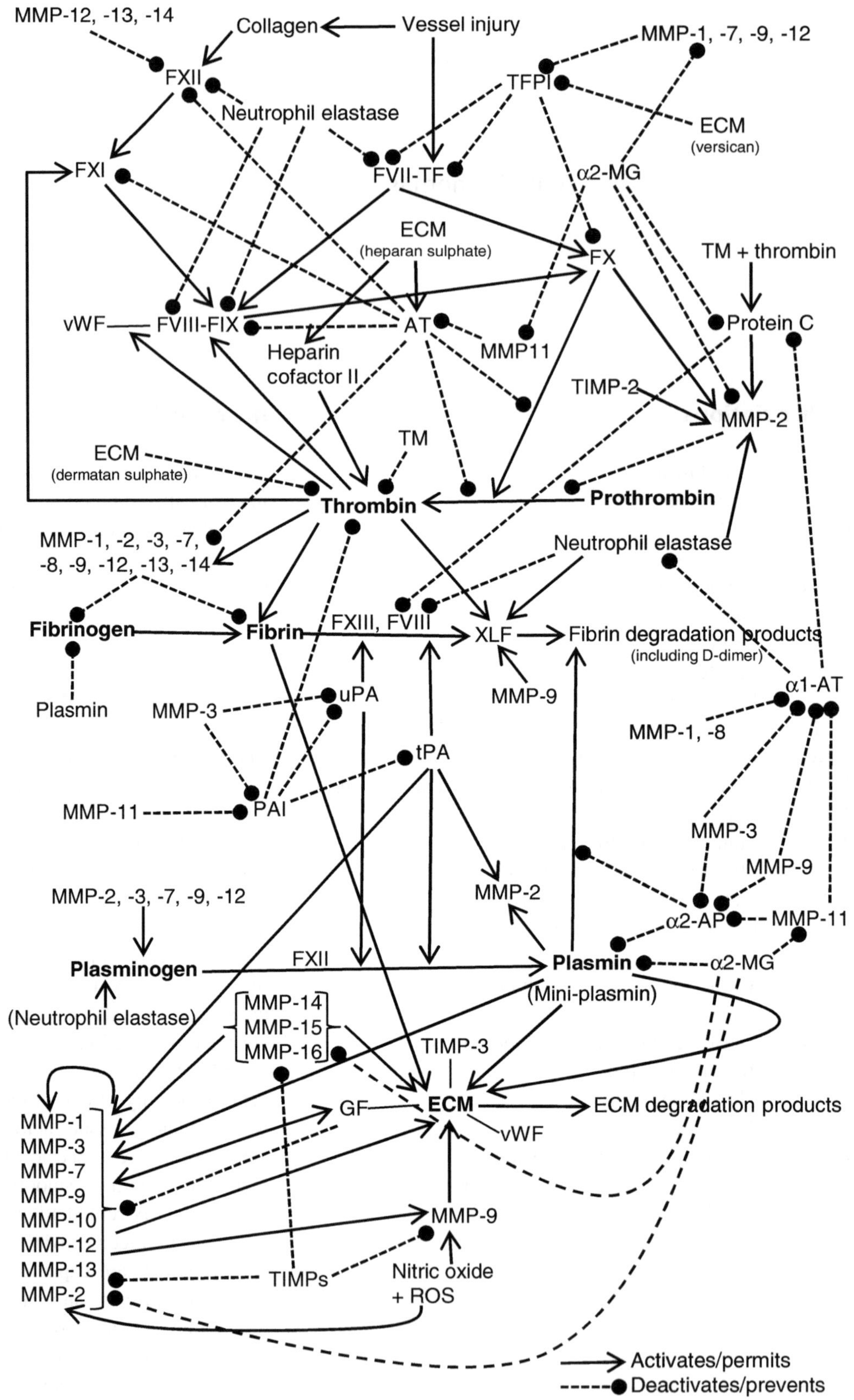

Fig. 19.1 Diagram outlining the considerable overlap between the coagulatory, fibrinolytic, and matrix metalloproteinase (MMP) systems

many of the complex relationships between the coagulatory, fibrinolytic, and MMP systems, while the various activities of MMPs are expanded in Table 19.1.

MMP activity is regulated at several levels: gene induction, vesicle trafficking, secretion (not all MMPs), and proform activation. MMPs are also regulated by their differential temporal and spatial expression. They can form complexes with their specific inhibitors, the tissue inhibitors of MMPs (TIMPs), but plasma proteases, including α2-macroglobulin (α2-MG), can also inhibit MMPs [2, 4, 11, 12]. While many MMPs are expressed as inactive preproforms, the membrane-type MMPs (MMP-14, -15, -16, -17) and MMP-11, -21, -23, and -27 are activated during processing along the endosomal pathway [2, 11]. Pro-MMPs can be activated by many processes, including chemical (via reactive oxygen species or nitric oxide, for example) and biological means (e.g., GFs, MMPs, or plasma proteinases) [2–4, 11].

MMPs in Peripheral Blood

Most of the components of blood and the vessel wall are capable of producing or interacting with MMPs. Culture studies suggest that MMP-1 expression may be increased during hyperglycemia, while diabetes is also associated with altered MMP gene expression [16, 17]. Patients with type 2 diabetes have elevated levels of MMP-2 and TIMP-1 protein, but not MMP-9, with MMP expression independent of age, duration of diabetes, blood pressure, or serum lipid concentration [16], while both MMP-2 and -9 are elevated in serum from patients with type 1 diabetes [17]. Several studies have measured MMP levels in plasma and serum, but since the absolute concentration of various MMPs is now known to be dependent on how the blood sample was collected and stored [18], the accuracy of many measurements is uncertain. Nevertheless, it seems that there are localized differences in MMP levels in plasma due to differences in the secretion of MMPs from the cells of the blood (predominantly platelets, neutrophils, monocytes) and the artery wall (endothelial cells, smooth muscle cells, macrophages, fibroblasts). These different concentrations of proteases, in conjunction with the differing numbers of platelets, neutrophils, and erythrocytes, result in differential lysis of the clot. Platelet-rich ("arterial" or "white") clots contain fibrin fiber that are more resistant to fibrinolysis and retract more strongly than platelet-poor ("venous" or "red") clots [19]. Both platelet-rich and platelet-poor clots can be found in veins [1]. Thus, fibrinolysis in venous thrombi may be heterogeneous, leaving channels in the clot ("recanalization") through the platelet-poor regions [19, 20].

Origin of MMPs in the Blood and Vasculature

Platelets contain the gelatinases MMP-2 and -9 in their cytoplasm and within platelet granules [21], but these MMPs can exhibit contradictory effects in thrombus formation. MMP-2 stimulates platelet aggregation, with maximal release at maximum platelet aggregation. MMP-9, however, opposes the MMP-2 effect by inhibiting aggregation. Its release from platelets is maximal at 30 % aggregation [22]. MMP-1 and -3 have also been identified in platelets, as have TIMP-1 and -4; the presence of MMP-1 is thought to prime the platelets for aggregation, while MMP-3 has no effect on aggregation [21, 23]. Platelet adhesion results in the release of MMP-1 and -2, with possible activation of the pro-MMP-1 by the platelets [21, 23]. During the onset of thrombosis, platelets release tissue factor (TF) from their α-granules to complex with FVIIa and initiate coagulation. However, platelets also secrete TFPI, which antagonizes the initiation of coagulation (Fig. 19.1). MMP-1, -7, -9, -13, and neutrophil surface proteases are all capable of degrading TFPI, thus allowing coagulation progression [2, 8, 13, 19].

Neutrophils secrete MMP-2, -8, and -9 from various storage granules, as well as cathepsins and other matrix proteases [2, 13, 19, 24]. MMP-2 and -9 are released from gelatinase granules within neutrophils [19] to become activated and influence coagulation and fibrinolysis (Fig. 19.1). MMP-2, -3, -7, -9, and -12 can cleave plasminogen to produce angiostatin, an angiogenesis inhibitor, while further angiogenesis inhibitors are produced from cleaved collagens. Other matrix components, released from the ECM after protease activity, can contribute to the inhibition of coagulation [4, 25, 26]. Neutrophil elastase, a serine protease, is also important in thrombus formation and resolution. It has the capacity to control fibrin generation (altering clot stability by inactivating TFPI) and to degrade fibrin (both directly and indirectly via its effect on plasminogen activation) [19, 24]. Neutrophil elastase cleaves plasminogen to form mini-plasminogen, which is readily activated to form mini-plasmin, without need of any cofactors. Mini-plasmin is more efficient at degrading cross-linked fibrin than normal plasmin and is considerably less sensitive to a2-antiplasmin (a2-AP) inhibition [19], but many MMPs can degrade fibrinogen independently of plasmin [4]. Plasmin-degraded clots disassemble abruptly, releasing large particles into the circulation, possibly resulting in thromboemboli. Elastase-degraded clots release soluble (not particulate) products into the blood [19, 20]. These differences in thrombus stability and plasmin activity will have a significant influence on thrombus resolution in blood vessels.

Monocytes rapidly upregulate their production of MMP-9 on contact with endothelial cells, matrix components (including collagen), fibrinogen, or inflammatory

Table 19.1 MMP production and activation and substrates

MMP	Alternative name	Produced by	Activated by	Substrate – vessel wall	Substrate – blood	Other	References
MMP-1	Collagenase-1, interstitial collagenase	Smooth muscle cells, endothelial cells, macrophages, monocytes, platelets	MMP-3, -7, -12, plasmin, activated platelets	Col1, col2, col3, col7, col8, col10, col11, gelatin, laminin, vitronectin, aggrecan, tenascin, fibronectin, perlican	TFPI, fibrin(ogen), α1-AT, α2-MG	(Pro-)IL-1β, pro-MMP-1, -2, pro-TNF-α, Complement 1q	[2–5, 7, 8, 11, 28, 33]
MMP-2	Gelatinase-A	Smooth muscle cells, endothelial cells, macrophages, monocytes, neutrophils, fibroblasts, platelets, cardiomyocytes	MMP-11, -14, -15, -16, ROS, thrombin, FXa, uPA, tPA, neutrophil elastase	Col1, col3 col4,col5, col7, col10, col11, laminin, elastin, gelatin, fibronectin, chondroitin sulphate, decorin, osteonectin, aggrecan, vitronectin	Fibrin(ogen), thrombin, α1-AT, plasminogen	(Pro)-IL-1β, IL-2 receptor-α, endothelin, adrenomedullin, platelet integrins, pro-TGF-β, pro-TNF-α, pro-MMP-1, -2, -13, Complement 1q, monocyte chemoattractant protein-3, fibroblast GF receptor	[2–7, 11, 12, 16, 19, 22, 23, 28, 33, 41, 50, 51]
MMP-3	Stromelysin-1	Smooth muscle cells, endothelial cells, macrophages, monocytes, cardiomyocytes	Plasmin, cathepsins, mast cell proteases	Broad range	Fibrin(ogen), PAI-1, α2-AP, uPA, plasminogen, α1-AT	Pro-MMP-1, -3, -7, -8, -9, -13, E-cadherin, pro-IL-1β, pro-heparin-binding EGF-like GF, pro-TNF-α, Complement 1q	[2–4, 6, 7, 9, 11, 33, 41, 50, 51]
MMP-7	Matrilysin-1, PUMP-1	Macrophages, monocytes, fibroblasts epithelial cells	Plasmin, cathepsins, mast cell proteases	Broad range	Fibrin(ogen), TFPI, plasminogen, α1-AT	Pro-α-defensin, Fas ligand, pro-TNF-α, E-cadherin, RANK ligand, heparin-binding EGF-like GF	[2, 3, 6, 8, 10, 11, 28]
MMP-8	Collaginase-2, neutrophil collagenase	Smooth muscle cells, endothelial cells, macrophages, monocytes, neutrophils		Col1, col2, col3, col7, col10, gelatin, tenascin, aggrecan	Fibrinogen, α1-AT, α2-MG	Pro-MMP-8, complement 1q	[2, 5, 6, 28, 51]
MMP-9	Gelatinase-B	Smooth muscle cells, endothelial cells, macrophages, monocytes, neutrophils, platelets	Plasmin MMP-3, -7, -11, -12, tissue kallikrein, nitric oxide, ROS, cathepsins, mast cell proteases, uPA, tPA	Col1, col4, col5, col7, col10, col11, col14, laminin, elastin, gelatin, osteonectin, galactin-3, fibronectin, aggrecan, vitronectin	TFPI, fibrin(ogen), α1-AT, plasminogen, other serpins, α2-MG	Angiogenic fragments, (pro)-IL-1β, IL-2 receptor-α, IL-10, vascular endothelial GF, (pro-) TGF-β, intercellular adhesion molecule-1, pro-TNF-α, Complement 1q, IL-2 receptor-α	[2–4, 7, 8, 11, 12, 22, 28]
MMP-10	Stromelysin-2	Endothelial cells, monocytes, fibroblasts, NK-cells, T-cells, chondrocytes	MMP-11, plasmin, plasma kallikrein, trypsin, neutrophil elastase	Broad range	Fibrinogen	Pro-MMP-1, -7, -8, -9	[2, 4, 5, 7, 11, 28]
MMP-11	Stromelysin-3	Smooth muscle cells, endothelial cells, macrophages[a], carcinomas, placenta, uterus	Activated intracellularly	Very weak	PAI, α2-AP, α2-MG, AT, other serpins		[2, 29, 51]

MMP-12	Macrophage metalloelastase	Macrophages, monocytes, chondrocytes, osteocytes	Plasmin, cathepsins, mast cell proteases	Col1, col4, elastin, fibronectin, laminin, aggrecan, gelatin	FXII, fibrinogen, TFPI, plasminogen, α2-MG, α1-AT	Pro-TNF-α	[2–6, 8, 11, 19, 28, 33, 51]
MMP-13	Collagenase-3	Smooth muscle cells, endothelial cells, macrophages, fibroblasts, cardiomyocytes	MMP-2, -14, -15, -16, plasmin, trypsin	Col1, col2, col3, col6, col7, col9, col10, col14, osteonectin, perlican, fibronectin, gelatin, aggrecan, tenascin	FXII, fibrinogen, α2-MG	Pro-MMP-9, -13, complement 1q	[2–7, 11, 41, 51]
MMP-14	MT1-MMP	Endothelial cells, macrophages, monocytes	Activated intracellularly	Col1, col2, col3, laminin, gelatin, fibronectin, vitronectin, aggrecan	FXII, fibrin(ogen), α2-MG, α1-AT	Pro-MMP-2, -13	[2–5, 10, 11, 28, 51]
MMP-15	MT2-MMP	Smooth muscle cells, endothelial cells, T-cells, NK-cells	Activated intracellularly	Gelatin, fibronectin, vitronectin, collagen, aggrecan, tenascin, perlican	Transglutaminase	Pro-MMP-2, (pro-)TNF-α, LRP	[2, 5]
MMP-16	MT3-MMP	Smooth muscle cells, endothelial cells, macrophages, T-cells	Activated intracellularly	Col3, gelatin, fibronectin, vitronectin, collagen, aggrecan	α2-MG, α1-AT, LRP	Pro-MMP-2	[2, 4, 5]
MMP-17	MT4-MMP	Endothelial cells, macrophages, monocytes, B-cells	Activated intracellularly	Gelatin	Fibrin(ogen), LRP	Pro-MMP-2	[2]
MMP-19	RASI (rheumatoid arthritis synovial inflammation)	Smooth muscle cells, endothelial cells, macrophages, monocytes, activated lymphocytes, keratinocytes		Col1, col4, laminin, basement membrane, fibronectin, aggrecan, cartilage oligomeric matrix protein, gelatin	Fibrin(ogen)		[3–5, 28]
MMP-20	Enamelysin	Tooth enamel		Amelogenin, aggrecan, cartilage oligomeric matrix protein			[5, 11]
MMP-23	Cysteine array (CA)-MMP	Monocytes, foam cells, fibroblasts, epithelial cells, chondrocytes		Laminin, gelatin			[5, 11, 28], personal observation
MMP-24	MT5-MMP	Brain specific	Activated intracellularly	Gelatin, fibronectin, vitronectin, collagen, aggrecan		pro-MMP-2	[3, 5, 11]
MMP-25	MT6-MMP	Peripheral blood leukocytes	Activated intracellularly	Col4, gelatin, laminin, fibronectin	Fibrin	Pro-MMP-2	[5, 11]
MMP-26	Matrilysin-2, endometase	Endometrium		Col4, fibronectin, gelatin	α1-AT, fibrinogen	MMP-9	[5, 11]
MMP-27	C-MMP, MMP-22	Fibroblasts		Gelatin, casein		Autolysis	[11]

[a]Not produced in monocytes

mediators [such as tissue necrosis factor-α (TNF-α), lipopolysaccharide (LPS), or oxidised low-density lipoprotein (LDL)] [2, 27, 28]. MMP-12, -14, and -16 (but not MMP-1 or -3) production in monocytes is also upregulated by inflammatory cytokines, while contact with CD40 ligand upregulates MMP-1, -3, -8, -9, and -11 expression [2, 29]. Interestingly, monocytes treated with an MMP-9 inhibitor lose the ability to aggregate upon contact with fibrinogen (despite fibrinogen's ability to activate proinflammatory pathways in monocytes), suggesting the presence of an autocrine mechanism in this process [27]. Monocytes also express MMP-10, -19, and -23 [2, 28]. These changes in monocyte MMP production are thought to facilitate entry of these cells into the vessel wall, where they can become macrophages. Tissue macrophages express MMP-13, -14, and -16, while foamy macrophages (macrophages that have migrated into the vessel wall and have become lipid-laden) have upregulated production of MMP-1, -3, -8, -9, -13, and -23. Both foamy and non-foamy macrophages constitutively secrete TIMP-1, -2, and -3 [2, 29–34] (also personal observations).

The vessel wall is lined by thrombo-resistant endothelial cells, which have constitutive MMP-2 expression. MMP-1, -3, -8, -9, and -11 levels are upregulated by inflammatory cytokines, or exposure to macrophages, oxidised LDL, or CD40 ligand [2, 29]. MMP-1 and -2 expression may also be upregulated by high glucose levels [2]. These results suggest that inflammation and immune mechanisms are associated with MMP production by endothelial cells. Endothelial cells also express MMP-13 and the inhibitors TIMP-1 and -2, which are not responsive to oxidised LDL. TIMP-2, however, may be upregulated in response to CD40 ligand [2, 35], while TIMP-1 is induced by prostaglandins and a wide variety of cytokines, including transforming GF (TGF)-β and platelet-derived growth factor (PDGF) [36].

Vascular smooth muscle cells constitutively express MMP-2, production of which is further upregulated by stretch and reactive oxygen species; MMP-9 expression can also be upregulated [2, 37, 38]. Smooth muscle cells appear to be subject to immune activation, as the presence of inflammatory cytokines such as interleukin-1 (IL-1), IL-4, and TNF-α, or contact with activated T-cell membranes (or CD40 ligand) induce the smooth muscle cells to produce MMP-1, -3, -8, and -9 [2, 29]. Smooth muscle cell expression of MMP-11 and TIMP-1, -2, and -3 appear to be upregulated by fibrogenic cytokines such as TGF-β and PDGF [2, 39].

There are several further cell types found in blood or the vasculature that are capable of secreting MMPs, including T-cells (MMP-1, -2, -3, -9), mast cells (MMP-2, -9, TIMP-1), and adventitial fibroblasts (MMP-2, -9, TIMP-1, -2) [2, 3].

Role of MMPs in Coagulation, Thrombosis Formation, and Fibrinolysis

Every member of the MMP family is capable of degrading components of the vascular ECM, but their substrates are not limited to matrix. Many MMPs are active in the propagation and resolution of thrombosis (Table 19.1).

MMPs in Haemorrhage

The gelatinases, MMP-2 and MMP-9, have been implicated in aneurysm formation, acute neurovascular events, and unstable atherosclerotic plaque structure [40]. Elevated MMP-9 levels in plasma have also been associated with cerebral haemorrhage and perihaematomal oedema, with a negative association of the MMP-9 inhibitor TIMP-1 [41]. Patients with acute intracerebral haemorrhage also have more MMP-3, which is associated with increased mortality [41]. This increase in MMP-3 production may occur through the interaction of tPA and low-density lipoprotein receptor-related protein (LRP) on endothelial cells [42]. Animal studies support these findings, as MMP-9 null mice also have increased incidence of cerebral haemorrhage and oedema, with increased mortality [43]. There is at least partial compensation for the missing MMP-9 in knockout animals by an increase in MMP-2 and MMP-3 levels in areas of cerebral haemorrhage. A similar compensatory increase in MMP-2 expression has also been observed in vein grafts in MMP-9 null mice [44].

MMPs in DVT Resolution

Venous thromboembolism [deep vein thrombosis (DVT) and pulmonary embolism] is a common cause of cardiovascular-associated mortality and is associated with thrombi that are rich in fibrin [1]. DVT resolution often involves re-canalisation (clot retraction, fibrinolysis, and angiogenesis) and infiltration by leukocytes and other cells [45, 46]. The first leukocytes to appear in the thrombi are neutrophils and monocytes, both which can express high levels of MMPs (particularly after activation) [12, 28]. Recently, a study was performed examining patients presenting with DVTs, with blood samples being taken immediately and 6 months later. Compared with healthy controls, patients with DVTs had four to fivefold more MMP in their blood, with an increase in inflammation (as indicated by increased Toll-like receptor-4 gene expression in leukocytes) [47]. Unsurprisingly, patients with thrombi also had more fibrin D-dimer (an indicator of ongoing thrombosis and fibrinolysis [46, 48]) and P-selectin (an indicator of endothelial cell activation [46]) in the initial blood sample [47]. *In vivo* studies suggest that DVT resolution involves the production of fresh matrix, requiring MMP production and activation and production of pro-fibrotic GF by invading leukocytes (from the blood) and smooth muscle cells and fibroblasts (from the vessel wall) [45, 46]. These results support two hypotheses: that thrombosis is linked to inflammation, and that DVT resolution, like wound healing, requires remodelling [12, 46]. While venous thrombolysis is predominantly mediated by plasminogen activation, at least part of the efficacy of plasmin is due to its ability to activate many MMPs [9, 12]. Thus, successful thrombus resolution is associated with active matrix remodelling consisting of early collagenolysis, elastolysis, and gelatinolysis (predominantly due to MMP-2, -8, -9, and -14 being produced by cells within the thrombus rather than from the circulation), followed by fibrosis [12, 45, 46].

Studies using genetically modified mice can give insight into the varying contributions of the various proteases. DVTs in uPA null mice have fewer neutrophils and monocytes than wild-type controls, even though the thrombi are similar in size. The thrombi have significantly more interferon-γ (IFNγ) (an inducer of MMP-2), plasminogen activator inhibitor-1 (PAI-1), and active MMP-2 and -14, with reduced plasmin activity. The thrombi also have less fibrinogen, possibly because of the increased MMP-2 production [49]. MMP-2 is known to inactivate fibrinogen, effectively limiting its availability for participation in the coagulation cascade [50]. MMP-8, -12, -13, and -14 can also inactivate fibrinogen [45, 51]. Interestingly, the efficiency of the enzymic action of MMP-2 on fibrinogen is similar to that of plasmin, both being lower than that of thrombin [50]. The ability of MMP-2 to inactivate fibrinogen is probably the reason for the large thrombi found in MMP-2 null mice, as there was no change in plasmin expression [49]. MMP-14 is the major cell surface activator of MMP-2, but MMP-2 may also be activated by proteases within the thrombus, including activated protein C and factor Xa [45]. MMP-2 reporter mice have more MMP-2 activity and increased MMP-14 expression in resolving DVTs, possibly mediated by an endothelial cell response to thrombin [45]. When uPA was inhibited using aprotinin rather than a genetic deletion, the size of the thrombus was increased, as was MMP-9 activity [14]. Taken together, these studies indicate that MMPs are important early thrombolytic agents, able to compensate for a reduction in plasmin or lack of uPA [14, 49].

The proportion of different MMP-positive cells within the DVT may give insight into the age of the DVT. Recently formed (1–5 day old) experimental DVTs produced in mice had a MMP-9/MMP-2 cell ratio of >2.0, while thrombi older than 7 days had a ratio of <2.0 [15], but it remains to be seen whether this method can be used clinically. The changes in MMP levels may be due to the altered venous pressure in the thrombus [52]. An elevated venous pressure (resulting in reduced shear stress) is known to induce elevated enzymic activity, including MMP-2 and -9 activity, which in turn produces venous dilation and further increases in venous pressure [52, 53]. In the rat, acute venous occlusion is immediately accompanied by an upregulation of MMP-1, -8, -9, and TIMP-1 and -2, with no early differences in MMP-2, -3, -9, and -12. The changes in blood pressure due to the thrombotic occlusion result in vein wall expansion, with upregulation of the expression and activity of the proteases [53].

MMPs in Varicose Veins

Varicose veins are dilated, elongated, and tortuous, often having areas of vein wall thickening or thinning and thrombosis, possibly due to changes in ECM content and altered levels of MMPs and plasminogen activators [13, 54, 55]. Varicose veins tend to have altered elastin content and structure, with increased collagen type I (col1) and laminin, and reduced col3, with altered collagen bundle orientation [13, 55]. They also have elevated levels of MMP-1, -3, -7, -12, and -13 and TIMP-1 and -3 and less TIMP-2 compared with normal veins [13, 36, 54–56]. The expression and activity of gelatinases is not clear, however. Some researchers have reported that varicose veins have less pro- and active MMP-2, pro-MMP-9, and PAI-1, but no difference in TIMP-2 levels [36, 54]. Others report that the expression of MMP-2 and -9 is elevated in varicose veins and that there are regions of increased pro-MMP-9 in the plasma in these vessels [13, 55, 56]. As varicose veins also have reduced levels of uPA and tPA [54], this may indeed result in regions of reduced *activation* of the gelatinases. These changes in fibrinolytic and matrix proteases will influence thrombosis and thrombus clearance within the vein, as demonstrated by the occurrence of regions of blood stagnation and thrombophlebitis in varicose veins [13, 56].

MMPs in Acute Vein Graft Thrombosis

The saphenous vein is commonly used for surgically bypassing blocked areas of coronary and peripheral arteries because of the use of multiple grafting procedures, technical ease of use, and increasing need of repeat surgery [57]. Although these surgical procedures have improved both patient mortality and quality of life, their success is limited by graft thickening resulting in partial or complete closure of the vessel in up to 50 % of cases by 10 years after the procedure [57–59]. Saphenous vein grafts have been used to bypass blockages in coronary arteries for almost 50 years, with the engraftment operation being performed over 500,000 times each year worldwide [57, 60]. However, vein grafts are subject to early closure due to thrombus formation and longer term occlusion as a consequence of neointimal formation and accelerated atherosclerosis, often with further thrombotic events [57–59]. Failure of the graft may result in angina, myocardial infarction, or gangrene of the extremities, and often leads to repeat revascularisation procedures with their associated morbidity and costs [60].

Up to 18 % of vein grafts occlude in the first few days because of acute thrombosis. This thrombosis is caused by harvesting, surgical trauma, mechanical stress, and exposure of the graft to the arterial environment [57, 60]. Vein preparation prior to implantation results in increased degradative enzymic activity, including MMPs and other matrix-degrading proteases [2, 37, 61]. Gross damage also occurs when the graft is suddenly exposed to pulsatile and high-pressure flow, increased wall tension, and shear stress, resulting in increased MMP activity and a loss of thrombomodulin (TM). The endothelium is sloughed away and individual cells damaged, allowing platelets and leukocytes to adhere to the vessel. Medial and adventitial ECM fractures and any remaining vasa vasorum thromboses. TF and von Willebrand factor (vWF) within the vessel wall, normally protected by the endothelium, are thus exposed to circulating fibrin(ogen) and platelets, allowing rapid formation of thrombi [19, 61–63].

Early thrombosis particularly affects grafts in arteries with a small diameter or poor distal runoff [57, 64] and is caused by alterations in the graft wall, changes in blood rheology, and altered flow caused by sudden exposure to the arterial environment. Anti-thrombotic treatments are used to reduce the risk of early thrombosis, but these can be associated with increased postoperative bleeding and do not completely prevent graft failure [57, 60, 64]. Many of the components of the thrombus contribute to the development of a neointimal thickening, either by becoming absorbed into the vessel wall or by contributing factors that stimulate cells to proliferate and produce matrix, thus promoting the longer term complications of vein graft disease [2, 65]. Monocyte adhesion and infiltration into the graft also occur early after graft implantation. These cells transform to become macrophages and take up lipid to become 'foam cells'. Both foamy and non-foamy macrophages alter their ECM environment by producing proteases, such as fibrinolytic enzymes, cathepsins, heparanase, and MMPs, which degrade the ECM, thus allowing graft remodelling [2, 34, 61, 66, 67].

The specific role of MMP-9 has been examined in experimental vein grafts. MMP-2 and -9 are not present in normal vein (or are present in very low amounts), but their expression is increased upon engraftment. Other MMPs, including MMP-1 and MMP-3, are also upregulated [37, 44, 68]. In mouse vein grafts over 70 % of the graft endothelium is removed in the first 24 h, and both thrombus and neointimal formation is observed within a few days [44, 63, 69]. Microthrombi are present on the graft by the day after surgery [63], but probably occur even earlier. Fibrin formation has been found on arteries as early as 10 min after injury [65], and it is likely that veins placed into the arterial environment would similarly be subject to very early fibrin deposition and thrombosis. By 1 week after engraftment, 12–13 % of experimental vein grafts in mice have thrombi (Fig. 19.2a), but there is no evidence of a link between thrombus formation and a lack of MMP-9. Some grafts rupture, and others become thrombosed at later time points (Fig. 19.2b–d). Many occluded grafts are re-canalised, ensuring that circulation is re-established after the thrombotic event [44]. Compensatory graft remodelling is found earlier in MMP-9 null mice than in wild-type mice, possibly because of an increase in MMP-2 [44], but graft thickening may be reduced by limiting endothelial loss and early thrombus formation using a localised aspirin treatment [63].

One way to prevent the serious complications associated with systemic anti-coagulatory and thrombolyic regimes is to target drugs specifically to the vein graft. A model of saphenous vein-carotid artery engraftment in the pig has been recently adapted to assess the effectiveness of treatments for targeted acute vein graft thrombosis [70]. To minimise systemic effects, the vein was exposed to local tPA gene therapy prior to implantation. After implantation, blood flow in the graft was continuously measured using transit time ultrasonography to determine blood flow and the frequency of production and resolution of flow-restricting thrombi (cyclic flow reductions). Even as early as the day after engraftment, endothelial cells (when present) and underlying smooth muscle cells in the graft expressed elevated levels of tPA (Fig. 19.2e–f). Blood flow was increased in the graft, and the cyclic flow reductions were less severe, indicating the efficacy of the treatment [70]. This model could also be of use in investigating the effects of altering local levels of MMP production either directly or by using tPA to influence plasminogen activation, thus affecting MMP activation.

Conclusion

Acute venous thrombosis can be a life-threatening event and may in part be due to factors in the blood other than coagulatory or fibrinolytic enzymes. It is now known that inflammation and thrombosis are intimately connected, with considerable reciprocal activation of the coagulatory, fibrinolytic, and MMP systems. While each pathway has been studied extensively, details concerning how the pathways interact are limited and require further examination. This would allow personalised novel therapies to be investigated, possibly involving effective prophylaxis based on circulating factor assessment. Alternatively, the use of combination therapies, common to two or three of the pathways, may enable the design of treatments to prevent coagulation without promoting bleeding. These investigations may give insight into providing an integrated approach for the study and prevention of acute venous thrombosis and other thrombotic diseases.

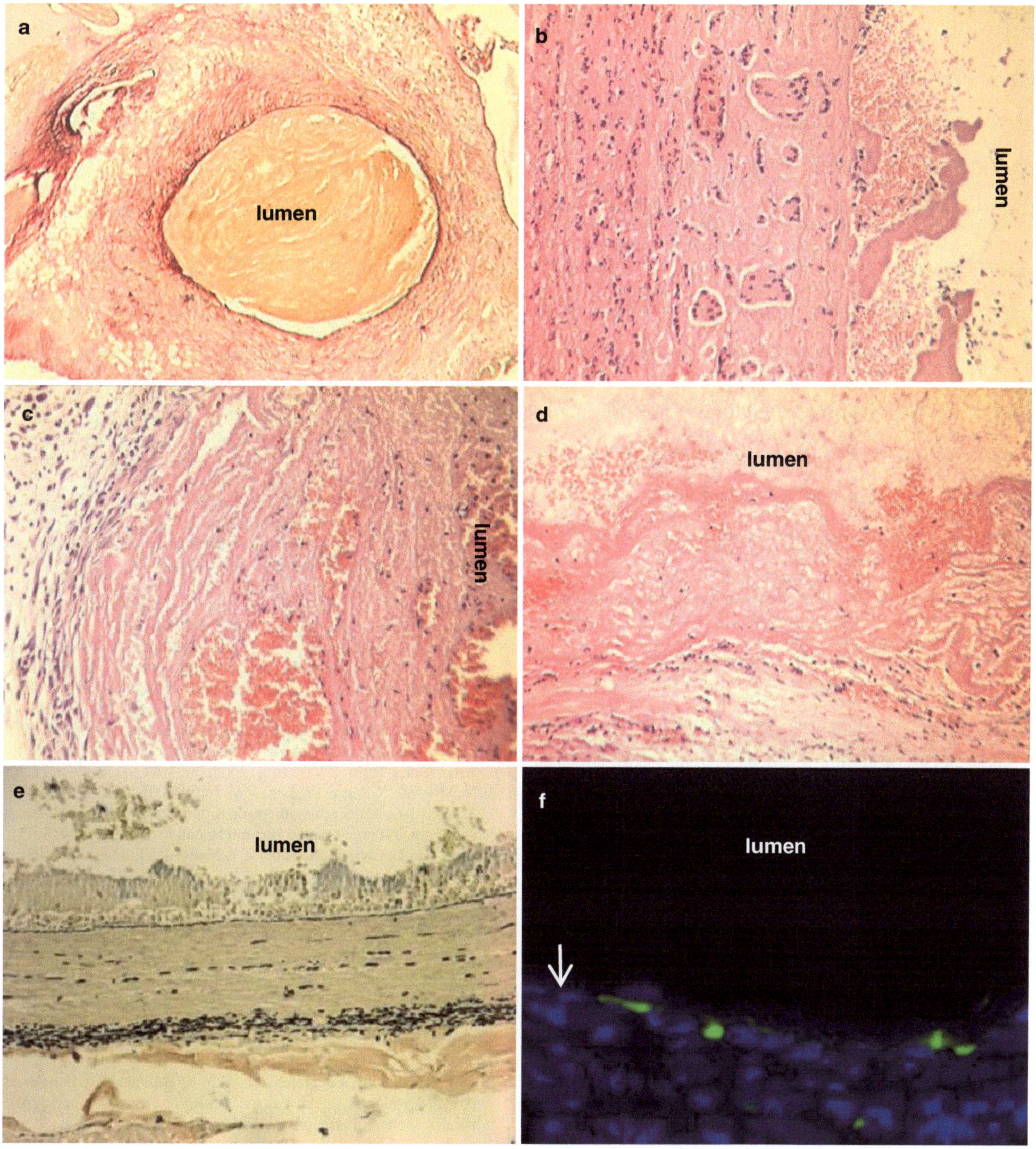

Fig. 19.2 Acute thrombosis in experimental vein grafts (**a**) Vena cava-carotid artery interposition graft in a MMP-9 null mouse 1 week after engraftment. The lumen is almost completely blocked by a fresh thrombus. (Elastin van Gieson stain, ×40.) (**b**) Vena cava-carotid artery interposition graft in a control mouse 4 weeks after engraftment, showing a recently formed thrombus on the luminal surface of the graft. (Haematoxylin and eosin stain, ×200.) (**c**) Vena cava-carotid artery interposition graft in a control mouse 5 weeks after engraftment. Acute rupture of the graft with infiltration of blood cells into the graft wall. The graft has relatively few cells. (Haematoxylin and eosin stain, ×200.) (**d**) Vena cava-carotid artery interposition graft in a MMP-9 null mouse, showing that acute thrombotic events can occur as late as 8 weeks after engraftment. (Haematoxylin and eosin stain, ×200.) (**e**) Propagation of a thrombus 1 day after engraftment of a control saphenous vein into the carotid artery of a pig. Thrombus caused by crush injury of the graft. (Elastin van Gieson stain, ×200.) (**f**) Pig saphenous vein-carotid artery interposition graft. The vein has been treated with tPA gene therapy prior to engraftment. tPA (*green*; anti-human tPA, no. 385R American Diagnostica, Inc., USA) is deposited along the luminal surface (*arrow*) or is found in cells within the graft, and its presence reduces the incidence and severity of thrombus formation, even after crush injury. (×1,000). (Nuclei appear blue (DAPI)).

References

1. Jerjes-Sanchez C. Venous and arterial thrombosis: a continuous spectrum of the same disease? Eur Heart J. 2005;26:3–4.
2. Newby AC. Dual role of matrix metalloproteinases (matrixins) in intimal thickening and atherosclerotic plaque rupture. Physiol Rev. 2005;85:1–31.
3. Nagase H, Visse R, Murphy G. Structure and function of matrix metalloproteinases and TIMPs. Cardiovasc Res. 2006;69:562–73.
4. Sternlicht MD, Werb Z. How matrix metalloproteinases regulate cell behaviour. Annu Rev Cell Dev Biol. 2001;17:463–516.
5. McCawley LJ, Matrisian LM. Matrix metalloproteinases: they're not just for matrix anymore. Curr Opin Cell Biol. 2001;13:534–40.
6. Ugwu F, Lemmens G, Collen D, Lijnen HR. Matrix metalloproteinase deficiencies do not impair cell-associated fibrinolytic activity. Thromb Res. 2001;102:61–9.
7. Lijnen HR. Matrix metalloproteinases and cellular fibrinolytic activity. Biochemistry. 2002;67:92–8.
8. Belaaouaj AA, Li A, Wun TC, Welgus HG, Shapiro SD. Matrix metalloproteinases cleave tissue factor pathway inhibitor. Effects on coagulation. J Biol Chem. 2000;275:27123–8.
9. Lijnen HR. Elements of the fibrinolytic system. Ann N Y Acad Sci. 2001;936:226–36.
10. Kluft C. The fibrinolytic system and thrombotic tendency. Pathophysiol Haemost Thromb. 2003;33:425–9.
11. Visse R, Nagase H. Matrix metalloproteinases and tissue inhibitors of metalloproteinases. Circ Res. 2003;92:827–39.
12. Deatrick KB, Eliason JL, Lynch EM, Moore AJ, Dewyer NA, Varma MR, et al. Vein wall remodeling after deep vein thrombosis involves matrix metalloproteinases and late fibrosis in a mouse model. J Vasc Surg. 2005;42:140–8.
13. Lim CS, Shalhoub J, Gohel MS, Shepherd AC, Davies AH. Matrix metalloproteinases in vascular disease – a potential therapeutic target? Curr Vasc Pharmacol. 2010;8:75–85.
14. Dewyer NA, Sood V, Lynch EM, Luke CE, Upchurch GR, Wakefield TW, et al. Plasmin inhibition increases MMP-9 activity and decreases vein wall stiffness during venous thrombosis resolution. J Surg Res. 2007;142:357–63.
15. Nosaka M, Ishida Y, Kimura A, Kondo T. Immunohistochemical detection of MMP-2 and MMP-9 in a stasis-induced deep vein thrombosis model and its application to thrombus age estimation. Int J Legal Med. 2010;124:439–44.
16. Lee SW, Song KE, Shin DS, Ahn SM, Ha ES, Kim DJ, et al. Alterations in peripheral blood levels of TIMP-1, MMP-2, and MMP-9 in patients with type-2 diabetes. Diabetes Res Clin Pract. 2005;69:175–9.
17. Gharagozlian S, Svennevig K, Bangstad HJ, Winberg JO, Kolset S. Matrix metalloproteinases in subjects with type 1 diabetes. BMC Clin Pathol. 2009;9:7.
18. Jung K, Klotzek S, Stephan C, Mannello F, Lein M. Impact of blood sampling on the circulating matrix metalloproteinases 1, 2, 3, 7, 8, and 9. Clin Chem. 2008;54:772–3.
19. Wohner N. Role of cellular elements in thrombus formation and dissolution. Cardiovasc Hematol Agents Med Chem. 2008;6:224–8.
20. Weisel JW, Litvinov RI. The biochemical and physical process of fibrinolysis and effects of clot structure and stability on the lysis rate. Cardiovasc Hematol Agents Med Chem. 2008;6:161–80.
21. Jurasz P, Chung AW, Radomski A, Radomski MW. Nonremodeling properties of matrix metalloproteinases: the platelet connection. Circ Res. 2002;90:1041–3.
22. Fernandez-Patron C, Martinez-Cuesta MA, Salas E, Sawicki G, Wozniak M, Radomski MW, et al. Differential regulation of platelet aggregation by matrix metalloproteinases-9 and –2. Thromb Haemost. 1999;82:1730–5.
23. Galt SW, Lindemann S, Allen L, Medd DJ, Falk JM, McIntyre TM, et al. Outside-in signals delivered by matrix metalloproteinase-1 regulate platelet function. Circ Res. 2002;90:1093–9.
24. Massberg S, Grahl L, von Bruehl ML, Manukyan D, Pfeiler S, Goosmann C, et al. Reciprocal coupling of coagulation and innate immunity via neutrophil serine proteases. Nat Med. 2010;16:887–96.
25. Bourin MC, Lindahl U. Glycosaminoglycans and the regulation of blood coagulation. Biochem J. 1993;289:313–30.
26. Zheng PS, Reis M, Sparling C, Lee DY, La Pierre DP, Wong CKA, et al. Versican G3 domain promotes blood coagulation through suppressing the activity of tissue factor pathway inhibitor-1. J Biol Chem. 2006;281:8175–82.
27. Kaneider NC, Mosheimer B, Gunther A, Feistritzer C, Wiedermann CJ. Enhancement of fibrinogen-triggered pro-coagulant activation of monocytes in vitro by matrix metalloproteinase-9. Thromb J. 2010;8:2.
28. Reel B, Sala-Newby GB, Huang WC, Newby AC. Diverse patterns of cyclooxygenase-independent metalloproteinase gene regulation in human monocytes. Br J Pharmacol. 2011;163:1679–90.
29. Schonbeck U, Mach F, Sukhova GK, Atkinson E, Levesque E, Herman M, et al. Expression of stromelysin-3 in atherosclerotic lesions: regulation via CD40-CD40 ligand signaling in vitro and in vivo. J Exp Med. 1999;189:843–53.
30. Chase AJ, Bond M, Crook MF, Newby AC. Role of nuclear factor-kB activation in metalloproteinase-1, -3, and -9 secretion by human macrophages in vitro and rabbit foam cells produced in vivo. Arterioscler Thromb Vasc Biol. 2002;22:765–71.
31. Luan Z, Chase AJ, Newby AC. Statins inhibit secretion of metalloproteinases-1, -2, -3, and -9 from vascular smooth muscle cells and macrophages. Arterioscler Thromb Vasc Biol. 2003;23:769–75.
32. Thomas AC, Sala-Newby GB, Ismail Y, Johnson JL, Pasterkamp G, Newby AC. Genomics of foam cells and nonfoamy macrophages from rabbits identifies arginase-I as a differential regulator of nitric oxide production. Arterioscler Thromb Vasc Biol. 2007;27:571–7.
33. Newby AC. Metalloproteinase expression in monocytes and macrophages and its relationship to atherosclerotic plaque instability. Arterioscler Thromb Vasc Biol. 2008;28:2108–14.
34. Newby AC, George SJ, Ismail Y, Johnson JL, Sala-Newby GB, Thomas AC. Vulnerable atherosclerotic plaque metalloproteinases and foam cell phenotypes. Thromb Haemost. 2009;101:1006–11.
35. Li D, Liu L, Chen H, Sawamura T, Mehta JL. LOX-1, an oxidized LDL endothelial receptor, induces CD40/CD40L signaling in human coronary artery endothelial cells. Arterioscler Thromb Vasc Biol. 2003;23:816–21.
36. Woodside KJ, Hu M, Burke A, Murakami M, Pounds LL, Killewich LA, et al. Morphologic characteristics of varicose veins: possible role of metalloproteinases. J Vasc Surg. 2003;38:162–9.
37. George SJ, Zaltsman AB, Newby AC. Surgical preparative injury and neointima formation increase MMP-9 expression and MMP-2 activation in human saphenous vein. Cardiovasc Res. 1997;33: 447–59.
38. Grote K, Flach I, Luchtefeld M, Akin E, Holland SM, Drexler H, et al. Mechanical stretch enhances mRNA expression and proenzyme release of matrix metalloproteinase-2 (MMP-2) via NAD(P)H oxidase-derived reactive oxygen species. Circ Res. 2003;92:e80–6.
39. Fabunmi RP, Baker AH, Murray EJ, Booth RF, Newby AC. Divergent regulation by growth factors and cytokines of 95 kDa and 72 kDa gelatinases and tissue inhibitors or metalloproteinases-1, -2, and -3 in rabbit aortic smooth muscle cells. Biochem J. 1996;315:335–42.
40. Hobeika MJ, Thompson RW, Muhs BE, Brooks PC, Gagne PJ. Matrix metalloproteinases in peripheral vascular disease. J Vasc Surg. 2007;45:849–57.
41. Alvarez-Sabin J, Delgado P, Abilleira S, Molina CA, Arenillas J, Ribo M, et al. Temporal profile of matrix metalloproteinases and

their inhibitors after spontaneous intracerebral hemorrhage. Stroke. 2004;35:1316–22.
42. Suzuki Y, Nagai N, Umemura K. Novel situations of endothelial injury in stroke – mechanisms of stroke and strategy of drug development: intracranial bleeding associated with the treatment of ischemic stroke: thrombolytic treatment of ischemia-affected endothelial cells with tissue-type plasminogen activator. J Pharmacol Sci. 2011;116:25–9.
43. Tang J, Liu J, Zhou C, Alexander JS, Nanda A, Granger DN, et al. MMP-9 deficiency enhances collagenase-induced intracerebral hemorrhage and brain injury in mutant mice. J Cereb Blood Flow Metab. 2004;24:1133–45.
44. Thomas AC, Newby AC. Effect of matrix metalloproteinase-9 knockout on vein graft remodelling in mice. J Vasc Res. 2010;47: 299–308.
45. Dahi S, Lee JG, Lovett DH, Sarkar R. Differential transcriptional activation of matrix metalloproteinase-2 and membrane type-1 matrix metalloproteinase by experimental deep venous thrombosis and thrombin. J Vasc Surg. 2005;42:539–45.
46. Wakefield TW, Myers DD, Henke PK. Mechanisms of venous thrombosis and resolution. Arterioscler Thromb Vasc Biol. 2008;28:387–91.
47. Deatrick KB, Elfline M, Baker N, Luke CE, Blackburn S, Stabler C, et al. Postthrombotic vein wall remodeling: preliminary observations. J Vasc Surg. 2011;53:139–46.
48. John MA, Elms MJ, O'Reilly EJ, Rylatt DB, Bundesen PG, Hillyard CJ. The simpliRED D dimer test: a novel assay for the detection of crosslinked fibrin degradation products in whole blood. Thromb Res. 1990;58:273–81.
49. Sood V, Luke CE, Deatrick KB, Baldwin J, Miller EM, Elfline M, et al. Urokinase plasminogen activator independent early experimental thrombus resolution: MMP2 as an alternative mechanism. Thromb Haemost. 2010;104:1174–83.
50. Monaco S, Gioia M, Rodriguez J, Fasciglione GF, Di PD, Lupidi G, et al. Modulation of the proteolytic activity of matrix metalloproteinase-2 (gelatinase A) on fibrinogen. Biochem J. 2007;402:503–13.
51. Hiller O, Lichte A, Oberpichler A, Kocourek A, Tschesche H. Matrix metalloproteinases collagenase-2, macrophage elastase, collagenase-3, and membrane type 1-matrix metalloproteinase impair clotting by degradation of fibrinogen and factor XII. J Biol Chem. 2000;275:33008–13.
52. Raffetto JD, Qiao X, Koledova VV, Khalil RA. Prolonged increases in vein wall tension increase matrix metalloproteinases and decrease constriction in rat vena cava: potential implications in varicose veins. J Vasc Surg. 2008;48:447–56.
53. Alsaigh T, Pocock ES, Bergan JJ, Schmid-Schonbein GW. Acute venous occlusion enhances matrix metalloprotease activity: implications on endothelial dysfunction. Microvasc Res. 2011;81:108–16.
54. Badier-Commander C, Verbeuren T, Lebard C, Michel JB, Jacob MP. Increased TIMP/MMP ratio in varicose veins: a possible explanation for extracellular matrix accumulation. J Pathol. 2000;192: 105–12.
55. Sansilvestri-Morel P, Fioretti F, Rupin A, Senni K, Fabiani JN, Godeau G, et al. Comparison of extracellular matrix in skin and saphenous veins from patients with varicose veins: does the skin reflect venous matrix changes? Clin Sci. 2007;112:229–39.
56. Kowalewski R, Sobolewski K, Wolanska M, Gacko M. Matrix metalloproteinases in the vein wall. Int Angiol. 2004;23:164–9.
57. Motwani JG, Topol EJ. Aortocoronary saphenous vein graft disease: pathogenesis, predisposition, and prevention. Circulation. 1998;97:916–31.
58. Dashwood MR, Loesch A. The saphenous vein as a bypass conduit: the potential role of vascular nerves in graft performance. Curr Vasc Pharmacol. 2009;7:47–57.
59. Lee MS, Park SJ, Kandzari DE, Kirtane AJ, Fearon WF, Brilakis ES, et al. Saphenous vein graft intervention. JACC Cardiovasc Interv. 2011;4:831–43.
60. Hagemeyer CE, Peter K. Ex-vivo thrombolytic gene therapy for vein graft patency: the frontier for development of selective, localised therapeutic approaches. Thromb Haemost. 2009;102: 3–4.
61. Johnson JL, van Eys GJ, Angelini GD, George SJ. Injury induces dedifferentiation of smooth muscle cells and increased matrix-degrading metalloproteinase activity in human saphenous vein. Arterioscler Thromb Vasc Biol. 2001;21:1146–51.
62. Sperry JL, Deming CB, Bian C, Walinsky PL, Kass DA, Kolodgie FD, et al. Wall tension is a potent negative regulator of in vivo thrombomodulin expression. Circ Res. 2003;92:41–7.
63. Torsney E, Mayr U, Zou Y, Thompson WD, Hu Y, Xu Q. Thrombosis and neointima formation in vein grafts are inhibited by locally applied aspirin through endothelial protection. Circ Res. 2004;94:1466–73.
64. Poston RS, Gu J, Brown JM, Gammie JS, White C, Nie L, et al. Endothelial injury and acquired aspirin resistance as promoters of regional thrombin formation and early vein graft failure after coronary artery bypass grafting. J Thorac Cardiovasc Surg. 2006;131:122–30.
65. Thomas AC, Campbell JH. Timecourse of fibrin deposition and removal after arterial injury. Thromb Res. 2003;109:65–9.
66. Kockx MM, De Meyer GRY, Bortier H, de Meyere N, Muhring J, Bakker A, et al. Luminal foam cell accumulation is associated with smooth muscle cell death in the intimal thickening of human saphenous vein grafts. Circulation. 1996;94:1255–62.
67. Fitzgerald M, Hayward IP, Thomas AC, Campbell GR, Campbell JH. Matrix metalloproteinase can facilitate the heparanase-induced promotion of phenotype change in vascular smooth muscle cells. Atherosclerosis. 1999;145:97–106.
68. Sharony R, Pintucci G, Saunders PC, Grossi EA, Baumann FG, Galloway AC, et al. Matrix metalloproteinase expression in vein grafts: role of inflammatory mediators and extracellular signal-regulated kinases-1 and -2. Am J Physiol Heart Circ Physiol. 2006;290:H1651–9.
69. Shi C, Patel A, Zhang D, Wang H, Carmeliet P, Reed GL, et al. Plasminogen is not required for neointima formation in a mouse model of vein graft stenosis. Circ Res. 1999;84:883–90.
70. Thomas AC, Wyatt MJ, Newby AC. Reduction of early vein graft thrombosis by tissue plasminogen activator gene transfer. Thromb Haemost. 2009;102:145–52.

Idiopathic Venous Thromboembolism

20

Crina Sinescu

Abbreviations

APLAS	Antiphospholipid antibody syndrome
CUS	Compression ultrasonography
DVT	Deep vein thrombosis
HDL	High density lipoprotein
IL	Interleukin
LDL	Low density lipoprotein
LMWH	Low molecular weight heparin
MDCT	Multi-detector computer tomography
PE	Pulmonary embolism
RV	Right ventricle
RVT	Residual vein thrombosis
SDCT	Single-detector computer tomography
VKAs	Vitamin K antagonists
VT	Venous thromboembolism
VTE	Venous thrombotic event

Introduction

Venous thromboembolism is a manifest disease that includes deep vein thrombosis (DVT) and pulmonary embolism (PE). It is the third most common cardiovascular disorder after coronary artery disease and stroke.

Definition

Annual incidence of venous thrombotic events (VTEs) is approximately 0.1 % among persons in early adulthood and increases to nearly 1 % among those who are at least 60 years old. Idiopathic or unprovoked venous thrombosis is defined as any VTE in the absence of an identifiable predisposing factor. The International Cooperative Pulmonary Registry evaluated the incidence of unprovoked PE at about 20 % of all VTEs [1].

Of patients diagnosed with proximal DVT, around 50 % have an associated PE; 70 % of patients with PE have a positive diagnosis for DVT. PE can be diagnosed 3–7 days after the occurrence of a DVT, can be fatal in 10 % of cases, and presents with shock or hypotension in 5–10 % of cases; 50 % of the remaining patients present with signs of right ventricular (RV) dysfunction. Chronic complications such as thromboembolic pulmonary hypertension can occur in 0.5–5 % of patients treated for PE. The complete list of factors that predispose to VTE is presented in Table 20.1.

Risk Factors for VTE

Apart from traditional risk factors (Table 20.1), it worth mentioning less usual risk factors for VTE, which correspond to the classic atherosclerotic cascade. Many risk factors for VTE, such as dyslipidemia, obesity, hypertension, diabetes, and smoking, overlap with those for atherothrombosis. As a consequence, VTE is starting to be considered a "full-time member" of the cardiovascular syndrome "club" that includes coronary artery disease, peripheral artery disease, and cerebrovascular disease.

More evidence describing the continuum between VTE and arterial disease has appeared in past years [3]. Stein et al. [4] found a 2.5 increased risk for VTE in obese patients. In a prospective study of 250 women, the authors investigated which factors predispose to VTE. They found an increase in risk of 2.9-fold for obese subjects (body mass index >29 kg/m^2), 1.9-fold for smokers, and 1.9-fold for those with hypertension [5]. Pradoni et al. [6] suggested a link between atherosclerosis and VTE; they discovered that patients with spontaneous veinous thrombosis had a higher incidence of carotid plaques than controls, translating into a 2.3-fold risk increase for VTE vs. controls. Subsequently, Spencer et al. [7] showed that idiopathic VTE is associated with increased

C. Sinescu, MD, PhD, FESC
Department of Cardiology,
Carol Davila University of Medicine,
Bucharest, Romania
e-mail: crinasinescu@gmail.com

E.A. Gabriel, S.A. Gabriel (eds.), *Inflammatory Response in Cardiovascular Surgery*,
DOI 10.1007/978-1-4471-4429-8_20, © Springer-Verlag London 2013

Table 20.1 Predisposing factors for VTE

Strong (risk increased by more than tenfold)	
	Fracture (hip or leg)
	Hip or knee prosthesis
	Major surgery (general)
	Major trauma
	Spinal cord injury
Moderate (risk increased by two to ninefold)	
	Arthroscopic knee surgery
	Central venous lines
	Chemotherapy
	Chronic heart or respiratory failure
	Hormone replacement therapy
	Malignancy
	Oral contraceptive therapy
	Paralytic stroke
	VTE in antecedents
	Thrombophilia
Weak (odds ratio < 2)	
	Bed rest > 3 days
	Immobility due to sitting (e.g., prolonged travel)
	Advanced age
	Laparoscopic surgery
	Obesity or overweight
	Pregnancy/postpartum
	Varicose veins

Modified from [2, 3]

risk of acute myocardial infarction among younger patient populations (ages 20–64 years). In addition, the risk of myocardial infarction and stroke was evaluated in a large population that included 25,199 patients with DVT, 16,925 patients with PE, and 163,566 controls [8]. During the subsequent 20 years of follow-up, presence of VTE was associated with a 20–40 % increase in risk for arterial cardiovascular events (for patients with DVT, the relative risks was 1.60 for myocardial infarction to 2.19 for stroke in the first year after the thrombotic event; for patients with PE, the relative risk was 2.60 for myocardial infarction and 2.93 for stroke). The fact that VTE and atherosclerosis are two analogous entities has recently been shown in a meta-analysis: patients with VTE have more asymptomatic atherosclerosis and more cardiovascular events than control subjects [9]. The risk of having a future VTE was 2.33 greater for obesity, 1.51 for hypertension, 1.42 for diabetes mellitus, 1.18 for smokers, and 1.16 for hypercholesterolemia. High-density lipoprotein (HDL) cholesterol was lower in subjects with events. Both low levels of HDL cholesterol and elevated fasting glucose have been found to double the risk of VTE in a cohort of 208 patients [10]. A large study of 20,374 middle-aged and elderly adults were followed for more than 12 years for incident VTE, and results showed that metabolic syndrome was associated with an 1.84-fold increased risk for VTE, a result largely attributable to abdominal obesity [11].

Diet also influences the occurrence of thrombotic events. A total of 14,962 middle-aged adults participated in a prospective trial to evaluate the role of dietary intake in the development of DVT or PE [12]. Surprisingly, a diet including more plant food and fish and less red and processed meat was associated with a lower incidence of VTE.

Hormonal replacement therapy and contraception have been linked to atherothrombotic events and venous thrombotic disease. Contraceptives, especially those that contain third-generation progestins, increase the risk of VTE [13]. The Women's Health Initiative randomized trial enrolled subjects receiving estrogen-plus-progestin hormone replacement therapy and showed a twofold increase in the risk of VTE compared with those in the placebo group [14].

An interesting question, that of whether venous thromboembolism is related to psychosocial factors, was answered in a study dating from 2008 [15]. The authors found that persistent stress and low occupational class were independently related to future PE but not to DVT.

Pathophysiology

The three keywords that describe both venous thrombosis and atherothrombosis are inflammation, systemic/local hypercoagulability, and endothelial dysfunction. Inflammation plays an important role in the pathogenesis of this entity; elevated C-reactive protein (a sensitive marker of systemic inflammation) has been linked to an increased risk of VTE. A total of 10,505 patients enrolled in the ARIC (Atherosclerosis Risk in Communities) study showed that elevated C-reactive protein is independently associated with increased risk of VTE [16]. Increased values of systemic inflammatory markers (C-reactive protein, fibrinogen, and factor VIII) are especially found in patients who had an unprovoked DVT or PE compared with those with secondary VTE [17]. Genetic anomalies of interleukin (IL)-1β and IL-10 genes also influence the risk of idiopathic VTE [18]. The JUPITER (Justification for the Use of statins in Prevention: an Intervention Trial Evaluating Rosuvastatin) trial showed that 20 mg/day of rosuvastatin reduced the rate of symptomatic VTE by 43 % in patients with elevated C-reactive protein and low-density lipoprotein (LDL) cholesterol levels <130 mg/dl compared with placebo [19].

Hypercoagulability anomalies (which together with endothelial lesions and venous stasis form Virchow's triad) include inherited thrombophilias (activated protein C resistance due to factor V Leiden mutation; prothrombin gene mutation; congenital dysfibrinogenemia; deficiencies of protein C, protein S, and antithrombin III), hyperhomocysteinemia (most often acquired because of dietary folate deficiency but also can be inherited because of a deficiency in methylenetetrahydrofolate reductase; has been associated with both VTE and atherothrombosis), and antiphospholipid antibody syndrome (APLAS; an acquired thrombophilia that increases the risk for both VTE and arterial thromboembolism).

Endothelial injury and dysfunction expressed as a traumatic injury of the vessel wall may also result in VTE [20]. For example, local endothelial injury from pacemaker leads and long-term indwelling venous catheters increases the risk of VTE [21].

Diagnosis

The initial assessment for determination of DVT is the clinical probability assessment. For suspected DVT, the Wells score has been validated and has well-established criteria (Table 20.2). A score ≥2 indicates that the probability of DVT is likely, and a score of <2 indicates that the probability of DVT is unlikely. For PE, a Wells score >4 indicates PE is likely, and a score of ≤4 indicates PE is unlikely (Table 20.3). We can also use the simplified or revised Geneva score (Table 20.4).

Symptoms such as dyspnea, cough, or chest pain are present in the majority of patients with PE. Additional symptoms include hemoptysis and syncope. Specific signs for PE are tachypnea (>20 respiratory cycles/min), tachycardia (>100 beats/min), signs of DVT, fever (>38.5 °C), and cyanosis.

Chest x-rays are nonspecific but can exclude other causes of dyspnea and chest pain. Electrocardiographic findings could show signs of RV overload such as inversion of T waves in V1-V4, QR pattern in V1, complete or incomplete right bundle branch block, or the classic S1Q3T3.

Negative highly sensitive D-dimer assays can exclude PE in patients with low or moderate clinical probability, whereas moderately sensitive arrays can exclude PE only in patients with a low clinical probability.

Compression ultrasonography (CUS) can be used either as a backup procedure to reduce a false-negative result when using single-detector computer tomography (SDCT) or can be used in patients that have contraindications to contrast dye or radiations (Fig. 20.1).

Ventilation-perfusion scintigraphy is very safe for excluding a PE if it is normal. A high probability of PE establishes the diagnosis with a high degree of probability; additional tests may be considered in selected patients with a low clinical probability.

Single-detector computer tomography (SDCT) and multidetector CT (MDCT) are diagnostic if a thrombus is evident at least at a segmental level, whereas incertitude exists regarding treatment of a sub-segmental defect (Figs. 20.2 and 20.3). Patients with non-high clinical probability can have only MDCT or combined SDCT plus CUS for diagnostic purposes. Further testing is needed in patients with negative MDCT and high clinical probability.

Among invasive diagnostic exams, even though pulmonary angiography is the gold standard in the diagnosis of PE,

Table 20.2 Wells score for DVT diagnosis

Clinical characteristics	Score
Active cancer	+1
Paralysis or plaster immobilization	+1
Bed rest >3 days or major surgery in the last 4 weeks	+1
Localized tenderness along the distribution of the deep venous system	+1
Entire leg swollen	+1
Calf swelling >3 cm when compared with asymptomatic leg	+1
Pitting edema	+1
Collateral superficial veins (nonvaricose)	+1
Previously documented deep vein thrombosis	+1
Alternative diagnosis at least as likely as deep vein thrombosis	−2
Clinical probability	
Unlikely	<2
Likely	≥2

Modified from [22, 23]

Table 20.3 Well's score for PE diagnosis

Clinical characteristics	Score
Hemoptysis	+1
Cancer	+1
Previous pulmonary embolism or deep venous thrombosis	+1.5
Heart rate >100/min	+1.5
Recent surgery or immobilization	+1.5
Clinical signs of deep venous thrombosis	+3
Alternative diagnosis less likely than that of pulmonary embolism	+3
Clinical probability	
Low	<2
Intermediate	2–6
High	>6

Modified from [24]

Table 20.4 Revised and simplified revised Geneva scores for PE diagnosis

Clinical characteristics	Revised score	Simplified score
Age >65 years	+1	+1
Active malignant condition	+2	+1
Surgery or fracture within 1 month	+2	+1
Hemoptysis	+2	+1
Previous deep vein thrombosis or pulmonary embolism	+3	+1
Unilateral lower-limb pain	+3	+1
Heart rate 75–94/min	+3	+1
Pain on lower deep venous palpation and unilateral edema	+4	+1
Heart rate >94/min	+5	+1
Clinical probability		
Low	0–3	0–1
Intermediate	4–10	2–4
High	>10	≥5

Modified from [25, 26]

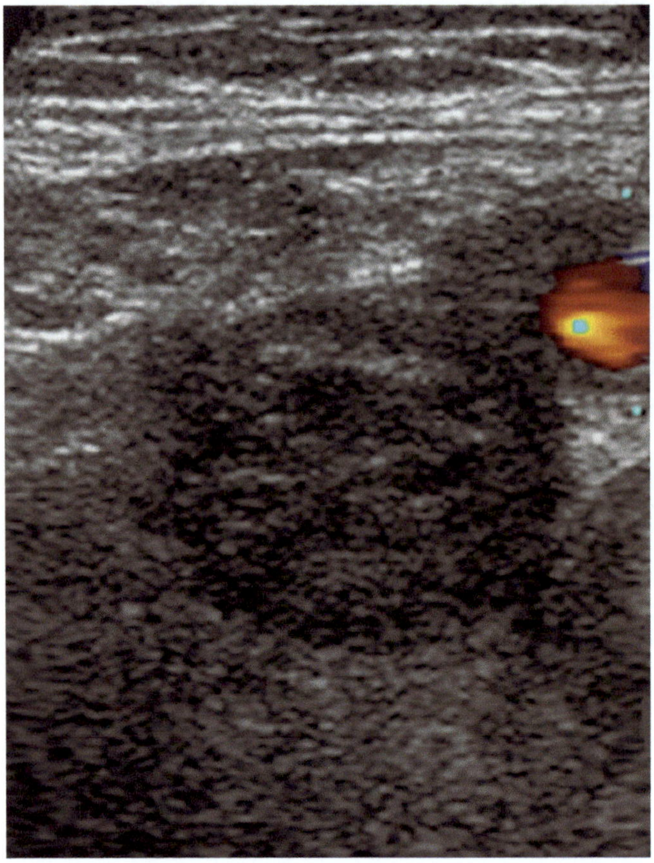

Fig. 20.1 Compression ultrasonography showing a thrombosed femural vein (*middle plane*) and patent femural artery (*right side*)

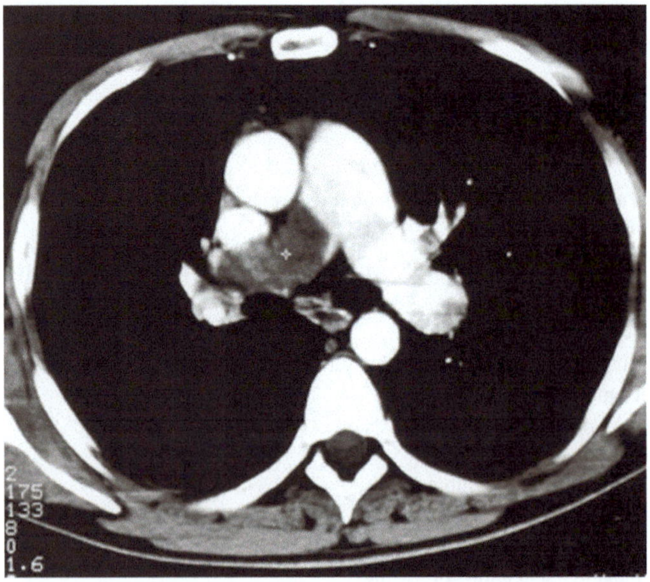

Fig. 20.2 Computer tomography plane showing a thrombosed proximal right pulmonary artery

it is rarely used because of its invasive nature. Diagnostic criteria for PE include direct evidence of a thrombus, visible filling defect, and other indirect signs (slow flow contrast, regional hypoperfusion, and delayed or diminished pulmo-

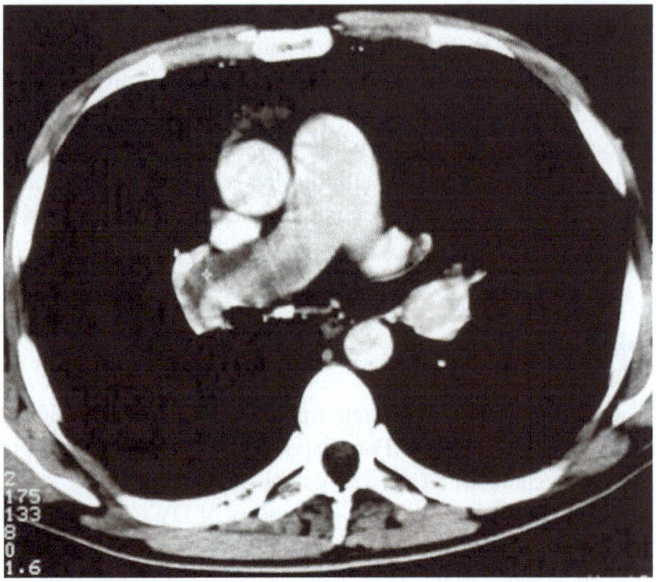

Fig. 20.3 Computer tomography plane showing a thrombosed proximal right pulmonary artery

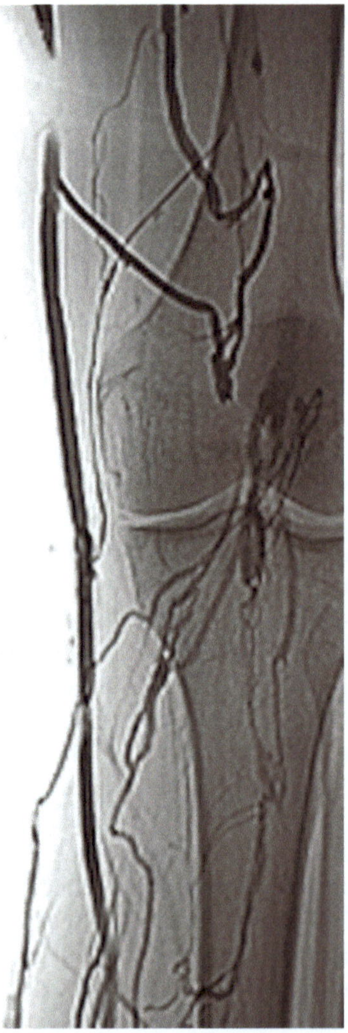

Fig. 20.4 Venography of the left thigh showing thrombosed great saphenous vein

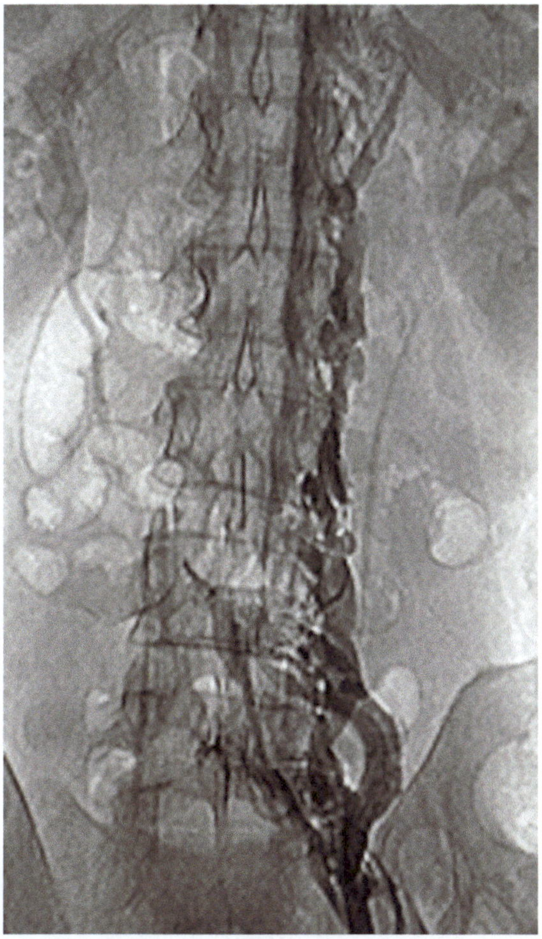

Fig. 20.5 Venography of an extended thrombosed iliac vein

nary venous flow). Venography is also less used today (Figs. 20.4 and 20.5).

Echocardiography is especially useful in emergency management decisions. The absence of RV overload/dysfunction excludes PE as a cause of hemodynamic instability in a patient with hypotension or shock (Figs. 20.6, 20.7, 20.8, 20.9, 20.10, and 20.11). It has a very important role in stratifying patients with non-high risk PE into intermediate and low-risk categories. Echocardiographic criteria of RV dysfunction include RV hypokinesis and dilatation, RV size >30 mm at annulus, tricuspid insufficiency of >2.8 m/s, a ratio of RV/left ventricle >1, paradoxical septal systolic motion, and a pulmonary acceleration time <90 ms.

Complications

(a) Complications of DVT include the post-thrombotic syndrome (Figs. 20.12 and 20.13) (evolves in 20–50 % of patients and could result in lifelong limb pain, swelling, heaviness, edema, and leg ulcers) [27] and PE.
(b) Complications of PE include RV dysfunction, hemodynamic instability, and chronic thromboembolic hypertension. In the acute phase, stratification of PE includes high-risk PE and non-high-risk PE.

High-risk PE is a life-threatening condition in which short-term mortality exceeds 15 %. It includes PE in association with shock or hypotension (systolic blood pressure

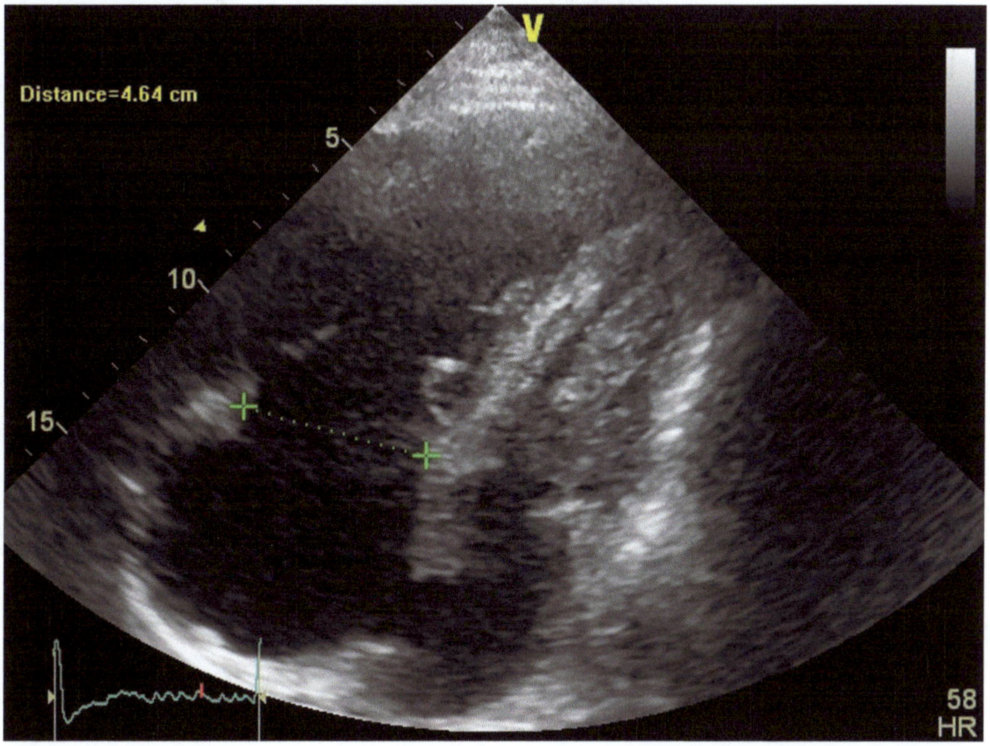

Fig. 20.6 Subcostal view of a dilated right ventricle in the context of chronic thromboembolic pulmonary hypertension

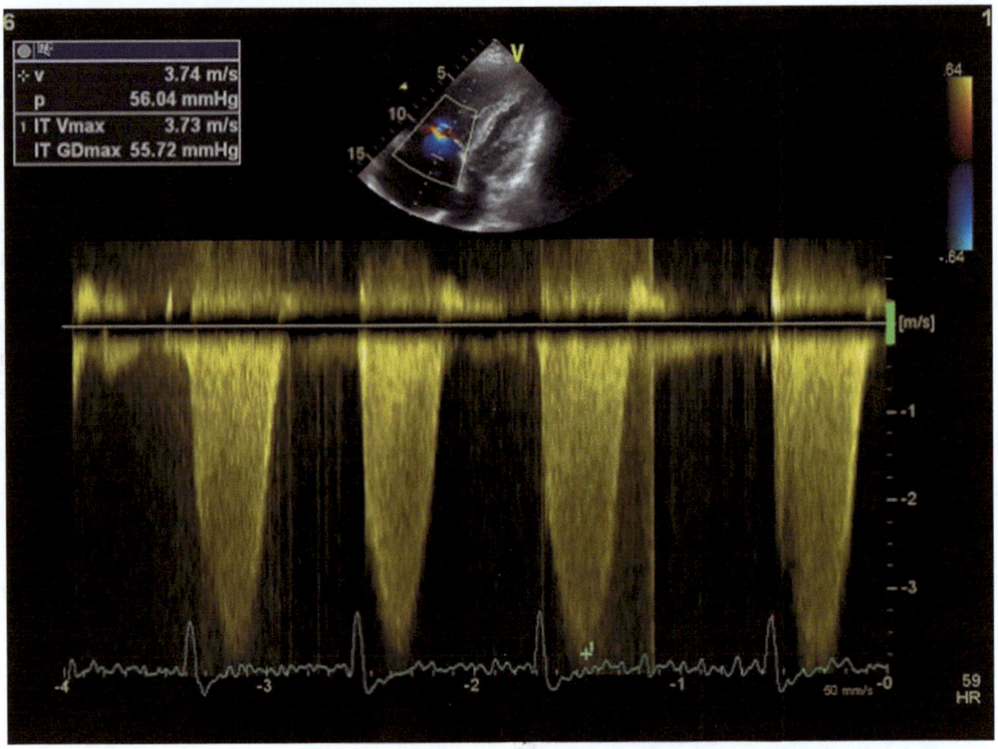

Fig. 20.7 CW Doppler on the tricuspid valve showing elevated right ventricle-right atrium gradient

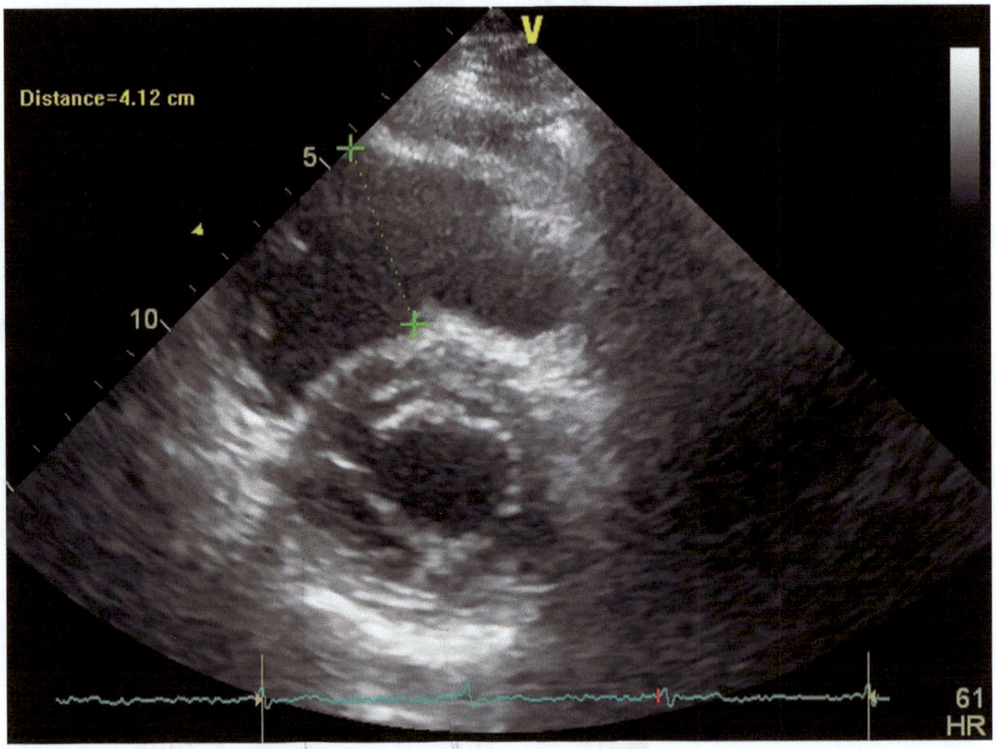

Fig. 20.8 Parasternal short-axis view at mitral valve level showing a dilated right ventricle in the context of a hemodinamic unstable pulmonary embolism

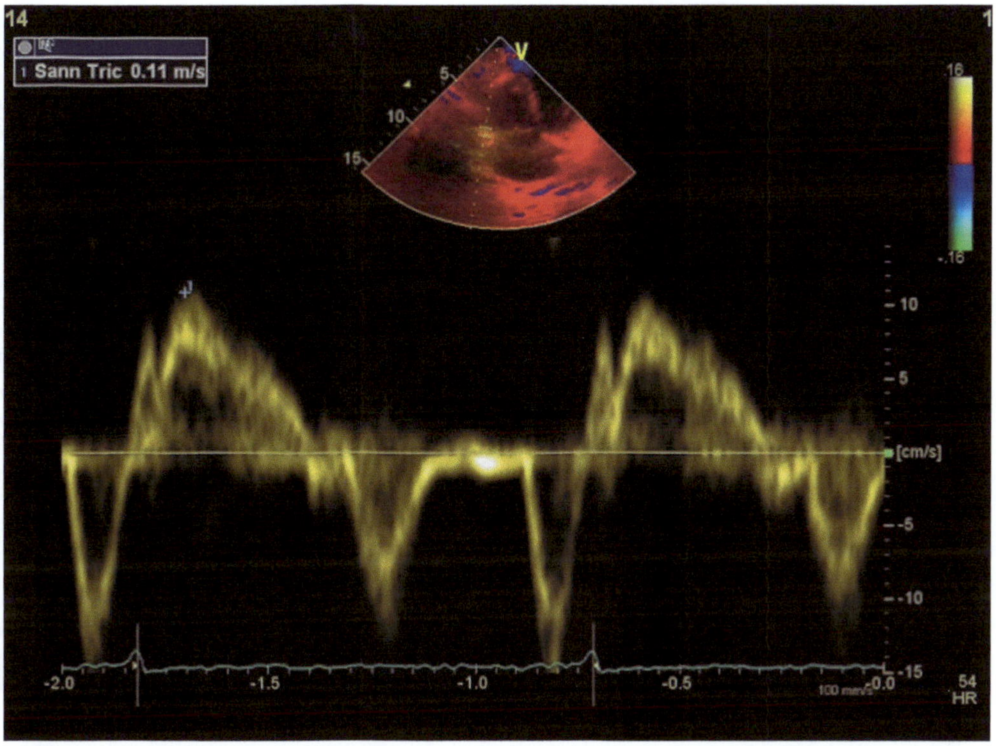

Fig. 20.9 Preserved systolic function using pulsed tissue doppler of the right ventricle free wall in the context of pulmonary embolism

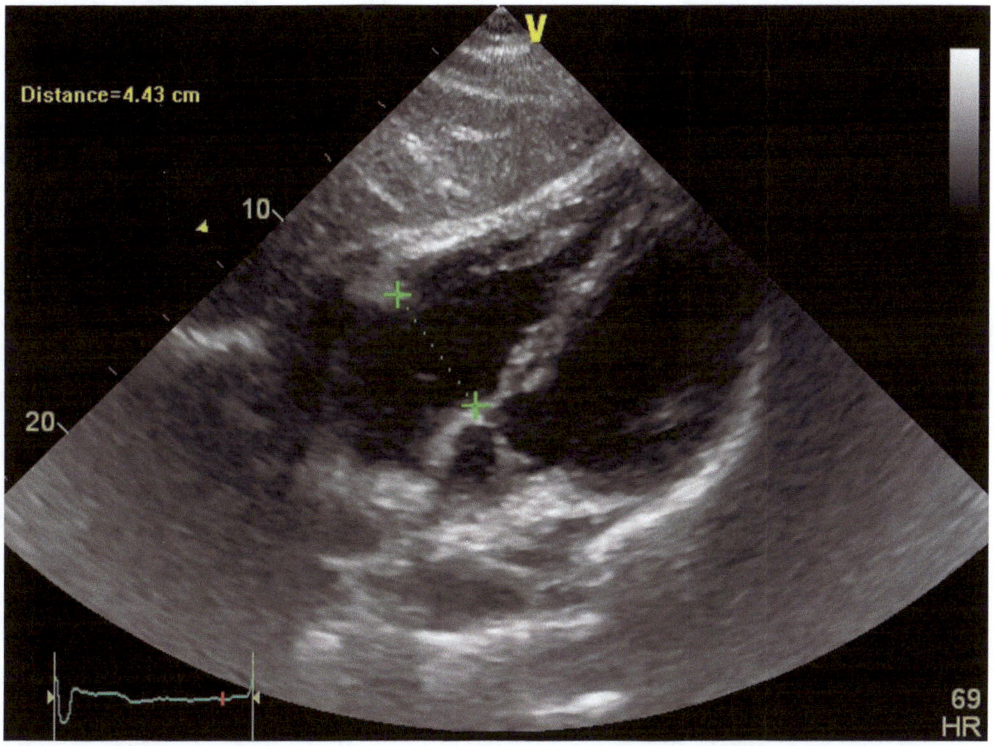

Fig. 20.10 Subcostal view showing a dilated right ventricle in the setting of a hemodinamic unstable pulmonary embolism

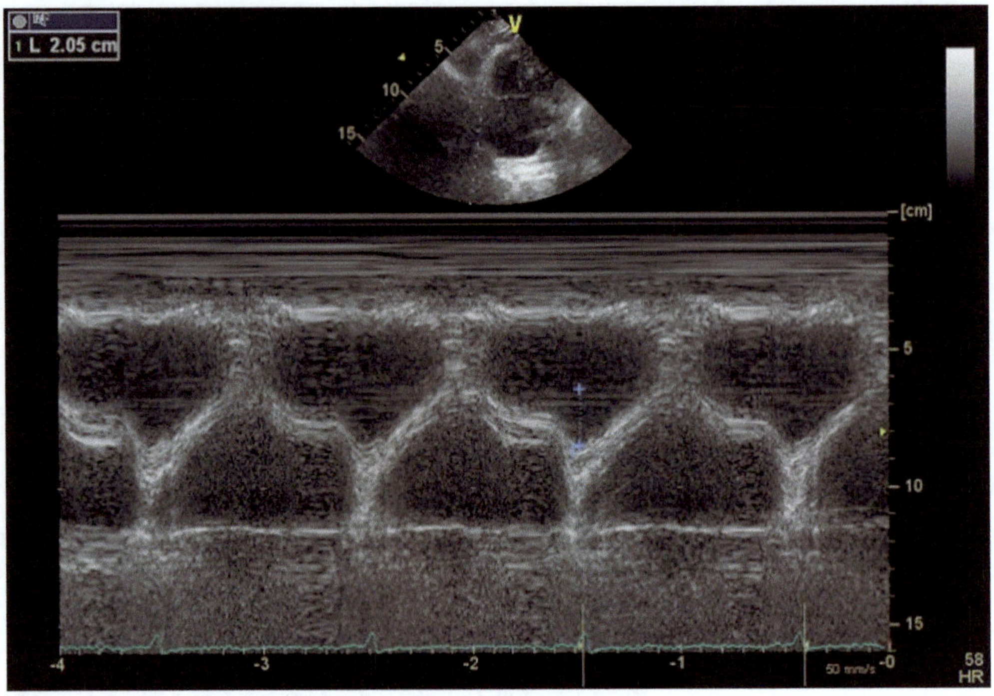

Fig. 20.11 Preserved systolic function using the tricuspid annular plane systolic motion (TAPSE) of the right ventricle free wall in the context of chronic thromboembolic disease

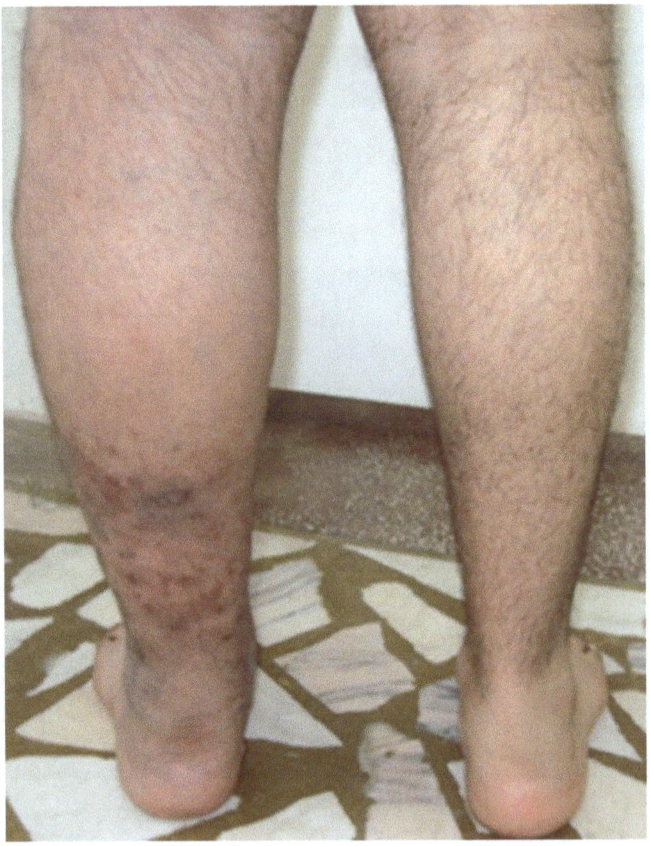

Fig. 20.12 Post-thrombotic syndrome associated with oedema and cutaneous trophic disorder (*left leg*)

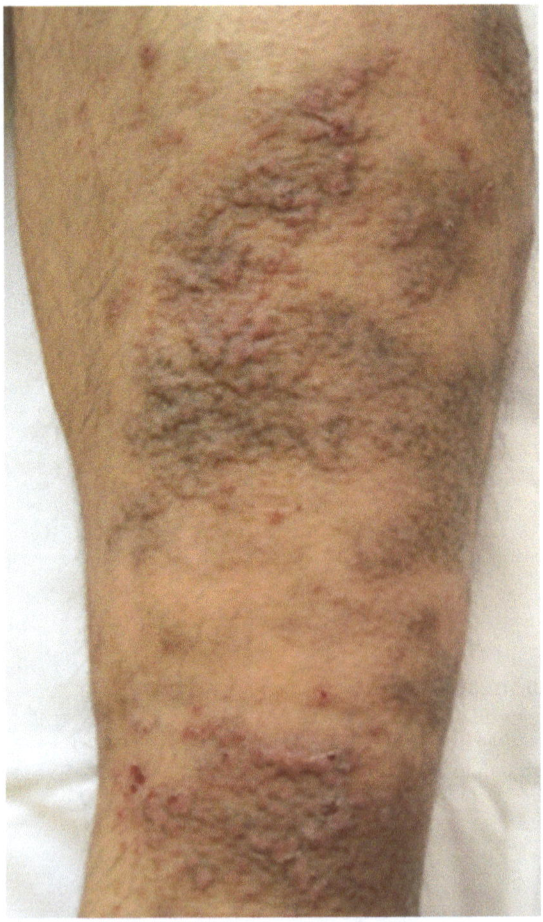

Fig. 20.13 Post-thrombotic syndrome associated with cutaneous trophic disorder

<90 mmHg or a pressure drop >40 mmHg for >15 min if not caused by new-onset arrhythmia, hypovolemia, or sepsis).

Non-high-risk PE is further categorized into intermediate (3–15 % short-term risk of mortality) and low-risk PE (<1 % short-term mortality). Intermediate-risk PE is defined by the presence of RV dysfunction defined by the presence of at least one of the following: echocardiographic findings (previously mentioned), RV dilatation at CT, BNP or NT-proBNP elevation, increased right heart pressure at right heart catheterization, and positive cardiac troponin T or I.

Treatment

Once DVT has been diagnosed, treatment goals are: symptom relief, prevention of embolization and recurrence, control of thrombus progression during the acute phase in order to clear away the risk of an immediate, possibly fatal pulmonary embolism, control of acute and chronic pulmonary and peripheral venous hypertension, and control of relapsing disease in the intermediate and long-term course. Treatment of VTE is composed of three periods: the acute phase (days), the intermediate phase (weeks or months), and the long-term period (months or years).

Acute Treatment

In patients with DVT or stable PE, either unfractionated heparin or low-molecular-weight heparin (LMWH) can be used safely (except in case of severe renal impairment for LWMH use). Monitoring anti-Xa activity is useful in patients with severe renal failure, in pregnancy, and in obese patients (to be done 4 h after the morning injection). Monitoring of unfractionated heparin is done 4–6 h after the bolus injection and 3 h after each adjustment, aiming for an activated partial thromboplastin time of 70–90 s. Table 20.5 shows standard doses of LMWH. There is no benefit of immobilization for the clinical outcome of patients with PE. Wearing stockings markedly reduces the incidence of post-thrombotic syndrome.

In patients with hemodynamic unstable PE, intravenous thrombolysis is mandatory, followed by unfractionated heparin (bolus of 80 U/kg and subsequent infusion of 15–18 U/kg/h). The most used thrombolytic protocols are shown in Table 20.6 [28–30]. Contraindications to thrombolysis are shown in Table 20.7. Thrombolysis could be used in patients with intermediate-risk PE after thorough consideration of conditions that increase bleeding risk. Surgical pulmonary embolectomy can be performed in patients who may need cardiopulmonary resuscitation, in patients with contraindications to thrombolysis, and in those with a patent foramen ovale and intracardiac thrombi. Hemodynamic support including vasopressors, and mechanical ventilation may be needed in severe cases.

Table 20.5 Curative doses of LMWH and fondaparinux for PE treatment

	Dose	Interval
Enoxaparin	1.0 mg/kg	Every 12 h
	or 1.5 mg/kg[a]	Once daily[a]
Tinzaparin	175 U/kg	Once daily
Fondaparinux	5 mg (body weight <50)	Once daily
	7.5 mg (body weight 50–100 kg)	
	10 mg (body weight>100 kg)	

Modified from [3]

[a]Approved for inpatient treatment of PE in the United States and in some European countries

Table 20.6 Thrombolytic doses for pulmonary embolism

Streptokinase [28]	250,000 IU as a loading dose over 30 min, followed by 100,000 IU/h over 12–24 h. Accelerated regimen: 1.5 million IU over 2 h
Urokinase [29]	4,400 IU/kg as a loading dose over 10 min, followed by IU/kg/h over 12–24 h
Recombinant tissue plasminogen activator [28–30]	Accelerated regimen: 3 million IU over 2,100 mg over 2 h or 0.6 mg/kg over 15 min (maximum dose 50 mg)

Table 20.7 Contraindications to fibrinolytic therapy

Absolute contraindications[a]
Hemorrhagic stroke
Stoke of unknown origin at any time
Ischemic stroke in preceding 6 months
Central nervous system damage or neoplasms
Recent major trauma/surgery/head injury (within preceding 3 weeks)
Gastrointestinal bleeding within the last month
Known bleeding
Relative contraindications
Transient ischemic attack in preceding 6 months
Oral anticoagulant therapy
Pregnancy or within 1 week postpartum
Non-compressible punctures
Traumatic resuscitation
Refractory hypertension (systolic blood pressure >180 mmHg)
Severe liver disease
Infective endocarditis
Active peptic ulcer

Modified from [3, 31]

[a]Absolute contraindications might become relative in a patient with life-threatening unstable PE

Table 20.8 Comparative properties of thrombin and factor Xa inhibitors in comparison to warfarin

	Warfarin	Rivaroxaban	Apixaban	Dabigatran	Edoxaban
Target	Vitamin K	Factor Xa	Factor Xa	Factor IIa	Factor Xa
Prodrug	No	No	No	Yes	No
Bioavailability (%)	>95	>57–86	>49	6.5	50
T (max) (h)	72–96	2–4	1–4	1.25–3	1–2
Half-life (h)	40	9–13	8–15	12–14	9–11
Monitoring	INR-adjusted	Not needed	Not needed	Not needed	Not needed
Administration in VTE	Once daily	15 mg bid for 3 weeks followed by 20 mg od	10 mg bid for 1 week followed by 5 mg bid	150 mg bid	60 mg od
Metabolism and elimination	CYP 2C9, 3A4, 1A2	CYP3A4; 33 % renal, 66 % fecal	CYP3A4; 75 % fecal, 25 % renal	80 % renal, 20 % fecal	35 % renal
Drug interactions	CYP 2C9, 1A2, and 3A4	CYP 3A4 inhibitor P-GP inhibitor	CYP 3A inhibitor P-GP inhibitor	P-GP inhibitor	P-GP inhibitor

Modified from [32]

T(max) indicates peak plasma levels, *h* hours, *P-gp* P-glycoprotein, *od* once daily, *bid* twice daily

Intermediate Phase Treatment and Chronic Treatment

After the acute phase, oral anticoagulation is mandatory. It can be done either by vitamin K antagonists (VKAs) or by newer anticoagulants. VKAs such as warfarin have several limitations, such as a slow onset of action, frequent monitoring of INR because of the limited therapeutic index, food and drug interactions, inter-individual dosing differences, and warfarin resistance. The only apparent advantages of VKAs over newer anticoagulants are the possibility to administer an antidote in case of overdose and its use independent of renal failure.

Newer anticoagulants are available and are ready to use in VTE (Table 20.8). The main advantages over VKAs include: fixed-dose administration, no INR testing, and no interactions with food or drugs.

Rivaroxaban is an oral direct inhibitor of factor Xa [33] that inhibits factor Xa in a concentration-dependent manner via a rapid and reversible binding. It reduces the rate of development of VTE in patients after total hip or knee arthroplasty vs. LMWH with no significant differences in risk of bleeding [34–37]. Compared with enoxaparin, it reduces the costs associated with drug administration for prophylaxis and treatment of VTE events. Also it reduces the incidence of symptomatic VTE [38].

Apixaban is a reversible active direct inhibitor of factor Xa that can also be administered orally (fixed oral dose may replace LMWH combined with vitamin K antagonists in the treatment of DVT) [39]. Compared with LMWH, apixaban was more effective for prevention of VTE as compared with LMWH without enhancing bleeding risk after knee and hip replacement [40, 41].

Dabigatran etexilate is a competitive reversible oral anticoagulant that inhibits thrombin directly. It has the potential to replace traditional anticoagulants for prevention of VTE in patients who have undergone elective total hip or knee replacement surgery [42, 43].

Table 20.9 Factors that increase recurrence risk in idiopathic VTE

Immobilization
Cancer
Chronic obstructive pulmonary disease
Family history
Male gender[a]
Overweight, obesity[a]
Low levels of apolipoprotein AI and high-density lipoprotein cholesterol[a]
Proximal DVT[a]
Symptomatic PE[a]
Elevated D-dimer levels after discontinuing anticoagulation[a]
Failure to recanalize leg veins after anticoagulation for DVT[a]

Modified after [44]

[a]Validated for idiopathic VTE

Oral anticoagulants should be started as soon as possible, preferably on the first day if a stable PE has been diagnosed, and should aim for a target INR (international normalized ratio) of 2–3 when VKAs are used.

Oral anticoagulants should be continued for 3 months if a reversible factor has been identified (surgery, trauma, medical illness, estrogen therapy, pregnancy, etc.; see Table 20.1).

Patients with thrombophilia (deficit of protein C or S, lupus anticoagulant, homozygous for factor V Leyden, or homozygous for PTG 20210A) are candidates for chronic oral anticoagulant treatment as recurrence is high. At this time, there is no clear benefit of chronic VKA treatment in patients heterozygous for factor V Leyden or heterozygous for PTG 20210A.

Patients with provoked or apparently unprovoked VTE should benefit from chronic oral anticoagulants treatment, *especially* if any of the factors in Table 20.9 are present. Also, if the bleeding risk is low, lifelong anticoagulation is advised.

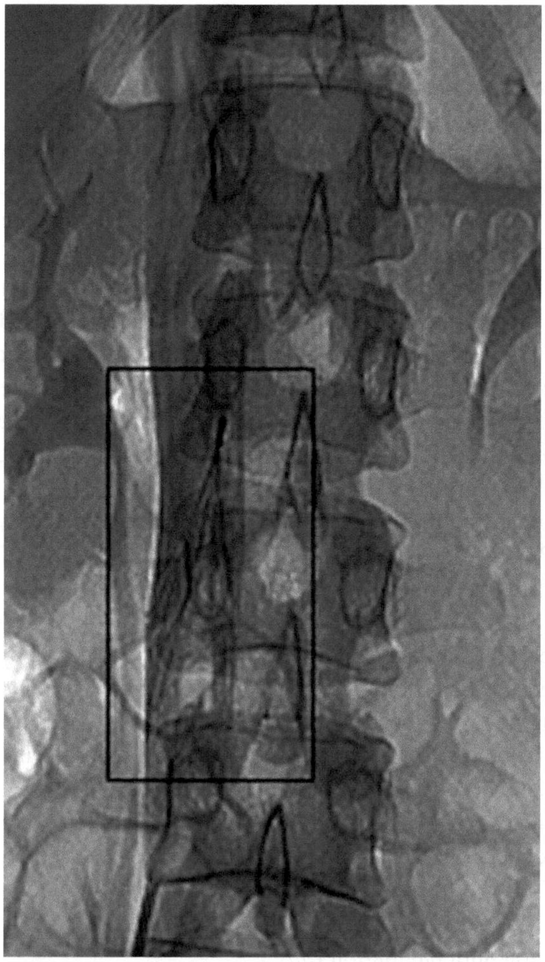

Fig. 20.14 Caval filter (*mid-plane*)

Treatment for chronic thromboembolic hypertension is pulmonary endarterectomy and should be advised when severe symptoms and RV failure occur.

For cancer patients, LMWH and especially dalteparin are indicated for the first 3–6 months of a proximal DVT and/or PE at an initial dose of 200 U/kg subcutaneously once daily; afterwards oral anticoagulants should be continued indefinitely or until cancer is cured.

The rationale for caval filter insertion (Fig. 20.14) is to lower the chance of pulmonary embolism originating from a proven proximal DVT (usually with dimensions more than 4 mm). According to the latest American Heart Association guidelines on VTE (2011), venous filters are indicated when there is an absolute contraindication to anticoagulation and when there is a high risk of VTE recurrence while on anticoagulation and evidence of active bleeding complications requiring termination of anticoagulation therapy. Relative contraindications include large, free-floating iliofemoral thrombus in high-risk patients, propagating iliofemoral thrombus while on anticoagulation, patients with significant fall risk, and chronic PE in

Table 20.10 The HASBLED score

Letter	Clinical characteristics[a]	Points awarded
H	Hypertension	1
A	Abnormal renal and liver function (I point each)	1 or 2
S	Stroke	1
B	Bleeding	1
L	Labile INRs	1
E	Elderly (e.g., age>65 years)	1
D	Drugs or alcohol (1 point each)	1 or 2
		Maximum 9 points

Modified from [45, 46]

[a]*Hypertension* – systolic blood pressure >160 mmHg, *Abnormal kidney function* – the presence of chronic dialysis or renal transplantation or serum creatinine ≥μmol/l, *Abnormal liver function* – chronic hepatic disease (e.g.. cirrhosis) or biochemical evidence of significant hepatic derangement (e.g., bilirubin >2× the upper limit of normal, in association with aspartame aminotransferase/alanine aminotransferase/alkaline phosphatase >3× the upper limit normal, etc.), *Bleeding* – history and/or predisposition to bleeding, e.g., bleeding diathesis, anemia, etc, *Labile INRs* unstable/high INRs or poor time therapeutic range (e.g., <60 %), *Drugs/alcohol* – concomitant use of drugs, such as antiplatelet agents, non-steroidal antiinflammatory drugs, or alcohol abuse, etc., *INR* – international normalized ratio

patients with pulmonary hypertension. As soon as oral anticoagulants can be introduced, they should be removed because of increased complication rates (insertion site thrombosis in 10 % of cases, recurrent DVT in 20 % of cases, post-thrombotic syndrome in 40 %, and occlusion of the inferior vena cava in 22 % of patients at 5 years). Whatever the reason for filter insertion, temporary filters should be favored over permanent filters.

In pregnancy, VKAs are not advised in the first and the third trimester, and they should be considered with caution in the second trimester. LMWHs are safe.

Thrombectomy in DVT may be indicated when the anticoagulation therapy is inefficient or contraindicated. It is rarely used nowadays in iliofemoral massive thrombosis (afterwards the caval vein must be interrupted for prevention of pulmonary embolism).

As with the catheter-guided approach, surgery is a treatment concept for descending iliac DVT or recent onset in young and otherwise healthy individuals, and it is rarely used.

Risk of Bleeding

Multiple parameters have been integrated into the HAS-BLED risk score [45] and have been validated on a population of 3,978 European subjects with atrial fibrillation from the EuroHeart Survey (Table 20.10). A score of ≥3 indicates high risk for bleeding; thus, anticoagulation should not be advised.

Recurrence of VTE

General Considerations

During 25 years of follow-up, Heit et al. [47] reported probable/definite cumulative percentages of VTE recurrence at 1 and 10 years of 12.9 %/5.6 % and 30.4 %/17.6 %. Independent predictors of first overall VTE recurrence included increasing age and body mass index, neurologic disease with paresis, malignant neoplasm, and neurosurgery. Independent predictors of a first probable/definite recurrence included the presence of a clear diagnostic and the presence of neurologic disease in patients with hospital-acquired VTE. Recurrence risk was increased by malignant neoplasm but varied with concomitant chemotherapy, patient age and sex, and study year.

Follow-up was also performed in 355 consecutive patients with a first episode of symptomatic DVT [48]. After 8 years, the cumulative incidence of recurrent venous thromboembolism was 30.3 %. Survival after 8 years was 70.2 %. The presence of cancer and impaired coagulation inhibition increased the risk for recurrent venous thromboembolism [hazard ratios, 1.72 (CI, 1.31–2.25) and 1.44 (CI, 1.02–2.01), respectively), and the cumulative incidence of the post-thrombotic syndrome was 29.1 % after 8 years (CI, 23.4–34.7 %). The development of ipsilateral recurrent deep venous thrombosis was strongly associated with the risk for the post-thrombotic syndrome (hazard ratio, 6.4; CI, 3.1–13.3). The presence of cancer increased the risk for death (hazard ratio, 8.1; CI, 3.6–18.1).

In the largest cohort with long-term follow-up, comprising 1,626 patients with either idiopathic or provoked thrombosis in whom anticoagulation had been stopped, follow-up was performed 10 years after the first event [49]. The cumulative incidence of recurrent VTE at 10 years was 39.9 % (if the population was dichotomized into idiopathic versus provoked initial events, the 10-year recurrence rate was 52 % for idiopathic DVT versus 22 % for provoked DVT). The adjusted hazard ratio for recurrent VTE was 2.02 (1.52–2.69) in those with thrombophilia, 2.30 (95 % CI, 1.82–2.90) in patients whose first VTE was unprovoked, 1.14 (1.06–1.12) for every 10-year increase of age, 1.44 (1.03–2.03) in those presenting with primary DVT, and 1.39 (1.08–1.80) for patients who received a shorter (up to 6 months) duration of anticoagulation. When the analysis was confined to patients with unprovoked VTE, the results did not change.

Clear evidence shows that a high rate of recurrence after provoked and especially unprovoked VTE exists. The numbers previously presented should change our habits in treating and preventing recurrences of this complex disease.

Searching for Hereditary Thrombophilia

Among patients with thrombophilia, certain populations, such as those who test positive for lupus anticoagulant, have a deficit of antithrombin, protein C, or S [50, 51], are homozygous for factor V Leyden (FVL), and are homozygous for PTG20210A [52, 53], should be provided with indefinite anticoagulation as recurrence is high. Deficiencies of antithrombin, protein C, or protein S are observed in fewer than 5 % of patients presenting with a first unprovoked VTE; if the patient is under the age of 50 and has a positive family history, the incidence increases up to about 15 %. The possibility of identifying more than one hereditary defect in patients presenting with an unprovoked VTE with a negative family history is between 1 and 3 %.

Regarding those heterozygous for FVL and heterozygous for PTG20210A, there is little evidence that prolonged anticoagulation would be of benefit. In a recent review [52], being heterozygous for FVL was associated with a 1.56-fold increased risk and being homozygous with a 2.65-fold increased risk compared with individuals without FVL. Being heterozygous for prothrombin G20210A was not predictive of recurrent VTE in probands compared with individuals without this anomaly. An older meta-analysis stated that heterozygous FVL and prothrombin G20210A are each associated with a significantly increased risk of recurrent VTE after a first event, but the magnitude of the increase in risk is modest and by itself is unlikely to merit extended-duration anticoagulation [53].

Some hemostatic abnormalities have been associated with increased VTE, such as homocysteine and increased factor VIII and VII. A study from 1995 [54] underlined that high factor VIII concentrations are common and represent a clear increase in the risk of thrombosis, similar to the risks conferred by deficiencies of the coagulation-inhibiting proteins and activated protein C resistance. Another paper [55] showed that the relative risk of recurrent venous thrombosis was 1.08 for each increase of 10 IU per deciliter in the plasma level of factor VII. Regarding hyperhomocysteine, it has been shown that treatment with vitamin B supplements did not reduce the risk of VTE in two clinical trials, even though it did reduce homocysteine levels [56, 57]. Because the results of these tests should not affect patient management, testing for these abnormalities is discouraged.

APLAS consists of the occurrence of venous or arterial thrombosis or recurrent fetal loss in association with a positive lupus anticoagulant or elevated β2-glycoprotein I antibody or cardiolipin levels. To conclude that APLAS is positive, these tests must remain persistently positive for a minimum of several months following the initial thrombotic event. Typically, an unexplained prolongation of the aPTT is found in approximately two-thirds of patients. APLAS is frequently identified in patients with systemic lupus erythematous in the context of certain drug intakes (i.e., thorazine, hydralazine). Other etiologies are infections, underlying malignancy, or idiopathic status.

In summary, hereditary hemophilia should be investigated in the following subgroups of population: patients with venous thromboembolism before the age of 40–45 years, recurrent VTE, patients with arterial thrombosis younger than 30 years old, idiopathic prolongation of the activated partial thromboplastin time, systemic lupus erythematous, repeated fetal loss, neonatal thrombosis, unusual site for thrombosis (e.g., mesenteric vein, cerebral sinus), idiopathic thrombocytopenic purpura, thrombophilic abnormalities in the same family, and family history of VTE.

Idiopathic VTE

Risk Factors for Recurrence (see also Table 20.9)

In 2007, Nijkeuter et al. [58] proved in their study that risk factors for recurrent VTE in secondary and idiopathic thrombosis were immobilization for>3 days and being an inpatient; COPD or malignancies were risk factors for bleeding. Malignancy, higher age and immobilization, and being an inpatient were risk factors for mortality.

Another paper showed that men have a 3.6-fold higher relative risk of recurrence of VTE compared to women [59].

Very interestingly, overweight seemed to predict the rate of VTE recurrence. A total of 1,107 patients were followed for an average of 46 months after a first unprovoked venous thromboembolism and withdrawal of anticoagulant therapy [60]. The authors excluded pregnant patients, those requiring long-term antithrombotic treatment, and those who had a previous or secondary thrombosis, natural coagulation inhibitor deficiency, lupus anticoagulant, or cancer. Four years after discontinuation of anticoagulant therapy, the probability of recurrence was 9.3 % among patients of normal weight and 17 % among patients with increased body mass index (overweight and obese patients).

Proof that patients with high levels of apolipoprotein AI and HDL have a decreased risk of recurrent venous thromboembolism comes from a study conducted in 772 patients after a first spontaneous venous thromboembolism (average follow-up 48 months) [61].

The same author investigated the risk of recurrence among patients with spontaneous symptomatic PE and those with DVT without symptoms of PE. He found that subjects with a first symptomatic PE not only have a higher risk of recurrent VTE than those with DVT without symptoms of PE, but are also at increased risk of symptomatic PE at recurrence [62].

A landmark trial that deserves special attention assessed the risk of recurrence in patients with unprovoked DVT or PE using a prediction model (the Vienna prediction model) [63]. The authors prospectively enrolled 929 patients with a first unprovoked VTE who had been treated with oral anticoagulants for at least 3 months, excluding patients with VTE provoked by surgery, trauma, pregnancy, female hormone intake, deficiency of antithrombin, protein C or protein S, and presence of the lupus anticoagulant or cancer. Patients entered the study at the time of discontinuation of oral anticoagulation. The study end point was recurrent symptomatic deep vein thrombosis confirmed by venography or color duplex sonography (in case of proximal thrombosis of the contralateral leg) or recurrent symptomatic pulmonary embolism confirmed by ventilation-perfusion scanning and/or spiral computed tomography. Follow-up had a median of 43.3 months after discontinuation of anticoagulation. Of the patients, 18.9 % had recurrent VTE, and the following factors were related to a higher recurrence risk: male sex (hazard ratio versus female sex 1.90, 95 % confidence interval 1.31–2.75), proximal DVT (hazard ratio versus distal 2.08, 95 % confidence interval 1.16–3.74), PE (hazard ratio versus distal thrombosis 2.60, 95 % confidence interval 1.49–4.53), and elevated levels of D-dimer determined by ELISA (hazard ratio per doubling 1.27, 95 % confidence interval 1.08–1.51). Subsequently, the authors developed a normogram that can be used to calculate risk scores and to estimate the cumulative probability of recurrence (Fig. 20.15).

D-dimers have been largely utilized to predict the rate of recurrence after an unprovoked venous embolic event. It is suggested that the results of quantitative D-dimer assays, measured at the end of warfarin therapy (3 or 6 months) and then 1 month after its discontinuation, can help stratify such patients with respect to recurrence risk. Seven studies totaling 1,888 patients with a first unprovoked VTE were included in a meta-analysis to clarify whether the D-dimer value is a predictor of recurrent disease in patients who have stopped anticoagulant therapy after a first unprovoked VTE. A D-dimer level of less than 500 ng/ml (a "negative test") was associated with a 3.5 % annual risk of recurrence, whereas a D-dimer over this level (a "positive test") was associated with an 8.9 % risk in each of the first 2 years (Table 20.11). As there is no D-dimer "standard" worldwide, practitioners have to rely on the manufacturer's cutoof point for a positive or negative D-dimer test to assess recurrence risk. In another landmark trial [65], D-dimer testing was performed 1 month after the discontinuation of anticoagulation in patients with a first unprovoked proximal deep-vein thrombosis or pulmonary embolism who had received a vitamin K antagonist for at least 3 months. Patients were divided in three groups and followed up for 1.4 years: those who had normal D-dimer values stopped the treatment and had a VTE recurrence of 6.2 %, those who had abnormal D-dimer values and continued treatment had a VTE recurrence of 2.9 %, and those who had abnormal D-dimer values but discontinued treatment had a VTE recurrence of 15 %. The authors

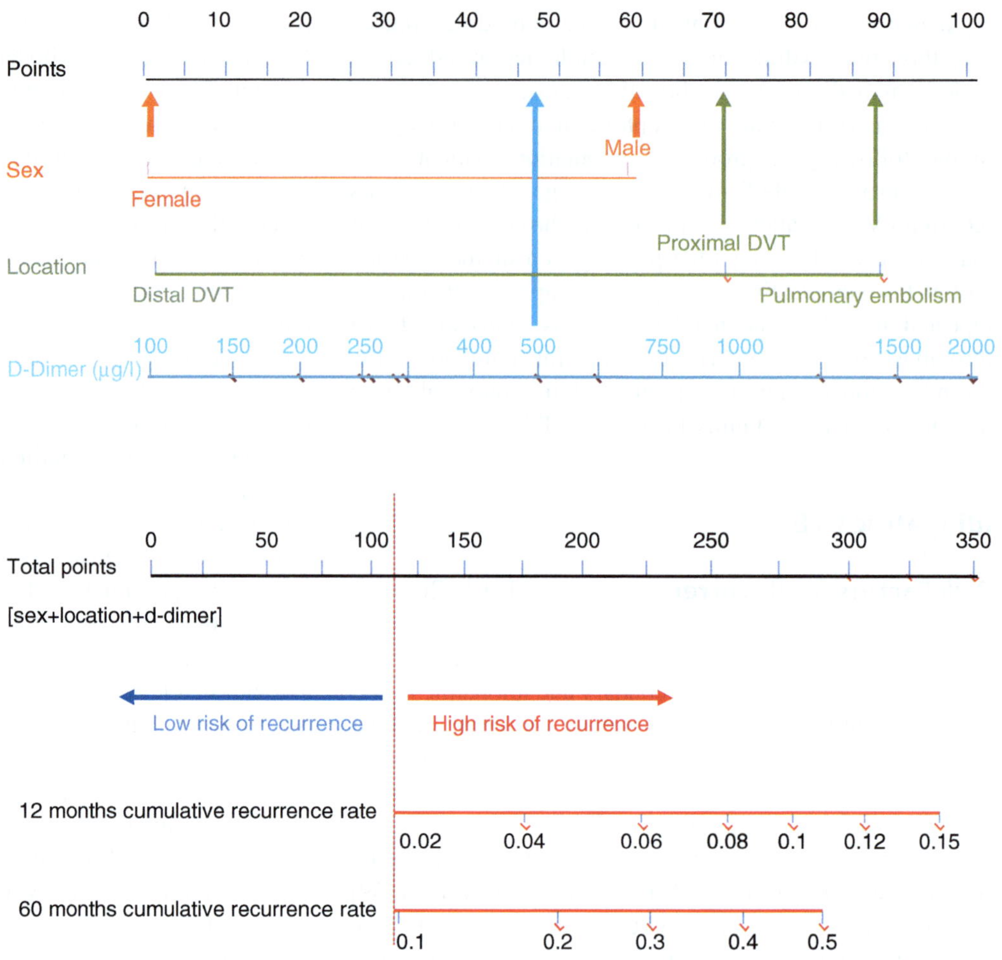

Fig. 20.15 The Vienna prediction model for VTE recurrence. Values of D-dimer, sex, and VTE location correspond to points on *upper panel* line. Value of total points (*lower line*) are assigned a VTE recurrence risk at 12 and 60 months (Modified from [62])

Table 20.11 D-Dimer values and VTE recurrence rate

Author/year/D-dimer assay	D-dimer level (ng/ml)	Actualized VTE rate (95 % CI)
Palareti, 2003, Vidas (ELISA)	>500	7.3 (4.3–10.3)
	≤500	2.8 (1.0–4.5)
Eichinger, 2003, Asserachrom (ELISA)	≥250	4.5 (3.4–5.6)
	<250	3.0 (1.5–4.4)
Paraleti, 2006, Simply Red(Qualitative)	Pos (>500)	10.9 (5.9–15.9)
	Neg (≤500)	4.4 (2.6–6.1)
Shrivastava, 2006, Liatest (Stago)	≥500	11.3 (0.0–24.1)
	<500	3.7 (0.0–8.7)
Tait, 2007, Vidas (ELISA)	≥500	14.4 (7.7–21.1)
	<500	3.7 (0.1–7.6)
Baglin, 2006, MDA, (Liatest)	≥500	8.8 (5.2–12.2)
	<500	4.8 (1.5–8.1)
Poli, 2008, IL- Test (Liatest)	≥250	10.8 (5.6–15.9)
	<250	3.8 (1.4–6.1)

Modified from [52, 64]

concluded that in patients with abnormal D-dimer values, anticoagulation should be continued, whereas in patients with a normal D-dimer level, the optimal course of anticoagulation is not clearly established. However, a more recent overview from the same authors stated that measurement of D-dimer in conjunction with clinical variables shows promise in being able to identify individuals at particularly low risk of recurrence, as women younger than age 65 with a normal D-dimer 1 month after stopping anticoagulation had a very low risk of recurrence (0.4 % per year) [66].

Residual Venous Thrombus on CUS

One of the advantages of obtaining an ultrasound at the completion of anticoagulation is to establish a baseline for distinguishing new from old thrombus in case the patient develops symptoms of a recurrent DVT. However, if thrombus is still present, there is an increased risk for recurrence if the treatment is stopped. In the "DACUS" study [67], subjects with a first episode of DVT, treated with anticoagulation for 3 months were randomized to either stop or continue anticoagulants for 9 additional months if there was residual vein thrombosis (RVT) at echo, whereas in those without RVT, anticoagulation was stopped. Recurrent events occurred in 27.2 % of those who discontinued and 19.3 % of those who continued anticoagulation and in 1.3 % in those without RVT. Major bleeding occurred in 1.1 % patients who stopped and in 2.3 % in those who continued anticoagulation.

Prandoni et al. [68] enrolled 538 consecutive outpatients with a first episode of acute proximal DVT at completion of an uneventful 3-month period of anticoagulation and randomized them to fixed-duration anticoagulation (no further anticoagulation for secondary thrombosis and an extra 3 months for unprovoked thrombosis) or flexible-duration ultrasonography-guided anticoagulation (no further anticoagulation in patients with recanalized veins and continued anticoagulation in all other patients for up to 9 months for secondary DVT and up to 21 months for unprovoked thrombosis); 17.2 % of patients allocated to fixed-duration anticoagulation and 11.9 % of patients allocated to flexible-duration anticoagulation developed recurrent VTE. For patients with unprovoked DVT, the adjusted HR was 0.61 (CI, 0.36–1.02) and 0.81 (CI, 0.32–2.06) for those with secondary DVT. Major bleeding occurred in 0.7 % of patients in the fixed-duration group and 1.5 % of patients in the flexible-duration group. The authors suggested that tailored anticoagulation therapy conducted by residual thrombosis at echo should be integrated into clinical practice. A Canadian study [69] analyzed the outcome of 646 participants with a first, unprovoked major VTE over a 4-year period. If women had none or one of the following characteristics of hyper-pigmentation, edema or redness of either leg, D-dimer≥ 250 μg/l while taking warfarin, body mass index ≥30 kg/m^2, or age ≥65 years, then they had a low annual risk of recurrence (1.6 %) and could safely abort anticoagulation, whereas women with two or more of these risk factors had an increased annual risk for recurrence (14.1 %). Conflicting results come from a study conducted by Cosmi et al. [70], which stated that RVO at the time of anticoagulation withdrawal is not a risk factor for recurrence of VTE.

Limitations in tailoring such a strategy include the standardization of ultrasound protocols and criteria for assessing residual thrombus.

Other Anticoagulation Strategies Used in the Treatment of Idiopathic VTE

Ridker et al. [71] recently analyzed outcomes of patients with idiopathic venous thromboembolisms who had received full-dose anticoagulation therapy for a median of 6.5 months and who were randomly assigned to placebo or low-intensity warfarin (target INR, 1.5–2.0). Follow-up at 4.3 years showed that low-intensity warfarin therapy was associated with a reduction in the risk of recurrent venous thromboembolism between 76 and 81 % (risk reductions were similar for all subgroups, including those with and those without inherited thrombophilia). Major hemorrhage occurred in two patients assigned to placebo and five assigned to low-intensity warfarin. Eight patients in the placebo group and four in the group assigned to low-intensity warfarin died. Another paper from 2003 [72] showed controversial results: after 3 months of conventional warfarin therapy for unprovoked venous thromboembolism, patients were randomized similarly to the previous study; however, the study started at 3 months after the initial event. At 2.4 years, the low-intensity warfarin regimen did not reduce the risk of clinically important bleeding and was not efficient in reducing recurrences. A new generation of anticoagulants might bring huge benefits in treating this entity.

Cancer-Related Consideration

The majority of patients diagnosed with unprovoked VTE are found to have a hereditary or acquired risk factor if detailed questionnaire and biology tests are performed. Around 10–20 % of patients aged over 50 will be diagnosed with an occult malignancy within 1–2 years from the initial VTE. We must keep in mind however that 66 % of these patients already have a diagnosis of cancer when they initially present with VTE [73].

At this time, there is insufficient evidence to recommend an aggressive investigation (for example, screening with computed tomography of the abdomen and pelvis) unless the patient is symptomatic (for example, bowel habits, weight loss, cough, etc.) or presents with objective findings that suggest the presence of an underlying malignancy. Even if an extensive etiological workup is made, up to one-third of cancers are missed. A thorough history questionnaire, physical examination, chest x-ray, and routine blood work (including a complete blood count, basic chemistries, liver function, and lactate dehydrogenase) accompanied by age-appropriate cancer screening along with ongoing clinical surveillance have been proved to be the best strategy.

A list with the most important papers regarding the incidence of occult malignancy detected with screening and during follow-up in patients with VTE is presented in Table 20.12.

Algorithm for the Treatment of Idiopathic VTE

Several treatment algorithms exist for current decision-making [3, 44, 75].

After reviewing all available data, we propose a new improved algorithm that could ease the risk stratification in VTE (Figs. 20.16 and 20.17).

The two ends of the VTE spectrum are secondary VTE without risk factors for recurrence (for which anticoagulation is mandated for 3–6 month) and idiopathic VTE (for which anticoagulation is mandated indefinitely if the bleeding score is low or medium). In between the two sit secondary VTE with temporary risk factors for

Table 20.12 Incidence of occult malignancy detected with screening and during follow-up in patients with venous thrombotic events

Author/year/study type	Patient no. and pathology	Duration of FU	Investigations done	Cancer diagnosed with screening/during FU	Comments
Monreal et al./1991/ prospective	113 pts with DVT of lower limbs	Mean 12–15 month	Initial screen: Hx, exam, CBC, LFTs, ESR, LDH, SPEP, CXR, blood smear, CEA, and abdo/pelvic US	11 pts (9.7 %)/1 pt (1.0 %)	Cancer was more commonly found in pts with idiopathic DVT compared to pts with known risk factors for DVT (7 of 31 pts vs. 5 of 82 pts; $p = 0.0127$) and in those pts with abnormal LDH levels (6 of 23 vs. 6 of 90; $P = 0.007$). the majority of cancers were identified with a CBC, LDH, CEA, CXR, and abdo US or CT
Monreal et al./1993/ prospective	78 pts with PE	Mean 9–21 month	Initial screen : Hx, exam, ESR, CBC, blood smear, LFTs, LDH, SPEP, CXR, CEA, and abdo/pelvic US Additional test if pt agreed or abnormalities found: UGI endoscopy, thoracic CT (if abnormal CXR), BM biopsy (if abnormal SPEP), colonoscopy (if abnormal CEA), and prostate biopsy (if abnormal node)	7 pts (9 %)/2 pts (2.6 %)	Cancer was more commonly found in pts with idiopathic PE as compared with pts with known risk factors for PE (6 of 27 pts vs. 3 of 51 pts; $p < 0.05$)
Bastounis et al./1996/ prospective	293 pts with 1st episode of DVT	2 years	A II pts underwent screening: Hx, exam, CBC, ESR, LFTs, creat, SPEP, UA, CXR, CEA, and in 222 pts, abdo/pelvic CT	22 pts (7.5 %)/7 pts (2.4 %)	Cancer was diagnosed in 25 % pts with idiopathic DVT as compared with 4 % pts with secondary DVT
Cailleux et al./1997/ prospective	148 pts with DVT or PE	3–6 months	A II pts underwent screening: Hx, exam, laboratory tests, CXR, and abdo/pelvic US	6 pts (4.1 %)/not reported	US was abnormal in 8 pts (5.4 %) but detected only 6 cancers. In 5 of the 6 cases, clinical exam and lab test suggested presence of underlying cancer
Enguidanos et al./2002/prospective	48 pts with unprovoked DVT	1 year	A II pts underwent screening: Hx, exam, laboratory tests, AFP, CEA, CA19-9, CA 125, SCA, NSE, beta2-microglobulin, PSA (for men), and CA 15–3 (for women)	6 pts (12.5 %)/2 pts (4.2 %)	Cancer was diagnosed in 8 pts (16 %) and a positive tumor marker was identified in 23 pts (48 %). This yielded a sensitivity of 12 %, a specificity of 52 %, a PPV of 5 %, and an NPV of 75 %. Pts who had negative tumor marker and were asymptomatic during admission had no subsequent cancer diagnosis
Monreal et al./2004/ prospective	864 pts with DVT or PE and no prior VTE within 2 years	1 year	Routine screen: Hx, exam, ESR, CBC, LFTs, creat, UA, SPEP, and CXR If routine screen neg, pts underwent additional limited w/u: Abdo/pelvic US, CEA, PSA, and CA 125 If routine screen or limited w/u abnormal, pts underwent additional extensive w/u: UGI endoscopy, colonoscopy, BM biopsy, abdo/pelvic CT, thoracic CT, bronchoscopy, and prostate US	34 pts (3.9 %) with routine screen, 13 pts (1.6 %) with additional screening/14 pts (out of 817 for FU = 1.7 %)	The routine screen identified almost half of the malignancies. Logistic regression analysis showed a statistically significant association with occult malignancies for idiopathic VTE (OR, 3.3; $P < 0.002$), as well as age above 70 years (OR, 4.0; $P < 0.001$)

Piccioli et al./2004/ randomized controlled trial	201 pts with unprovoked and 1st episode of DVT or PE	2 years	Limited screen: Hx, exam, CBC, LFTs, calcium, UA and CXR Extensive screen: abdo/pelvis US, abdo/pelvis CT, gastroscopy or barium swallow, colonoscopy or sigmoidoscopy plus BE, stool guaiac, sputum cytology, tumors markers (CEA, AFP, CA 125), mammogram and Pap smear for women, and transabdominal US of the prostate and PSA for men	Limited 0 pts (0 %), Extensive: 13 pts (13.1 %) / Limited: 10 pts (9.8 %), Extensive : 1 pt (1 %)	Extensive screen had short delay in diagnosis of cancer (1 vs. 11.6 months, [$P<0.001$]) and cancer detection at earlier stages. Lower cancer-related mortality was not statistically significant (2.0 % vs. 3.9 %; [absolute difference, 1.9 % (95 % CI, -5.5-10.9)]). Trial was stopped prematurely because of recruitment issues
Van Doormaal et al./2009/center controlled study	630 pts with unprovoked VTE	Median 30 months	Limited screen: Hx, exam, laboratory tests, and CXR. Extensive screen: limited screen plus thoracic CT, abdo Ct, and mammogram (in women)	Limited: 7 pts (2.4 %) Extensive: 12pts (3.5 %)/ Limited: 15 pts (5.3 %)	No differences in cancer detection or deaths during the study (8.3 % in limited screen vs. 7.6 % in extensive screen) were observed
Jara–Palomares et al./2010/prospective cohort	107 pts with PE	2 years	All patients underwent initial screen: Hx, exam, routine blood chemistries, CBC, tumor markers (CEA, AFP, CA 19-9, CA 125, and in men, PSA),CXR, and abdo/pelvic US. If any abnormalities found, appropriate diagnostic procedures performed	5 pts (4.7 %)/4 pts (3.9 %)	Overall sensitivity of screening program was 55.5 % in pts with idiopathic PE. Number needed to screen was 12.1 (6.1 in idiopathic PE, 58 in secondary PE) Idiopathic PE (OR: 12.82; $p=0.03$) was an independent risk factor for occult cancer in these pts with logistic regression analysis

Modified from [74]

Abdo abdomen, *AFP* alpha-fetoprotein, *BE* barium enema, *BM* bone marrow, *CA* carbohydrate antigen, *CEA* carcinoembryonic antigen, *CBC* complete blood count, *CI* confidence interval, *creat* creatinine, *CRP* C-reactive protein, *CXR* chest radiography, *DVT* deep vein thrombosis, *ESR* erythrocyte sedimentation rate, *FU* follow-up, *Hx* history, *LDH* lactic dehydrogenase, *LFTs* liver function tests, *LN* lymph node, *mos* months, *neg* negative, *No.* number, *NSE* neuron-specific enolase, *OR* odds ratio, *PE* pulmonary embolus, *NPV* negative predictive value, *PPV* positive predictive value, *PSA* prostate-specific antigen, *pt* patient, *pts* patients, *SCC* squamous-cell antigen, *SPEP* serum protein electrophoresis, *UA* urinanalysis, *UGI* upper gastrointestinal, *US* ultrasound, *vs.* versus, *VTE* venous thromboembolism, *w/u* work up, *yrs* years

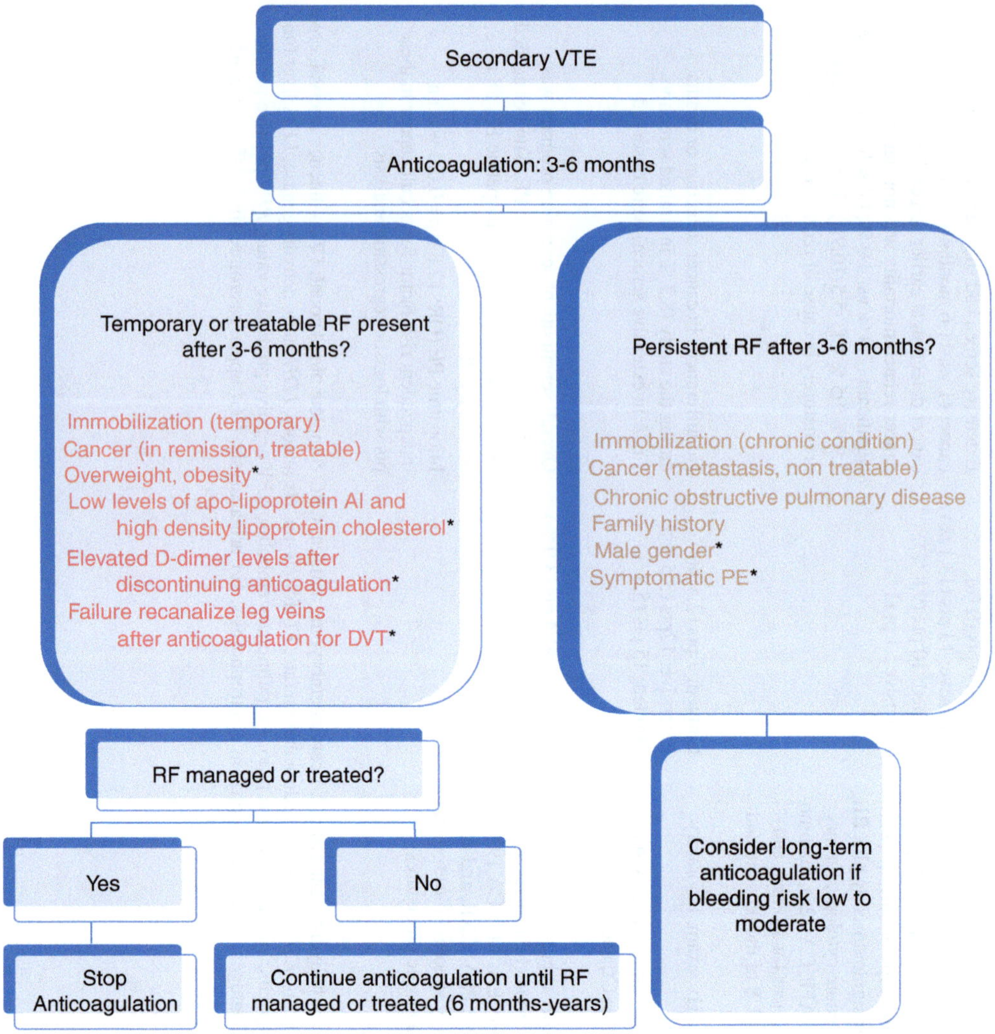

Fig. 20.16 Treatment algorithm for secondary VTE. *RF* risk factors for recurrence of VTE, * validated for idiopathic VTE (RF-risk factors)

recurrence and secondary VTE with permanent risk factors for recurrence. In the first case, anticoagulation is mandatory until the risk factor disappears or has been cured (3–6 months to several years). In the latter situation, long-term anticoagulation is mandatory for low or medium bleeding risk.

Nonetheless, we should not forget that patient preference is crucial for tailoring anticoagulation therapy. This being said, we strongly recommend the algorithm from Figs. 20.16 and 20.17 for medical decisions, even though in selected cases the most effective treatment protocol could be decided on a case-by-case basis, accounting for the risk-benefit ratio in each situation.

Fig. 20.17 Treatment algorithm for idiopathic VTE. *RF* risk factors for recurrence of VTE, * validated for idiopathic VTE (RF-risk factors)

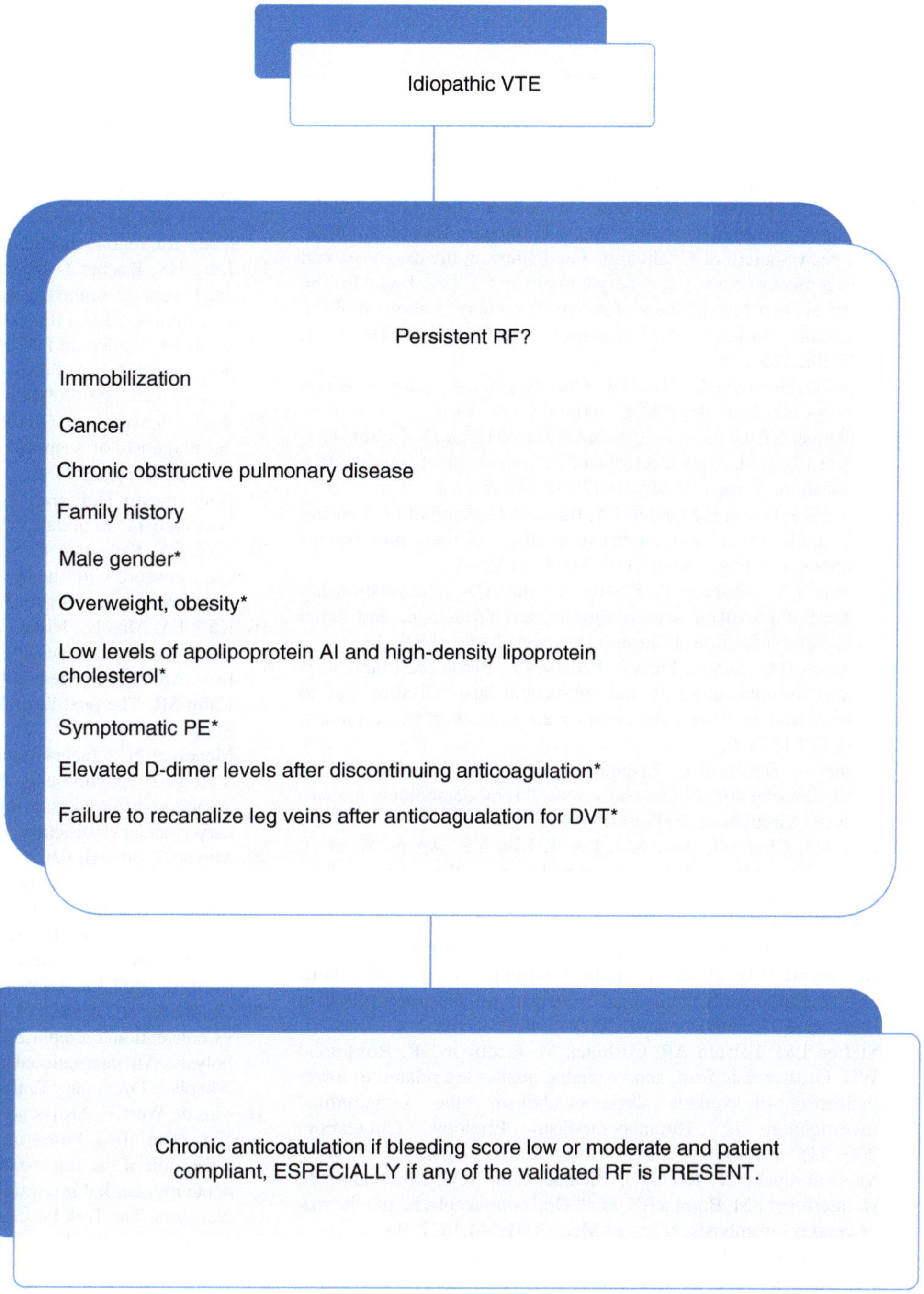

References

1. Goldhaber SZ, Visani L, De Rosa M. Acute pulmonary embolism: clinical outcomes in the International Cooperative Pulmonary Embolism Registry (ICOPER). Lancet. 1999;353(9162):1386–9.
2. Anderson Jr FA, Spencer FA. Risk factors for venous thromboembolism. Circulation. 2003;107(23 Suppl 1):I9–16.
3. Torbicki A, Perrier A, Konstantinides S, et al. Task Force for the Diagnosis and Management of Acute Pulmonary Embolism of the European Society of Cardiology. Guidelines on the diagnosis and management of acute pulmonary embolism: the Task Force for the Diagnosis and Management of Acute Pulmonary Embolism of the European Society of Cardiology (ESC). Eur Heart J. 2008;29:2276–315.
4. Stein PD, Beemath A, Olson RE. Obesity as a risk factor in venous thromboembolism. Am J Med. 2005;118:978–80.
5. Goldhaber SZ, Grodstein F, Stampfer MJ, Manson JE, Colditz GA, Speizer FE, et al. A prospective study of risk factors for pulmonary embolism in women. JAMA. 1997;277:642–5.
6. Prandoni P, Bilora F, Marchiori A, Bernardi E, Petrobelli F, Lensing AW, et al. An association between atherosclerosis and venous thrombosis. N Engl J Med. 2003;348(15):1435–41.
7. Spencer FA, Ginsberg JS, Chong A, Alter DA. The relationship between unprovoked venous thromboembolism, age, and acute myocardial infarction. J Thromb Haemost. 2008;6:1507–13.
8. Sorensen HT, Horvath-Puho E, Pedersen L, Baron JA, Prandoni P. Venous thromboembolism and subsequent hospitalisation due to acute arterial cardiovascular events: a 20-year cohort study. Lancet. 2007;370:1773–9.
9. Ageno W, Becattini C, Brighton T, Selby R, Kamphuisen PW. Cardiovascular risk factors and venous thromboembolism: a meta-analysis. Circulation. 2008;117:93–102.
10. Jang MJ, Choi WI, Bang SM, Lee T, Kim YK, Ageno W, et al. Metabolic syndrome is associated with venous thromboembolism in the Korean population. Arterioscler Thromb Vasc Biol. 2009;29:311–5.
11. Steffen LM, Cushman M, Peacock JM, Heckbert SR, Jacobs Jr DR, Rosamond WD, et al. Metabolic syndrome and risk of venous thromboembolism: Longitudinal Investigation of Thromboembolism Etiology. J Thromb Haemost. 2009;7:746–51.
12. Steffen LM, Folsom AR, Cushman M, Jacobs Jr DR, Rosamond WD. Greater fish, fruit, and vegetable intakes are related to lower incidence of venous thromboembolism: the Longitudinal Investigation of Thromboembolism Etiology. Circulation. 2007;115:188–95.
13. Vandenbroucke JP, Rosing J, Bloemenkamp KW, Middeldorp S, Helmerhorst FM, Bouma BN, et al. Oral contraceptives and the risk of venous thrombosis. N Engl J Med. 2001;344:1527–35.
14. Rossouw JE, Anderson GL, Prentice RL, LaCroix AZ, Kooperberg C, Stefanick ML, et al. Risks and benefits of estrogen plus progestin in healthy postmenopausal women: principal results from the Women's Health Initiative randomized controlled trial. JAMA. 2002;288:321–33.
15. Rosengren A, Freden M, Hansson PO, Wilhelmsen L, Wedel H, Eriksson H. Psychosocial factors and venous thromboembolism: a long-term follow-up study of Swedish men. J Thromb Haemost. 2008;6:558–64.
16. Folsom AR, Lutsey PL, Astor BC, Cushman M. C-reactive protein and venous thromboembolism: a prospective investigation in the ARIC cohort. Thromb Haemost. 2009;102:615–9.
17. Luxembourg B, Schmitt J, Humpich M, Glowatzki M, Dressler D, Seifried E, et al. Cardiovascular risk factors in idiopathic compared to risk-associated venous thromboembolism: a focus on fibrinogen, factor VIII, and high-sensitivity C-reactive protein (hs-CRP). Thromb Haemost. 2009;102:668–75.
18. Zee RY, Glynn RJ, Cheng S, Steiner L, Rose L, Ridker PM. An evaluation of candidate genes of inflammation and thrombosis in relation to the risk of venous thromboembolism: the Women's Genome Health Study. Circ Cardiovasc Genet. 2009;2:57–62.
19. Glynn RJ, Danielson E, Fonseca FA, Genest J, Gotto Jr AM, Kastelein JJ, et al. A randomized trial of rosuvastatin in the prevention of venous thromboembolism. N Engl J Med. 2009;360:1851–61.
20. van Stralen KJ, Rosendaal FR, Doggen CJ. Minor injuries as a risk factor for venous thrombosis. Arch Intern Med. 2008;168:21–6.
21. Joffe HV, Kucher N, Tapson VF, Goldhaber SZ. Upper-extremity deep vein thrombosis: a prospective registry of 592 patients. Circulation. 2004;110:1605–11.
22. Wells PS, Anderson DR, Bormanis J, et al. Value of assessment of pretest probability of deep-vein thrombosis in clinical management. Lancet. 1997;350(9094):1795–8.
23. Wells PS, Anderson DR, Rodger M, et al. Evaluation of D-dimer in the diagnosis of suspected deep-vein thrombosis. N Engl J Med. 2003;349(13):1227–35.
24. Bounameaux H, Perrier A, Righini M. Diagnosis of venous thromboembolism: an update. Vasc Med. 2010;15(5):399–406.
25. Klok FA, Kruisman E, Spaan J, et al. Comparison of the revised Geneva score with the Wells rule for assessing clinical probability of pulmonary embolism. J Thromb Haemost. 2008;6(1):40–4.
26. Klok FA, Mos IC, Nijkeuter M, et al. Simplification of the revised Geneva score for assessing clinical probability of pulmonary embolism. Arch Intern Med. 2008;168(19):2131–6.
27. Kahn SR. The post thrombotic syndrome. Thromb Res. 2011;127 Suppl 3:S89–92.
28. Meneveau N, Schiele F, Vuillemenot A, Valette B, Grollier G, Bernard Y, et al. Streptokinase vs alteplase in massive pulmonary embolism. A randomized trial assessing right heart haemodynamics and pulmonary vascular obstruction. Eur Heart J. 1997;18(7):1141–8.
29. Meyer G, Sors H, Charbonnier B, Kasper W, Bassand JP, Kerr IH, et al. Effects of intravenous urokinase versus alteplase on total pulmonary resistance in acute massive pulmonary embolism: a European multicenter double-blind trial. The European Cooperative Study Group for Pulmonary Embolism. J Am Coll Cardiol. 1992;19(2):239–45.
30. Goldhaber SZ, Agnelli G, Levine MN. Reduced dose bolus alteplase vs conventional alteplase infusion for pulmonary embolism thrombolysis. An international multicenter randomized trial. The Bolus Alteplase Pulmonary Embolism Group. Chest. 1994;106(3):718–24.
31. Van de Werf F, Ardissino D, Betriu A, Cokkinos DV, Falk E, Fox KA, et al. Task Force on the Management of Acute Myocardial Infarction of the European Society of Cardiology. Management of acute myocardial infarction in patients presenting with ST-segment elevation. The Task Force on the Management of Acute Myocardial Infarction of the European Society of Cardiology. Eur Heart J. 2003;24(1):28–66.
32. Eriksson BI, Quinlan DJ, Weitz JI. Comparative pharmacodynamics and pharmacokinetics of oral direct thrombin and factor xa inhibitors in development. Clin Pharmacokinet. 2009;48(1):1–22. doi:10.2165/0003088-200948010-00001.
33. Perzborn E, Roehrig S, Straub A, Kubitza D, Mueck W, Laux V. Rivaroxaban: a new oral factor xa inhibitor. Arterioscler Thromb Vasc Biol. 2010;30(3):376–81.
34. Eriksson BI, Borris LC, Dahl OE, et al. Dose-escalation study of rivaroxaban (BAY 59-7939)—an oral, direct Factor Xa inhibitor—for the prevention of venous thromboembolism in patients undergoing total hip replacement. Thromb Res. 2007;120(5):685–93.
35. Eriksson BI, Borris L, Dahl OE, et al. Oral, direct Factor Xa inhibition with BAY 59-7939 for the prevention of venous thromboembolism after total hip replacement. J Thromb Haemost. 2006;4(1):121–8.
36. Eriksson BI, Borris LC, Dahl OE, et al. A once-daily, oral, direct Factor Xa inhibitor, rivaroxaban (BAY 59-7939), for thrombopro-

phylaxis after total hip replacement. Circulation. 2006;114(22): 2374–81.
37. Turpie AG, Fisher WD, Bauer KA, et al. BAY 59-7939: an oral, direct Factor Xa inhibitor for the prevention of venous thromboembolism in patients after total knee replacement. A phase II dose-ranging study. J Thromb Haemost. 2005;3(11):2479–86.
38. Kwong LM. Cost-effectiveness of rivaroxaban after total hip or total knee arthroplasty. Am J Manag Care. 2011;17(1):S22–6.
39. Buller H, Deitchman D, Prins M, Segers A. Efficacy and safety of the oral direct factor Xa inhibitor apixaban for symptomatic deep vein thrombosis. The Botticelli DVT doseranging study. J Thromb Haemost. 2008;6(8):1313–8.
40. Lassen MR, Raskob GE, Gallus A, Pineo G, Chen D, Hornick P. Apixaban versus enoxaparin for thromboprophylaxis after knee replacement (ADVANCE-2): a randomized double-blind trial. Lancet. 2010;375(9717):807–15.
41. Lassen MR, Gallus A, Raskob GE, Pineo G, Chen D, Ramirez LM. Apixaban versus enoxaparin for thromboprophylaxis after hip replacement. N Engl J Med. 2010;363(26):2487–98.
42. Eriksson BI, Dahl OE, Rosencher N, et al. Dabigatran etexilate versus enoxaparin for prevention of venous thromboembolism after total hip replacement: a randomised, double-blind, non-inferiority trial. Lancet. 2007;370(9591):949–56.
43. Eriksson BI, Dahl OE, Rosencher N, et al. Oral dabigatran etexilate vs. subcutaneous enoxaparin for the prevention of venous thromboembolism after total knee replacement: the RE-MODEL randomized trial. J Thromb Haemost. 2007;5(11):2178–85.
44. Goldhaber SZ, Piazza G. Optimal duration of anticoagulation after venous thromboembolism. Circulation. 2011;123(6):664–7.
45. Pisters R, Lane DA, Nieuwlaat R, de Vos CB, Crijns HJ, Lip GY. A novel userfriendly score (HAS-BLED) to assess one-year risk of major bleeding in atrial fibrillation patients: the Euro Heart Survey. Chest. 2010;138(5):1093–100.
46. Camm AJ, Kirchhof P, Lip GY, Schotten U, Savelieva I, Ernst S, et al. Guidelines for the management of atrial fibrillation: the Task Force for the Management of Atrial Fibrillation of the European Society of Cardiology (ESC). Eur Heart J. 2010;31(19):2369–429. Epub 2010 Aug 29.
47. Heit JA, Mohr DN, Silverstein MD, Petterson TM, O'Fallon WM, Melton III LJ. Predictors of recurrence after deep vein thrombosis and pulmonary embolism: a population-based cohort study. Arch Intern Med. 2000;160:761–8.
48. Prandoni P, Lensing AW, Cogo A, Cuppini S, Villalta S, Carta M, et al. The long-term clinical course of acute deep venous thrombosis. Ann Intern Med. 1996;125:1–7.
49. Prandoni P, Noventa F, Ghirarduzzi A, Pengo V, Bernardi E, Pesavento R, et al. The risk of recurrent venous thromboembolism after discontinuing anticoagulation in patients with acute proximal deep vein thrombosis or pulmonary embolism: a prospective cohort study in 1,626 patients. Haematologica. 2007;92:199–205.
50. Vossen CY, Walker ID, Svensson PJ, et al. Recurrence rate after a first venous thrombosis in patients with familial thrombophilia. Arterioscler Thromb Vasc Biol. 2005;25:1992–7.
51. Lijfering WM, Brouwer JL, Veeger NJ, et al. Selective testing for thrombophilia in patients with first venous thrombosis: results from a retrospective family cohort study on absolute thrombotic risk for currently known thrombophilic defects in 2479 relatives. Blood. 2009;113:5314–22.
52. Segal JB, Brotman DJ, Necochea AJ, et al. Predictive value of factor V Leiden and prothrombin G20210A in adults with venous thromboembolism and in family members of those with a mutation: a systematic review. JAMA. 2009;301:2472–85.
53. Ho WK, Hankey GJ, Quinlan DJ, Eikelboom JW. Risk of recurrent venous thromboembolism in patients with common thrombophilia: a systematic review. Arch Intern Med. 2006;166:729–36.
54. Koster T, Blann AD, Briët E, Vandenbroucke JP, Rosendaal FR. Role of clotting factor VIII in effect of von Willebrand factor on occurrence of deep-vein thrombosis. Lancet. 1995;345:152–5.
55. Kyrle PA, Minar E, Hirschl M, et al. High plasma factor VIII and the risk of recurrent venous thromboembolism. N Engl J Med. 2000;343:457–62.
56. den Heijer M, Willems HP, Blom HJ, et al. Homocysteine lowering by B vitamins and the secondary prevention of deep vein thrombosis and pulmonary embolism: a randomized, placebo-controlled, double-blind trial. Blood. 2007;109:139–44.
57. Ray JG, Kearon C, Yi Q, et al. Homocysteine-lowering therapy and risk for venous thromboembolism: a randomized trial. Ann Intern Med. 2007;146:761–7.
58. Nijkeuter M, Sohne M, Tick LW, Kamphuisen PW, Kramer MH, Laterveer L, et al. The natural course of hemodynamically stable pulmonary embolism: clinical outcome and risk factors in a large prospective cohort study. Chest. 2007;131:517–23.
59. Kyrle PA, Minar E, Bialonczyk C, Hirschl M, Weltermann A, Eichinger S. The risk of recurrent venous thromboembolism in men and women. N Engl J Med. 2004;350:2558–63.
60. Eichinger S, Hron G, Bialonczyk C, Hirschl M, Minar E, Wagner O, et al. Overweight, obesity, and the risk of recurrent venous thromboembolism. Arch Intern Med. 2008;168: 1678–83.
61. Eichinger S, Pecheniuk NM, Hron G, Deguchi H, Schemper M, Kyrle PA, et al. High-density lipoprotein and the risk of recurrent venous thromboembolism. Circulation. 2007;115: 1609–14.
62. Eichinger S, Weltermann A, Minar E, Stain M, Schonauer V, Schneider B, et al. Symptomatic pulmonary embolism and the risk of recurrent venous thromboembolism. Arch Intern Med. 2004;164:92–6.
63. Eichinger S, Heinze G, Jandeck LM, Kyrle PA. Risk assessment of recurrence in patients with unprovoked deep vein thrombosis or pulmonary embolism: the Vienna Prediction Model. Circulation. 2010;121:1630–6.
64. Verhovsek M, Douketis JD, Yi Q, et al. Systematic review: D-dimer to predict recurrent disease after stopping anticoagulant therapy for unprovoked venous thromboembolism. Ann Intern Med. 2008;149:481–90.
65. Palareti G, Legnani C, Cosmi B, et al. Predictive value of D-dimer test for recurrent venous thromboembolism after anticoagulation withdrawal in subjects with a previous idiopathic event and in carriers of congenital thrombophilia. Circulation. 2003;108: 313–8.
66. Cosmi B, Legnani C, Tosetto A, et al. Sex, age, and normal post-anticoagulation D-dimer as risk factors or recurrence after idiopathic venous thromboembolism in the PROLONG study extension. J Thromb Haemost. 2010;8(9):1933–42.
67. Siragusa S, Malato A, Anastasio R, et al. Residual vein thrombosis to establish duration of anticoagulation after a first episode of deep vein thrombosis: the Duration of Anticoagulation based on Compression UltraSonography (DACUS) study. Blood. 2010; 112:511–5.
68. Prandoni P, Prins MH, Lensing AW, et al. Residual thrombosis on ultrasonography to guide the duration of anticoagulation in patients with deep venous thrombosis: a randomized trial. Ann Intern Med. 2009;150:577–85.
69. Rodger MA, Kahn SR, Wells PS, et al. Identifying unprovoked thromboembolism patients at low risk for recurrence who can discontinue anticoagulant therapy. Can Med Assoc J. 2008;179:417–26.
70. Cosmi B, Legnani C, Iorio A, et al. Residual venous obstruction, alone and in combination with D-dimer, as a risk factor for recurrence after anticoagulation withdrawal following a first idiopathic deep vein thrombosis in the Prolong Study. Eur J Vasc Endovasc Surg. 2010;39:356–65.

71. Ridker PM, Goldhaber SZ, Danielson E, et al. Long-term, low-intensity warfarin for the prevention of recurrent venous thromboembolism. N Engl J Med. 2003;348:1425–34.
72. Kearon C, Ginsberg JS, Kovacs MJ, et al. Comparison of low-intensity warfarin therapy with conventional-intensity warfarin therapy for long-term prevention of recurrent venous thromboembolism. N Engl J Med. 2003;349:631–9.
73. Carrier M, Le Gal G, Wells PS, Fergusson D, Ramsey T, Rodger MA. Systematic review: the Trousseau syndrome revisited: should we screen extensively for cancer in patients with venous thromboembolism? Ann Intern Med. 2008;149:323–33.
74. Rosovsky R, Lee AY. Evidence-based mini-review: should all patients with idiopathic venous thromboembolic events be screened extensively for occult malignancy? Hematology Am Soc Hematol Educ Program. 2010;2010:150–2.
75. Bauer KA. Duration of anticoagulation: applying the guidelines and beyond. Hematology Am Soc Hematol Educ Program. 2010;2010:210–5.

Inflammation, Thrombogenesis, Fibrinolysis, and Vein Wall Remodeling After Deep Venous Thrombosis

21

Jose Antonio Diaz and Daniel Durant Myers Jr.

Introduction

Venous thromboembolism and its sequelae, postthrombotic syndrome and chronic thromboembolic pulmonary hypertension, affect millions of people worldwide. The purpose of this chapter is to present recent and current research focused on defining the mechanism that drives vein wall remodeling after venous thrombosis.

Epidemiology

VTE includes both deep vein thrombosis (DVT) and pulmonary embolism (PE). After acute coronary syndrome and stroke, VTE is the third most common cardiovascular disease. VTE occurs worldwide, in any age group and all socioeconomic groups in North America and Western Europe [1]. In a recent study by Silverstein et al. [2] the estimated total annual number of VTE events in the United States exceeded 900,000. Symptomatic VTE accounted for two-thirds of the cases reported. Interestingly, no changes in the incidence of VTE were noted during the 25-year cohort study.

The incidence of VTE varies among ethnic groups, with a higher incidence among Whites and African Americans compared with Asians and Native Americans [2]. VTE is more frequent among women during childbearing years and men after the age of 45 [2]. However, the incidence rates increase exponentially with age for both men and women and for both DVT and PE. The overall age-adjusted incidence rate is higher for men (114 per 100,000 person-years) than women (105 per 100,000 person-years); the male:female ratio is 1.2:1 [2, 3].

J.A. Diaz, MD(✉) • D.D. Myers Jr., DVM, MPH, DACLAM
Section of Vascular Surgery, Department of Surgery,
School of Medicine, University of Michigan,
2800 Plymouth Rd, North Campus Research Complex,
B26, Room 251N, 48105 Ann Arbor, MI, USA
e-mail: josediaz@med.umich.edu; ddmyers@med.umich.edu

The overall mortality associated with VTE is 30 % [4]. Of note, the annual number of PE-related deaths in the USA may exceed myocardial infarction–related and stroke-related deaths [4]. Almost 60 % of PE is diagnosed postmortem, and sudden death after symptomatic PE occurs in approximately 35 % of patients [4]. Thus, it is not surprising that PE is an independent risk factor for poor outcome at 3-month follow-up [4].

The factors that could lead to or interact with one another to lead to VTE were first described by Rudolph Virchow in 1856 [5] and include: (1) endothelial injury, (2) blood stasis or turbulent flow, and (3) and blood hypercoagulability. Vessel wall endothelial damage initiates a local inflammatory response, which promotes a prothrombotic state driven by tissue factor, adhesion molecules, and proinflammatory cytokines [5]. Stewart et al. [6] in 1974 first established the link between vascular inflammation and veinous thrombosis (VT). This process promotes thrombosis via rolling, adherence, and migration of the activated leukocytes [6]. Current research in vascular biology supports this hypothesis.

Multiple independent risk factors for VTE have been identified, including advanced patient age, surgery, trauma, prolonged bed confinement or immobility, active malignancy with or without concurrent chemotherapy, central vein catheterization or transvenous pacemaker, history of superficial vein thrombosis, varicose veins, and neurological disease with leg paresis [1].

The genetic predisposition to VTE has been demonstrated in association with deficiencies or abnormalities of specific plasma proteins such as protein S and protein C, or downregulation of the anticoagulant system (activated protein C [APC] resistance, factor V Leiden), and increased plasma concentrations of procoagulant factors (fibrinogen, prothrombin; factors VIII, IX, and XI). More recently, increased basal innate immunity activity and reactivity have added new paradigms to the list of inherited or acquired disorders predisposing to thrombosis [7].

Approximately 30 % of the time, VTE will recur within 10 years of the initial episode, with most recurrences

E.A. Gabriel, S.A. Gabriel (eds.), *Inflammatory Response in Cardiovascular Surgery*,
DOI 10.1007/978-1-4471-4429-8_21, © Springer-Verlag London 2013

occurring within the first 6–12 months [8]. Independent predictors of recurrence include male gender [9], increasing patient age and body mass index, neurological disease with leg paresis, and active cancer [10]. Other predictors include idiopathic VTE; a lupus anticoagulant or antiphospholipid antibody; deficiencies of antithrombin, protein C, or protein S; and, as recently reported, persistently increased plasma fibrin D-dimer and residual venous thrombosis [4].

The two major complications associated with VTE are post-thrombotic syndrome and chronic thromboembolic pulmonary hypertension [8]. Approximately 12 % of all cases of post-thrombotic syndrome in the community are related to VTE [8].

Pathophysiology

Endothelium

The endothelium forms the inner cell lining of all blood vessels in the body and is a spatially distributed organ. On average, the total endothelium in a person weighs approximately 1 kg and covers a total surface area of 4,000–7,000 square meters [1]. The endothelium is involved in most if not all disease processes, either as a primary determinant of pathophysiology or as a target of collateral damage [1]. Endothelial cells play a critical role in hemostasis. In a healthy individual, there is a balance between procoagulant and anticoagulant mechanisms. The anticoagulant effect involves the endothelial cells supporting local fibrinolysis in which coagulation (platelet adhesion and activation) and inflammation (leukocyte activation) remain suppressed [11] (Fig. 21.1). In contrast, a procoagulant effect is observed during states of endothelial disturbance, e.g., physical (vascular trauma) or functional (sepsis) [11] (Fig. 21.1).

It is widely known that, under normal conditions, cellular blood components interact with the vessel wall in order to promote normal vascular repair.

The effect of the thrombus on the cellular components of the vein wall is not well defined; however, post thrombosis, the vein wall increases in stiffness and thickness and loses compliance [13]. The non-injured vein wall at rest is characterized by a continuous endothelium, a thin and compliant structure with scattered vascular smooth muscle cells (VSMCs) (Fig. 21.2). In contrast, the post-thrombotic vein wall is thickened, with loss of endothelium (early) and disrupted matrix and proliferative VSMC. The longer an occlusive or partially occlusive thrombus is in contact with the vein wall, the greater the inflammatory response and damage to the vein wall as defined in a recent review by DeRoo et al. [13] (Fig. 21.2).

Inflammation and Thrombogenesis

There is evidence to suggest that inflammation and thrombosis interact and have mechanisms in common. Selectins are glycoproteins that are expressed by leukocytes, activated endothelial cells, and platelets. The role of selectins is to mediate the initial adhesion interactions of leukocytes stimulated by physiological changes in blood flow at sites of vascular endothelial injury. Three selectins have currently been identified: P-selectin, E-selectin, and L-selectin [14]. P- and E-selectins are cell adhesion molecules with critical roles in thrombogenesis. Animal studies using rat and mouse venous thrombosis models demonstrated upregulation of P-selectin and E-selectin in the vein wall 6 h and 6 days after thrombus induction, respectively [14] (Fig. 21.1). P-selectin is involved in leukocyte rolling and adhesion, an early inflammatory mechanism that facilitates leukocyte transmigration. The P-selectin receptor, P-selectin glycoprotein ligand 1 (PSGL-1), is a glycoprotein expressed on the surface of leukocytes and platelets that plays a critical role in the recruitment of leukocytes and platelets into inflamed tissue. The interaction of PSGL-1 with P-selectin (the endothelial cell P-selectin: PSGL-1-leukocyte complex) promotes rolling and adhesion of leukocytes and platelets, which ultimately result in increased vein wall cell infiltration [15] (Fig. 21.1).

A study by Wagner et al. showed that the increase in the number of P-selectin molecules present on the endothelial cell surface is due to the release from the Weibel-Palade body (WPB). WPBs are the endothelial-specific storage organelle for regulated secretion of von Willebrand factor (vWF) and P-selectin onto its membrane [15]. Thus, the exocytosis of WPB initiates a rapid translocation of P-selectin to the endothelial surface, resulting in augmented endothelial adhesiveness for leukocytes and platelets. Soluble P-selectin (sP-sel) is released from activated platelets and endothelial cells, and levels rise significantly during pathologic conditions. The function of sP-sel has been shown to be an endogenous activator of coagulation via generation of plasma microparticles in addition to its ability to bind to PSGL-1, leading to leukocyte recruitment and rolling [16].

Circulating cell-derived microparticles (MP) contribute to the coagulation and amplification of thrombosis (Fig. 21.1). They are present in the blood of healthy individuals. These MPs are small vesicles (less than 1 μm) consisting of a plasma membrane surrounding a small amount of cytoplasm with cell-specific surface molecules [17]. Endothelial cells, leukocytes, and platelets have a very well-structured plasma membrane characterized by a controlled transverse lipid distribution termed "rafts." The activation of these cells promotes a general membrane content redistribution during which rafts concentrate in areas of the cell that will ultimately

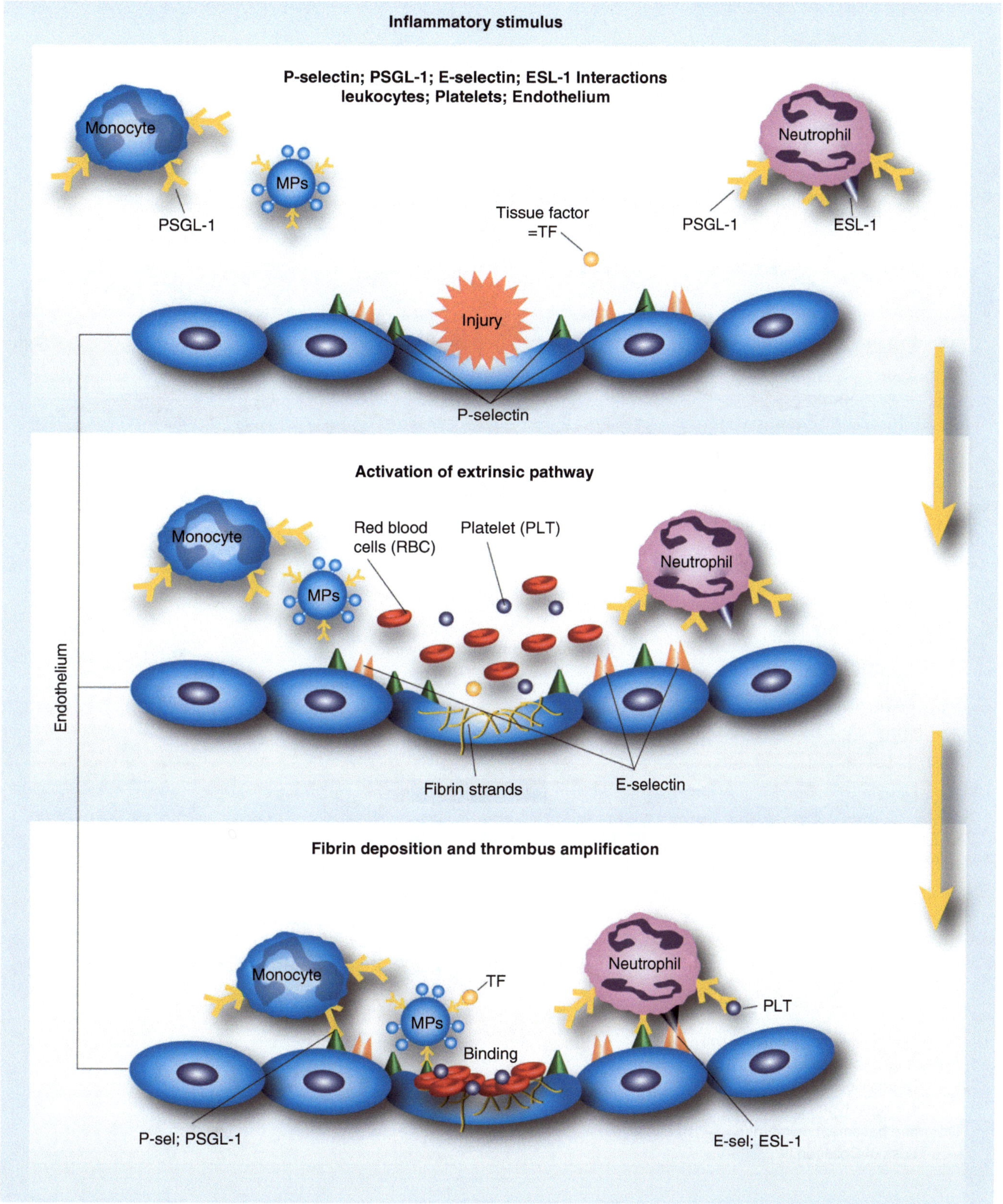

Fig. 21.1 Hypothesized mechanisms of acute venous thrombosis post activation of the venous endothelium. The activation of tissue factor, P-selectin and E-selectin, platelets, inflammatory cells, and microparticles lead to thrombus formation and amplification (From Stanley et al. [12] with permission)

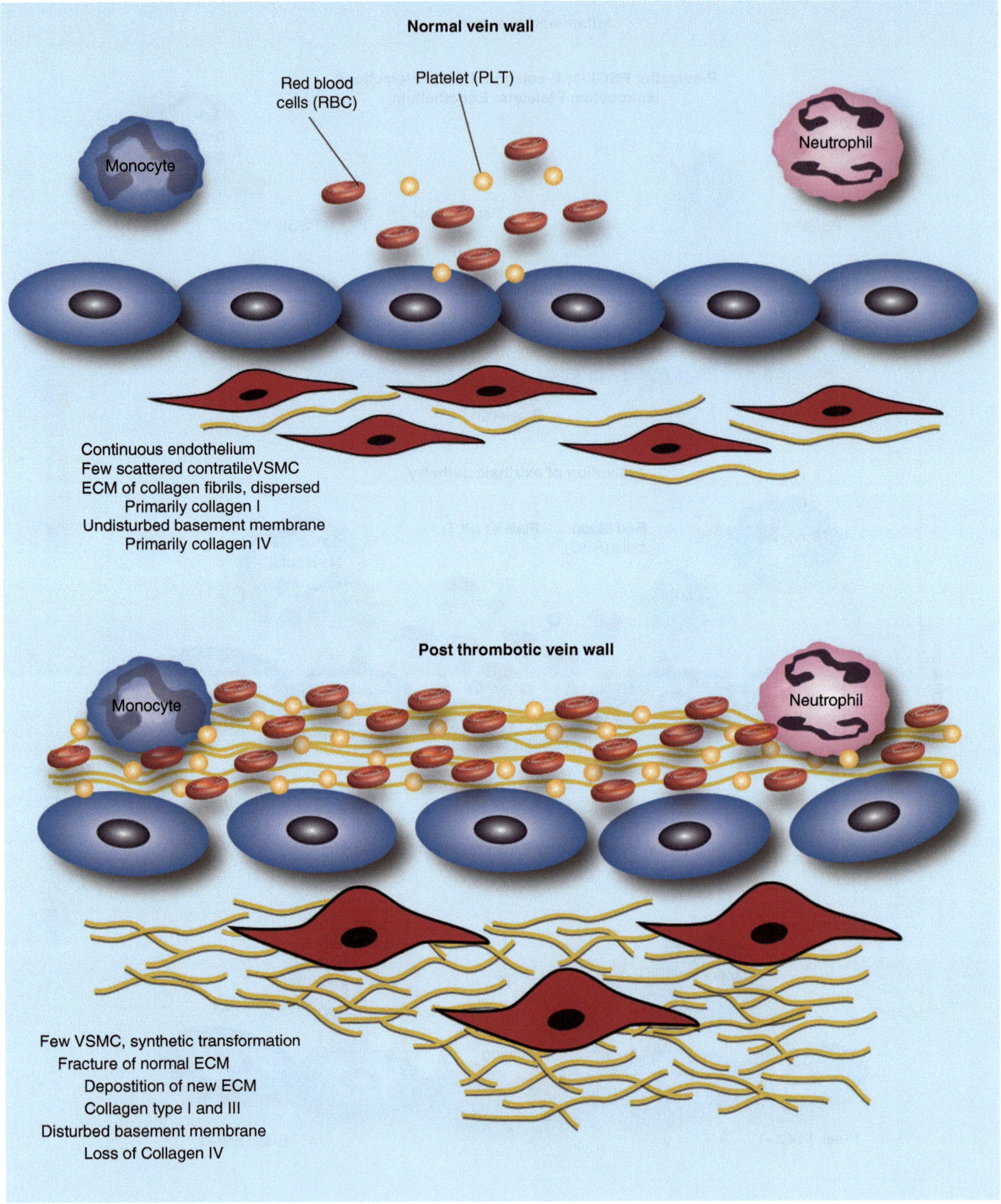

Fig. 21.2 Vein wall matrix changes post venous thrombosis (Modified from DeRoo et al. [13] with permission)

derive in MP. Therefore, the MP membrane is rich in lipid rafts. These MPs concentrate tissue factor (TF) in caveolae where it is stored with the tissue factor pathway inhibitor (TFPI). The fusion of MP with activated platelets promotes thrombus formation in a TF-dependent manner. In addition to TF, the expression of prothrombinase activity on the membrane [18] and PSGL-1 [11] are involved in the procoagulant activity of MPs (Fig. 21.1).

During inflammation, activation of endothelial cells upregulates surface expression of P-selectin, leading to formation of the endothelial cell-P-selectin: PSGL-1-leukocyte complexes. These complexes stimulate the production of MPs from leukocytes, particularly monocytes, along with platelets and endothelial cells. In addition, the accumulation of leukocyte markers expressed on the surface of MPs in the growing thrombus is mediated by the P-selectin-PSGL-1 complex [11]. Therefore, MP concentration increases dramatically at the area of vein wall injury and inflammation [19]. MPs also possess a phosphatidylserine-rich anionic surface capable of assembling complexes of the coagulation cascade. Another molecule expressed on the MP membrane surface is PSGL-1, which then can bind to upregulated P-selectin on platelet surfaces in the thrombus. There is even evidence that macrophage-1 (Mac-1) on leukocyte-derived MPs can allow interactions between MPs and inactivated platelets using glycoprotein 1b alpha (GP1ba), resulting in further platelet activation with P-selectin upregulation [20, 21]. All these events occurring in the area of thrombus formation lead to thrombus amplification. The increase of circulating MPs with the onset of inflammation adds to the proposed mechanisms linking vein wall inflammation and thrombogenesis (Fig. 21.1).

Circulating inhibitory mechanisms regulating the process of thrombogenesis include anti-thrombin III (ATIII), protein C, protein S, TFPI, and glycocalyx-associated glycosaminoglycans, such as heparin sulfate, endothelial protein C receptor, and thrombomodulin (TM), which facilitates inhibitory activity of thrombin by anti-thrombin III and APC by TM.

Anti-thrombin III, a plasma glycoprotein synthesized in the liver, is a serine protease inhibitor (SERPIN) structurally related to other plasma protease inhibitors, such as alpha 1-antichymotrypsin, alpha 2-antiplasmin, and heparin cofactor II. Anti-thrombin III acts as a pseudo-substrate for the inhibition of the intrinsic pathway (factors IIa [thrombin], IXa, Xa, XIa, XIIa) and the extrinsic pathway (factor VII), kallikrein, and plasmin. Other targets of anti-thrombin III include trypsin and the C1s subunit, which are involved in the classical complement pathway. The anti-thrombin III plasma half-life is 60–70 h, while the thrombin-antithrombin (TAT) complex is cleared by the liver, and its inhibitory activity is increased by heparin [1].

Protein C, a vitamin K-dependent plasma glycoprotein, is synthesized as a single chain and cleaved prior to secretion by the liver. Plasma protein C is a two-chain molecule, consisting of a light and heavy chain. Its half-life is 6–7 h. Once protein C binds to its receptor, endothelial protein C receptor, it is cleaved (activated) by the thrombin-thrombomodulin complex on the endothelial surface, resulting in activated protein C (APC). In the presence of calcium and protein S, APC inactivates factor Va and factor VIIIa of the "protein C anticoagulant pathway."

Protein S, a vitamin K-dependent plasma glycoprotein, is synthesized by the liver, the endothelial cells, and the megakaryocytes. Protein S is a cofactor of APC in the protein C anticoagulant pathway. In addition, protein S exhibits APC-independent anticoagulant activity by binding to factors Va, VIIIa and Xa [1]. In serum, protein S is found in two forms: free (active) and protein bound (inactive). Almost 70 % of circulating protein S is bound to a complement protein (C4b-binding protein). The remaining 30 % circulates as "free protein S," which has a half-life of 96 h. It is the free protein S that acts as a cofactor for protein C [1].

TFPI is a single-chain plasma polypeptide that inhibits factor Xa and TF-factor VIIa complex catalytic activity. Plasma only contains 20–30 % of the intravascular minor fraction of TFPI, and it is largely bound to lipoproteins. The majority of TFPI (60–70 %) is normally bound to the vascular endothelium. This pool of TFPI is released into circulation after heparin injection [1].

Prostacyclin and nitric oxide (NO) are secreted by endothelial cells. These compounds synergistically contribute to vessel homeostasis by reducing vascular smooth muscle cells tone and growth, platelet aggregation, leukocyte adhesion to endothelium, and susceptibility to thrombosis. Interestingly, Osanai et al. demonstrated that vessel homeostasis might be maintained through an increase in prostacyclin production in vascular endothelial cells when NO synthesis is impaired [22].

We recently used our mouse inferior vena cava (IVC) ligation model to generate venous thrombosis in order to study the role of interleukin-6 (IL-6) in thrombus development. Specifically, an antibody (anti-IL-6) was administered to mice pre-thrombus induction that leads to in vivo neutralization [23]. We found that IL-6 had an acute and a chronic effect. During the acute phase (2 days post-thrombosis), C-C motif chemokine ligand 2 or CCL-2 (the mouse equivalent to human monocyte chemotactic protein-1 [MCP-1]) was significantly decreased in the group where circulating IL-6 was blocked. This was demonstrated by the gene expression and protein level [23]. The decrease in CCL-2 caused a reduction in the number of monocytes recruited into the injured area at an intermediate time point (6 days post thrombosis), indicating a dynamic and linked process. At the chronic time point (14 days post thrombosis), a statistically significant decrease in fibrosis was observed in the group treated with anti-IL6 vs. control [23]. This was demonstrated using several methods, including Masson's stain quantification of fibrosis. In summary, we have shown a relationship between IL-6/CCL-2/monocyte recruitment and fibrosis for the first time in the context of VT, exhibiting a potential pathway that started early on in venous thrombosis (VT) and continued to have an impact on chronic VT as well [23]. This is an important step in understanding the link between inflammation and thrombosis in the context of VT and indeed a recent insight into the molecular and cellular contributions to venous thrombosis.

The role of neutrophil extracellular traps (NETs) in acute inflammation was recently described. In addition to their phagocytic and bactericidal functions, activated neutrophils have been shown to release chromatin deoxyribonucleic acid (DNA) and histone containing granular antimicrobial proteins, which form extracellular matrices or traps [24]. The mechanisms regarding neutrophil cell death and the formation of NETs appear to be separate from apoptosis and necrosis and appear to rely upon the formation of intracellular reactive oxygen species [25]. NETs have been shown to kill bacteria while forming a microbial containment barrier [26, 27]. In addition, NETS have been reported to form during sepsis and in inflammatory non-infectious disease states such as small-vessel vasculitis [28, 29].

It was demonstrated that NETs were associated with DVT when using an experimental baboon model of occlusive balloon-induced iliac deep vein thrombosis [30]. Plasma DNA samples collected at baseline were significantly lower than plasma DNA samples collected at 2 and 6 days post-DVT ($p<0.01$) [30]. Furthermore, the rise in plasma DNA kinetics was similar to our previous findings of plasma D-dimers in the same experimental model [31]. In addition to plasma DNA, histologic samples of iliac veins (6 days post-DVT) and controls were stained using an antibody directed toward DNA histone complexes (nuclear origin) and evaluated for the presence of DNA nuclei and extracellular DNA or NETs. Affected vessels demonstrated punctate staining of nuclear DNA and diffuse staining of extracellular DNA compared to controls. Furthermore, immunocolocalization of VWF strings were dispersed within the DNA core and between the DNA core and the vessel wall [30]. These are the first reported results demonstrating that markers of NETs were present in both the plasma and thrombus in experimental DVT. These results provide early evidence regarding the interactions and roles of NETs (DNA and histones), vWF, and platelet binding in venous thrombosis.

Plasminogen Activators and Thrombolysis

Venous thrombosis is a dynamic process with thrombus formation (thrombogenesis) and dissolution (thrombolysis) occurring almost simultaneously under normal conditions in a healthy individual [1]. Thrombolysis depends on multiple physiological processes, including fibrinolysis. In response to thrombus formation, natural anticoagulants such as protein C and protein S have roles in thrombolysis. Similarly, circulating plasminogen is activated to plasmin, which is the main fibrinolytic enzyme [11]. Plasmin's main substrates include fibrin, fibrinogen, and other coagulation factors. In addition, plasmin interferes with vWF-mediated platelet adhesion by proteolysis of GpIb receptor complex [32].

Plasminogen activators are serine proteases that activate plasminogen by the proteolytic cleavage of a single arginine-valine peptide bond. Plasminogen activator inhibitor type 1 (PAI-1) is the primary inhibitor of the plasminogen activators, both tissue type plasminogen activator (t-PA) and urokinase type plasminogen activator (u-PA), and hence fibrinolysis [11]. PAI-1 is produced by the endothelium but is also secreted in an active form by the liver and adipose tissue. Increased PAI-1 levels are found in various disease states such as cancer, obesity and metabolic syndrome. Thus, the increased occurrence of thrombosis in patients with these conditions has been suggested to be associated with elevated PAI-1 levels. PAI-1 elevation appears to synergize with factor V Leiden genetic abnormalities [11]. It is possible that elevated PAI-1 levels could suppress fibrinolysis and increase thrombosis, hence increasing the clinical manifestations of DVT. However, studies on the role of elevated levels of PAI-1 to venous thrombosis have been contradictory [33].

Polymorphism in the PAI-1 gene has been suggested to be associated with an increased risk of VTE. Human studies have evaluated the role of genetic polymorphisms, particularly the 4 G/5 G insertion/deletion in the promoter region, which affects transcription rates. The highest levels of PAI-1 have been noted in those individuals carrying the 4 G/4 G polymorphism. Akar et al. reported an increased risk of DVT (odds ratio 5.5) in individuals with the 4 G allele polymorphism. This risk of DVT was even greater when the 4 G polymorphism coexisted with factor-V-Leiden deficiency [34]. Another study by Zoller et al., showed an increased risk of PAI-1 elevation (odds ratio 8.14) in individuals carrying the 4 G polymorphism in combination with other thrombophilic markers. The risk of PE development was increased in individuals with the 4 G/4 G polymorphism and protein S deficiency (odds ratio 4.5) [35].

Fibrin degradation products (FDPs) result from the action of plasmin on deposited fibrin. FDPs include fragments E and fragment D, which, during physiological thrombolysis, are released as a covalently linked dimer, the D-dimer [11]. Clinically, testing of circulating D-dimer is used as a surrogate maker for diagnosis of ongoing DVT and/or PE. In addition, the presence of elevated D-dimer levels after successful treatment of DVT has a high positive predictive value for recurrent DVT [11]. In patients with suspected disseminated intravascular coagulation, D-dimer levels may also aid in the diagnosis.

Platelet-activating factor (PAF) and endothelin-1 (ET-1) play a role in thrombogenesis. PAF, also known as PAF-acether or acetyl-glyceryl-ether-phosphorylcholine (AGEPC), is a potent phospholipid activator and mediator of many leukocyte functions, including platelet aggregation, inflammation, and anaphylaxis. In addition, ET-1 is a 21-amino-acid peptide produced in a variety of tissues including endothelial and smooth muscle cells. Functions of ET-1 include binding to ET-1 receptors on the vascular smooth muscle, which are Gq-proteins, inducing increased inositol 1,4,5 phosphate levels, leading to calcium release and subsequent muscle contraction. Although an association between ET-1 and platelet activation has been suggested, the data remain unclear [36].

Thrombus Resolution and Vein Wall Remodeling

DVT resolution is a fibrotic process that mimics wound healing. This process involves profibrotic growth factors, collagen deposition, and matrix metalloproteinase (MMP) expression and activation [13, 37]. The kinetics of the leukocyte in the vein wall follows the same pattern of that observed in the thrombus. Thus, immediately after thrombus formation, an early influx of polymorphonuclear (PMN) cells is followed by monocyte migration. Leukocyte migration from the vein lumen into the wall and into the thrombus follows a specific sequence of events leading to thrombus resolution [11].

The first cell type that migrates into the thrombus is the PMN leukocyte. PMNs are essential for early thrombus resolution as they promote both fibrinolysis and collagenolysis [11]. In support of this concept, a study using a rat model of stasis DVT showed that neutropenia was associated with increased thrombus size at 2 and 7 days, increased intrathrombus collagen deposition, and significantly low intrathrombus levels of both uPA and MMP-9 [38].

The second cell type observed in the thrombus is the monocyte. Monocytes are important cells in later thrombus resolution. Monocyte influx into the thrombus is detected at day 8 after thrombus generation and correlates with elevated MCP-1 levels, a CC chemokine that promotes monocyte chemotaxis and activation. MCP-1 has been associated with DVT resolution [11]. In a study using a mouse model of stasis-induced thrombosis, late thrombus resolution was tested using target-deleted CC receptor-2 (CCR-2 KO) mice. In this study, late impairment of thrombus resolution appeared to be due to impaired MMP-2 and MMP-9 activity [11]. This situation was reversible with the administration of exogenous interferon gamma (INF-γ), in part attributable to recovery of MMP-2 and MMP-9 activities without an increase in thrombus monocyte influx [39].

Thrombus resolution involves a number of proinflammatory factors that are released into the local environment. These factors include IL-1 beta (IL-1β) and tumor necrosis factor (TNF)-alpha [11]. It has been suggested that these mediators are released by leukocytes and smooth muscle cells found within the resolving thrombus, although the specific mechanisms involved in this process are yet to be elucidated [13]. Henke et al. observed that elastinolysis occurred at early time points in a mouse model of stasis-induced DVT. In this model, the occurrence of elastinolysis was determined by an increase in vein wall stiffness. Elastinolysis persisted for 14 days, along with elevated MMP-2 and MMP-9 activities. In the same model, early vein wall collagenolysis was observed within the first 7 days, representing an acute response to injury [39].

The elevation of profibrotic mediators, including transforming growth factor (TGF)-beta, IL-13, and MCP-1, has been associated with early biomechanical injury during DVT. These mediators are present in the vein wall and thrombus and may drive the fibrotic response. Exogenous MCP-1 may accelerate DVT resolution, but it also promotes organ fibrosis in vivo. TGFβ is also present in the thrombus and is activated during thrombolysis. This factor appears to be a key mechanism promoting vein wall fibrosis. In mice, late fibrosis has been associated with a significant increase in vein wall collagen after stasis thrombogenesis [40]. Increased gene expression and activity of collagen I and III, MMP-2, and MMP-9 have also been observed. Thus, vein wall injury is associated with active matrix remodeling, which seems to promote net fibrosis [40].

We demonstrated that inhibition of the inflammatory response can decrease vein wall fibrosis [23]. These data add to the evidence of the close interaction between inflammation and fibrosis [23]. In another study using an IVC stenosis model in rats, animals were treated with either low-molecular-weight heparin or an oral P-selectin inhibitor 2 days after thrombus initiation. In this study, the P-selectin inhibitor significantly decreased vein wall injury (independent of thrombus size), which was assessed by vein wall tensiometry (stiffness), intimal thickness score, IL-13 levels, MCP-1 levels, and platelet-derived growth factor-β (PDGFβ) levels [41].

In addition, we recently demonstrated a link between hyperlipidemia and DVT and its effects in both fibrinolysis and vein wall remodeling [37]. An association was found between hyperlipidemia and high levels of PAI-1 in ApoE KO mice, leading to the production of a larger thrombus compared to controls [37]. Also, decreased levels of uPA production in ApoE KO mice was noted, leading to decreased levels of MMP-2 and 9, MCP-1 and monocyte recruitment, which are all key participants in vein wall remodeling [37]. These results are the first to demonstrate that hyperlipidemia and DVT are linked and, in the context of hyperlipidemia, both fibrinolysis and vein wall remodeling are impaired [37].

Furthermore, we found that levels of PAI-1 (circulating PAI-1, vein wall PAI-1 and Liver PAI-1) were significantly decreased in ApoE KO hylperlipidemic mice treated with rosuvastatin compared to controls, suggesting a profibrinolytic effect of rosuvastatin [42] and might be responsible for the protective effect of rosuvastatin on DVT positive patients [43].

In summary, thrombus resolution and vein wall remodeling are complex processes that vary with the degree of thrombus burden and age (chronicity). Novel therapeutic approaches aimed at alleviating post-thrombotic cell wall damage will need to be directed at the sequence of events occurring at the vein wall:thrombus interface over time.

Acknowledgments The author's would like to thank Dr. Katherine Shuster for her careful edits of this book chapter. Financial support was obtained from the Jobst Foundation Grant (to JAD and DDM).

Conflicts of Interest The authors have no conflicts of interest to disclose.

References

1. Kitchens CS, Alving BM, Kessler CM. Consultative hemostasis and thrombosis. Philadelphia: W.B. Saunders Co.; 2002.
2. Silverstein MD, Heit JA, Mohr DN, Petterson TM, O'Fallon WM, Melton 3rd LJ. Trends in the incidence of deep vein thrombosis and pulmonary embolism: a 25-year population-based study. Arch Intern Med. 1998;158(6):585–93.
3. Heit JA. The epidemiology of venous thromboembolism in the community: implications for prevention and management. J Thromb Thrombolysis. 2006;21(1):23–9.
4. Heit JA, Cohen AT, Anderson Jr FA, on Behalf of the VTE Impact Assessment Group. Estimated annual number of incident and recurrent, non-fatal and fatal Venous Thromboembolism (VTE) Events in the US (abstract). Blood. 2005;106(11):910.
5. Virchow R. Gesammelte Abhandlungen zur Wissenschaftlichen Medicin, vol. 520–525. Frankfurt: A M Von Meidinger Sohn; 1856.
6. Stewart GJ, Ritchie WG, Lynch PR. Venous endothelial damage produced by massive sticking and emigration of leukocytes. Am J Pathol. 1974;74(3):507–32.
7. Sacher RA. Thrombophilia: a genetic predisposition to thrombosis. Trans Am Clin Climatol Assoc. 1999;110:51–60; discussion 61.
8. Schulman S, Lindmarker P, Holmstrom M, Larfars G, Carlsson A, Nicol P, et al. Post-thrombotic syndrome, recurrence, and death 10 years after the first episode of venous thromboembolism treated with warfarin for 6 weeks or 6 months. J Thromb Haemost. 2006;4(4):734–42.
9. McRae S, Tran H, Schulman S, Ginsberg J, Kearon C. Effect of patient's sex on risk of recurrent venous thromboembolism: a meta-analysis. Lancet. 2006;368(9533):371–8.
10. Cushman M, Tsai AW, White RH, Heckbert SR, Rosamond WD, Enright P, et al. Deep vein thrombosis and pulmonary embolism in two cohorts: the longitudinal investigation of thromboembolism etiology. Am J Med. 2004;117(1):19–25.
11. Wakefield TW, Myers DD, Henke PK. Mechanisms of venous thrombosis and resolution. Arterioscler Thromb Vasc Biol. 2008;28(3):387–91.
12. Stanley JC, Veith FJ, Wakefield TW (editors) Current Therapy in Vascular and Endovascular Surgery, 5th edition. Elsevier (in press).
13. Deroo S, Deatrick KB, Henke PK. The vessel wall: a forgotten player in post thrombotic syndrome. Thromb Haemost. 2010;104(4):681–92.
14. Myers Jr D, Farris D, Hawley A, Wrobleski S, Chapman A, Stoolman L, et al. Selectins influence thrombosis in a mouse model of experimental deep venous thrombosis. J Surg Res. 2002;108(2):212–21.
15. Wagner DD, Frenette PS. The vessel wall and its interactions. Blood. 2008;111(11):5271–81.
16. Andre P, Hartwell D, Hrachovinova I, Saffaripour S, Wagner DD. Pro-coagulant state resulting from high levels of soluble P-selectin in blood. Proc Natl Acad Sci USA. 2000;97(25):13835–40.
17. Ahn ER, Lander G, Jy W, Bidot CJ, Jimenez JJ, Horstman LL, et al. Differences of soluble CD40L in sera and plasma: implications on CD40L assay as a marker of thrombotic risk. Thromb Res. 2004;114(2):143–8.
18. Satta N, Toti F, Feugeas O, Bohbot A, Dachary-Prigent J, Eschwege V, et al. Monocyte vesiculation is a possible mechanism for dissemination of membrane-associated procoagulant activities and adhesion molecules after stimulation by lipopolysaccharide. J Immunol. 1994;153(7):3245–55.
19. Myers DD, Wakefield TW. Inflammation-dependent thrombosis. Front Biosci. 2005;10:2750–7.
20. Pluskota E, Woody NM, Szpak D, Ballantyne CM, Soloviev DA, Simon DI, et al. Expression, activation, and function of integrin alphaMbeta2 (Mac-1) on neutrophil-derived microparticles. Blood. 2008;112(6):2327–35.
21. Andrews RK, Berndt MC. Microparticles facilitate neutrophil/platelet crosstalk. Blood. 2008;112(6):2174–5.
22. Osanai T, Akutsu N, Fujita N, Nakano T, Takahashi K, Guan W, et al. Cross talk between prostacyclin and nitric oxide under shear in smooth muscle cell: role in monocyte adhesion. Am J Physiol Heart Circ Physiol. 2001;281(1):H177–82.
23. Wojcik BM, Wrobleski SK, Hawley AE, Wakefield TW, Myers Jr DD, Diaz JA. Interleukin-6: a potential target for post-thrombotic syndrome. Ann Vasc Surg. 2011;25(2):229–39.
24. Brinkmann V, Reichard U, Goosmann C, Fauler B, Uhlemann Y, Weiss DS, et al. Neutrophil extracellular traps kill bacteria. Science. 2004;303(5663):1532–5.
25. Fuchs TA, Abed U, Goosmann C, Hurwitz R, Schulze I, Wahn V, et al. Novel cell death program leads to neutrophil extracellular traps. J Cell Biol. 2007;176(2):231–41.
26. Papayannopoulos V, Zychlinsky A. NETs: a new strategy for using old weapons. Trends Immunol. 2009;30(11):513–21.
27. Wartha F, Henriques-Normark B. ETosis: a novel cell death pathway. Sci Signal. 2008;1(21):e25.
28. Kessenbrock K, Krumbholz M, Schonermarck U, Back W, Gross WL, Werb Z, et al. Netting neutrophils in autoimmune small-vessel vasculitis. Nat Med. 2009;15(6):623–5.
29. Clark SR, Ma AC, Tavener SA, McDonald B, Goodarzi Z, Kelly MM, et al. Platelet TLR4 activates neutrophil extracellular traps to ensnare bacteria in septic blood. Nat Med. 2007;13(4):463–9.
30. Fuchs TA, Brill A, Duerschmied D, Schatzberg D, Monestier M, Myers Jr DD, et al. Extracellular DNA traps promote thrombosis. Proc Natl Acad Sci USA. 2010;107(36):15880–5.
31. Meier TR, Myers Jr DD, Wrobleski SK, Zajkowski PJ, Hawley AE, Bedard PW, et al. Prophylactic P-selectin inhibition with PSI-421 promotes resolution of venous thrombosis without anticoagulation. Thromb Haemost. 2008;99(2):343–51.
32. Adelman B, Michelson AD, Loscalzo J, Greenberg J, Handin RI. Plasmin effect on platelet glycoprotein Ib-von Willebrand factor interactions. Blood. 1985;65(1):32–40.

33. Crowther MA, Roberts J, Roberts R, Johnston M, Stevens P, Skingley P, et al. Fibrinolytic variables in patients with recurrent venous thrombosis: a prospective cohort study. Thromb Haemost. 2001;85(3):390–4.
34. Akar N, Yilmaz E, Akar E, Avcu F, Yalcin A, Cin S. Effect of plasminogen activator inhibitor-1 4G/5G polymorphism in Turkish deep vein thrombotic patients with and without FV1691 G-A. Thromb Res. 2000;97(4):227–30.
35. Zoller B, Garcia de Frutos P, Dahlback B. A common 4G allele in the promoter of the plasminogen activator inhibitor-1 (PAI-1) gene as a risk factor for pulmonary embolism and arterial thrombosis in hereditary protein S deficiency. Thromb Haemost. 1998;79(4): 802–7.
36. Gresele P. Platelets in thrombotic and non-thrombotic disorders: pathophysiology, pharmacology, and therapeutics. Cambridge/New York: Cambridge University Press; 2002.
37. Diaz JA, Ballard-Lipka NE, Farris DM, Hawley AE, Wrobleski SK, Myers DD, et al. Impaired fibrinolytic system in ApoE gene-deleted mice with hyperlipidemia augments deep vein thrombosis. J Vasc Surg. 2012;55:815–22.
38. Varma MR, Moaveni DM, Dewyer NA, Varga AJ, Deatrick KB, Kunkel SL, et al. Deep vein thrombosis resolution is not accelerated with increased neovascularization. J Vasc Surg. 2004;40(3): 536–42.
39. Henke PK, Pearce CG, Moaveni DM, Moore AJ, Lynch EM, Longo C, et al. Targeted deletion of CCR2 impairs deep vein thrombosis resolution in a mouse model. J Immunol. 2006;177(5): 3388–97.
40. Deatrick KB, Eliason JL, Lynch EM, Moore AJ, Dewyer NA, Varma MR, et al. Vein wall remodeling after deep vein thrombosis involves matrix metalloproteinases and late fibrosis in a mouse model. J Vasc Surg. 2005;42(1):140–8.
41. Myers Jr DD, Henke PK, Bedard PW, Wrobleski SK, Kaila N, Shaw G, et al. Treatment with an oral small molecule inhibitor of P selectin (PSI-697) decreases vein wall injury in a rat stenosis model of venous thrombosis. J Vasc Surg. 2006;44(3):625–32.
42. Patterson KA, Zhang X, Wrobleski SK, Hawley AE, Lawrence DA, Wakefield TW, et al. Rosuvastatin reduced deep vein thrombosis in ApoE gene deleted mice with hyperlipidemia through non-lipid lowering effects. Thromb Res. 2012 Dec 28 (in press).
43. Glynn RJ, Danielson E, Fonseca FA, Genest J, Gotto AM, Jr, Kastelein JJ, et al. A randomized trial of rosuvastatin in the prevention of venous thromboembolism. N Engl J Med. 2009;360(18): 1851–1861.

Varicose Veins: Venous Wall Changes, Inflammation, and Matrix Metalloproteinases

22

Joseph D. Raffetto

Introduction

Varicose veins are superficial vessels that are abnormally twisted, lengthened, or dilated, and they are usually caused by inefficient or defective valves within the vein. Varicose veins are part of the spectrum of chronic venous diseases (CVDs), which affect millions of people throughout Western populations [1]. There is significant evidence in the literature that wall dysfunction consisting of alterations in the endothelium and smooth muscle cells (SMCs) are a principal cause for varicose veins [2]. In addition, matrix metalloproteinases (MMPs) are present in varicose veins and can be found in the endothelium, smooth muscle, and adventitial layers of the vein wall [3]. However, it is unclear whether the presence of MMPs is a result of chronic inflammation and venous wall remodeling or whether MMPs actually functional in veins, causing biochemical changes in the venous wall leading to early dilation and chronic irreversible changes typified by varicose veins [2]. Furthermore, the role of venous wall dysfunction appears to precede valve dysfunction, is linked to MMPs [2], and is tightly regulated by hypoxia inducible factor.

Basic Scientific Evidence for Primary Vein Wall Changes

In an early study, investigators evaluated the collagen and elastin content of the nonthrombophlebitic greater saphenous varicose vein and normal-appearing saphenous vein in proximity to the same segment of vein containing the varicose vein, and they compared the varicose vein to normal control saphenous veins. The study found an increase in collagen, a significant decrease in elastin, and an increased collagen:elastin ratio in both varicose veins and competent "normal" saphenous vein segments that were adjacent to the varicosities compared with the normal control saphenous vein. This study demonstrated that in patients with varicose veins, collagen and elastin changes were present, but, importantly, normal-appearing saphenous veins in proximity to varicose veins also demonstrated connective tissue changes in the venous wall. These findings support the notion that vein wall changes precede valvular insufficiency [4]. Other human studies have corroborated these findings. In an interesting study using duplex ultrasound-evaluated segments of varicose veins of the greater saphenous vein, saphenous vein segments had a dilated varicosity that was proximal to a competent venous valve and adjacent to a normal-appearing distal vein segment. The study evaluated the rigidity of the vein wall, matrix fibers, and elastin in the varicose vein and compared it to the continuous normal-appearing vein. It was demonstrated that the rigidity was the same in both the proximal varicose vein and normal distal saphenous vein, and both vein segments had increased matrix fibers and fragmented elastin. It was concluded that the role of the venous valve dysfunction leading to reflux in varicose veins is secondary to the primary changes that occur in the wall [5]. The same investigators evaluated the matrix proteins in the wall of varicose veins in 372 specimens and compared them to normal control veins in 36 specimens. The varicose veins demonstrated a significant increase in wall matrix proteins, including collagen, laminin, and tenascin, and a nearly significant increase in fibronectin (Table 22.1). Importantly, in patients with varicose vein, the normal-appearing segments of vein just inferior to the varicose vein had the same biochemical profile as the adjacent varicose vein [6]. This study provided further evidence that alterations of structural proteins in the vein wall occur in normal-appearing veins taken from contiguous segments of a varicose vein and precede the changes of venous valve reflux during varicose vein formation.

J.D. Raffetto, MD, MS, FACS, FSVM
Division of Vascular and Endovascular Surgery, Brigham and Women's Hospital, Harvard Medical School, Boston, MA, USA

Department of Surgery, 112, VA Boston Healthcare System, 1400 VFW Parkway, West Roxbury, MA 02132, USA
e-mail: joseph.raffetto@med.va.gov

E.A. Gabriel, S.A. Gabriel (eds.), *Inflammatory Response in Cardiovascular Surgery*,
DOI 10.1007/978-1-4471-4429-8_22, © Springer-Verlag London 2013

Table 22.1 Structural protein alterations in varicose vein wall and in the smooth muscle cells (SMC) of varicose veins

Protein	Varicose vein[a]
Vein wall collagen	Increased
Vein wall elastin	Decreased
Vein wall laminin	Increased
Vein wall tenascin	Increased
Vein wall fibronectin	Similar
SMC collagen type I	Increased
SMC collagen type III	Decreased
SMC collagen type IV	Similar
SMC fibronectin	Decreased

[a]Indicates relative to normal control veins

Vein Wall Inflammation, SMC Dysfunction, MMP Expression, and Venous Dilation

A significant finding in varicose veins is the role of inflammation as a consequence of inflammatory cell infiltrate. Several studies have evaluated inflammatory cells and activation in varicose veins and normal control veins. In human saphenous vein specimens from patients with CVD, an increased number of monocytes/macrophage infiltration in the venous wall and valves was demonstrated. The inflammatory invasion is an important step in the events leading to inflammation, cytokine and proteinase production, and structural changes in the vein wall architecture. Elevated intercellular adhesion molecule-1 (ICAM-1), a marker of activation of leukocytes to adhere to the endothelium, has also been detected in CVD vein specimens, but not in normal veins [7]. This would suggest that certain predisposing factors and/or stimuli cause the vein endothelium to express ICAM-1, leading to leukocyte activation and infiltration, with further inflammatory responses that initiate the release of cytokines and MMPs. In fact, a study evaluating patients with venous hypertension demonstrated that there was sequestration of activated neutrophils and monocytes in the microcirculation. This persisted even after elevating the limbs and decreasing the venous hypertension, which indicated that leukocytes were adhering to the endothelium [8]. In another interesting study, plasma collected from patients with CVD caused significant granulocyte activation, which was more prominent in advanced stages of CVD (skin changes and ulcer). In addition, there was increased hydrogen peroxide production from activated granulocytes in the patient's plasma than the control patient plasma [9]. These data suggested the presence of a circulating activating factor in the plasma of patients with CVD, which could activate the ICAM-1 on endothelium, initiating the early events that may be important in the pathophysiology of CVD and varicose veins.

Immunohistochemical studies of SMC cultured from varicose veins were found to have a decreased number of cells staining for collagen type III and fibronectin compared to control veins, although the transcriptional products (same amount of mRNA product) of these two proteins were not dissimilar in varicose veins versus control vein. In addition, the synthesis and deposition of collagen type III but not type I were significantly lower in varicose veins. When matrix metalloproteinases (MMPs) -1, -2, and -9 and the natural tissue inhibitors of MMPs (TIMPs) -1 and -2 were analyzed from the supernatant of confluent SMC, no differences were observed. These data suggested that the regulation as well as changes for both collagen type III and fibronectin in SMC was a post-transcriptional event [10]. Although there was no difference in MMP and TIMP in the supernatant tested, this did not exclude the possibility that altered expression, activity and other types of MMPs exist in whole tissues including TIMP. Further work in this area demonstrated that varicose greater saphenous vein had a smaller spiraled collagen distribution specifically in the intima and media. To investigate the latter findings, the same investigators demonstrated that inhibition of MMP with marimastat (BB-2516, non-selective MMP inhibitor) resulted in partial restoration in the production of collagen type III in smooth muscle cells from varicose veins. In addition, MMP-3, which degrades fibronectin, was elevated in both its transcription product and protein expression. It was concluded that the mechanism involved in collagen type III and fibronectin degradation in the smooth muscle cells cultured from varicose veins is likely linked to the expression of MMP-3 and its proteinase activity [11]. The important properties of type III collagen in blood vessels is the ability to provide elasticity and distensibility. The abnormal production of type III collagen in both SMC cultured from varicose veins and fibroblasts cultured from dermal biopsies of patients with CVD raises the possibility that varicose veins' pathology may arise from abnormal matrix collagen deposition and is likely a systemic disease [12]. Furthermore, to identify factors involved in abnormal elasticity and distensibility in varicose veins, a study evaluated the content of hydroxyproline and quantified collagen types I, III, and V. It was found that in both SMC and fibroblast of patients with varicose veins, as compared to control, had an increase in hydroxyproline content, indicating increased collagen; however, the proportion of collagen type III was significantly reduced despite normal mRNA transcript. These data were consistent with previous reports and offered an explanation for the loss of distensibility and elasticity in varicose veins; they suggested that the defect is generalized, supporting a genetic basis for the alterations observed in patients' varicose veins [13]. Taken together, these findings suggest that at least in cultured SMC from varicose vein, there is an imbalance of collagen production with dysregulation and increased type I collagen but reduced type III collagen production. Because of normal expression of mRNA for type III collagen, the reduction in synthesis is related to post-transcriptional events. The inhibition of type III collagen synthesis could be a result of degradation/inhibition by MMP-3 and may explain changes in the mechanical properties of the vein wall leading to inappropriate elasticity and distensibility, which results in varicose vein formation. Finally, the similar abnormalities found in dermal cultured fibroblasts indicate that the problem of varicose veins is a systemic disease, likely with genetic factors involved.

Localization of MMPs and Significance, Models of Venous Hypertension and MMP Activation, MMP Modulation by Flavonoids

A possible explanation for venous dilation and tortuosity may be the influences of MMPs and TIMPs, which lead to venous wall remodeling and subsequent dilatation and valve incompetence. Several authors have found an increased expression, localization, and activity of MMPs in the venous segments of varicose veins and in veins with thrombophlebitis compared to control veins [3, 14, 15]. It is unclear whether MMPs are present because of a secondary process due to cellular inflammatory infiltration and wall remodeling or directly involved in the formation of varicose veins. The question is how MMPs cause venous dilation and varicose vein formation. The role of MMPs in varicose vein has largely been attributed to their proteolytic effects on extracellular matrix (ECM), degradation of the valve leaflets, and weakening of vein wall structure [16, 17]. The localization of MMPs in the varicose vein wall adventitia and fibroblast is consistent with a role in ECM degradation [15]. However, in varicose veins, MMPs have also been localized in the vicinity of the endothelium and SMC [15, 18], raising the possibility of additional effects of MMPs on these cell types. Other studies have investigated the ratio of TIMP-1/MMP-2 and found a threefold ratio increase in varicose veins compared to normal veins, concluding that proteolytic inhibition and ECM accumulation may account for the pathogenesis of varicose veins [19].

Animal models of venous hypertension utilizing a femoral artery and vein fistula in the rat have demonstrated an increased sustained venous pressure above 90 mmHg with significant abnormal structural changes in the vein valve and wall. In addition, there was significant expression of MMP-2 and MMP-9 at 6 weeks [20]. In a similar animal model, untreated veins developed venous hypertension with reflux and morphologic changes in the vein wall and valve, but in veins treated with the flavonoid Dalfon, which reduces inflammation by modulating inflammatory cells, there were reduced physiologic and anatomic changes in the vein wall and valves as a response to venous hypertension [21]. Importantly, these two latter studies demonstrated the feasibility of a venous hypertensive model, the implications of MMPs, and how certain drugs may alter the effects of inflammation on the vein wall to maintain valve function and reduced venous wall destruction.

MMPs and Effects on Endothelial and SMC Venous Function

It is possible that MMPs may have acute and chronic effects on the vein wall. Early changes may cause functional and metabolic changes to the vein wall, while the later effects of MMPs may alter wall matrix composition to such an extent that dilation and tortuousity becomes the prominent morphological feature [2]. In recent studies, evidence for how MMPs acutely influence venous wall dilation was determined. In a rat inferior vena cava (IVC) model where exogenous MMP-2 was added, changes in vein wall contraction resulting in relaxation was recorded. MMP-2 caused time-dependent venous relaxation in phenylephrine-contracted IVC. However, MMP-2-induced venous relaxation was essentially abolished in 96 mmol/l KCl depolarizing solution, which prevents outward movement of K^+ ions from the cell through K^+ channels, which is necessary during venous relaxation in hyperpolarized vascular tissue. In order to define which K^+ channels were involved, the investigators tested the effects of K^+ channel agonists and antagonists on MMP-2-induced venous relaxation. MMP-2 caused further relaxation of vein segments in the presence of activators of the ATP-sensitive potassium (K_{ATP}) channel, indicating that MMP-2 was not working through the K_{ATP} channel during cell hyperpolarization (a condition of negative membrane potential caused by outward potassium ion movement leading to smooth muscle cell relaxation and resulting in venous relaxation). In contrast, blockade of the large conductance Ca^{2+}-dependent K^+ channels (BK_{Ca}) with iberiotoxin significantly inhibited the MMP-2 effect on venous relaxation, suggesting that MMP-2 actions in part involve hyperpolarization by activation of BK_{Ca}. MMP-2 induced activation of K^+ channels likely causes SMC hyperpolarization and leads to decreased Ca^{2+} influx through voltage-gated channels [22]. In addition, it was determined that nitric oxide (NO) was abundant in acetylcholine-stimulated IVC. However, in the presence of MMP-2, there was no measurable increase of NO, indicating that the NO-cGMP pathway was not stimulated by MMP-2-induced relaxation. In addition, using inhibitors of the NO-cGMP (L-NAME) and PGI_2-cAMP (indomethicin) pathways did not cause inhibition of MMP-2-induced relaxation of phenylephrine-contracted IVC, indicating that the MMP-2 mechanism likely involves hyperpolarization, resulting in venous dilation [22, 23]. Taken together, these data demonstrated a novel effect of MMPs on venous tissue function and suggest that protracted MMP-2 induced venous relaxation could lead to progressive venous dilatation, possibly influencing the venous wall before changes in the valve occur, and leading to varicose vein formation [22].

In the same rat IVC and venous isometric contraction apparatus, it was determined that MMP-2 attenuates $[Ca^{2+}]_e$-dependent vascular smooth muscle (VSM) contraction (by inhibiting Ca^{2+} entry into the smooth muscle) without affecting Ca^{2+} release from intracellular Ca^{2+} stores. In addition, in an effort to determine the mechanism of MMP-2 induced vasorelaxation, it was found that MMP-2 induced VSM relaxation does not involve the generation of RGD or activation of $\alpha_v\beta_3$ integrin receptor (RGD contains the Arg-Gly-Asp tripeptide known to activate integrin receptors and lead to membrane hyperpolarization). From this study, it was concluded that MMP-2-induced inhibition of the Ca^{2+} entry mechanism of VSM contraction may play a role in the venous dilation associated with varicose vein formation [24].

From previous data, it is known that MMPs are found in the wall of varicose vein [3, 14, 15] and that MMP-2 can cause venous relaxation by hyperpolarization [2]. However, the relation among venous pressure, MMP expression, and venous dysfunction is unclear. A study to test the hypothesis that prolonged increases in vein wall tension cause overexpression of MMPs and decreased contractility, which in turn promote venous dilation, was performed in rat IVC. The results demonstrated that increases in the magnitude and duration (2-g for 24 h) of wall tension were associated with reduced contraction and overexpression of MMP-2 and -9. There was a direct correlation between the expression of MMP-2 and -9 with a decrease vein contractile function. These responses were partially reversible with MMP inhibitors. Importantly, the key factor was the amount of tension applied since tissues exposed to 0-g tension for 24 h had normal contraction. Taken together, MMP-2 (as well as MMP-9) promotes IVC relaxation, indicating that protracted increases in venous pressure and wall tension increase MMPs expression, which in turn reduces venous contraction and leads to progressive venous dilation (Fig. 22.1) [25].

An important question is what regulates the induction of MMPs during venous stretch and dilation. A possible mechanism may involve hypoxia-inducible factors (HIF), which are nuclear transcriptional factors of heterodimeric protein consisting of α and β subunits. HIF expression may be oxygen or non-oxygen dependent including mechanical stretch. The importance of HIFs is that they regulate the transcription of several target genes of oxygen homeostasis including remodeling of the ECM [26, 27]. In a recently published study evaluating rat IVC and an ex-vivo model of stretch and the induction of HIF and MMPs, the main study findings were that phenylephrine-induced and KCl-induced contraction was restored in IVCs exposed to prolonged 2-g tension plus the HIF inhibitor (UO126 and echinomycin). However, treatment with DMOG, which stabilizes the HIF molecule, further reduced phenylephrine-induced and KCl-induced contraction in veins subjected to prolonged 2-g tension. HIF-1α and HIF-2α mRNA was overexpressed in IVC exposed to

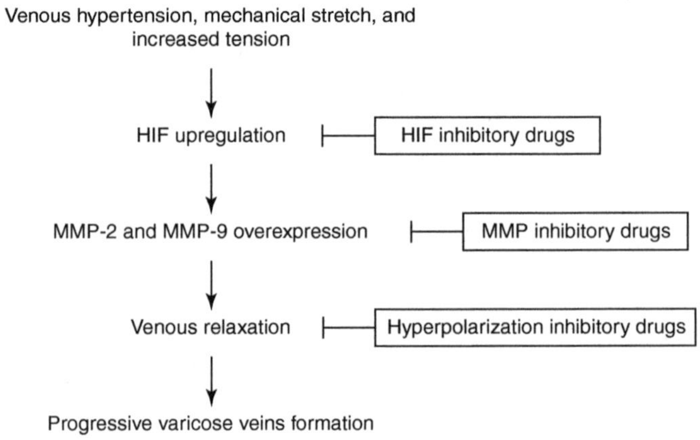

Fig. 22.1 Progressive venous hypertension causing increased mechanical stretch and tension on the vein wall induces overexpression of HIF-1α and HIF-2α. HIF molecule via non-hypoxic conditions promotes MMP-2 and MMP-9 mRNA and protein levels to increase. MMP-2 causes venous relaxation via hyperpolarization. At different stages of the venous-hypertension cascade, a variety of inhibitors (|—) are available that may have potential as therapeutic targets for preventing varicose vein formation

prolonged 2-g tension, and the overexpression was reversed by the inhibitors (UO126, echinomycin, and 17-DMAG) of HIF. In addition, the overexpression of HIF-1α and HIF-2α stretched IVC was associated with increased MMP-2 and MMP-9 mRNA and protein in IVC subjected to prolonged 2-g wall tension, but was reversed by the inhibitors (UO126, echinomycin, and 17-DMAG) of HIF, with a decrease in expression of MMP-2 and MMP-9. The authors concluded from the study that prolonged increases in vein wall tension are associated with overexpression of HIF-1α and HIF-2α, increased MMP-2 and MMP-9 expression, and reduced venous contraction in rat IVCs (Fig. 22.1). This study elucidated the mechanism and relation of HIF and MMPs, indicating that increased vein wall tension induces HIF overexpression and causes an increase in MMP expression and reduction of venous contraction, leading to progressive venous dilation, and it may be a cause in varicose vein formation. As with targeting MMPs and hyperpolarization-induced relaxation, specific inhibitors aiming at HIF regulation may be important in the future study of varicose veins [28].

Drugs for the Treatment of Varicose Veins

Because MMPs and the HIF pathway are linked to the pathogenesis of varicose veins, interest in modulating drugs for possible clinical treatment is an area of research. There are a number of selective and non-selective inhibitory drugs against MMPs. The drugs classes consists of tissue inhibitors of MMPs (TIMP-1,2,3,4), hydroxamates (Batimastat [BB-94], Marimastat [BB-2516]), carboxylates (BAY12-9566, compound 12c,d, compound 22, PGE-2909492), thiols (compound 4a–k, compound 5a–c, compound 36a,b), aminomethyl benzimidazole analogs, tetraclyclines (doxycycline, minocycline), monoclonal antibodies (REGA-3G12, REGA-2D9, REGA-2F9, REGA-1G8), siRNA, and other synthetic drugs (Ro 28-2653, Ro 32-3555 [Trocade]). The affinity of these drugs to substrate are moderate/high (tetracylines, hydroxamates, thiols) to very high (TIMPs), and the effective dose concentrations are in the micromolar to picomolar range, respectively. The major limitations of these drugs is broad-spectrum inhibition, low specificity, toxicity, and cross reactivity with other proteins [29]. Many of these drugs are used in the laboratory for research purposes, and very few have been tried clinically (tretracycline in venous ulcer treatment) given their limitations. Although saponosides (horse chestnut seed extract, escin) and flavonoids (Daflon), which have anti-inflammatory properties, have been used clinically to treat patients with active venous disorders, to date no studies evaluating these drugs have been carried out with the intention to actually prevent de-novo, progression, or recurrent varicose veins [29].

Inhibitors of HIF (U0126, 17-[2-(dimethylamino)ethyl] amino-17-desmethoxygeldanamycin [17-DMAG], or echinomycin), which target different levels of HIF activation, stabilization and translocation into the nucleus, and DNA binding, are exclusively used in laboratory experimentation [28].

Various K^+ channel agonists leading to hyperpolarization and smooth muscle relaxation have been used to treat hypertension both experimentally and clinically [30]. However, the spectrum of K^+ channels is found in both arteries and veins, and given that we want to reverse the process of venous relaxation, non-selective K^+ channel inhibitors would affect both systems in non-hypertensive patients with varicose veins with possible unwanted and dangerous side effects. To date, no studies have evaluated the effectiveness of K^+ channel blockade to treat varicose vein disease, and future studies to identify selective venous K^+ channels blockers are required before treatment of varicose veins can occur clinically.

Conclusions

Varicose vein SMCs have an important abnormality in collagen type III and fibronectin protein production, and the events are related to post-transcription events involving MMP-3. Importantly, patients with varicose veins have a systemic abnormality in collagen synthesis that not only affects the SMC of the vein but also the fibroblast from dermis. These findings suggest a genetic cause for varicose vein development and certainly are consistent with cross-sectional population based studies suggesting that varicose veins have an underlying yet unidentified genetic cause [31]. The endothelium plays an important part and likely initiates the early events with inflammation and expression of ICAM-1 leading to infiltration of leukocytes in the venous wall. These events have been studied in an AV-fistula rat model with important findings of venous wall and valve degeneration, with expression of both MMP-2 and MMP-9. Flavonoids may offer therapeutic benefit with decreasing venous wall changes, but further investigation is necessary to evaluate long-term use of these drugs. MMPs play a critical role in ECM turnover, but also have variable functions both early and late in the venous wall vasodilatory effects and degradation of venous wall, respectively. Basic scientific study has elucidated one possible mechanism involving MMP-2 in venous dilation, which involves hyperpolarization. The distension of veins is associated with the overexpression of MMPs and is tightly regulated by HIF molecules. The understanding of the molecular mechanism involving MMPs and venous wall dilation provides an avenue for new pharmacologic therapies. Future studies to define preventative drugs in patients at risk for varicose vein formation, progression, and recurrences will offer important advantages in the treatment of a disease that affects millions of people worldwide.

References

1. Bergan JJ, Schmid-Schonbein GW, Coleridge Smith PD, Nicolaides AN, Boisseau MR, Eklof B. Chronic venous disease. N Engl J Med. 2006;355:488–98.
2. Raffetto JD, Khalil RA. Mechanisms of varicose vein formation: valve dysfunction and wall dilation. Phlebology. 2008;23:85–98.
3. Kowalewski R, Sobolewski K, Wolanska M, Gacko M. Matrix metalloproteinases in the vein wall. Int Angiol. 2004;23:164–9.
4. Gandhi RH, Irizarry E, Neckman GB, Halpern VJ, Mulcare RJ, Tilson MD. Analysis of the connective tissue matrix and proteolytic activity of primary varicose veins. J Vasc Surg. 1993;20:814–20.
5. Kirsch D, Wahl W, Bottger T, Junginger T. Primary varicose veins – changes in the venous wall and elastic behavior. Chirurg. 2000;71:300–5.
6. Kirsch D, Dienes HP, Kuchle R, et al. Changes in the extracellular matrix of the vein wall – the cause of primary varicosis? Vasa. 2000;29:173–7.
7. Takase S, Bergan JJ, Schmid-Shonbein G. Expression of adhesion molecules and cytokines on saphenous veins in chronic venous insufficiency. Ann Vasc Surg. 2000;14:427–35.
8. Saharay M, Shields DA, Porter JB, Scurr JH, Coleridge Smith PD. Leukocyte activity in the microcirculation of the leg in patients with chronic venous disease. J Vasc Surg. 1997;26:265–73.
9. Takase S, Schmid-Shonbein GW, Bergan JJ. Leukocyte activation in patients with venous insufficiency. J Vasc Surg. 1999;30:148–56.
10. Sansilvestri-Morel P, Nonotte I, Fournet-Bourguignon MP, et al. Abnormal deposition of extracellular matrix proteins by cultured smooth muscle cells from human varicose veins. J Vasc Res. 1998;35:115–23.
11. Sansilvestri-Morel P, Rupin A, Jullien ND, et al. Decreased production of collagen type III in cultured smooth muscle cells from varicose vein patients is due to a degradation my MMPs: possible implication of MMP-3. J Vasc Res. 2005;42:388–98.
12. Sansilvestri-Morel P, Rupin A, Jaisson S, Fabiani JN, Verbeuren TJ, Vanhoutte PM. Synthesis of collagen is dysregulated in cultured fibroblasts derived from skin of subjects with varicose veins as it is in venous smooth muscle cells. Circulation. 2002;106:479–83.

13. Sansilvestri-Morel P, Rupin A, Badier-Commander C, Fabiani JN, Verbeuren TJ. Chronic venous insufficiency: dysregulation of collagen synthesis. Angiology. 2003;54 Suppl 1:S3–8.
14. Gillespie DL, Patel A, Fileta B, et al. Varicose veins possess greater quantities of MMP-1 than normal veins and demonstrate regional variation in MMP-1 and MMP-13. J Surg Res. 2002;106:233–8.
15. Woodside KJ, Hu M, Burke A, et al. Morphologic characteristics of varicose veins: possible role of metalloproteinases. J Vasc Surg. 2003;38:162–9.
16. Pascarella L, Penn A, Schmid-Schonbein GW. Venous hypertension and the inflammatory cascade: major manifestations and trigger mechanisms. Angiology. 2005;56:S3–10.
17. Herouy Y, Nockowski P, Schopf E, Norgauer J. Lipodermatosclerosis and the significance of proteolytic remodeling in the pathogenesis of venous ulceration (review). Int J Mol Med. 1999;3:511–5.
18. Thulesius O. The venous wall and valvular function in chronic venous insufficiency. Int Angiol. 1996;15:114–8.
19. Badier-Commander C, Verbeuren T, Lebard C, Michel JB, Jacob MP. Increased TIMP/MMP ratio in varicose veins: a possible explanation for extracellular matrix accumulation. J Pathol. 2000;192:105–12.
20. Takase S, Pascarella L, Bergan JJ, Schmid-Schonbein GW. Hypertension-induced venous valve remodeling. J Vasc Surg. 2004;39:1329–34.
21. Takase S, Pascarella L, Lerond L, Bergan JJ, Schmid-Shonbein GW. Venous hypertension, inflammation and valve remodeling. Eur J Vasc Endovasc Surg. 2004;28:484–93.
22. Raffetto JD, Ross RL, Khalil RA. Matrix metalloproteinase-2 induced venous dilation via hyperpolarization and activation of K+channels. Relevance to varicose vein formation. J Vasc Surg. 2007;45:373–80.
23. Feletou M, Vanhoutte PM. Endothelium-derived hyperpolarizing factor: where are we now? Arterioscler Thromb Vasc Biol. 2006;26:1215–25.
24. Raffetto JD, Khalil RA. MMP-2 induced vein relaxation via inhibition of [Ca2+]e dependent mechanisms of venous smooth muscle contraction. Role of RGD peptides. J Surg Res. 2010;159:755–64.
25. Raffetto JD, Qiao X, Koledova VV, Khalil RA. Prolonged increases in vein wall tension increase matrix metalloproteinases and decrease constriction in rat vena cava. Potential implications in varicose veins. J Vasc Surg. 2008;48:447–56.
26. Semenza GL. Regulation of oxygen homeostasis by hypoxia-inducible factor 1. Physiology (Bethesda). 2009;24:97–106.
27. Semenza GL. Vascular responses to hypoxia and ischemia. Arterioscler Thromb Vasc Biol. 2010;30:648–52.
28. Lim CS, Qiao X, Reslan OM, Xia Y, Raffetto JD, Paleolog E, et al. Prolonged mechanical stretch is associated with upregulation of hypoxia-inducible factors and reduced contraction in rat inferior vena cava. J Vasc Surg. 2011;53:764–73.
29. Raffetto JD, Khalil RA. Matrix metalloproteinases in venous tissue remodeling and varicose vein formation. Curr Vasc Pharmacol. 2008;6:158–72.
30. Feletou M, Kohler R, Vanhoutte PM. Endothelium-derived vasoactive factors and hypertension: possible roles in pathogenesis and as treatment targets. Curr Hypertens Rep. 2010;12:267–75.
31. Cornu-Thenard A, Boivin P, Baud MM, et al. Importance of the familial factor in varicose disease: clinical study of 134 families. J Dermatol Surg Oncol. 1994;20:318–26.

Part VII

Visceral Vasculopathy

Management of Aneurysms in Takayasu's Arteritis

23

Christian Espinoza Silva, Diego Soto Valdés, and Vania Rozas Almeida

Introduction

Takayasu's arteritis (TA) is a chronic inflammatory vascular disease of unknown etiology that affects the aorta, proximal parts of its major branches, and the pulmonary arteries. It is a typical "large-vessel" nonatherosclerotic vasculitis, which can produce vascular stenosis, aneurysm formation, and other presentations in the aorta or affected vessels.

History

Dr. Mikito Takayasu (1860–1938) was the first to describe retinal vascular abnormalities in association with aortitis in 1905 (Fig. 23.1) [1]. The original work, presented by Takayasu at the Annual Meeting of the Japan Ophthalmology Society [2], showed peculiar vessels in the retinal fundus characterized by arteriovenous anastomosis around the papilla in a 22-year-old woman. The curious thing is that Takayasu did not describe the absence of a radial pulse. This sign was described at the same meeting by two other ophthalmologists, Onishi and Kagoshima, who also described patients with ocular findings similar to those of Takayasu, adding that their patients had no radial pulses [3]. In 1761, Morgagni described a 40-year-old woman with multiple stenoses and aneurysms of the great vessels, also reporting the absence of a radial pulse [4].

C.E. Silva, MD, PhD (✉)
Cardiovascular and Heart Transplant Surgeon, Servicio Cardiovascular, National Institute of Thorax, José Manuel Infante 717, Providencia, Santiago, Chile
e-mail: cardiocirugia@gmail.com

D.S. Valdés
Resident of General Surgery, Department of Surgery, University of Santiago of Chile, Santiago, Chile

V.R. Almeida
Servicio Cardiovascular, National Institute of Thorax, José Manuel Infante 717, Providencia, Santiago, Chile

Epidemiology

TA is an uncommon chronic inflammatory vasculitis, with an incidence of 2–3 cases per million population. It mostly young women, with a 9:1 female predominance [3, 5–7], usually Asian women [8]. In fact, TA is responsible for about 5 % of all vascular diseases in India and Japan [9].

Although TA was first described in Asia and is undoubtedly more prevalent among patients in India, Africa, and South America, this disease has a worldwide distribution, with an increasing incidence in Western countries [10].

Pathophysiology

TA most commonly involves the aortic arch and its major branches, but may involve any segment of the aorta. This condition affects the vessel walls, producing medial destruction of the aortic wall with stenosis, occlusion, or aneurysm formation. Although TA usually produces obstructive lesions, it may have a dilative component in 15 % of cases [11], and it is usually associated with disease elsewhere. However, different reports suggest a wide spectrum of prevalence, with aneurysm formation varying from 0 to 87.5 % [12, 13].

Although TA is widely known as a chronic vasculitis that affects large vessels, the intimate processes of the pathophysiology in this clinical picture remain only partially explained because they have not been completely elucidated. For this reason, TA is considered to be a multifactorial disease, with autoimmune mechanisms undoubtedly involved. In 2004, Seko et al. [14] postulated an interesting pathogenic sequence, which we will analyze in more depth. This pathologic sequence may implicate the stimulation from an antigen of unknown nature, possibly infectious, that triggers heat shock protein 65 expression in aortic tissue. This, in turn, would induce the human major histocompatibility complex class I chain-related gene A (MICA) [15].

E.A. Gabriel, S.A. Gabriel (eds.), *Inflammatory Response in Cardiovascular Surgery*, DOI 10.1007/978-1-4471-4429-8_23, © Springer-Verlag London 2013

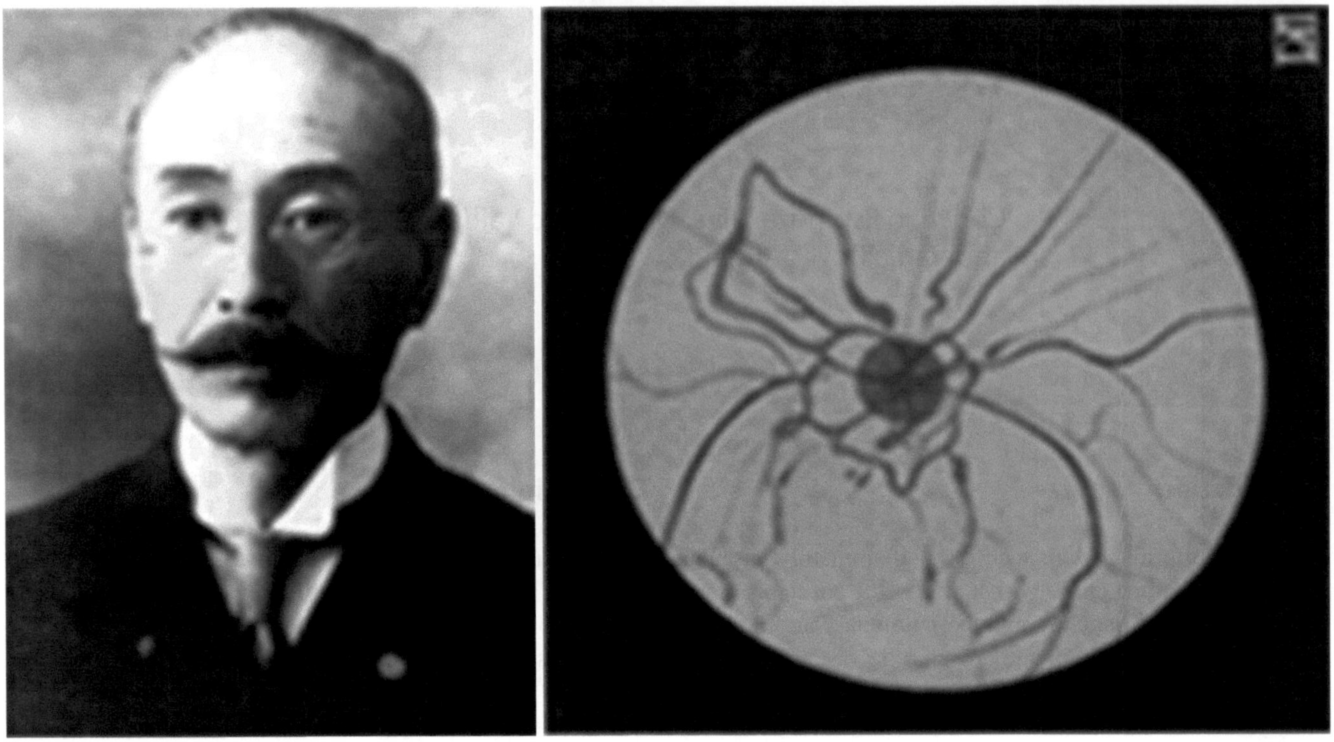

Fig. 23.1 Juzenkai Zasshi, vol. 50, 1908, photograph courtesy of the Collections of the Department of Ophthalmology, Kanazawa University

As a response to this process, inflammatory cells, such as T-cells and natural killer (NK) cells, which express NKG2D receptors, could recognize MICA, resulting in acute inflammation. This process is increased and self-perpetuated.

Cellular Immunity

TA clearly seem to be an autoimmune disease in which cellular immunity plays a major role and humoral immunity participates in a form that still remains to be clarified. In fact, immunohistochemical studies have shown different cell strains involved in the aortoarteritis process, suggesting a critical role in the onset of the disease. Gamma-delta T cells, NK cells, cytotoxic T cells, T-helper cells, and macrophages are some of the cells found in the aortic wall. This process does not seem to start in the endothelium of the aortic wall. The pathogenesis implies the stimulation of an antigen of unknown nature. T cells, NK cells, and cytotoxic T cells express and release massive amounts perforin (a membrane-disrupting protein) through the recognition of MICA, which is directly placed on the surface of arterial vascular cells [14]. This way, the endothelial cells of the vasa vasorum are activated to allow the lymphocytes to gain access to the media and adventitia of the arterial wall [16], thus amplifying the inflammatory response, recruiting especially mononuclear cells.

Immature dendritic cells (DCs) are vastly distributed migratory cells in charge of sampling the antigens in the environment. Once activated, the profile of their chemokine receptor is modified, migrating to lymphoid tissues. Here they express a mature chemokine-producing DC profile and costimulatory molecules that interact with antigen-specific T cells.

In giant cell arteritis (also called Horton's arteritis), DCs are activated and produce chemokines (CCL18, CCL19, and CCL21) that bind the chemokine receptor (CCR7) they express, leading to the entrapment of DC within the vascular wall [17]. The co-localization of DC near T-cells indicates that they are probably involved in the physiopathology of the TA by a similar mechanism.

Study of the cellular composition within the adventitia in Takayasu's arteritis has shown inflammatory infiltrates containing T-cells colocalizing with dendritic cells (DC) [18, 19]. This fact is essential in the development and maintenance of inflammation in the vascular wall.

The antigens (of unknown nature) are presented to killer T-cells by an epitope associated with the major histocompatibility complex (MHC) on the activated DCs, which facilitates the cytotoxic reaction present within the vascular wall.

Humoral Immunity

Although the existence of a humoral role is not known, specific immunologic markers for aortoarteritis, rheumatoid factor, and antinuclear antibodies have been identified, supporting the role of an autoimmune component [20, 21] in the establishment of the disease.

The presence of immune complexes in the sera and receptors of lymphocytes has been reported, but the results differ among authors [22].

Anti-aorta antibodies have long been reported in TA [23–28], but in the study by Baltazares [29], reactive antibodies against a total human aorta extract were searched for, including their main protein components, elastin, fibronectin, and collagen, but no difference was found compared with controls. However, in the same trial, the immunoblot technique showed an immunoprecipitate of a 45 kDa protein in the sera of TA patients significantly more frequently than in the sera of the control group [29]. In the same line of research, Eichhorn [30] suggested that an antigen to these antibodies was stored within the cytoplasm when they found that healthy cells exposed to sera from patients with TA had a bright, homogeneous, and specific immunofluorescent cytoplasm stain and weak membrane stain.

There are reports about the presence of antiphospholipid antibodies in a significant proportion of patients with TA [31–33], anticardiolipin antibodies and antimonocyte antibodies [34]. These were correlated with disease activity, suggesting a pathogenic role in TA. Finally, alpha-beta T-cells would then infiltrate the arterial wall and specifically recognize one or a few autoantigens presented by a shared epitope associated with a specific MHC on the DCs.

The participation of other proinflammatory mediators, such as interleukin (IL)-6, mainly synthesized by macrophages and T-cells, is also known. Functions of the IL-6 are to activate B-cells, enhance T-cell cytotoxicity [35] and NK cell activity [36], stimulate fibroblast proliferation, and induce acute-phase protein synthesis. Other proinflammatory molecules, such as RANTES chemokine (regulated on activation, normal T-cell-expressed and secreted) and IL-8 cytokine, are potent chemoattractants for most mononuclear cells, including those that constitute the majority of the inflammatory infiltrate of the vascular wall in TA. Interleukin-6 and RANTES can also induce the production of metalloproteinases (MMP) in the matrix from mononuclear cells and smooth muscle cells. These proteolytic enzymes degrade elastin and collagen, which are structural components of the arterial wall [37].

These findings have been reinforced by several studies in patients with TA that showed higher serum concentrations of IL-6 [38], RANTES [39], IL-8 [40], MMP-2, MMP-3, and MMP-9. The levels of these latter two MMPs are correlated with disease activity [41]. However, studies of mRNA of proinflammatory cytokines showed increased gene expression of TNF-alpha, IFN-gamma, IL-2, IL-3, and IL-4 and higher expression of IL-12 mRNA after stimulation of cells with lipopolysaccharide and lower mRNA expression of IL-10 than in controls. These results suggest a chronic establishment of the inflammatory response in Takayasu's arteritis [42].

In conclusion, notwithstanding numerous studies, the physiopathology of TA remains unknown and is probably multifactorial, involving several actors.

The data strongly implicate of autoimmune processes, mainly led by cellular immunity, whose role remains to be elucidated. The 2004 study by Seko et al. linked some of the previously discussed data [43]. Therefore, the model proposed in Fig. 23.2 is valid for the understanding the pathogenesis of the disease. The pathologic sequence may implicate the stimulation from an unknown antigen, triggering the expression of heat shock protein 65 in the aortic wall, which in turn would induce the expression of MICA. Inflammatory cells recognize MICA and secrete perforin, disrupting the endothelial membrane of the vasa vasorum and gaining access to the arterial wall.

Inflammatory mediators, such as cytokines and chemokines, are released, allowing inflammatory cells to amplify the process and entrap DCs within the arterial wall.

Alpha-beta T-cells would specifically recognize one or a few autoantigens presented by a shared epitope associated with a specific MHC on the DCs. These DC could simultaneously cooperate to some extent with the B-cells and determine a humoral immunity mainly consisting of anti-endothelial cell autoantibodies that could trigger complement-dependent cytotoxicity against endothelial cells (though this last pathogenic mechanism remains very controversial). This condition would produce medial destruction of the aortic wall with stenosis, occlusion, or aneurysm formation.

Clinical Presentation

The clinical presentation of Takayasu's arteritis is varied and not specific. In fact, it usually develops in a very insidious way, leading the physician to consider other diagnoses, especially when the disease develops in children. Classically, this condition has two distinguishable phases, acute and chronic, and recent studies have also divided it into early (prepulseless) and late (pulseless) phases [44].

In the acute phase, the symptoms are related to the severity of the vascular inflammation. It can cause constitutional symptoms, such as weight loss, fatigue, night sweats, anorexia, malaise [45], and fever (which is more frequent in pediatric patients).

Children can present also joint pain or arthritis and extremities pain. When these symptoms are present, the differential diagnosis must be performed considering other autoimmune diseases, such as rheumatic fever and juvenile rheumatoid arthritis [46].

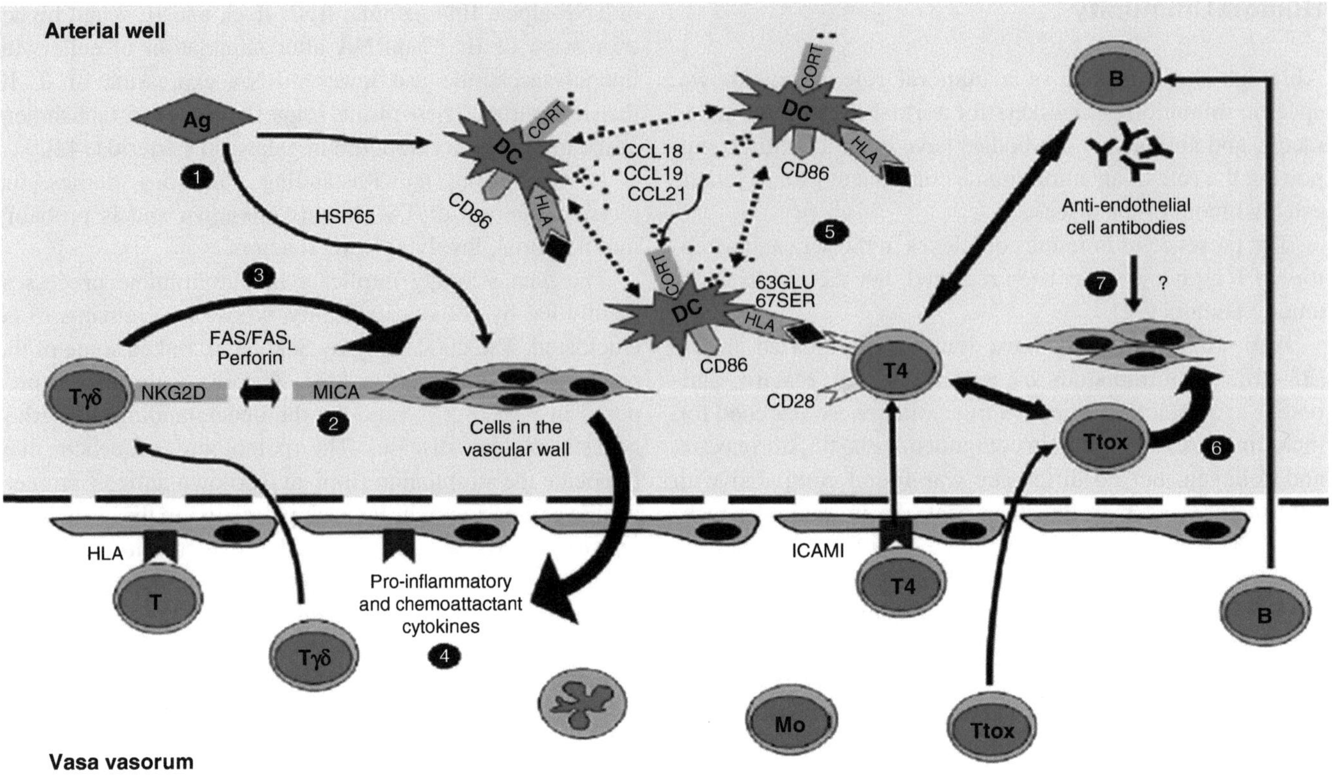

Fig. 23.2 Overview of the physiopathology of TA (brief explanation of different immunological interactions proposed by Seko's investigations published by Arnaud in 2006) [1]. (*1*) Stimulation by an antigen of unknown nature triggers heat shock protein 65 expression, which in turn induces MICA. (*2*) Infiltrating gamma-delta T cells and NK cells expressing NKG2D receptors recognize MICA and release perforin. (*3*) Proinflammatory cytokines amplify the inflammatory response, inducing more MHC antigen and costimulatory molecule expression on vascular cells and thus recruiting more mononuclear cells. (*4*) One or a few (auto)antigens are presented to killer T-cells by a shared epitope associated with specific MHC on the activated dendritic cells trapped within the vascular wall. (*5*) This leads to a cytotoxic reaction of the cells within the vascular wall. (*6*) These dendritic cells simultaneously cooperate with B lymphocytes and induce anti-endothelial cell autoantibodies, whose role is controversial

In the chronic phase, patients report symptoms referable to the organs involved. In a large published experience, more than half of all patients experienced upper extremity claudication, 50 % presented symptoms associated with cerebrovascular insufficiency (vision loss, lightheadedness, stroke), and a third reported carotid artery pain [13]. Less frequently, other symptoms have been reported, such as instability, vertigo, orthostatism, syncope [4], and hypertension (as a result of renal artery involvement, which was the most common presenting sign in an Indian trial) [47].

Laboratory Tests

Markers of inflammation, such as C reactive protein levels and the erythrocyte sedimentation rate, are elevated, which may help make the diagnosis, despite being very nonspecific. Multiple studies indicate that C-reactive protein levels and the erythrocyte sedimentation rate are elevated in approximately 70 % of patients in the acute phase and 50 % in the chronic phase of disease [4]. Leukocytosis and anemia may also be present, although, like the other markers, they are very nonspecific variables [48].

Imaging Study

For decades, angiography was considered the "gold standard" to confirm the diagnosis of Takayasu's arteritis (Fig. 23.3). Although this technique can show the location and grade of the stenotic or aneurysmatic lesion [49], it is an invasive method with several limitations (radiation exposure, adverse reactions to contrast media, and arterial damage [50]). Therefore, it will probably be replaced by multiple less invasive techniques that also provide information about changes in the wall, such as ultrasonography, contrast CT scan, and MRI.

Ultrasonographic study can show the stenotic or aneurysmatic lesions and may contribute to the diagnostic process as well as to the evaluation of the grade and progress of the disease [51]. Patients with Takayasu's arteritis can present an homogeneous, midechoic, circumferential wall thickening with luminal stenosis on carotid echo-Doppler imaging [52]. These findings have been described as pathognomonic of Takayasu's arteritis and have been called the "macaroni sign" (Fig. 23.4) [53].

The CT scan may have some advantages over angiography, allowing demonstration of the mural changes of the affected vessels, such as wall thickening, calcification, or thrombus, which are not seen with conventional angiography [54], but in order to determine the degree and extension of the damage to the vessels more accurately, the use of magnetic resonance imaging (MRI) may be more helpful than CT scans. MRI has other technical advantages: paramagnetic contrast media rarely cause anaphylactic reactions and are non-nephrotoxic (which can be a determinant in the pediatric patients), ionizing radiation is not used, and soft-tissue differentiation is better [55]. However, some disadvantages of MRI are that it is less available, costs more, and has more technical difficulties than CT scans.

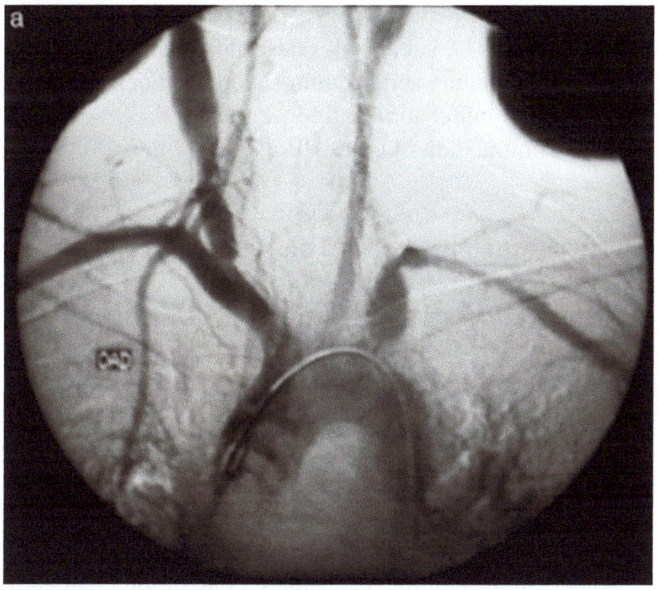

Fig. 23.3 Angiographic imaging: aneurysmal dilations of the right common artery and left intrathoracic subclavian artery

Another diagnostic advantage of MRI compared to the CT scan is an increased sensitivity in detecting mural edema, a finding that is present in almost all acute-phase patients. However, some studies question the use of MRI as a single follow-up imaging technique because of the contradictory findings of disease activity in patients with Takayasu's arteritis [56].

The use of 18F-FDG PET and enhanced CT has also been described to determine the inflammatory status of the vessels. Parallel studies show that these tests can show the distribution of the inflammation in the aorta, its branches, and the pulmonary artery, suggesting that the 18F-FDG accumulation observed in Takayasu's arteritis patients directly indicates the inflammation in the vascular wall [57].

Diagnostic Criteria and Classification

Several diagnostic criteria models have been proposed in the literature [58, 59]. In 1988, Ishikawa [60] published his clinical criteria to establish the diagnosis of Takayasu's arteritis. These proposed criteria were based on clinical and angiographic data from 96 patients with Takayasu's disease.

- One obligatory criterion: age ≤40 years.
- Two major criteria: left and right mid-subclavian artery lesions.
- Nine minor criteria: high erythrocyte sedimentation rate, common carotid artery tenderness, hypertension, aortic regurgitation, annuloaortic ectasia, lesions of the pulmonary artery, left mid common carotid artery, distal brachiocephalic trunk, thoracic aorta, and abdominal aorta.

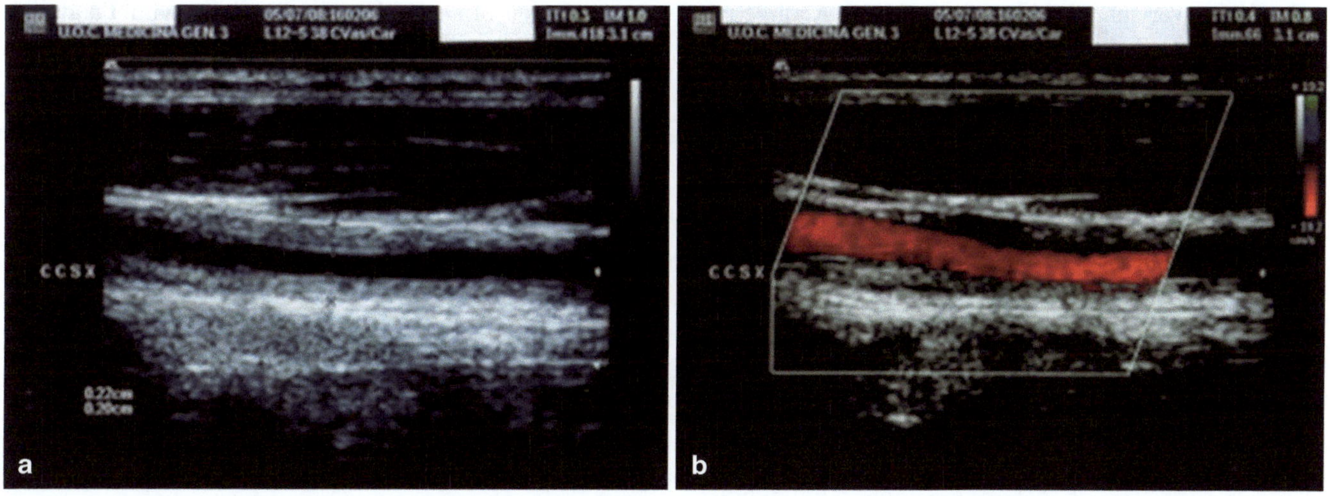

Fig. 23.4 Ultrasound B-mode (**a**) and color-duplex (**b**) flow imaging of the left common carotid artery (longitudinal section): homogeneous, midechoic, circumferential wall thickening ("macaroni sign") with luminal stenosis. CCSX indicates the left common carotid artery. Intima-media thickness is 0.20–0.22 cm (the maximal normal value is 0.06 cm) [1]

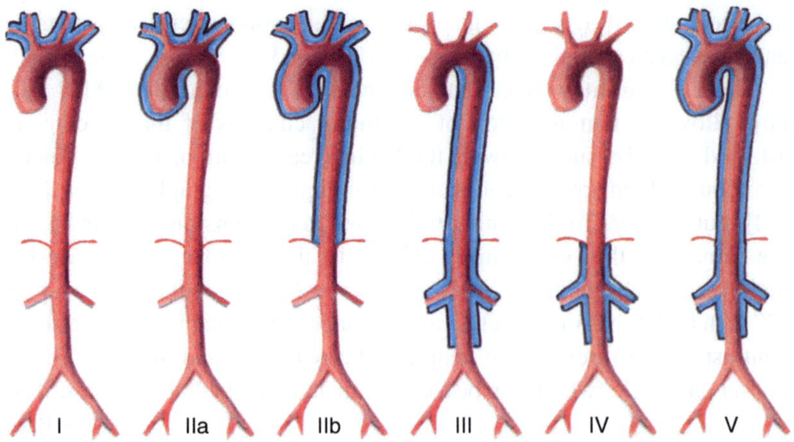

Fig. 23.5 Classification of Takayasu's arteritis according to the anatomic site of involvement

In addition to the obligatory criteria, the presence of two major criteria, one major plus two or more minor criteria, or four or more minor criteria suggests a high probability of the presence of Takayasu's disease. The criteria had 84 % sensitivity in 96 patients with this disease.

In 1990, The American College of Rheumatology [61] established the current and most widely used diagnostic criteria. They proposed that three or more criteria must be present to make the diagnosis:

1. Age of onset of illness 40 years or less. Development of symptoms or findings related to Takayasu's arteritis at age 40 or less.
2. Claudication of extremities. Development and worsening of fatigue and discomfort in the muscles of one or more limbs with activity, especially the upper extremities.
3. Decreased brachial artery pulse. Decreased pulsation of one or both brachial arteries.
4. Differential blood pressure greater than 10 mmHg. Differential pressure greater than 10 mmHg systolic between arms.
5. Murmur over subclavian arteries or aorta. Audible murmur on auscultation on one or both subclavian arteries or abdominal aorta.
6. Abnormal arteriography. Arteriographic narrowing or occlusion of all primary aortic branches or large arteries in the proximal upper and lower extremities not due to arteriosclerosis, fibromuscular dysplasia, or similar causes: changes usually focal or segmental.

Three or more criteria provide a sensitivity and specificity for diagnosis of 90.5 % and 97.8 %, respectively [13].

Concerning the classification of TA, in 1996 Hata et al. [62] published the classification currently used, which grouped the different presentations into five types depending on the affected segments, adding two subtypes depending on the involvement of the pulmonary or coronary artery.

In 2004, Nastri [63] published a diagram of this new classification.

Type I. Aortic arch vessels
Type IIA. Ascending Aorta, aortic arch, and branches
Type IIB. Type IIA vessels plus descending aorta
Type III. Descending and abdominal aorta and/or renal artery
Type IV. Abdominal aorta and renal artery
Type V. Combination of types IIB and IV (Fig. 23.5)

Aneurysmal Disease of Takayasu's Arteritis

The specific incidence of aneurysmal presentation is not known, but it is more frequent in Japan, India, Thailand, Mexico, and Africa [64, 65], compared with occlusive disease, which is more prevalent in the United States and Europe. It is not quite clear why there is such a difference. Frequently, aneurysm formation develops in the descending aorta, followed by the abdominal aorta, and, less frequently, the ascending aortic segments.

Aneurysm formation is considered one of the main complications in Takayasu's arteritis and is an extreme marker of disease activity, usually present in patients with a long history of disease, implying a poor prognosis. Miyata published a comparison of survival rates of patients with Takayasu's arteritis based on the presence or absence of aneurysms, showing a 66.5 % survival rate in patients with aneurysms versus a 79.5 % survival rate in patients without them [66] in 15 years of follow-up.

Although the incidence of aneurysmal presentation of Takayasu's disease is unknown, some authors have provided information on small groups of patients. These studies show a moderately high incidence of aneurysms.

Matsumura in 1991 showed an incidence of saccular or fusiform aneurysms in 31.9 % (36/113) of patients with Takayasu's arteritis. Multiple aneurysms were found in 15 patients. In their study, most patients were over 40 years old, and most of the aneurisms were located in the ascending aorta [65]. In 1994, Kerr et al. [45] published a series of 60 patients with Takayasu's arteritis from the National Institute of Health. Twenty-three percent had aortic aneurysm formation. In 2000, Sueyoshi, from Omura Hospital, showed 17 aortic aneurysms in 14 (45.2 %) of 31 patients [67].

It' is curious that Nakao [25], in his series of 84 patients, revealed no cases of aneurysmal dilatation of the aorta, describing only 6 cases of moderate post-stenotic dilatation in the angiographic findings. In Chile, Krämer reported that the incidence of aneurysm formation was less than 10 % [68].

Thoracic and Abdominal Aortic Aneurysms

Thoracic and abdominal aneurysms are the most common aneurysm presentations in Takayasu's arteritis [69]. Matsumura showed a markedly high frequency in the thoracic area (29 thoracic and 7 abdominal, respectively) [65]. However, Sueyoshi [13] showed a proportional distribution between the thorax and abdomen (9 and 8 patients, respectively). In 2004, Kieffer et al. in Paris [70] published a series of 27 years' experience, including 10 thoracic and 23 thoracoabdominal aneurysms. Six patients had associated aneurysms of the proximal aorta.

Extracranial Supraaortic Aneurysm

Aneurysms also occur in the subclavian [71], innominate, and carotid arteries (Regina et al., 1998 [72]), but extracranial carotid aneurysms caused by Takayasu's arteritis are extremely rare [73]. Tabata et al. [74] reported six cases of extracranial carotid aneurysm among 106 cases in 50 years.

These anatomical presentations may have surgical difficulties in the resection and replacement of the arteries, with a relatively high incidence of stroke. Therefore, decision-making in these cases must be tailored to the individual, depending upon the extent of involvement and the symptoms, and also evaluating the possibility of hybrid intervention with the use of endovascular stent grafts [75] (Fig. 23.6).

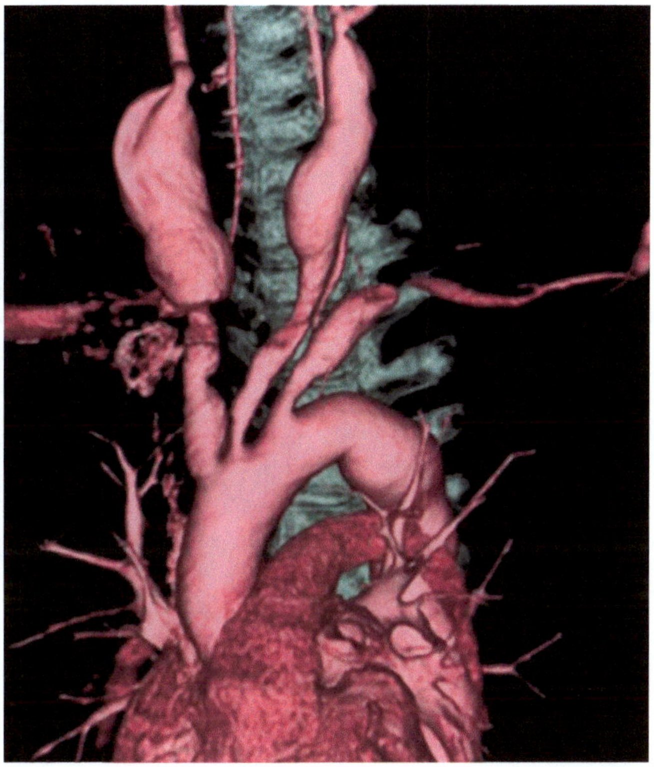

Fig 23.6 Bilateral common carotid artery aneurysm in Takayasu"s arteritis: Tochii M. Asian Cardiovasc Thorac Ann. 2008;16:185–186

Coronary Lesions

Coronary artery involvement in Takayasu's arteritis was first described by Frovig in 1951, and the first coronary artery bypass grafting was performed by Young [76] in 1973.

Endo et al. [3] in 2003 published their experience in coronary angiography in 130 patients with Takayasu's arteritis. Thirty-one had coronary artery lesions, and only four had aneurysmal coronary ectasia (Fig. 23.7). In their experience, aneurysms were not treated surgically because they were diffuse and the patients had no angina.

The incidence of coronary lesions complicating Takayasu's arteritis is relatively low. Nasu [77] in 1976 reported coronary lesions complicating Takayasu's arteritis in 10.5 % (8/76 autopsy cases). More recently, Amano and Zuzuki [78] reported 45 % of coronary lesions, of which 73 % are occlusive coronary lesions localized around the coronary ostia as a result of the extension of inflammation-induced intimal proliferation and fibrous contraction from the ascending aorta.

Treatment and Management

As mentioned earlier, Takayasu's arteritis is a chronic disease, which in its initial phase has only nonspecific symptoms, making the differential diagnosis difficult. This is the challenge for the clinician, because in the chronic phase, the symptoms are actually signs of a long process of complications, such as stenosis or aneurysmal formations.

According to the study published by Koide [79] about the therapeutic approach in Japan in the 1980s, the vast majority of patients received drug therapy alone (75 %), and surgery was a viable option in 12 % of patients. With the current technical advances, especially the development of different endovascular techniques, surgery has become a more popular therapy [80].

At present, a more profound understanding of the immunological mechanisms of the pathogenesis responsible for vascular injury allows a better treatment approach, trying to diminish the inflammatory process [81] with more specific therapies.

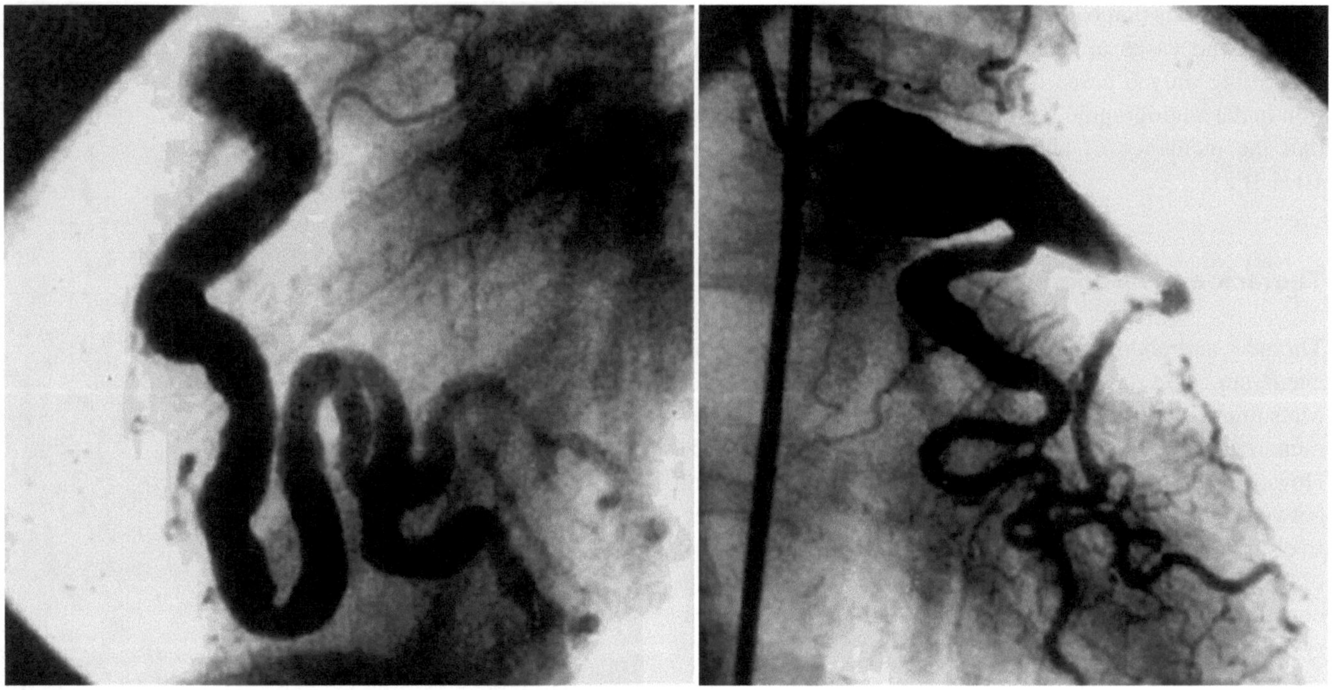

Fig. 23.7 Diffuse dilatation of the right and left coronaries arteries in a patient with Takayasu's arteritis. Endo M: J Tho Card Surg 2003;125(3): 570–7

Medical Treatment

Anti-inflammatory and immunosuppressive agents are the main medical therapy strategy for Takayasu's arteritis. Corticosteroids are still used in the active phase. Several reports have claimed that long-term prednisolone therapy contributes to angiographic improvement [82, 83]. Guidelines of the Health Ministry of Japan (1992) recommend 30 mg/day of corticosteroids as the initial dose for adult patients in the active phase. The initial dose is tapered at a rate of 5 mg every 2 weeks down to 10 mg and thereafter at a rate of 2.5 mg every 2 weeks until withdrawal or the minimum dose required to control inflammation [84].

Some patients in whom withdrawal from corticosteroids is difficult may require additional immunosuppressive drugs such as cyclophosphamide or azathioprine [84]. The use of other drugs, such as methotrexate, mycophenolate mofetil, and infliximab, has been reported [80]. These agents are usually continued for at least 1 year after remission and are then tapered until discontinuation in addition to a long-term low-dose corticosteroid therapy.

When patients are started on corticosteroids, other preventive measures are necessary, such as osteoporosis prevention. Management of traditional cardiovascular risk factors (such as dyslipidemia and hypertension includes calcium antagonists, beta-blockers, hypotensive diuretics, cardiac glycoside, coronary vasodilator agents [80]), and lifestyle changes, as well as long-term aspirin therapy to prevent thrombosis in the affected vessels with stenotic or occlusive lesions or embolism from aneurysms.

Future treatments, such as anti-TNF therapy, are showing promising results. For example, Hoffman [85] reported a sustained remission in TA. This indicates that the road ahead will include immune therapies targeted to a very specific phenomenon.

Surgical Treatment

Takayasu's arteritis primarily affects large arteries (the aorta and its branches). It can produce stenotic, occlusive, and aneurysmal lesions. As the disease progresses, the great vessels grow thicker, developing focal and raised plaques that produce stenosis and aneurysms in the major branches of the thoracic aorta. These plaques are usually found in the distal thoracic and abdominal aorta. It has been suggested that the growth rate and risk of rupture of aneurysms in Takayasu's arteritis is lower than the risk of atherosclerotic aneurysms [86]. The formation of aortic hematomas, dissection, and rupture in both the ascending and descending arch and the abdominal aortic aneurysms has been described.

In adults, less than 20 % of patients require surgical treatment [87, 88], which is completely different from what happens in pediatric patients, where nearly 80 % undergo some type of surgical treatment of stenotic lesions [89].

Different studies and reports have shown low morbidity and mortality rates for surgical treatment of different lesions of Takayasu's arteritis, except for aortic aneurysm surgery. In fact, although patients with Takayasu's arteritis are younger, the involvement of multiple arterial segments, such as kidney or cardiac, may increase the risks, which may affect the overall outcome of surgery.

For this reason, it may be important to maintain a conservative approach in the management of patients with Takayasu's disease, with a complete preoperative and multidisciplinary evaluation being indispensable [90].

Several studies have suggested that surgery should be performed only if there is a condition that could affect the prognosis of a patient and should be avoided during the acute illness, with steroid therapy being preferred as a first treatment approach before surgery [91] to prevent progression of the disease and complications. Moreover, the AHA/ACC guidelines do not distinguish the surgical approach for Takayasu's arteritis from that for other diseases of the thoracic aorta. Revascularization for aortic stenosis or aneurysm occurs for the same indications as in non-inflammatory disorders: secondary organ vascular insufficiency or risk of rupture [92].

However, emergency surgery is not usually necessary since the lesions are made in the chronic phase of the disease [93], permitting the development of collateral circulation. Currently, percutaneous angioplasty has become an effective alternative to occlusive lesions, and possibly the indications for this technique will increase with time.

Surgical treatment for Takayasu's arteritis is difficult. It is very important not to forget the main pathological feature, extensive destruction of the medial elastic fibers that maintain the strength of the aortic wall. Therefore, during the procedure, fragile and inflamed tissues are manipulated, and complications such as hemorrhage, pseudoaneurysm, and detachment of the prosthetic graft develop postoperatively [94]. This is why surgeons must always be aware of the anastomotic fragility and the risk of graft failure due to complications of the suture line, which may have stenosis, aneurysm, or pseudoaneurysm [86].

In the aneurysmal presentation, the surgical priority should be determined based on the lesion's diameter, morphology, and propensity for dilatation. Different authors do not distinguish between surgical indications of Takayasu's arteritis and other diseases of the thoracic aorta, and taking into account the different results published in the literature, the surgical approach tends to be less aggressive.

Treatment consists of replacing dilated lesions, preferably in single-stage surgery, especially for aortic arch or descending thoracic aorta aneurysms, but multi-stage surgery sometimes must be performed to reduce the surgical invasiveness, especially when the damage is very extensive or multiple locations are affected.

The surgical team's experience is fundamental to obtain good results in any complex disease, and Takayasu's arteritis is not an exception. This is especially the case when conditions involve additional technical complications, such as the fragility of tissues and presence of microscopic disease that has not been detected, which has been widely demonstrated in Takayasu's disease aneurysms, where the operative mortality is higher, indicating that this presentation is a marker of disease severity.

Robbs et al. [86] from South Africa reported an operative mortality of 3–4 % in their patients with Takayasu's arteritis, most of whom had aneurysms. The mortality was related to ruptured aneurysms. In 2004, Kieffer in Paris [70] reported an operative mortality of 9 %, paraplegia in 9 %, and satisfactory postoperative outcomes with open surgery of descending thoracic and thoracoabdominal aortic aneurysms in 33 patients with Takayasu's arteritis [95].

After surgery for Takayasu's arteritis, anastomotic false aneurysms (anastomotic detachment) can occur at any time in the long term, although the incidence seems to be low even in the active phase of the disease.

It is unclear what the phenomenon is that occurs in this area. Some authors suggest the possibility of recurrence of arteritis in areas with disease-free margins during resection. Others raised the possibility of development of the disease in an area not resected without macroscopic or angiografic involvement, but with microscopic signs of disease [90].

Miyata reported an incidence of anastomotic aneurysms of the suture line in 8.5 % of the sutures performed in 14 patients (22 of 259 anastomoses). No association was found between the incidence of aneurysms and increased activity of arteritis or the use of corticosteroids, but this process indeed presented more frequently in patients with aneurysm disease compared with those with anastomotic disease [96].

Therefore, constant vigilance is necessary in patients who have undergone replacement of a segment, since we know that although the segments may appear normal on angiography, the participation of microscopic disease occurs in 44 % of cases [97].

The reported incidence of anastomotic aneurysm among patients with atherosclerosis ranges widely from 1.7 to 15 % per anastomosis. It has been speculated that the variation in incidence is caused by differences in the types of arterial reconstruction, sites of anastomosis, methods of diagnosis, and differences in the length and completeness of the follow-up study. To prevent this complication, it is recommended to reinforce the sutures with Teflon felt strips and/or suppression of active or persisting inflammation with corticosteroids. In addition, if possible, sites of normal tissue without inflammatory changes should be chosen as anastomotic sites [97].

Surgery or Endovascular Repair for Aortic Aneurysm

In surgical repair of aortic aneurysms due to Takayasu's arteritis, the outcome has been improved with endovascular techniques. Recently, successful endovascular aneurysmal repair (stent grafting) for dilated lesions was reported in a small series [98]. However, reintervention for ruptured aneurysms after endovascular treatment was also reported [99]. The long-term efficacy of endovascular aneurysmal repair remains uncertain even for atherosclerotic pathology, but the new endovascular approach may provide an interesting alternative for patients with thoracic or abdominal aortic aneurysms.

References

1. Famous historical figures in the Japanese ophthalmology. http://www.nichigan.or.jp/english/ophthalmology.jsp. Accessed on Dec 29, 2011.
2. Takayasu M. A case with peculiar changes of the central retinal vessels. Acta Soc Ophthalmol Jap, Tokyo. 1908;12:554.
3. Endo M, Tomizawa Y, Nishida H, Aomi S, Nakazawa M, Tsurumi Y, et al. Angiographic findings and surgical treatments of coronary artery involvement in Takayasu arteritis. J Thorac Cardiovasc Surg. 2003;125:570–7.
4. Miranda H, Blanco JL, Moreno F. Arteritis de Takayasu. Acta Med Colomb. 2011;36:93–7.
5. Weyand C, Goronzy J. Medium- and large-vessel vasculitis. N Engl J Med. 2003;349:160–9.
6. Maksimowicz-mckinnon K, Hoffman G. Takayasu arteritis: what is the long-term prognosis? Rheum Dis Clin N Am. 2007;48:777–86.
7. Lupi-Herrera E, Sanchez-Torres G, Horwitz S, Gutierrez FE. Pulmonary artery involvement in Takayasu's arteritis. Chest. 1975; 67:69–74.
8. American College of Cardiology Foundation, American Heart Association Task Force et al. on Practice Guidelines, American Association for Thoracic Surgery, American College of Radiology, American Stroke Association, Society of Cardiovascular Anesthesiologists, Society for Cardiovascular Angiography and Interventions, Society of Interventional Radiology, Society of Thoracic Surgeons, Society for Vascular Medicine, North American Society for Cardiovascular Imaging, Hiratzka LF, Bakris GL, Beckman JA, Bersin RM, Carr VF, et al. ACCF/AHA/AATS/ACR/ASA/SCA/SCAI/SIR/STS/SVM Guidelines for diagnosis and management of patients with thoracic aortic disease. J Am Coll Cardiol. 2010;55:e53–54.
9. Regina G, Angiletta D, Bortone A, et al. Aortic aneurysms in Takayasu arteritis. Diagnosis, screening and treatment of abdominal, thoracoabdominal and thoracic aortic aneurysms. 2011:309–28.
10. Regina G, Angiletta D, Bortone A, Fullone M, Marinazzo D, Pulli R. Aortic Aneurysm in Takayasu Arteritis. In Grundmann R. Editor, Diagnosis, Screening and Treatment of Abdominal, Toracoabdominal and Thoracic Aortic Aneurysms. InTech. 311–328.
11. Isselbacher EM, Eagel KA, Desanctis RW. Diseases of the aorta. In: Braunwald E, editor. Heart disease: a textbook of cardiovascular medicine, vol. 2. Philadelphia: WB Saunders; 1997. p. 1546.
12. Kumar S, Subramanyan R, Ravi Mandalam K, et al. Aneurysmal form of aortoarteritis (Takayasu's disease): analysis of thirty cases. Clin Radiol. 1990;42:342–7.
13. Sueyoshi E, Sakamoto I, Hayashi K. Aortic aneurysms in patients with Takayasu's arteritis: CT evaluation. AJR Am J Roentgenol. 2000;175:1727–33.
14. Seko Y, Minota S, Kawasaki A, Shinkai Y, Maeda K, Yagita H, et al. Perforin-secreting killer cell infiltration and expression of a 65-kDheat-shock protein in aortic tissue of patients with Takayasu's arteritis. J Clin Invest. 1994;93(2):750–8.
15. Choy MK, Phipps ME. MICA polymorphism: biology and importance in immunity and disease. Trends Mol Med. 2010; 16(3):97–106. Epub 2010 Feb 12.
16. Hotchi M. Pathological studies on Takayasu arteritis. Heart Vessels Suppl. 1992;7:11–7.
17. Krupa WM, Dewan M, Jeon MS, Kurtin PJ, Younge BR, Goronzy JJ, et al. Trapping of misdirected dendritic cells in the granulomatouslesions of giant cell arteritis. Am J Pathol. 2002;161(5):1815–23.
18. Inder SJ, Bobryshev YV, Cherian SM, Wang AY, Lord RS, Masuda K, et al. Immunophenotypic analysis of the aortic wall in Takayasu's arteritis: involvement of lymphocytes, dendritic cells and granulocytesin immuno-inflammatory reactions. Cardiovasc Surg. 2000;8(2):141–8.
19. Inder SJ, Bobryshev YV, Cherian SM, Lord RS, Masuda K, Yutani C. Accumulation of lymphocytes, dendritic cells, and granulocytes in the aortic wall affected by Takayasu's disease. Angiology. 2000;51(7):565–79.
20. Arnaud L, Kahn JE, Girszyn N, Piette AM, Bletry O, et al. Takayasu's arteritis: an update on physiopathology. Eur J Intern Med. 2006;17:241–6.
21. Toure' MK, Pasquier G, Herreman F, Bonnin A, Fouchard J, Houille F. Anévrysmes au cours de la maladie de Takayasu. Arch Mal Coeur. 1982;75:695–700.
22. Gyotoku Y, Kakiuchi T, Nonaka Y, Saito Y, Ito I, Murao S. Immune complexes in Takayasu's arteritis. Clin Exp Immunol. 1981;45(2): 246–52.
23. Ito I. Aortitis syndrome with reference to the detection of antiaorta antibody from patients' sera. Jpn Circ J. 1966;30:75–9.
24. Ito I, Saito Y, Nonaka Y. Immunological aspects of aortitis syndrome. Jpn Circ J. 1975;39(4):459–62.
25. Nakao K, Ikeda M, Kimata S, Niitani H, Niyahara M. Takayasu's arteritis. Clinical report of eighty-four cases and immunological studies of seven cases. Circulation. 1967;35(6):1141–5.
26. Ueda H, Ito I, Saito Y. Autoantibodies in cardiovascular disease. Jpn J Clin Med. 1964;22:1271–8.
27. Dhingra R, Talwar KK, Chopra P, Kumar R. An enzyme linked immunosorbent assay for detection of anti-aorta antibodies in Takayasu arteritis patients. Int J Cardiol. 1993;40(3):237–42.
28. Dhingra R, Chopra P, Talwar KK, Kumar R. Enzyme-linked immunosorbent assay and immunoblot study in Takayasu's arteritis patients. Indian Heart J. 1998;50(4):428–32.
29. Baltazares M, Mendoza F, Dabague J, Reyes PA. Antiaorta antibodies and Takayasu arteritis. Int J Cardiol. 1998;66 Suppl 1:S183; discussion S189.
30. Eichhorn J, Sima D, Thiele B, Lindschau C, Turowski A, Schmidt H, et al. Anti-endothelial cell antibodies in Takayasu arteritis. Circulation. 1996;94(10):2396–401.
31. Misra R, Aggarwal A, Chag M, Sinha N, Shrivastava S. Raised anticardiolipin antibodies in Takayasu's arteritis. Lancet. 1994; 343(8913):1644–5.
32. Yokoi K, Akaike M, Shigekiyo T, Saito S. An elderly patient with Takayasu's arteritis associated with antiphospholipid antibodies. Nippon Ronen Igakkai Zasshi. 1994;31(9):716–9.
33. Yokoi K, Hosoi E, Akaike M, Shigekiyo T, Saito S. Takayasu's arteritis associated with antiphospholipid antibodies. Report of two cases. Angiology. 1996;47(3):315–9.
34. Tripathy NK, Sinha N, Nityanand S. Antimonocyte antibodies in Takayasu's arteritis: prevalence of and relation to disease activity. J Rheumatol. 2003;30(9):2023–6.

35. Okada M, Kitahara M, Kishimoto S, Matsuda T, Hirano T, Kishimoto T. IL-6/BSF-2 functions as a killer helper factor in the in vitro induction of cytotoxic T cells. J Immunol. 1988;141(5):1543–9.
36. Luger TA, Krutmann J, Kirnbauer R, Urbanski A, Schwarz T, Klappacher G, et al. IFN-beta 2/IL-6 augments the activity of human natural killer cells. J Immunol. 1989;143(4):1206–9.
37. Kishimoto T. Interleukin-6 and its receptor in autoimmunity. J Autoimmun. 1992;5(Suppl A):123–32.
38. Schall TJ, Bacon K, Toy KJ, Goeddel DV. Selective attraction of monocytes and T lymphocytes of the memory phenotype by cytokine RANTES. Nature. 1990;347(6294):669–71.
39. Noris M, Daina E, Gamba S, Bonazzola S, Remuzzi G. Interleukin-6 and RANTES in Takayasu arteritis: a guide for therapeutic decisions? Circulation. 1999;100(1):55–60.
40. Tripathy NK, Sinha N, Nityanand S. Interleukin-8 in Takayasu's arteritis: plasma levels and relationship with disease activity. Clin Exp Rheumatol. 2004;22(6 Suppl 36):S27–30.
41. Matsuyama A, Sakai N, Ishigami M, Hiraoka H, Kashine S, Hirata A, et al. Matrix metalloproteinases as novel disease markers in Takayasu arteritis. Circulation. 2003;108(12):1469–73.
42. Tripathy NK, Chauhan SK, Nityanand S. Cytokine mRNA repertoire of peripheral blood mononuclear cells in Takayasu's arteritis. Clin Exp Immunol. 2004;138(2):369–74.
43. Seko Y, Sugishita K, Sato O, Takagi A, Tada Y, Matsuo H, et al. Expression of costimulatory molecules (4-1BBL and Fas) and major histocompatibility class I chain-related a (MICA) in aortic tissue with Takayasu's arteritis. J Vasc Res. 2004;41(1):84–90.
44. Forsey J, Dhandayuthapani G, Hamilton MCK, Tizard EJ, Ramanan AV. Takayasu arteritis: key clinical factors for early diagnosis. Arch Dis Child Educ Pract Ed. 2011;96:176–82.
45. Kerr GS, Hallahan CW, Giordano J, et al. Takayasu arteritis. Ann Intern Med. 1994;120:919–29.
46. Zapata A, Arruda L, Lourdes B, Marino JC, Kiss MHB, Almeida C. Arteritis de Takayasu. An Pediatr. 2003;58(3):211–6.
47. Sharma BK, Sagar S, Singh AP, et al. Takayasu arteritis in India. Heart Vessels Suppl. 1992;7:37–43.
48. Nakau K, Ikeda M, Kimata S, Niitani H, Miyahara M, Ishimi Z, et al. Takayasu's arteritis. Clinical report of eighty-four cases and immunological studies of seven cases. Circulation. 1967;35:1141–55.
49. Tabaee AS, Mali S, Vahedian J, Arefi S. Aortic aneurysm in Takayasu's syndrome. Iran Heart J. 2008;9(2):55–8.
50. Agarwal V. Imaging in Takayasu's arteritis. J Indian Rheumatol Assoc. 2005;13:41–2.
51. Chaubal N, Dighe M, Shah M. Sonographic and color doppler findings in aortoarteritis (Takayasu arteritis). J Ultrasound Med. 2004;23(7):937–44.
52. Meini S, De Franco V, Auteri A, Pieragalli D. Takayasu's arteritis. The macaroni sign. Circulation. 2006;114:e544.
53. Maeda H, Handa N, Matsumoto M, Hougaku H, Ogawa S, Oku N, et al. Carotid lesions detected by B-mode ultrasonography in Takayasu's arteritis: "macaroni sign" as an indicator of the disease. Ultrasound Med Biol. 1991;17:695–701.
54. Yamada I, Nakagawa T, Himeno Y, Numano F, Shibuya H. Takayasu arteritis: evaluation of the thoracic aorta with CT angiography. Radiology. 1998;209:103–9.
55. Sueyoshi E, Sakamoto I, Uetani M. MRI of Takayasu's arteritis: typical appearances and complications. AJR Am J Roentgenol. 2006;187:W569–75.
56. Tso E, Flamm SD, White RD, Schvartzman PR, Mascha E, Hoffman GS. Takayasu arteritis: utility and limitations of magnetic resonance imaging in diagnosis and treatment. Arthritis Rheum. 2002;46:1634–42.
57. Kobayashi Y, Ishii K, Oda K, Nariai T, Tanaka J, Ishiwata K, et al. Aortic wall inflammation due to Takayasu arteritis imaged with 18F-FDG PET coregistered with enhanced CT. J Nucl Med. 2005;46:917–22.
58. Fiessinger JN, Tawfik-Taher S, Capron L, Laurian C, Cormier JM, Camilleri JP, et al. Maladie de Takayasu. Criteres diagnostiques. Nouv Presse Med. 1982;11:583Y–6.
59. Bletry O, Aime P, Degoulet J, Cosserat J, Piette A, Becour B. Validation de nouveaux criteres diagnostiques de l_arterite deTakayasu. Rev Med Interne. 1995;16(S1):70.
60. Ishikawa K. Diagnostic approach and proposed criteria for the clinical diagnosis of Takayasu's arteriopathy. J Am Coll Cardiol. 1988;12:964–72.
61. Arend WP, Michel BA, Bloch DA, et al. The American College of Rheumatology 1990 criteria for the classification of Takayasu arteritis. Arthritis Rheum. 1990;33:1129–34.
62. Hata A, Noda M, Moriwaki R, Numaño F. Angiographic findings of Takayasu arteritis: New classification. Int J Cardiol. 1996;54:S155–63.
63. Nastri M, Baptista L, Baroni R, Blasbalg R, de Ávila L, Leite C, et al. Gadolinium-enhanced three-dimensional MR angiography of Takayasu arteritis. Radiographics. 2004;24:773–86.
64. Desiron Q, Zeaiter R. Takayasu's arteritis. Acta Chir Belg. 2000;100:1–6.
65. Matsumura K, Hirano T, Takeda K, Matsuda A, Nakagawa T, Yamaguchi N, et al. Incidence of aneurysms in Takayasu's arteritis. Angiology. 1991;42:308–15.
66. Miyata TT, Sato O, Koyama H, Shigematsu H, Tada Y. Long-term survival after surgical treatment of patients with Takayasu's arteritis. Circulation. 2003;3:1474–80.
67. Sueyoshi E, Sakamoto I, Hayashi K. Aortic aneurysms in patients with Takayasu's arteritis: CT evaluation. Am J Roentgenol. 2000;175:1727–33.
68. Krämer A. Enfermedad de Takayasu en Chile. Reumatologia. 2001;17(3):119–20.
69. Giordano JM. Surgical treatment of Takayasu's arteritis. Int J Cardiol. 2000;75 Suppl 1:123.
70. Kieffer E, Chiche L, Bertal A, Koskas F, Bahnini A, Blã Try O, et al. Descending thoracic and thoracoabdominal aortic aneurysm in patients with Takayasu's disease. Ann Vasc Surg. 2004;18(5):505–13. Epub 2004 Aug 6.
71. Chiou A, Fantini G. Subclavian artery aneurysm: an unusual manifestation of Takayasu's arteritis. Cardiovasc Surg. 1999;7(3):310–4.
72. Regina G, Fullone M, Testini M, Todisco C, Greco L, Rizzi R, et al. Aneurysms of the supra-aortic trunks in Takayasu's disease. Report of two cases. J Cardiovasc Surg (Torino). 1998;39(6):757–60.
73. Funiu H, Kokubo Y, Kondo R, Saino M, Ohki M, Kayama T, et al. A case of bilateral extracranial carotid artery aneurysms caused by Takayasu's arteritis. No To Shinkei. 2004;56(11):971–5.
74. Tabata M, Kitagawa T, Saito T, Uozaki H, Oshiro H, Miyata T, et al. Extracranial carotid aneurysm in Takayasu's arteritis. J Vasc Surg. 2001;34(4):739–42.
75. Angiletta D, Impedovo G, Pestrichella F, Martiradonna F, Fullone M, Marotta V, et al. Endovascular treatment of two rare cases of aneurysms of the supra-aortic trunks. Ital J Vasc Endovasc Surg. 2004;11(3):139–42.
76. Young JA, Sengupta A, Khaja FU. Coronary arterial stenosis, angina pectoris and atypical coarctation of the aorta due to nonspecific arteritis. Treatment with aortocoronary bypass graft. Am J Cardiol. 1973;32:356–60.
77. Nasu T. Takayasu's truncoarteritis in Japan. A statistical observation of 76 autopsy cases. Pathol Microbiol (Basel). 1975;43:140–6.
78. Amano J, Suzuki A. Coronary artery involvement in Takayasu's arteritis. Collective review and guideline for surgical treatment. J Thorac Cardiovasc Surg. 1991;102:554–60.
79. Koide K. Takayasu arteritis in Japan. Heart Vessels Suppl. 1992;7:48–54.
80. Ogino H, Matsuda H, Minatoya K, Sasaki H, Tanaka H, Matsumura Y, et al. Overview of late outcome of medical and surgical treatment for Takayasu arteritis. Circulation. 2008;118:2738–47.

81. Liang P, Hoffman GS. Advances in the medical and surgical treatment of Takayasu arteritis. Curr Opin Rheumatol. 2005;17(1):16–24.
82. Kulkarny TP, D'Cruz IA, Gandhi MJ, Dadhich DS. Reversal of neovascular hypertension caused by nonspecific aortitis after corticosteroid therapy. Br Heart J. 1974;36:114–6.
83. Ishikawa K, Yonekawa Y. Regression of carotid stenosis after corticosteroid therapy in occlusive thromboarotopathy (Takayasu's disease). Stroke. 1987;18:677–9.
84. Ito I. Medical treatment of Takayasu arteritis. Heart Vessels Suppl. 1992;7:133–7.
85. Hoffman GS, Merkel PA, Brasington RD, Lenschow DJ, Liang P. Anti-tumor necrosis factor therapy in patients with difficult to treat Takayasu arteritis. Arthritis Rheum. 2004;50(7):2296–304.
86. Robbs JV, Abdool-Carrim AT, Kadwa AM. Arterial reconstruction for non-specific arteritis (Takayasu's disease): medium to long term results. Eur J Vasc Surg. 1994;8:401–7.
87. Ishikawa K, Maetani S. Long-term outcome for 120 Japanese patients with Takayasu's disease. Clinical and statistical analyses of related prognostic factors. Circulation. 1994;90:1855–60.
88. Fields CE, Bower TC, Cooper LT, Hoskin T, Noel AA, Panneton JM, et al. Takayasu's arteritis: operative results and influence of disease activity. J Vasc Surg. 2006;43:64–71.
89. Kalangos A, Christenson JT, Cikirikcioglu M, Vala D, Buerge A, Simonet F, et al. Long-term outcome after surgical intervention and interventional procedures for the management of Takayasu's arteritis in children. J Thorac Cardiovasc Surg. 2006;132: 656–64.
90. Giordano J, Leavitt RY, Hoffman G, Fauci AS. Experience with surgical treatment of Takayasu's disease. Surgery. 1991; 109:252.
91. Song M-H, Nakayama T, Hattori K, Tokuda Y, Mabuchi Y, Ueda Y. Aortic root aneurysm in Takayasu arteritis syndrome: exploration in active phase and repair in inactive phase. J Thorac Cardiovasc Surg. 2008;136:1084–5.
92. American College of Cardiology Foundation, American Heart Association Task Force et al. on Practice Guidelines, American Association for Thoracic Surgery, American College of Radiology, American Stroke Association, Society of Cardiovascular Anesthesiologists, Society for Cardiovascular Angiography and Interventions, Society of Interventional Radiology, Society of Thoracic Surgeons, Society for Vascular Medicine, North American Society for Cardiovascular Imaging, Hiratzka LF, Bakris GL, Beckman JA, Bersin RM, Carr VF, et al. ACCF/AHA/AATS/ACR/ASA/SCA/SCAI/SIR/STS/SVM guidelines for the diagnosis and management of patients with thoracic aortic disease. J Am Coll Cardiol. 2010;55:e27–129.
93. Giordano J. Surgical treatment of Takayasu's arteritis. Cleve Clin J Med. 69(Supp II);2002:146.
94. Matsuura K, Ogino H, Matsuda H, Minatoya K, Sasaki H, Yagihara T, et al. Surgical outcome of aortic arch repair for patients with Takayasu arteritis. Ann Thorac Surg. 2006;81:178–82.
95. Arnaud L, Haroche J, Limal N, Toledano D, Gambotti L, Costedoat Chalumeau N, et al. Takayasu arteritis in France: a single-center retrospective study of 82 cases comparing white, North African, and black patients. Medicine (Baltimore). 2010;89(1):1–17.
96. Miyata T, Sato O, Deguchi J, et al. Anastomotic aneurysms after surgical treatment of Takayasu's arteritis: a 40-year experience. J Vasc Surg. 1998;27:438–45.
97. Kerr GS, Hallahan CW, Giordano J, Leavitt RY, Fauci AS, Rottem M, et al. Takayasu's arteritis. Ann Intern Med. 1994;120:919.
98. Baril DT, Carroccio A, Palchik E, Ellozy SH, Jacobs TS, Teodorescu V, et al. Endovascular treatment of complicated aortic aneurysms in patients with underlying arteriopathies. Ann Vasc Surg. 2006;20:464–71.
99. Regina G, Bortone A, Impedovo G, De Cillis E, Angiletta D, Marotta V. Endovascular repair of thoracic stent-graft bulging rupture in a patient with multiple thoracic aneurysms due to Takayasu disease. J Vasc Surg. 2007;45:391–4.

Mesenteric Vasculitis

24

Mateus Picada-Correa and Gustavo S. Oderich

Introduction

Vasculitis is a rare disease associated with inflammatory response of vessel walls, with or without associated necrosis and granulomata. It affects 20 individuals per million a year. Chronic inflammation can weaken or thicken the arterial wall, leading to aneurysm, stenoses, and occlusions. Systemic vasculitides have varied etiologies and pathogenetic mechanisms, yet most have not been well defined. Vasculitides are classified according to the vessel size and presence or absence of necrosis, granulomas, or both (Table 24.1).

Large-vessel vasculitis affects the aorta and its branches, medium-size vessel vasculitis has a predilection for the visceral arteries, and small-vessel vasculitis affects arterioles, venules, and capillaries. Although vasculitis of the mesenteric arteries is rare, accounting for less than 5 % of all cases of mesenteric ischemia [2], it can lead to bowel gangrene and death if not immediately recognized and treated. This chapter summarizes the clinical features, diagnostic approaches and treatment of mesenteric vasculitis (MV).

Clinical Presentation

MV usually presents with bleeding or ischemic symptoms. Upper and lower gastrointestinal bleeding is the most common presentation and is associated with mucosal lesions or rupture of small branch artery aneurysms. Mesenteric ischemia presents with symptoms that are indistinguishable from those of atherosclerotic or embolic origin. The classic symptoms include abdominal pain, postprandial pain, "food fear," and weight loss. In patients with medium-size vessel vasculitis, such as polyarteritis nodosa (PAN), inflammation may lead to aneurysm formation and vessel rupture with either intra-abdominal or gastrointestinal hemorrhage. If the smaller arteries are involved, ulceration, perforation, and stricture formation can occur. In addition to bleeding and ischemic symptoms, patients often manifest other constitutional symptoms such as weight loss, malaise, fever, night sweats, arthralgias, myalgia, peripheral weakness, and headache.

Other less frequent manifestations include hepatitis, gastritis, esophagitis, pancreatitis, cholecystitis, and appendicitis [1, 3–10]. Nausea and vomiting are present in one-third of patients, and 27 % present with diarrhea.

Table 24.1 Most common causes of vasculitis

Classification of vasculitis
Large-vessel vasculitis
Takayasu arteritis
Giant cell arteritis
Medium-sized-vessel vasculitis
Poliarteritis nodosa
Kawasaki disease
Primary granulomatous central nervous system vasculitis
Small-vessel vasculitis
Antineutrophil cytoplasmic autoantibody
Wegener's granulomatosis
Churg-Strauss syndrome
Microscopic angiitis
Immune complex small-vessel vasculitis
Henoch-Schonlein purpura
Cryoglobulinemic vasculitis
Lupus vasculitis
Rheumatoid vasculitis
Sjogren syndrome vasculitis
Hypocomplementemic urticarial vasculitis
Behoet's syndrome
Goodpasture's syndrome
Serum sickness vasculitis
Inflammatory bowel disease vasculitis

Adapted from Ha et al. [1]

M. Picada-Correa, MD • G.S. Oderich, MD (✉)
Division of Vascular and Endovascular Surgery, Mayo Clinic, Rochester, MN, USA
e-mail: oderich.gustavo@mayo.edu

E.A. Gabriel, S.A. Gabriel (eds.), *Inflammatory Response in Cardiovascular Surgery*,
DOI 10.1007/978-1-4471-4429-8_24,

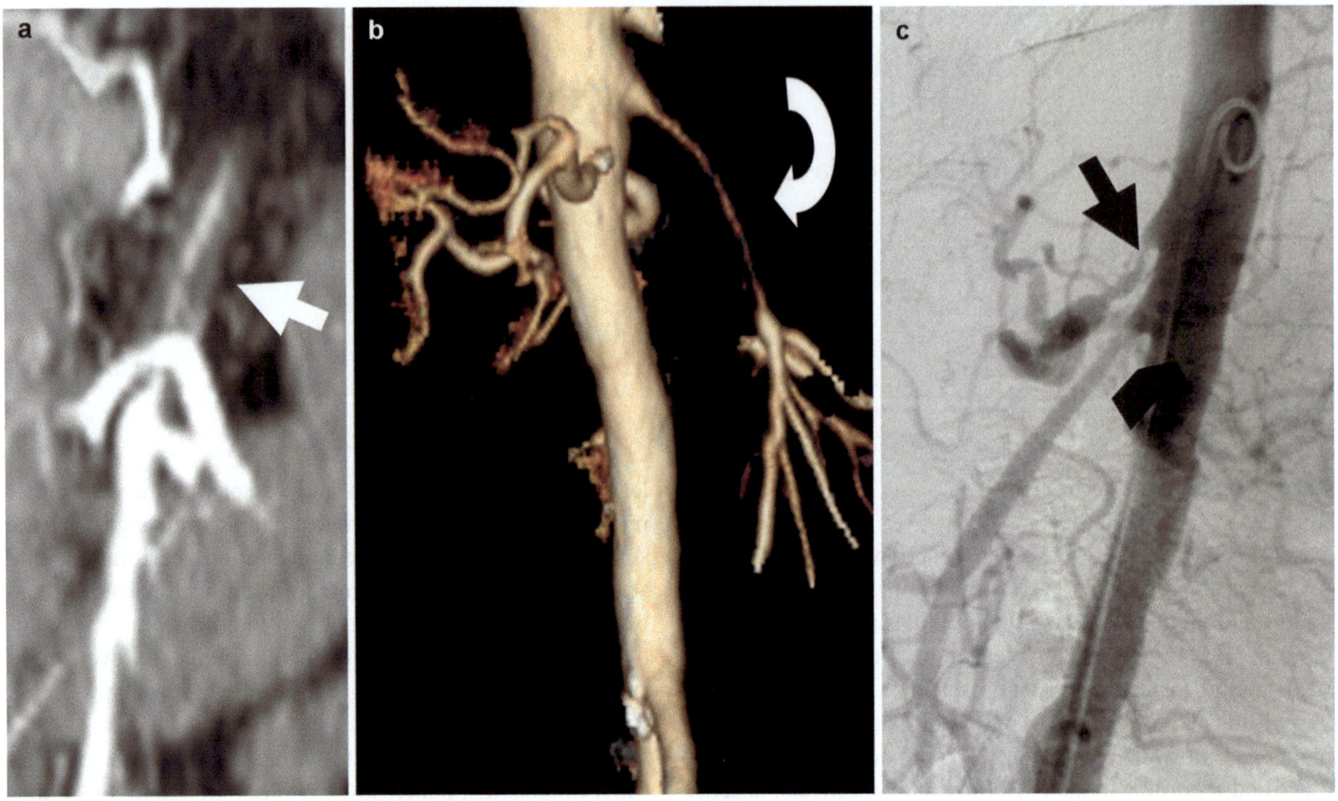

Fig. 24.1 Imaging findings consistent with mesenteric vasculitis includes arterial wall thickening (**a**, *white arrow*) and long and smooth tapered lesions (**b**, *curved white arrow*). Angiography remains the gold standard diagnostic study. Panel **c** shows a lateral aortography with high-grade celiac (**c**, *straight black arrow*) and superior mesenteric artery stenoses (**c**, *black arrowhead*)

Diagnostic Imaging

Duplex ultrasound is used to screen test and evaluate patency of the visceral arteries and presence of hemodynamically significant stenoses or occlusions. The criteria to identify a high-grade stenosis include peak systolic velocity >275 cm/s for the superior mesenteric artery (SMA) and >200 cm/s for the celiac axis [11]. Selective mesenteric angiography remains the gold standard for diagnosis of mesenteric vasculitis. The classic finding includes long, tapered, smooth lesions without stigmata of atherosclerosis, such as calcifications or atheromatous plaque (Fig. 24.1). Multiple and small aneurysms are also frequently seem. Barium enema may show thumbprinting due to submucosal edema or hemorrhage. Computed tomography angiography (CTA) is an excellent imaging study to diagnose and plan the intervention. It allows greater spatial resolution and is useful to diagnose other potential causes of abdominal pain and weight loss (e.g., malignancy). Specific findings consistent with mesenteric vasculitis include vessel wall thickening, periarterial edema or stranding, and long, smooth lesions with or without concomitant aneurysms or pseudoaneurysms (Fig. 24.1). This study is useful to plan open surgical reconstruction, allowing selection of a diseased-free site for inflow and outflow of bypass procedures. In addition, evaluation of bowel wall thickening (e.g., the target sign), increased attenuation of mesenteric fat, pneumatosis intestinalis, or pneumoperitoneum is consistent with complicated acute ischemia, bowel gangrene, and perforation.

Specific Disorders

A variant of specific vasculitis can manifest with symptoms of mesenteric ischemia or bleeding complications (Table 24.2).

Takayasu's Arteritis. Takayasu's arteritis or "pulseless disease" is a large-vessel granulomatous vasculitis characterized by ocular disturbances and decreased extremity pulses. Gastrointestinal manifestations include non-specific symptoms, such as anorexia, nausea, vomiting, and weight loss. Mesenteric ischemia can result from aortic narrowing and/or involvement of the visceral arteries. Diagnosis is confirmed by arteriography and/or CTA. Imaging findings include irregular thickening of the aortic wall or its main branches, with intimal wrinkling, stenosis, post-stenotic dilatation, aneurysm formation, or occlusion with subsequent luxurious collateral circulation [1, 3, 12].

Giant Cell Arteritis. Giant cell arteritis (GCA) is the most common systemic vasculitis. It occurs in the elderly and is characterized by inflammation involving large and

Table 24.2 Differential diagnosis of mesenteric ischemia

Arterial Occlusion	Venous Occlusion	Non-Occlusive Disease
Thromboembolism	Venous thrombosis	Narcotics
Left atrial origin	Infiltrative conditions	*Cocaine*
Aortic origin	*Neoplasm*	*Heroin*
Myxoma	Inflammatory conditions	Shock Bowel
Endocarditis	*Abdominal infectious diseases*	Familial dysautomia
Cholesterol	Hypercoagulable conditions	Pheochromocytoma
Atherosclerosis	*Polycitemia vera*	High-endurance athletes
SMA thrombosis	*Sickle cell disease*	Chronic renal failure
Arterial dissection	*Thrombocytosis*	Trauma
Aortic surgery	*Thrombophilia*	Corrosive injury
Stent placement	*Carcinoma*	
Therapeutic embolization	*Pregnancy drugs*	
Antiphospholipid antibody syndrome	Systemic vasculitis	Iatrogenic
Systemic vasculitis	*Wegener's granulomatosis*	*Radiation*
Takayasu's arteritis	*Systemic lupus erytematous*	*Prostraglandins antagonist Immunotherapy*
Giant cell arteritis	*Behçet's syndrome*	*Chemotherapy*
Polyarteritis nodosa	Complicated bowel obstruction	*Vasoconstriction*
Systemic lupus erytematous	*Strangulated hernia*	*Digitalis*
Henoch-Shonlein purpura	*Strangulated closed loop obstruction*	*Ergotamine*
Wegener's granulomatosis	*Volvulus*	*Vasopressin*
Churg-Strauss syndrome	*Intussusception*	*Epinephrine*
Thromboangiitis obliterans	*Intestinal overdistention*	*Hypotension*
Rheumatoid vasculitis	Enterocolic lymphocitic phlebitis	*Diuretics*
Behçet's syndrome		*Antidepressants*
Thrombotic thrombocytopenic purpura		
Hemolytic-uremic syndrome		
Fybromuscular dysplasia		
Diabetes mellitus		
Oxalosis		
Amyloidosis		

medium-sized arteries. The classic pathologic finding is the presence of giant cells (Fig. 24.2). GCA most frequently affects the aortic arch and its branches. GI symptoms include diffuse abdominal pain, typical intestinal angina, and bowel occlusion. CTA and duplex scans evidenced SMA or IMA occlusive disease and periarterial wall halo resulting from arterial wall inflammation. MRA is particularly helpful in determining wall thickness [9].

Polyarteritis Nodosa. PAN is a fibrinoid necrotizing vasculitis that mainly involves small and medium-sized arteries. The disease causes multiple aneurysms (50–60 %) with a predilection for the renal (80–90 %), mesenteric (50–70 %), hepatic (50–60 %), splenic (45 %),, and pancreatic branches (25–35 %). In addition to ischemic complications, hemorrhage occurs in 6 % of cases and bowel perforation in 5 % [1–4, 6]. Characteristic imaging findings include <1-cm aneurysms within the renal, mesenteric, and hepatic vasculature.

Wegener's Granulomatosis. Wegener granulomatosis (WG) is a medium- and small-size vessel granulomatous vasculitis of the upper and lower respiratory tract, added to glomerulonephritis. Ten percent of patients manifest gastrointestinal symptoms such as abdominal pain, diarrhea, and bleeding.

Microscopic Polyangiitis. Microscopic polyangiitis (MP), also know as hypersensivity vasculitis or leukocytoclastic angiitis, is a necrotizing small-vessel vasculitis, identical to PAN, except for presenting in smaller vessels. Unlike PAN, angiographic findings are usually normal and do not reveal microaneurysms.

Henoch-Schönlein Syndrome. Henoch-Schönlein syndrome (HSS) is a hypersensitivity-related acute small-vessel vasculitis occurring mainly in children up to 10 years. The most common cause is group A *Streptococcus Beta-hemolytic* accounting for 75 % of cases. Gastrointestinal bleeding is related to intramural hemorrhage and may precede skin lesions. The disease is confined to the mucosa and submucosa, and full-thickness necrosis and bowel perforation are rare.

Systemic Lupus Erythematous. Systemic lupus erythematous (SLE) is an autoimmune disorder that affects the musculoskeletal system, kidneys, GI tract, or skin. Small blood vessel inflammation of the gut produces a variety of complications, including intestinal ischemia, hemorrhage, ileus, ulceration, infarction, and perforation. Visceral artery involvement has a predilection for the SMA territory.

Behçet's Syndrome. Behçet's syndrome (BS) is a necrotizing vasculitis that involves multiple organ systems. The gastrointestinal tract is involved in 10–40 % of patients, predominantly the terminal ileum. BS appears with large, deeply penetrating ulcerations of the submucosa, muscle layer, or entire intestinal wall. As a result, a large prevalence

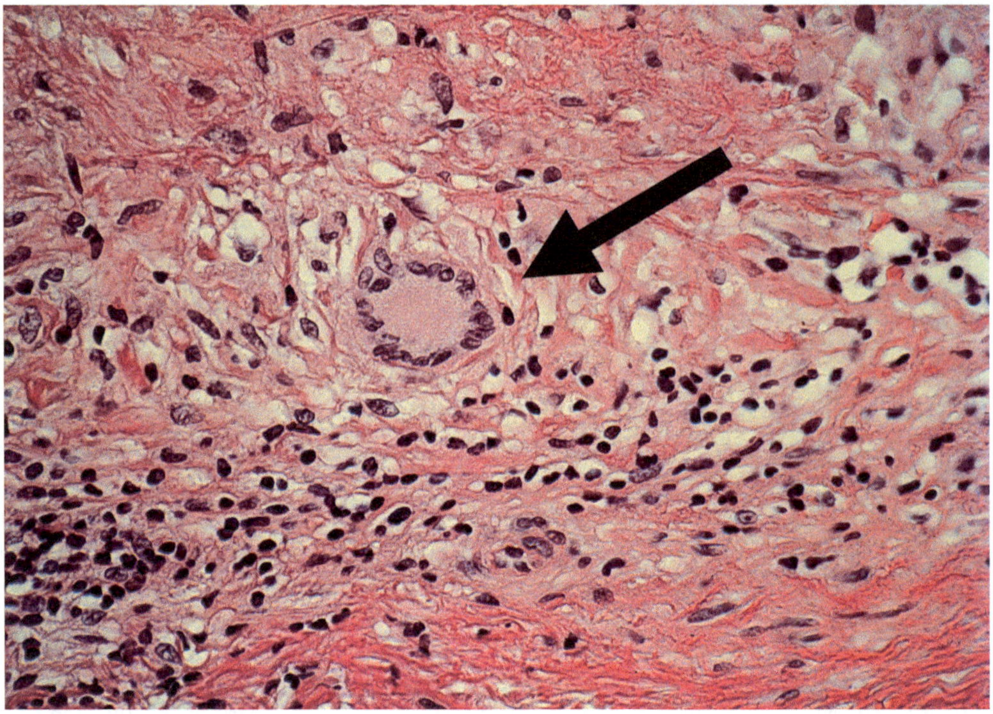

Fig. 24.2 Microscopic examination demonstrating a giant multinucleated cell (*black arrow*) in a patient with giant cell arteritis causing bilateral renal and superior mesenteric artery stenoses (H and E staining)

of complications such as hemorrhage, perforation, fistula, and peritonitis has been reported. The vasculitic process affects primarily small veins rather than arteries; hence, thrombophlebitis of superficial and deep veins and arterial thrombosis are common. Arterial involvement with aneurysmal disease involves pulmonary (50 %), aortic, and other large vessels. The presence of severe perienteric or pericolic infiltration raises the possibility of complications such as microperforation or localized peritonitis. [3, 4, 13]

Thromboangiitis Obliterans. Thromboangiitis obliterans (TAO), or Buerger's disease, is a distinct disease characterized by segmental, thrombosing, acute or chronic inflammation of small and intermediate-sized arteries and veins. Although it is not a classic vasculitis, the disease is considered one because of the intense inflammatory response. GI tract manifestations are rare.

Management

Medical Treatment

Because vasculitides are primarily inflammatory processes, corticosteroids alone or combined with other immunosuppressants are the basis of medical therapy [2]. Even in the presence of severe GI vasculitis, medical therapy should be initiated [4]. The medical regimen in the Mayo Clinic is based on previous work published in our institution [14, 15], which includes a daily dose of 40–60 mg of prednisone, which is preferred over a lower dose or alternate day corticosteroid therapy and aspirin. Prednisone is maintained at this dosage for approximately 4–6 weeks, after which it is tapered by 10 % every 2–4 weeks, depending on the absence of symptoms and level of inflammatory markers. The addition of an anti-metabolic or steroid-sparing agent may allow reduction of the prednisone dose, although these medications are reserved for patients without initial response to prednisone. The medical treatment resolved mesenteric symptoms in >87 % of our patients [2].

Open Surgical Reconstruction

Open surgery is indicated in patients who fail medical therapy because of persistent symptoms or intolerance of medications and in those who present with life-threatening acute mesenteric ischemia or bleeding. Levine et al. (2002) reported a lower (23 %) overall mortality for surgical patients presenting with less severe GI involvement. However, severe GI involvement has been associated with high mortality [16]. According to uni- and multivariate survival analysis of 62 patients presenting with GI vasculitidis, peritonitis, bowel perforation, GI ischemia, or infarction and intestinal occlusion were the only high-mortality predictors [4].

Mesenteric revascularization is indicated in patients with acute or chronic mesenteric ischemia (Fig. 24.3). Ritz and associates reported the Mayo Clinic experience with interventions for mesenteric vasculitis. Among 7,514 patients evaluated for vasculitis for 24 years, 120 had symptoms of mesenteric ischemia. Of these, 15 patients (4 %) required

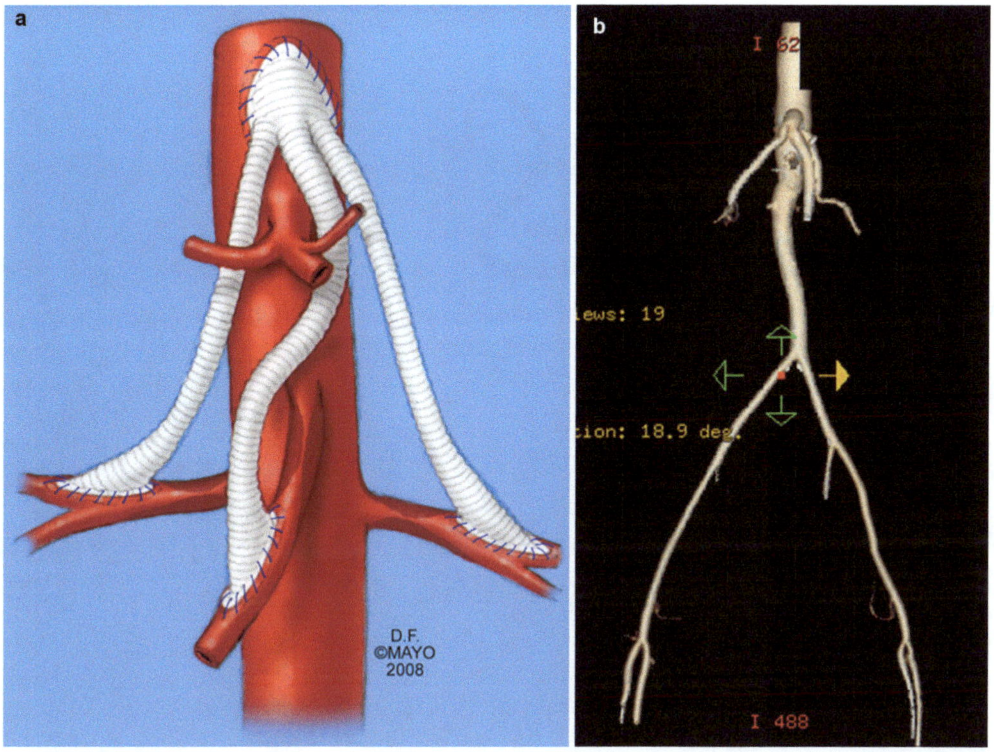

Fig. 24.3 Illustration of a supraceliac aorta to superior mesenteric artery and bilateral renal artery bypass (**a**) in a patient with Giant cell arteritis who presented with symptoms of chronic mesenteric ischemia and had difficult to control renovascular hypertension. Follow up computed tomography angiography (**b**) reveals widely patent grafts (b)

open or endovascular treatment for occlusive vasculitis. During the same period, 323 other patients required open surgery for atherosclerotic visceral disease. Procedures performed for mesenteric vasculitis included open revascularization in 14 patients and percutaneous transluminal angioplasty (PTA) in one. Twenty-two mesenteric arteries were treated. There were no early deaths and only three complications, which included GI bleeding and ileus and superior mesenteric vein thrombosis. There were no late deaths after a mean follow-up of 41 months; 14 patients (93 %) remained asymptomatic.

The most common etiologies were large- and medium-vessel vasculitides: Takayasu's arteritis due to aortic involvement proximal to or at the ostia of the mesenteric arteries in seven patients, polyarteritis nodosa in four patients, and giant cell arteritis in one. Three patients had indeterminate vasculitis.

The Mayo Clinic experience on surgical reconstructions performed for Takayasu's arteritis [12] included 42 (17 %) patients treated over 27 years. Fields and associates reviewed outcomes of 60 operations on 116 arteries. The survival rate was 100 % at 1 year and 97 % at both 5–10 years, similar to age- and gender-matched controls. The only death was unrelated to the initial procedure. Eleven patients underwent graft revision because of stenosis. Ten patients were reoperated during the first year of follow-up, related to disease activity. Freedom from graft revision in 5–10 years was 100 %.

There are no guidelines for how to approach open mesenteric reconstruction in mesenteric vasculitis. The general principal is to select the inflow and outflow anastomotic sites in noninflamed arteries. Similar to patients with atherosclerotic mesenteric disease, we favor an antegrade bypass from supraceliac aorta whenever possible. If the patient is older or has cardiac disease or a calcified aorta, a retrograde iliac-based mesenteric bypass with straight or C-shaped configuration is an excellent alternative and avoids aortic cross clamping. Both the celiac and SMA arteries are reconstructed, which may reduce rates of late failure if one of the graft limbs narrows or occludes. Finally, although renal or aortic concomitant reconstructions are avoided in patients with atherosclerotic disease, these patients may require more extensive reconstructions if the disease affects other visceral branches (Fig. 24.3). In our report on mesenteric vasculitis, 7 of 15 patients (47 %) had refractory renovascular hypertension and required concomitant renal bypasses [2, 12, 17].

Endovascular Treatment

Endovascular treatment of stenotic lesions should be reserved for focal and isolated lesions, or it can be used as a bridge to open surgery. The durability of endovascular therapy has not been demonstrated but likely does not match the results obtained with open surgery. Issues include the young age, the normal life expectancy, and the fact that vasculitis lesions are not favorable for angioplasty and stenting. These lesions are long, prone to recoil, and often involve branches; the technical result therefore is often suboptimal. In addition, angioplasty and stent placement contradict the basic principle

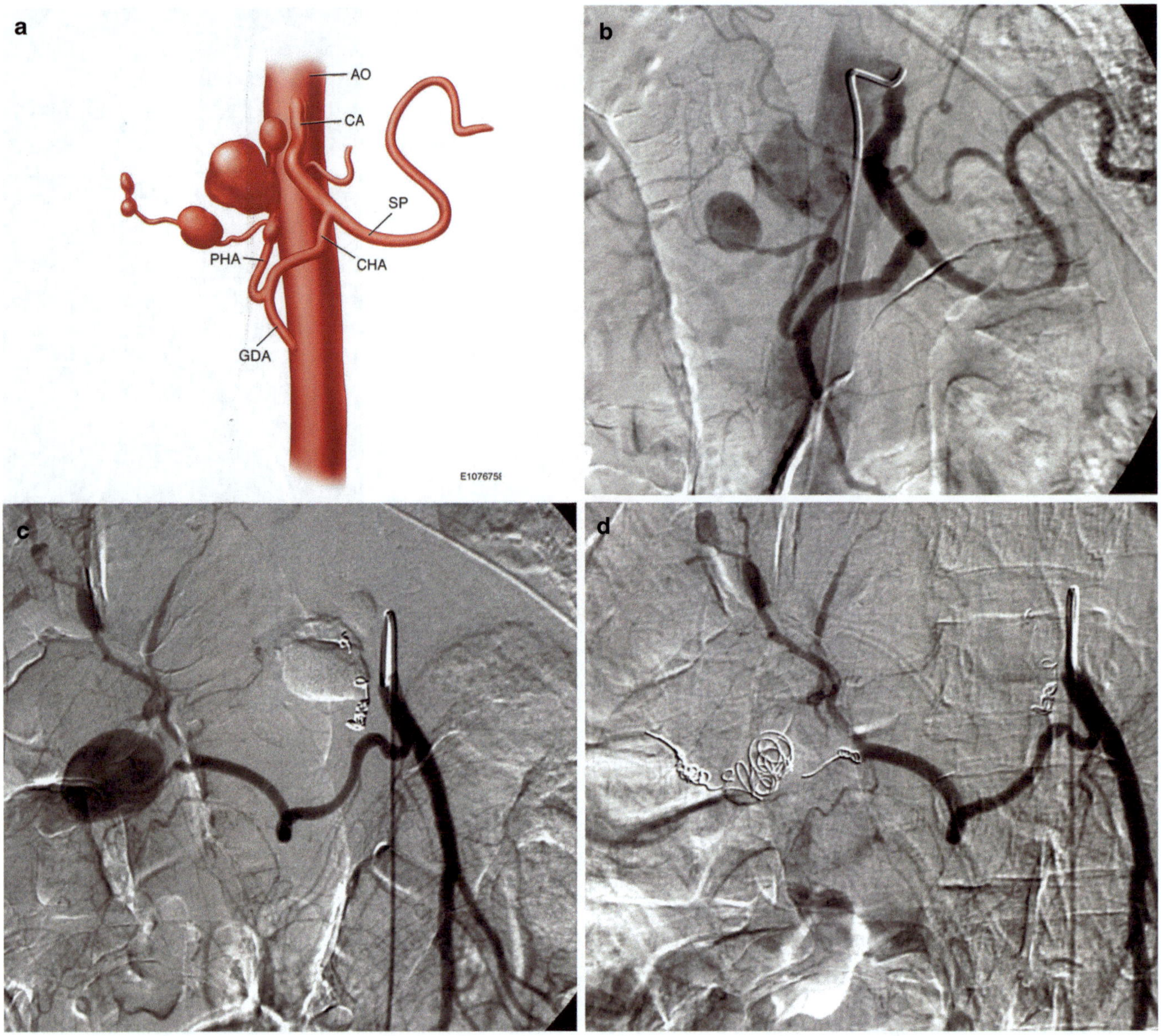

Fig. 24.4 Illustration depicts multiple hepatic artery branch aneurysms (**a**) in a patient who presented with ruptured intra-hepatic aneurysm associated with polyarteritis nodosa (PAN). Selective celiac axis (*CA*, **b**) and superior mesenteric artery (SMA, **c** and **d**) demonstrates several visceral aneurysms affecting the proper hepatic artery (*PHA*) and replaced right hepatic artery (**c**, **d**). The patient was successfully treated by coil embolization. *AO aorta*, *SP splenic artery*, *CHA common hepatic artery*, *GDA gastroduodenal artery*

of avoiding the inflammatory bed, especially in patients with active disease, acute inflammation, or those with chronic disease still on corticosteroids [16–19].

Percutaneous transcatheter embolization (PTE) of visceral aneurysms (Fig. 24.4) is an ideal technique to deal with small complicated visceral aneurysms and has lower complication rates. In a 10-year period, 176 patients with 185 visceral aneurysms were treated at the Mayo Clinic for a variety of causes. The overall 30-day mortality was 6.2 %, and immediate technical success was 98 %. After a mean follow-up of 24 months, there were ten late deaths, which were not related to the aneurysm.

Conclusion

Mesenteric vasculitis is a rare manifestation of systemic vasculitis. Most patients have involvement of other vascular territories. Clinical manifestations can range from mild discomfort to life-threatening bleeding or ischemia. Patients with vasculitis who present with abdominal pain and weight loss should be investigated for mesenteric ischemia. Medical therapy is the first line of treatment. Open surgical and/or endovascular reconstruction is indicated in patients who fail medical therapy or have life-threatening bowel ischemia.

References

1. Ha HK, Lee SH, Rha SH, et al. Radiologic features of vasculitis involving the gastrointestinal tract. Radiographics. 2000;20: 779–94.
2. Rits Y, Oderich GS, Bower TC, et al. Interventions for mesenteric vasculitis. J Vasc Surg. 2010;51:392–400.
3. Ahn E, Luk A, Chetty R, et al. Vasculitides of the gastrointestinal tract. Semin Diagn Pathol. 2009;26:77–88.
4. Pagnoux C, Mahr A, Cohen P, et al. Presentation and outcome of gastrointestinal involvement in systemic necrotizing vasculitides. Medicine (Baltimore). 2005;84:115–28.
5. Hunder CG, Arend WP, Bloch DA, et al. The American College of Rheumatology 1990 criteria for the classification of vasculitis. Arthritis Rheum. 1990;33:1065–7.
6. Watts RA, Scott DG. Vasculitis mimics. In: Watts RA, Scott DG, editors. Vasculitis in clinical practice. London: Springer; 2010. p. 143–54.
7. Krupski WC, Selzman CH, Whitehill TA. Unusual causes of mesenteric ischemia. Surg Clin North Am. 1997;77:471–502.
8. Tian XP, Zhang X. Gastrointestinal involvement in systemic lupus erythematosus: insight into pathogenesis, diagnosis and treatment. World J Gastroenterol. 2010;16(24):2971–7.
9. Sujobert P, Fardet L, Marie I, et al. Mesenteric ischemia in giant cell arteritis: 6 cases and a systematic review. J Rheumatol. 2007; 34:1727–32.
10. Hassoun Z, Lacrosse M, Ronde TD. Intestinal involvement in Buerger's disease. J Clin Gastroenterol. 2001;31(1):85–9.
11. Moneta GL, Lee RW, Yeager RA, et al. Mesenteric duplex scanning: a blinded prospective study. J Vasc Surg. 1993;17: 79–84.
12. Fields CE, Bower TC, Cooper LT, et al. Takayasu's arteritis: operative results and influence of disease activity. J Vasc Surg. 2006;43: 64–71.
13. Ragab G. Vasculitic manifestations in the gastrointestinal tract. In: Ball GV, Bridges Jr SL, editors. Vasculitis. 2nd ed. New York: Oxford University Press; 2008. p. 181–98.
14. Warrington KJ, Matteson EL. Management guidelines and outcome measures in giant cell arteritis (GCA). Clin Exp Rheumatol. 2007; 25:137–41.
15. Hunder GG, Sheps SG, Allen GL, et al. Daily and alternate-day corticosteroidregimensintreatmentofgiantcellsarteritis:comparision in a prospective study. Ann Intern Med. 1975;82:613–8.
16. Levine SM, Hellmann DB, Stone JH. Gastrointestinal involvement in polyarteritis nodosa (1986–2000): presentation and outcomes in 24 patients. Am J Med. 2002;112:386–91.
17. Park WM, Gloviczki P, Kj Jr C, et al. Contemporary management of acute mesenteric ischemia: factors associated with survival. J Vasc Surg. 2002;35:445–52.
18. Ozdil E, Parikh DK, Kracjer Z, et al. Stent placement in a patient with takayasu's arteritis. Cathet Cardiovasc Diagn. 1996;38: 373–6.
19. Tyagi S, Jolly N, Khalilullah M. Multivessel angioplasty in takayasu's arteritis. Indian Heart J. 1993;45:215–27.
20. Guillevin L, Le THD, Godeau P, et al. Clinical findings and prognosis of polyarteritis nodosa and Churg-Strauss angiitis: a study of 165 patients. Br J Rheumatol. 1988;27:258–64.
21. Guillevin L, Lhote F, Gayraud M, et al. Prognostic factors in polyarteritis nodosa and Churg-Strauss syndrome: a prospective study in 342 patients. Medicine (Baltimore). 1996;75:17–28.
22. Casella G, Bonzino B, Cutrino L, et al. Vasculitis and gastrointestinal involvement. Minerva Gastroenterol Dietol. 2006;52:195–214.

Part VIII

Peripheral Aneurysms

Inflammatory Peripheral Arterial Aneurysms

25

Gianluca Faggioli, Rodolfo Pini, Mauro Gargiulo, Antonio Freyrie, Raffaella Mauro, and Andrea Stella

Introduction

The inflammatory changes occurring in the wall of arterial aneurysms have been extensively studied in the abdominal aorta since the first description by While in 1972. However, similar aspects of atherosclerotic aneurysms located in other sites of the arterial system, such as the popliteal and femoral arteries, have been reported only exceptionally. To our knowledge, after an extensive search of PubMed using the terms *inflammatory aneurysms, peripheral inflammatory aneurysms, peripheral aneuysms,* and *popliteal aneurysms,* only two papers were found in the English language literature, and one of them is a case report [1, 2].

The fact that an inflammatory infiltrate has been described in a series of anatomical locations, such as the coronary arteries and the thoracic aorta, leads to the assumption that similar pathological processes occur more frequently than reported for "atherosclerotic" aneurysms of any anatomical district.

Peripheral Aneurysms and Inflammation

Atherosclerotic aneurysms of the lower limb arteries are rare compared to aortic aneurysms. Specifically, aneurysms of the popliteal artery, which are the most frequent among peripheral aneurysms (70 %), are tenfold rarer than abdominal aortic aneurysms (AAAs), and those of the femoral artery are rarer still, affecting 2.8–6.7 % of patients with AAAs [3, 4]. Similar to aortic aneurysms, the pathological process leading to peripheral aneurysm formation is not completely clear. Atherosclerosis is part of this process in the majority of cases; however, many authors have proposed the definition of "nonspecific degenerative aneurysms." However, the terminology of atherosclerotic aneurysms has remained commonly used [5].

The clinical features of these aneurysms, together with the recommendations for their treatment, are well discussed in the literature. However, no extensive analysis of the wall characteristics is available, and studies on the inflammatory parietal changes are lacking, with little or no histological data on the inflammatory involvement of the tunica media and adventitia.

In the work of our group published many years ago [1], 18 consecutive cases of peripheral artery atherosclerotic aneurysms were histologically examined and compared with a group of atherosclerotic femoral artery specimens obtained from the cadavers of a similar population in order to evaluate the prevalence of medial and adventitial inflammation, its type, and the amount. These findings could be useful for evaluating pathogenetic hypotheses.

Data from the Study

Eighteen consecutive patients [16 male (88.8 %), 47–79 years old; mean age 66.5] undergoing revascularization for aneurysms of the peripheral arteries were included. Symptoms included claudication of <300 meters in six cases (33.4 %) and rest pain in two cases (11.1 %). Ten patients (55.5 %) were asymptomatic. Pain was not present at the aneurysm site in any of the cases. Arteries involved were the popliteal artery, common femoral artery, and deep femoral artery, as reported in Table 25.1. A diagnosis of popliteal entrapment, cystic medionecrosis, or other non-atherosclerotic causes of aneurysm was excluded in each case, and an elevated ESR, leukocytosis, or autoimmune disease was not present in any of the

G. Faggioli, MD (✉)
Chirurgia Vascolare, Policlinico S. Orsola,
Via Massarenti 9, 40138 Bologna, Italy

Department of Vascular Surgery,
University of Bologna, Bologna, Italy
e-mail: gianluca.faggioli@unibo.it

R. Pini, MD • M. Gargiulo, MD • A. Freyrie, MD
R. Mauro, MD • A. Stella, MD
Department of Vascular Surgery,
University of Bologna, Bologna, Italy
e-mail: rudypini@gmail.com; mauro.gargiulo2@unibo.it; antonio.freyrie@unibo.it; raffaella.mauro1@gmail.com; andrea.stella2@unibo.it

E.A. Gabriel, S.A. Gabriel (eds.), *Inflammatory Response in Cardiovascular Surgery*,
DOI 10.1007/978-1-4471-4429-8_25, © Springer-Verlag London 2013

Table 25.1 Clinical and morphological characteristics according the histological findings

	Group I	Group II	Group III
Patients	9	5	4
Clinic			
Age	63.4	62.2	70.7
Males (%)	88.8	60	100
Smoking (%)	77.7	80	75
Diabetes (%)	22.2	40	25
Hypertension (%)	33.3	20	25
Leukocytosis	–	–	–
Increased ESR	–	–	–
Pain at aneurysm site	–	–	–
Morphology			
Aneurysm location			
Common femoral	–	2	–
Profunda femoris	–	–	1
Popliteal	9	3	3
Wall thickness	0.21 ± 0.03	0.36 ± 0.02	0.55 ± 0.05*
Number of inflammatory cells/2,116 um²	2.2 ± 0.3	9.2 ± 0.5	13.2 ± 0.3

*Group I and group II: $p<0.01$, group II and group III: $p<0.02$

Table 25.2 Patient characteristics in the PAAA and control groups

Parameters	PAAA	Control
Age	64.5	68.3
Males (%)	83.3	86.6
Smoking (%)	77.7	73.3
Diabetes (%)	27.7	13.3
Hypertension (%)	27.7	20.0
Wall thickness	0.33 ± 0.047	0.23 ± 0.02*
Atherosclerosis	+	+
Macroscopic signs of inflammation	–	–
Numbers of inflammatory cell	6.6 ± 1.14	1.48 ± 0.24**

*p = ns; **p = <0.001

patients. The intraoperative macroscopic examinations did not reveal the morphological aspects typical of inflammatory abdominal aneurysms or the inflammatory variants of AAA (perianeurysmatic fibroses with adherence to the neighboring structures, pearly white color) in any of the cases. In all the cases, gross evidence of atherosclerosis was present.

A segment of the aneurysm wall was harvested and then fixed in 10 % formalin and stained with hematoxylin & eosin, van Geison + elastic fibers, PTAH, and Alcian Pas. Ten specimens were also obtained from the atherosclerotic non-aneurysmatic femoral arteries of ten autopsies of patients with similar demographic characteristics (Table 25.2) and submitted to the same procedure for histological examination. Clinical history and laboratory examinations of all patients were reviewed with particular attention to infections, autoimmune diseases, arteritis, and the presence of non-specific leukocitosis.

Histological features of inflammation were classified according to the criteria proposed by Rose and Dent for

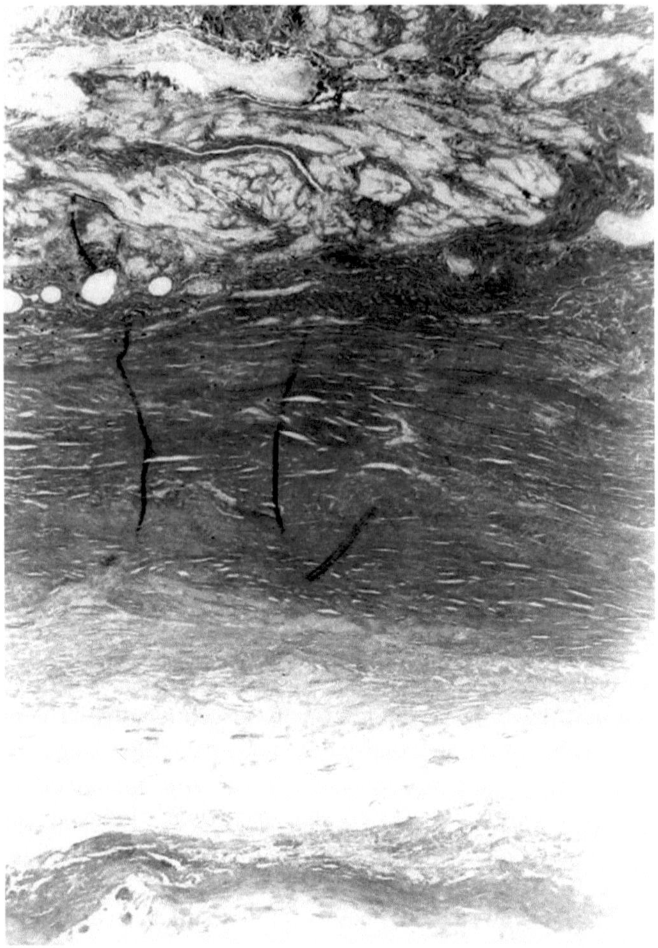

Fig. 25.1 Histological appearance of group I aneurysmatic wall showing absence of lymphomonoplasmocytic infiltrate (<4 cells/2,116 μm²)

abdominal aortic aneurysm (AAA) [6]: group I, scarce inflammatory infiltrate; group II, moderate inflammation; group III, severe degree of inflammatory infiltrate. Quantitatively, the number of inflammatory cells present within a 2,116 μm² square in 100 random fields was calculated. Group I was composed of specimens with <4 cells/2,116 μm², group II of specimens with 4–11 cells/2,116 μm², and group III of specimens with more than 11 cells. The mean wall thickness was calculated as a mean of three different random measurements in the same specimen and expressed in centimeters. The distribution of the specimens into the three groups was treated with the Kolmogorov-Smirnov test. Correlation between peripheral atherosclerotic artery aneurysms and control specimens and among the three different groups were evaluated by Mann-Whitney U test. Histological findings of cholesterol clusters, fibrohyaline degeneration, and internal elastic lamina disruption were always evident. In the media and adventitia, histological evidence of a slight lymphomonoplasmocytic infiltrate (<4 cells/2,116 μm²) was found in nine aneurysmatic walls (group I) (Fig. 25.1). In five cases (27.7 %), a moderate quantity (from 4 to 11 cells/2,116 μm²)

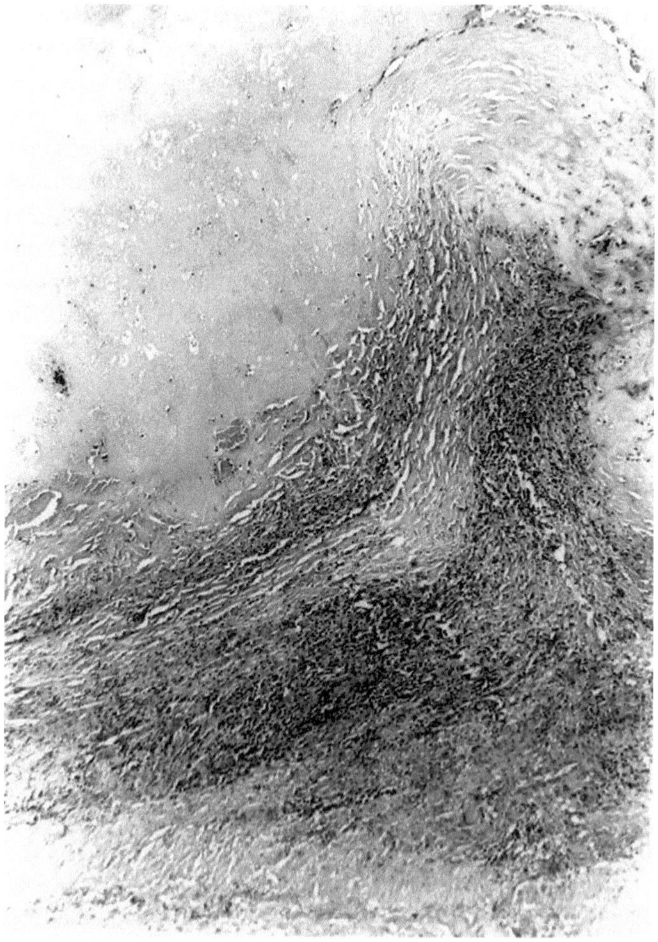

Fig. 25.2 Histological appearance of group II aneurysmatic wall. In this case, a moderate lymphomonoplasmocytic infiltrate can be seen in the tunica media and adventitia (from 4 to 11 cells/2,116 μm^{2}4 cells/2,116 μm^2)

of lymphomonoplasmocytic infiltrate was found in the tunica media and adventitia (group II) (Fig. 25.2). In the four remaining cases (22.2 %), the inflammatory infiltrate showed a high number (>11 cells/2,116 μm^2) of lymphomonoplasmocytic elements (group III) (Fig. 25.3). In this group of cases, it was possible to observe a different arrangement of the infiltrate: in pseudo-follicles in three cases and widespread in one case. In one case the lumen of the aneurysm was almost completely occupied by recent thrombus. In the ten control specimens, histology did not reveal moderate or severe inflammation in any of the cases. Mild changes were found in all of the cases. The mean number of inflammatory cells was 1.47 ± 0.24, and they were distributed mainly in the adventitia (Table 25.2).

In two of ten cases (20 %) of peripheral aneurysms with inflammatory histopathological features, an associated aortic aneurysm was present; however, the AAA did not show any macro- or microscopic features of the inflammatory forms.

While the distribution of the specimens in the three groups was not significantly different from the theoretical uniform distribution (Kolmogorov-Smirnov's test), when all the

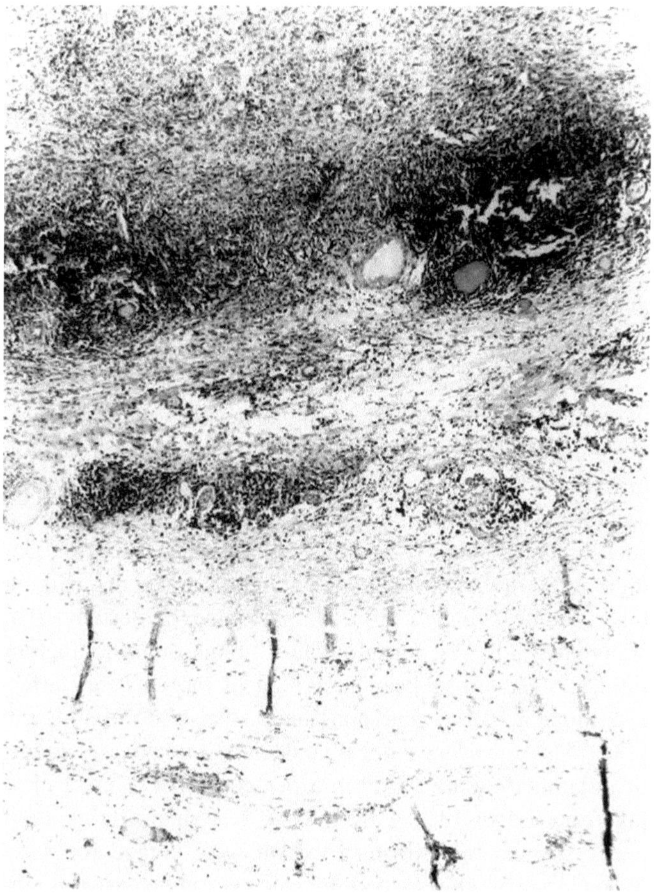

Fig. 25.3 The inflammatory infiltrate of patients in GIII shows a substantial number (>11 cells/2,116 μm^2) of lymphomonoplasmocytic elements, which sometimes are arranged in pseudo-follicles

aneurysm specimens were considered together, the number of inflammatory cells was significantly higher than that of atherosclerotic controls ($p<0.001$, Mann-Whitney U test). There was no statistical difference in wall thickness between these two groups; however, the difference in the wall thickness of the three groups of PAAA was significant (group I and II: $p<0.01$; group II and group III: $p<0.02$, Mann-Whitney U test).

Inflammatory Peripheral Aneurysms

The pathogenesis of peripheral arterial aneurysms is thought to be atherosclerotic in the majority of cases (99.1 %), even if the exact etiology is not known, especially at the femoral level [5, 6]. While the most appropriate definition for these forms should be "non-specific aneurysms," the terminology of "atherosclerotic aneurysms" is commonly used. Various etiopathogenetic hypotheses have been examined in the literature: in particular the vibration of the arterial wall due to the turbulence in the collateral breaching areas and the trauma caused by the inguinal ligament during flexing of the thigh [7]. Revascularization, either surgical or endovascular, is indicated because of the high percentage of complications (70 %) caused by thrombosis, peripheral emboli, and rupture. Different techniques are available nowadays, from the replacement of the aneurysmal segment with the insertion of a vein or prosthetic graft to endoluminal devices [8, 9].

The only report of a clinically evident popliteal inflammatory aneurysm has been published recently [2]. In that case, local and systemic symptoms of inflammation were present, such as swelling, redness with pain, and fever. Laboratory tests also showed signs of active inflammation, such as elevated leukocytes and CRP levels. Similarly to the findings of aortic inflammatory aneurysms, CT scans showed the typical arterial wall thickening and a surrounding hyperdense region [10]. The findings of inflammation are usually grossly evident in the abdominal aorta because of the fibrotic and inflammatory involvement of the surrounding structures, such as the ureters, left renal vein, vena cava, and duodenum. Very rarely, severe wall inflammation occurs without macroscopic evidence of wall thickening or periadvetitial adherence [11, 12]. Histological findings or inflammatory infiltrates have also been described in the coronary arteries, thoracic aorta, and non-aneurysmal abdominal aorta [13, 14]. However, clinical and morphological elements of inflammation are found in a percentage of AAAs, varying from 2.4 to 18.1 % of cases. The terms inflammatory aneurysm and inflammatory variant were coined for these forms [15, 16]. Our analysis of 18 consecutive cases of atherosclerotic peripheral aneurysms did not reveal any clinical or morphological features able to distinguish inflammatory from noninflammatory cases, similarly to the aorta and the fact that only recently a single case has been reported consistent with our findings. The arterial wall was never affected by periadventitial fibrotic phenomena causing adherences to neighboring structures. However, in a significant percentage of our cases (50 %), histology revealed a greater inflammatory infiltrate than is normally found in atherosclerotic arteries at this level or at the aortic level. Due to the different amount of inflammation, it was possible to make a distinction among three groups of aneurysms according to the number of inflammatory cells seen. According to these criteria, a total of nine atherosclerotic aneurysms (50 %) were divided between group II and group III. This result is rather surprising if compared with data obtained at the level of the abdominal aorta. This is especially true when considering the absence of clinical and macroscopic signs of inflammation, which correspond indeed to the absence of fibrosis.

The literature provides a large amount of data on the nonspecific inflammation in atherosclerotic arteries, referring mainly to the role of monocytes and macrophages in the genesis of foam cells. Activated T lymphocytes have been demonstrated within the atherosclerotic plaques. The cellular reaction of inflammatory aortic aneurysms has been shown to be mainly B lymphocytes, with an associated T4/T8 process. This process is supposed to be active and proliferating, as demonstrated by the presence of IL2 receptors, HLA-DR antigens, IgG, and IgM and by the activation of complement [1, 17–21]. Unfortunately, we could not perform any immunochemistry in this group of specimens, and we cannot be sure that the nature of the inflammation was identical to that seen in the aorta. Further prospective studies are therefore needed. The antigens that are able to trigger this process are unknown; the role of atheromatous components and of the fragmented elastin and collagen fibers needs to be evaluated.

Different hypotheses have been proposed to explain this phenomenon; most of them have been discounted by successive papers.

The development of the entire process and the significance for the interpretation of atherosclerotic disease are still obscure and require further investigation. These forms are not correlated with the presence of parietal fibrosis, and the surrounding tissues in the limb would not be as dangerously involved as the structures around the aorta (i.e., ureters); therefore, the significance of these findings is only for their pathogenetic implications. It would be interesting to understand the exact pathogenesis of fibrosis, which is almost always absent in these forms but is common in inflammatory AAAs, also determining differences in their postoperative evolution.

The recognition that the inflammatory process can involve arteries other than the abdominal aorta and that it is usually associated with aneurysmal forms may lead to a better understanding of its evolution.

References

1. Faggioli GL, Gargiulo M, Bertoni F, Bacchini P, Gessaroli M, Stella A. Parietal inflammatory infiltrate in peripheral aneurysms of atherosclerotic origin. J Cardiovasc Surg. 1992;33:331–6.
2. Akamatsu D, Fujishima F, Sato A, et al. Inflammatory popliteal aneurysm. Ann Vasc Surg. 2011;25:698.e13–6.
3. Szilagyi DE, Schwartz RL, Reddy DJ. Popliteal arterial aneurysms. Their natural history and management. Arch Surg. 1981;116(5):724–8.
4. Mahmood A, Salaman R, Sintler M, Smith SR, Simms MH, Vohra RK. Surgery of popliteal artery aneurysms: a 12-year experience. J Vasc Surg. 2003;37(3):586–93.
5. Johnston KW, Rutherford RB, Tilson MD, Shah DM, Hollier L, Stanley JC. Gested standards for reporting on arterial aneurysms. Subcommittee on Reporting Standards for Arterial Aneurysms, Ad Hoc Committee on Reporting Standards, Society for Vascular Surgery and North American Chapter, International Society for Cardiovascular Surgery. Vasc Surg. 1991;13(3):452–8.
6. Rose AG, Dent DM. Inflammatory variant of abdominal atherosclerotic aneurysm. Arch Pathol Lab Med. 1981;105(8):409–13.
7. Graham LM, Zelenock GB, Whitehouse Jr WM, Erlandson EE, Dent TL, Lindenauer SM, et al. Clinical significance of arteriosclerotic femoral artery aneurysms. Arch Surg. 1980;115(4):502–7.
8. Antonello M, Frigatti P, Battocchio P, Lepidi S, Cognolato D, Dall'Antonia A, et al. Open repair versus endovascular treatment

for asymptomatic popliteal artery aneurysm: results of a prospective randomized study. J Vasc Surg. 2005;42:185–93.
9. Sarcina A, Bellosta R, Luzzani L, Agrifoglio G. Surgical treatment of popliteal artery aneurysm. A 20 year experience. J Cardiovasc Surg (Torino). 1997;38(4):347–54.
10. Stella A, Gargiulo M, Faggioli GL, Gessaroli M, Bertoni F, Cenacchi G. Inflammatory abdominal aortic aneurysms: does an early stage exist? J Cardiovasc Surg. 1991;32:732–5.
11. Stella A, Gargiulo M, Pasquinelli G, Preda P, Faggioli GL, Cenacchi G, et al. The cellular component in the parietal infiltrate of inflammatory abdominal aortic aneurysms (IAAA). Eur J Vasc Surg. 1991;5:65–70.
12. Stella A, Gargiulo M, Faggioli GL, Bertoni F, Cappello I, Brusori S, et al. Postoperative course of inflammatory abdominal aortic aneurysms. Ann Vasc Surg. 1993;7:229–38.
13. Kniemeyer HW, Kolvenbach R, Rohde E, Godehardt E, Sandmann W. "Inflammatory aneurysm" of the aorta. Diagnosis, therapy, results. Chirurg. 1990;61(1):27–31.
14. Hoffmeister AW. Inflammatory aneurysm of the infrarenal aorta. Chirurg. 1990;61(3):168–70.
15. Miller DV, Maleszewski JJ. The pathology of large-vessel vasculitides. Clin Exp Rheumatol. 2011;29(1 Suppl 64):S92–8. Epub 2011 May 11. Review.
16. Mikami Y. Inflammatory abdominal aortic aneurysm. Ryoikibetsu Shokogun Shirizu. 2000;32:544–6. Review.
17. Kasashima S, Zen Y, Kawashima A, Endo M, Matsumoto Y, Kasashima F. A new clinicopathological entity of IgG4-related inflammatory abdominal aortic aneurysm. J Vasc Surg. 2009;49(5):1264–71; discussion 1271. Epub 2009 Feb 14.
18. Sakata N, Tashiro T, Uesugi N, Kawara T, Furuya K, Hirata Y, et al. IgG4-Positive plasma cells in inflammatory abdominal aortic aneurysm: the possibility of an aortic manifestation of IgG4-related sclerosing disease. Am J Surg Pathol. 2008;32(4):553–9.
19. Sasaki S, Yasuda K, Takigami K, Yamauchi H, Shiiya N, Sakuma M. Inflammatory abdominal aortic aneurysms and atherosclerotic abdominal aortic aneurysms – comparisons of clinical features and long-term results. Jpn Circ J. 1997;61(3):231–5.
20. Spina M, Degani AM, Stella A, Gargiulo M, Faggioli GL, Preda P, et al. Modifications and turnover of extracellular matrix components in human abdominal aortic atherosclerotic and inflammatory aneurysms. Eur J Histochem. 1992;32:13–4 (IF 1,041).
21. Gargiulo M, Stella A, Spina M, Faggioli GL, Cenacchi G, Degani A, et al. Content and turnover of extracellular matrix protein turnover in human non-specific and inflammatory abdominal aortic aneurysms. Eur J Vasc Surg. 1993;7:546–53.

Endovascular Femoropopliteal Interventions: Evolving Devices

26

Cassidy Duran and Jean Bismuth

Introduction

Peripheral arterial disease (PAD) is caused by systemic atherosclerosis and is strongly associated with cardiovascular and cerebrovascular disease. Important risk factors for PAD include age > 70, history of smoking, diabetes, hypertension, and hyperlipidemia, all known markers for cardiovascular disease [1]. While medical management in conjunction with an exercise regimen is the recommended initial approach, according to the American Heart Association/American College of Cardiology guidelines for the management of PAD, patients with lifestyle-compromising pain, nonhealing ulcers, or critical limb ischemia require invasive endovascular or surgical intervention [2]. There is some disagreement about the appropriate management of femoral-popliteal lesions among various groups of interventionalists, but the Inter-Society Consensus for the Management of PAD (TASC) provides a general approach. Because of the rapidly changing technology, for many interventionalists the endovascular option is the first line of therapy, despite very poor evidence for many of the products currently on the market.

According to the 2007 TASC II updated guidelines, TASC A and B lesions requiring intervention should be managed with endovascular intervention. TASC C lesions in patients who can tolerate open surgery should receive open bypass, but many patients will have comorbid conditions that limit surgical options, and in that case endoluminal intervention is appropriate [3]. These recommendations are supported with only level C evidence, meaning no randomized or well-conducted clinical trials have been performed and the evidence is based on solely expert opinion. According to the BASIL trial, the only multi-center randomized controlled trial (RCT) of angioplasty versus open surgical bypass for infrainguinal disease, the angioplasty first strategy was associated with similar amputation-free survival and decreased costs [4]. This, however, did not take into account the early endovascular failure rate of 20 % that required re-intervention. It is estimated that the reason endovascular interventions looked so good was that patients often go on to have a surgical bypass later, and so probably overall surgical results are better in spite of short-term drawbacks. In practice, interventions have moved far beyond the scope of the consensus guidelines (which in 2000 addressed only percutaneous transluminal angioplasty (PTA), bare metal stents, and open surgical bypass). Since first being introduced, widespread development of new technologies for peripheral endovascular interventions has occurred. This is true not only for the therapeutic device, but also for the platform that provides access to and the ability to treat the pathology. Flexible robotics offers the ability to reliably provide a stable platform through which one can deliver a variety of therapeutic devices. This has been demonstrated in a recent first-in-man study in which the technical success rate was 100 % for the navigation of 20 iliofemoral lesions and 95 % for successful delivery of therapeutic interventions (the only failure occurring when a surgeon with no previous endovascular experience was unable to cross the lesion). Safety of the device was demonstrated with no peri-procedural complications (Duran et al., article in press). In this chapter, we describe the pathophysiology of femoral atherosclerosis and restenosis, followed by an overview of current endovascular therapies for femoral-popliteal atherosclerotic disease and the role of inflammation in the durability of endovascular interventions.

Pathophysiology of PAD

PAD results from atherosclerosis of the aortoiliac and lower extremity vasculature. It occurs concurrently with atherosclerotic processes throughout the body, including the extracerebral and coronary vasculature, and is associated with the same risk factors. Atherosclerosis develops slowly over time

C. Duran, MD • J. Bismuth, MD (✉)
The Methodist DeBakey Heart and Vascular Center,
The Methodist Hospital, 6550 Fannin St. Smith Tower 1400,
Houston 77030, TX, USA
e-mail: jbismuth@tmhs.org

E.A. Gabriel, S.A. Gabriel (eds.), *Inflammatory Response in Cardiovascular Surgery*,
DOI 10.1007/978-1-4471-4429-8_26, © Springer-Verlag London 2013

and in the majority of individuals will not become symptomatic. The initial step in the development of atherosclerotic plaques involves diffuse initimal thickening and formation of a fatty streak of lipid-filled macrophages and smooth muscle cells (SMCs). These lesions are not pathologic, but retain the potential to develop into fibrous plaques that contain lipids and fibrous connective tissues. These fibrous plaques become calcified and can rupture, erode into the endothelium, or hemorrhage within the plaque, all processes that are associated with clinical sequelae. Ultimately, the plaques develop a necrotic core that is surrounded by inflammatory cells and SMCs, which are prone to rupture, intraplaque hemorrhage, and occlusion [5]. Not all plaques are created equal, however, and atheromatous lesions are known to differ by vascular bed [6]. Examination of plaque morphology demonstrates that fibrous cap atheromas predominate in the carotid arteries, while fibrocalcific plaques form in the femoral arteries [7]. The implication is that lesions with higher levels of inflammatory cells, while unstable, are less prone to recurrent stenosis, while more stable plaques are highly calcified and prone to restenosis. However, because the time between the initial insult of lower extremity ischemia and intervention is prolonged compared to cerebral ischemia resulting from carotid disease, it is unclear if these differing plaque characteristics represent differing linear progressions of disease.

Restenosis Following Infrainguinal Intervention

Rates of recurrent stenosis following endovascular interventions are significantly different in the femoral system as compared to the carotid and coronary arteries. Histopathologic evaluation of atherosclerotic plaques suggests that following intervention; stable plaques are actually more susceptible to restenosis [8]. In the carotid arteries, unstable, inflammatory plaques with high levels of macrophages and lipid cores were associated with lower restenosis rates, presumably related to extensive remodeling of the tissue induced by the inflammatory cells [9]. As opposed to the extensive remodeling induced by inflammatory mediators, which appears to result in positive remodeling in the carotid system, the fibrotic characteristics of femoral plaques lead to constrictive remodeling and progressive vessel occlusion [10], and constrictive remodeling may be the primary driver for luminal compromise in patients with recurrent disease [11]. Understanding this process may ultimately guide the choice of intervention or device.

Percutaneous Transluminal Angioplasty

The primary endovascular intervention for treatment of flow-limiting femoropopliteal atherosclerosis is balloon angioplasty or PTA. According to a 2008 Cochrane Database review, mortality and amputation rates did not differ significantly between bypass surgery and PTA. Primary patency was significantly higher in the bypass group after 12 months (OR 1.6) but not after 4 years ($P=0.14$) [12]. The outcomes for PTA, however, depend on lesion characteristics, and the best results are seen in the group with short, focal lesions [3]. A 2008 meta-analysis of PTA found a pooled estimate of success was 89.0 ± 2.2 % for immediate technical results. Results at 1–36 months were 77.4 ± 4.1 % and 48.6 ± 8.0 % for primary patency, 83.3 ± 1.4 % and 62.9 ± 11.0 % for secondary patency, 93.4 ± 2.3 % and 82.4 ± 3.4 % for limb salvage, and 98.3 ± 0.7 % and 68.4 ± 5.5 % for patient survival, respectively [13]. Outcomes following PTA depend on a number of known factors, including lesion length, presence of total occlusion, size of vessel, vessel overdilation, residual stenosis, and dissection, all parameters that influence the degree of vessel disruption and resultant inflammation following angioplasty. Following PTA, the resultant injury to the vascular intima and media leads to proliferation of vascular smooth muscle cells and induces local and systemic inflammatory responses [14–16]. Though the process has been more extensively studied in coronary interventions, the phenomenon has been shown to occur in peripheral vasculature as well [17]. Sheer stress during PTA induces a vascular inflammatory process in which polymorphonuclear neutrophils (PMNs) and monocytes are localized to the injured endothelium. These inflammatory mediators induce the migration of smooth muscle cells (SMC) from the medial layer of the vessel to the subendothelium. In turn, SMCs induce proliferation of extracellular matrix proteins and myofibroblasts that are responsible for neointimal hyperplasia, negative vascular remodeling, and ultimately restenosis [18].

Alternative Modalities for Angioplasty (Table 26.1)

Cryoplasty

Because of the high restenosis rates following PTA alone, alternative endovascular modalities have been developed to improve patency rates. One approach designed to limit the inflammatory response following angioplasty is endovascular cryoplasty in which cold thermal energy is delivered simultaneously inside an angioplasty balloon. Experimentally, cryotherapy induces SMC apoptosis, which would theoretically halt the inflammatory response to vessel injury during balloon angioplasty. However, a single-center experience with 86 patients failed to demonstrate improved outcomes over expected patency rates from PTA (48–37 % at 12–24 months, respectively) [19]. Schmidt published a series in which 109 infrapopliteal lesions (the most challenging of the lower extremity lesions) were treated and reported

Table 26.1 Outcomes following traditional PTA and alternative angioplasty approaches for femoropopliteal lesions

Intervention	Study type	Technical success (%)	Amputation free (%)	Survival (%)	Primary patency (%)	Secondary patency (%)	Time to f/u (months)
PTA	Meta-analysis	95.8	93.4	98.3	77.4	83.3	1
			82.4	68.4	48.6	62.9	36
	RCT (BASIL)	80	NR	78	50	NR	12
Cryoplasty	Prospective	88	NR	NR	47	NR	12
					38		24
	RCT (COLD)	35	NR	NR	79	NR	9
CBA	Prospective	91	100	NR	88	NR	3
	RCT	NR	93	100	38	NR	6
Subintimal angioplasty	Prospective	87	75	99	45	76	12
					25	50	36
Drug-coated balloon	RCT	NR	95.6	83.6	96	NR	12
					91.5		24
	Prospective	NR	96	84.6	91.7	NR	12

NR = not reported

improvement in 94 %, healing in 74 %, and a limb salvage rate of 95 % [20]. The single RCT of comparing cryotherapy to balloon angioplasty (COLD trial) demonstrated a mean patency of 79 % in the cryoplasty arm versus 67 % in the PTA arm ($P = 14$) at 9 months and a 30 % rate of stent placement for residual stenosis or dissection following cryoplasty versus 39 % in the PTA group [21]. Long-term results are pending, but at this time cryoplasty does not appear to offer significant advantages over PTA.

Cutting Balloon Angioplasty (CBA)

Cutting balloons are designed with atherotome blades that score atherosclerotic plaques. This technique treats lesions while limiting overdilation of the vessel and therefore elastic recoil as well as distal dissection. Reports on their use in the coronary, pulmonary and peripheral vasculature indicated that there is in fact a reduction in vessel trauma and elastic recoil during CBA, with a positive impact in remodeling [22–28]. Initial results of this technology in femoropopliteal lesions demonstrated high rates of technical success (93 %), limb salvage (100 %), and primary patency (88 %) [29]. However, in a RCT of CBA versus PTA in short (<10 cm) SFA stenosis, CBA yielded increased restenosis rates at 6 months (62 %) compared to PTA (38 %) [30].

Subintimal Angioplasty

The theories on the precise role of endovascular interventions in femoropopliteal chronic total occlusions are in flux. Open surgical bypass remains the de facto gold standard, but dedicated re-entry catheters designed for subintimal angioplasty have been shown to be safe and the procedure technically feasible [31]. In light of the improvements in endovascular tools for subintimal navigation and vessel re-entry, as well as high rates of morbidity and mortality following open surgery in a subset of high-risk patients, increasing numbers of threatened limbs are being treated percutaneously [32]. Scott and colleagues published their single-center experience with 506 infrainguinal occlusions. Primary patency at 12–36 months was 45 % (SE 3.0 %) and 25 % (SE 3.6 %), respectively, and secondary patency was 76 % (SE 2.6 %) and 50 % (SE 4.8 %) at 12–36 months. Patients with femorotibial occlusions and critical limb ischemia had worse outcomes. Limb salvage in patients with CLI was 75 %, and open surgical bypass was avoided in 77 % at 36 months [33]. These results indicate that in experienced hands, subintimal angioplasty is a reasonable first-line therapy for patients with infrainguinal occlusions. The aforementioned results are unlikely to be a true representation of the outcomes to be expected in the average interventional community practice, as the procedure is anecdotally plagued by being extremely operator dependent.

Stents (Table 26.2)

Disappointing long-term patency rates following PTA in the femoropopliteal segment prompted the use of stents following angioplasty. Balloon angioplasty leads to thrombus formation, recoil, intimal hyperplasia, and ultimately negative remodeling, while stents are impacted only by thrombus formation and inflammatory-mediated intimal hyperplasia [34, 35]. Additionally, stents in the muscular infrainguinal arteries are subject to stresses that result in stent fracture, which also induces intimal hyperplasia and in-stent stenosis.

In the early years of infrainguinal endovascular interventions, stainless-steel stents were deployed with disappointing results. Studies failed to demonstrate improved outcomes over angioplasty alone, and the indication for stents was

Table 26.2 Outcomes following standard and alternative stent deployment and atherectomy for femoropopliteal lesions

Intervention	Study type	Technical success (%)	Amputation free (%)	Survival (%)	Primary patency (%)	Secondary patency (%)	Time to f/u (months)
Nitinol stent	RCT (RESILIENT)	95.8	100	92.8 (30 day)	87.3	100	12
	RCT	NR	NR	95.8	66.6	NR	12
Stent-graft	RCT	100	98	92	72	83	12
					63	74	24
DES	RCT	100	NR	NR	100	NR	6
Atherectomy	Prospective	100	100	98	80	100	6

NR = not reported

limited to bail-out for residual stenosis or arterial dissection following PTA [36]. The role of primary stent placement has been revisited using nitinol stents. Second generation nitinol stents have spirally oriented interconnections, which have reduced rates of stent fracture and the resultant stenosis [37]. Recently, the RESILIENT trial demonstrated that primary deployment of self-expanding nitinol stents in moderate length femoral and popliteal lesions yielded better results than angioplasty alone [38]. Overall, studies examining the role of nitinol stents have yielded variable results, with moderate improvement in outcomes over PTA alone, and results varying significantly based on lesion specifics (TASC classification, lesions length, outflow vessel status) [39, 40].

Stent-Grafts

Efforts to overcome the challenges of percutaneous interventions in the femoropopliteal segment have led interventionalists to consider a role for covered stents. The idea is that covered stents will slow tissue in-growth and delay in-stent re-stenosis. In 2000, Lammer and colleagues established feasibility in a multicenter, international trial [41]. In 2005, ePTFE-covered stent-grafts (Viabahn, WL Gore and Associates, Flagstaff, AZ) were approved for deployment in the superficial femoral artery, and in 2007, approval was extended to a heparin-bonded Viabahn for SFA lesions. A 2007 single-center randomized study of Viabahn versus surgical bypass in 100 limbs showed that primary and secondary patency rates were comparable at 12 months [42], and in 4-year follow-up of patients randomized to surgical bypass versus stent-graft for SFA lesions, differences in primary and secondary patency rates were not statistically significant. Additionally, stent-grafts were much less likely to fracture, making them less vulnerable to failure from in-stent stenosis at the fracture site, and unlike bare-metal stents, successful outcomes were not dependent on lesion length [43]. Therefore, it is likely preferable to treat long lesions with stent-grafts, and these results indicate that stent-grafts should be considered a viable alternative to bypass in these patients.

Drug-Eluting Stents

Drug-eluting stents (DES) have been used with great success in the coronary vasculature, and their use is now well defined [44]. The utility of DES use in the infrainguinal arteries has begun to be explored. In a non-randomized, single-arm trial, everolimus-eluting stents use was found to be feasible with success rates comparable to established endovascular approaches [45]. The SIROCCO II trial randomized 57 patients to sirolimus-eluting stents versus nitinol bare metal stents for treatment of SFA disease. Despite a trend toward improved outcomes in the DES group, there were no statistically significant differences in outcomes between the two groups [46]. Given the significant cost of DES stents, currently treatment with DES cannot be recommended, although more data are on the way, which may very well influence that.

Drug-Coated Balloons

Local administration of the antiproliferative drug paclitaxel has also been found to effectively reduce rates of re-stenosis following PTA, but unlike DES, drug-coated balloons are effective in both the coronary and peripheral vessels. In a multicenter randomized trial of 154 patients with femoral or popliteal artery stenosis/occlusions, at 12 months 20 of 54 (37 %) lesions in the control group required revascularization compared with 2 of 48 (4 %) in the group treated with paclitaxel-coated balloons ($P<0.001$ vs. control); at 24 months, the re-intervention rates increased to 28 of 54 (52 %) in the control group and 7 of 48 (15 %) in the paclitaxel group [47]. These early results are promising, but require further investigation before definitive recommendations can be made. Currently, two large European studies are recruiting patients to further elucidate the role of drug-coated balloons in the treatment of peripheral vascular lesions.

Atherectomy

In contrast to the aforementioned devices, atherectomy devices aim to treat peripheral lesions through excision of an atherosclerotic plaque using percutaneous means. The SilverHawk directional atherectomy device (EV3, Minneapolis, MN) has a highspeed carbide cutting disc that cuts ribbons of atheroma and stores the excised plaque in the nose cone of the device. In 2004, Zeller reported his initial experience in 52 patients using the SilverHawk device. Although <50 % stenosis was found in 96 % and <30 % in 78 % of patients following atherectomy, additional percutaneous procedures were performed in 58 % of the patients. The device was safe, and rates of recurrent disease were not higher in the atherectomy-only group compared to the group in which additional procedures were performed [48]. Recently, the group with the largest experience (579 infrainguinal lesions) reported on their outcomes. The primary patency at 12–18 months was 59.1–49.4 % with a limb-salvage rate of 87.9 % at 18 months for patients with critical limb ischemia and 100 % limb salvage in patients with claudication [49]. At this time, no RCTs have compared atherectomy to angioplasty and stenting in the setting of lower extremity atherosclerotic disease. In our experience, atherectomy has been marred by distal embolization, and as we recently showed, distal embolization has the ultimate of consequence, limb loss [50].

Medical Management

Endovascular interventions permit interventionalists to treat the consequences of atherosclerosis, which are an important corollary for limb salvage, wound healing, and overall quality of life. However, interventional procedures do not target the underlying disease process itself, and as illustrated above, likely intensify the inflammatory process that underlies the atherosclerotic process. Furthermore, these patients are at high risk of cardiac or cerebrovascular death due to their systemic disease, with 25 % 1-year mortality from myocardial infarction or stroke among patients with CLI [51]. As such, irrespective of the type of intervention employed in treating these patients, appropriate medical management of their systemic atherosclerotic disease is of paramount importance. This includes aggressive management of LDL cholesterol (<100 for all PAD patients, <70 for PAD with diabetes) using HMG-CoA reductase inhibitors, maintenance of blood pressure <140/90 (or 130/80 for diabetics) using beta-blockade and ACE-inhibitors, anti-platelet therapy with aspirin or clopidogrel, and smoking cessation [52].

Conclusion

Infrainguinal atherosclerosis resulting in lifestyle-altering limb ischemia is a challenging entity to treat. Formerly open surgical bypass was the only option available for restoration of flow to the extremities, but the rapid pace of technologic advances in endovascular interventions has led to a paradigm shift in disease management. While there is no silver bullet for treating these complex lesions, increasingly endovascular interventions are being utilized as a first line therapy in even the most diseased segments. Interventionalists should closely scrutinize their approach to devices as clearly not all devices and techniques are created equal. Expectations often need to be tempered as the few and relatively poor studies are generally performed in centers with vast experience. Furthermore, the key to any success in the interventional space is the understanding that we are managing the complications of an inflammatory disease and long-term success is in great part based on the continued management of the medical aspects of this disease.

References

1. Hirsch AT, Criqui MH, Treat-Jacobson D, et al. Peripheral arterial disease detection, awareness, and treatment in primary care. JAMA. 2001;286(11):1317–24.
2. Hirsch AT, Haskal ZJ, Hertzer NR, et al. ACC/AHA 2005 practice guidelines for the management of patients with peripheral arterial disease (lower extremity, renal, mesenteric, and abdominal aortic): a collaborative report from the American Association for Vascular Surgery/Society for Vascular Surgery, Society for Cardiovascular Angiography and Interventions, Society for Vascular Medicine and Biology, Society of Interventional Radiology, and the ACC/AHA Task Force on Practice Guidelines (Writing Committee to Develop Guidelines for the Management of Patients with Peripheral Arterial Disease): endorsed by the American Association of Cardiovascular and Pulmonary Rehabilitation; National Heart, Lung, and Blood Institute; Society for Vascular Nursing; TransAtlantic Inter-Society Consensus; and Vascular Disease Foundation. Circulation. 2006;113(11):e463–654.
3. Lyden SP, Smouse HB. TASC II and the endovascular management of infrainguinal disease. J Endovasc Ther. 2009;16(2 Suppl 2): II5–18.
4. Adam DJ, Beard JD, Cleveland T, et al. Bypass versus angioplasty in severe ischaemia of the leg (BASIL): multicentre, randomised controlled trial. Lancet. 2005;366(9501):1925–34.
5. Owens C. Chapter 4: Atherosclerosis. In: Rutherford's vascular surgery. 7th ed. Philadelphia: Elsevier; 2010.
6. Bianda N, Di Valentino M, Périat D, et al. Progression of human carotid and femoral atherosclerosis: a prospective follow-up study by magnetic resonance vessel wall imaging. Eur Heart J. 2011. Available at: http://www.ncbi.nlm.nih.gov/pubmed/21920966. Accessed 18 Dec 2011.
7. Herisson F, Heymann M-F, Chétiveaux M, et al. Carotid and femoral atherosclerotic plaques show different morphology. Atherosclerosis. 2011;216(2):348–54.
8. Derksen WJM, de Vries J-PPM, Vink A, et al. Histologic atherosclerotic plaque characteristics are associated with restenosis rates after endarterectomy of the common and superficial femoral arteries. J Vasc Surg. 2010;52(3):592–9.
9. Hellings WE, Moll FL, De Vries J-PPM, et al. Atherosclerotic plaque composition and occurrence of restenosis after carotid endarterectomy. JAMA. 2008;299(5):547–54.
10. Pasterkamp G, Wensing PJ, Post MJ, et al. Paradoxical arterial wall shrinkage may contribute to luminal narrowing of human atherosclerotic femoral arteries. Circulation. 1995;91(5):1444–9.

11. Vink A, Schoneveld AH, Borst C, Pasterkamp G. The contribution of plaque and arterial remodeling to de novo atherosclerotic luminal narrowing in the femoral artery. J Vasc Surg. 2002;36(6):1194–8.
12. Fowkes F, Leng GC. Bypass surgery for chronic lower limb ischaemia. Cochrane Database Syst Rev. 2008;(2):CD002000.
13. Romiti M, Albers M, Brochado-Neto FC, et al. Meta-analysis of infrapopliteal angioplasty for chronic critical limb ischemia. J Vasc Surg. 2008;47(5):975–81.
14. Mendall MA, Patel P, Ballam L, Strachan D, Northfield TC. C reactive protein and its relation to cardiovascular risk factors: a population based cross sectional study. BMJ. 1996;312(7038):1061–5.
15. Forrester JS, Fishbein M, Helfant R, Fagin J. A paradigm for restenosis based on cell biology: clues for the development of new preventive therapies. J Am Coll Cardiol. 1991;17(3):758–69.
16. Serrano Jr CV, Ramires JA, Venturinelli M, et al. Coronary angioplasty results in leukocyte and platelet activation with adhesion molecule expression. Evidence of inflammatory responses in coronary angioplasty. J Am Coll Cardiol. 1997;29(6):1276–83.
17. Schillinger M, Exner M, Mlekusch W, et al. Balloon angioplasty and stent implantation induce a vascular inflammatory reaction. J Endovasc Ther. 2002;9(1):59–66.
18. Joviliano EE, Piccinato CE, Dellalibera-Joviliano R, Moriya T, Évora PRB. Inflammatory markers and restenosis in peripheral percutaneous angioplasty with intravascular stenting: current concepts. Ann Vasc Surg. 2011;25(6):846–55.
19. Samson RH, Showalter DP, Lepore Jr M, Nair DG, Merigliano K. CryoPlasty therapy of the superficial femoral and popliteal arteries: a reappraisal after 44 months' experience. J Vasc Surg. 2008;48(3):634–7.
20. Schmidt A, Piorkowski M, Werner M, et al. First experience with drug-eluting balloons in infrapopliteal arteries: restenosis rate and clinical outcome. J Am Coll Cardiol. 2011;58(11):1105–9.
21. Jahnke T, Mueller-Huelsbeck S, Charalambous N, et al. Prospective, randomized single-center trial to compare cryoplasty versus conventional angioplasty in the popliteal artery: midterm results of the COLD study. J Vasc Interv Radiol. 2010;21(2):186–94.
22. Barath P, Fishbein MC, Vari S, Forrester JS. Cutting balloon: a novel approach to percutaneous angioplasty. Am J Cardiol. 1991; 68(11):1249–52.
23. Vorwerk D, Adam G, Müller-Leisse C, Guenther RW. Hemodialysis fistulas and grafts: use of cutting balloons to dilate venous stenoses. Radiology. 1996;201(3):864–7.
24. Ito S, Suzuki T, Suzuki T. Adjunctive use of cutting balloon after rotational atherectomy in a young adult with probable Kawasaki disease. J Invasive Cardiol. 2003;15(5):297–300.
25. Bergersen LJ, Perry SB, Lock JE. Effect of cutting balloon angioplasty on resistant pulmonary artery stenosis. Am J Cardiol. 2003; 91(2):185–9.
26. De Giovanni JV. Balloon angioplasty for branch pulmonary artery stenosis – cutting balloons. Catheter Cardiovasc Interv. 2007;69(3):459–67.
27. Nakamura M, Yock PG, Kataoka T, et al. Impact of deep vessel wall injury on acute response and remodeling of coronary artery segments after cutting balloon angioplasty. Am J Cardiol. 2003;91(1):6–11.
28. Kawaguchi K, Kondo T, Shumiya T, et al. Reduction of early elastic recoil by cutting balloon angioplasty as compared to conventional balloon angioplasty. J Invasive Cardiol. 2002;14(9):515–9.
29. Rabbi JF, Kiran RP, Gersten G, Dudrick SJ, Dardik A. Early results with infrainguinal cutting balloon angioplasty limits distal dissection. Ann Vasc Surg. 2004;18(6):640–3.
30. Amighi J, Schillinger M, Dick P, et al. De novo superficial femoropopliteal artery lesions: peripheral cutting balloon angioplasty and restenosis rates – randomized controlled trial. Radiology. 2008;247(1):267–72.
31. Aslam MS, Allaqaband S, Haddadian B, et al. Subintimal angioplasty with a true reentry device for treatment of chronic total occlusion of the arteries of the lower extremity. Catheter Cardiovasc Interv. 2010. Available at: http://www.ncbi.nlm.nih.gov/pubmed/20824749. Accessed 4 Dec 2011.
32. Markose G, Miller FNAC, Bolia A. Subintimal angioplasty for femoro-popliteal occlusive disease. J Vasc Surg. 2010;52(5):1410–6.
33. Scott EC, Biuckians A, Light RE, et al. Subintimal angioplasty: our experience in the treatment of 506 infrainguinal arterial occlusions. J Vasc Surg. 2008;48(4):878–84.
34. Virmani R, Farb A. Pathology of in-stent restenosis. Curr Opin Lipidol. 1999;10(6):499–506.
35. Moreno PR, Palacios IF, Leon MN, et al. Histopathologic comparison of human coronary in-stent and post-balloon angioplasty restenotic tissue. Am J Cardiol. 1999;84(4):462–6, A9.
36. Cejna M, Thurnher S, Illiasch H, et al. PTA versus Palmaz stent placement in femoropopliteal artery obstructions: a multicenter prospective randomized study. J Vasc Interv Radiol. 2001;12(1):23–31.
37. Minar E, Schillinger M. New stents for SFA. J Cardiovasc Surg (Torino). 2009;50(5):635–45.
38. Laird JR, Katzen BT, Scheinert D, et al. Nitinol stent implantation versus balloon angioplasty for lesions in the superficial femoral artery and proximal popliteal artery: twelve-month results from the RESILIENT randomized trial. Circ Cardiovasc Interv. 2010;3(3):267–76.
39. Dick P, Wallner H, Sabeti S, et al. Balloon angioplasty versus stenting with nitinol stents in intermediate length superficial femoral artery lesions. Catheter Cardiovasc Interv. 2009;74(7):1090–5.
40. Mewissen MW. Primary nitinol stenting for femoropopliteal disease. J Endovasc Ther. 2009;16(2 Suppl 2):II63–81.
41. Lammer J, Dake MD, Bleyn J, et al. Peripheral arterial obstruction: prospective study of treatment with a transluminally placed self-expanding stent-graft. International Trial Study Group. Radiology. 2000;217(1):95–104.
42. Kedora J, Hohmann S, Garrett W, et al. Randomized comparison of percutaneous Viabahn stent grafts vs prosthetic femoral-popliteal bypass in the treatment of superficial femoral arterial occlusive disease. J Vasc Surg. 2007;45(1):10–6; discussion 16.
43. McQuade K, Gable D, Pearl G, Theune B, Black S. Four-year randomized prospective comparison of percutaneous ePTFE/nitinol self-expanding stent graft versus prosthetic femoral-popliteal bypass in the treatment of superficial femoral artery occlusive disease. J Vasc Surg. 2010;52(3):584–90. discussion 590–591, 591.e1-591.e7.
44. Zeller T, Macharzina R, Tepe G. The potential role of DES in peripheral in-stent restenosis. J Cardiovasc Surg (Torino). 2010; 51(4):561–5.
45. Lammer J, Bosiers M, Zeller T, et al. First clinical trial of nitinol self-expanding everolimus-eluting stent implantation for peripheral arterial occlusive disease. J Vasc Surg. 2011;54(2):394–401.
46. Duda SH, Bosiers M, Lammer J, et al. Sirolimus-eluting versus bare nitinol stent for obstructive superficial femoral artery disease: the SIROCCO II trial. J Vasc Interv Radiol. 2005;16(3):331–8.
47. Tepe G, Zeller T, Albrecht T, et al. Local delivery of paclitaxel to inhibit restenosis during angioplasty of the leg. N Engl J Med. 2008;358(7):689–99.
48. Zeller T, Rastan A, Schwarzwälder U, et al. Percutaneous peripheral atherectomy of femoropopliteal stenoses using a new-generation device: six-month results from a single-center experience. J Endovasc Ther. 2004;11(6):676–85.
49. McKinsey JF, Goldstein L, Khan HU, et al. Novel treatment of patients with lower extremity ischemia: use of percutaneous atherectomy in 579 lesions. Ann Surg. 2008;248(4):519–28.

50. Davies MG, Bismuth J, Saad WE, et al. Implications of in situ thrombosis and distal embolization during superficial femoral artery endoluminal intervention. Ann Vasc Surg. 2010;24(1): 14–22.
51. Weitz JI, Byrne J, Clagett GP, et al. Diagnosis and treatment of chronic arterial insufficiency of the lower extremities: a critical review. Circulation. 1996;94(11):3026–49.
52. Hirsch AT, Haskal ZJ, Hertzer NR, et al. ACC/AHA 2005 guidelines for the management of patients with peripheral arterial disease (lower extremity, renal, mesenteric, and abdominal aortic): executive summary a collaborative report from the American Association for Vascular Surgery/Society for Vascular Surgery, Society for Cardiovascular Angiography and Interventions, Society for Vascular Medicine and Biology, Society of Interventional Radiology, and the ACC/AHA Task Force on Practice Guidelines (Writing Committee to Develop Guidelines for the Management of Patients with Peripheral Arterial Disease) endorsed by the American Association of Cardiovascular and Pulmonary Rehabilitation; National Heart, Lung, and Blood Institute; Society for Vascular Nursing; TransAtlantic Inter-Society Consensus; and Vascular Disease Foundation. J Am Coll Cardiol. 2006;47(6): 1239–312.

Part IX

Cardiopulmonary Bypass

27 Modulation of Inflammatory Response in Cardiopulmonary Bypass

Shahzad G. Raja

Introduction

Cardiac surgery with cardiopulmonary bypass provokes a systemic inflammatory response syndrome (SIRS). Contact of the blood components with the artificial surface of the bypass circuit, ischemia-reperfusion injury, endotoxemia, and operative trauma are all possible causes of SIRS [1, 2]. This inflammatory reaction may contribute to the development of postoperative complications, including myocardial dysfunction, respiratory failure, renal and neurologic dysfunction, bleeding disorders, altered liver function, and, ultimately, multiple organ failure [1, 2].

The incidence, severity, and clinical outcome of SIRS are influenced by a large number of factors that can be broadly classified as biomaterial-dependent and biomaterial-independent (Table 27.1). The precise role of each of these factors and the reasons why certain patients develop life-threatening perioperative complications are currently the focus of considerable research. Diverse therapeutic strategies to modulate the systemic inflammatory response after cardiac surgery are being examined in experimental and clinical studies [2]. Currently available strategies can be broadly classified as (1) avoiding CPB altogether (off-pump surgery), (2) technical strategies (including modifying perfusion techniques and circuitry), (3) pharmaceutical strategies, and (4) endotoxemia-reducing strategies (Table 27.2). This chapter provides an overview of these strategies and focuses on their evidence-based potential and actual impact in reducing the systemic inflammatory response.

S.G. Raja, BSc, MBBS, MRCS, FRCS(C-Th)
Department of Cardiac Surgery,
Harefield Hospital, London, UK
e-mail: drrajashahzad@hotmail.com

Avoiding Cardiopulmonary Bypass

Off-Pump Coronary Artery Bypass Surgery

A radical and effective way of counteracting the effects of SIRS may be the omission of CPB itself. This idea provided the impetus for reintroduction of off-pump coronary artery

Table 27.1 Factors influencing systemic inflammatory response

Biomaterial-dependent factors[a]
Type of extracorporeal circuit
Type of oxygenator and pump
Biomaterial-independent factors
Extracorporeal perfusion factors
Composition of the priming solution
Cardioplegia
Pulsatile or non-pulsatile perfusion
Temperature during CPB
Preoperative factors
Morbid conditions[b]
Perioperative hemodynamic factors
Low cardiac output
Splanchnic hypoperfusion
Anesthetic techniques
Thoracic epidural anesthesia
Anesthetic agents and drugs
Lung management during CPB
Surgical factors
Incision and approach
Duration
Cardiotomy blood management
Shear stress
Transfusion
Postoperative factors
Continuous renal replacement therapies
Mechanical ventilation

CPB cardiopulmonary bypass
[a]Related to the composition of the synthetic surface of the circuit
[b]Such as poor left ventricular function or diabetes

E.A. Gabriel, S.A. Gabriel (eds.), *Inflammatory Response in Cardiovascular Surgery*,
DOI 10.1007/978-1-4471-4429-8_27, © Springer-Verlag London 2013

Table 27.2 Strategies to modulate inflammatory response

Cardiopulmonary bypass avoidance	
	Off-pump coronary artery bypass grafting
Technical strategies	
	Miniaturized extracorporeal circulation
	Heparin-bonded circuits
	Hemofiltration
	Leukocyte depletion
	Centrifugal pumps
	Cardiopulmonary bypass temperature
Pharmacologic strategies	
	Corticosteroids
	Aprotinin[a]
	Antioxidants
	Mannitol
	Allopurinol
	N-acetyl cysteine
	Vitamin C
	Vitamin E
	Complement inhibitors
	Monoclonal C5 antibody
	Compstatin
	C1 inhibitor
	Recombinant soluble inhibitor-1
	Monoclonal C3 antibody
	Monoclonal C5a antibody
	Phosphodiesterase inhibitors
	Milrinone
	Dopexamine
	Cyclooxygenase inhibitors
Endotoxemia-reducing strategies	
	Antimediator and antiendotoxin therapies
	Selective digestive decontamination
	Enteral nutrition & immunonutrition

[a]FDA restriction on routine use

bypass (OPCAB) surgery—a technique that predates CPB but was rapidly off-staged by on-pump coronary artery bypass graft (CABG) soon after the invention of the heart-lung machine because of the attraction of operating on a still heart in a bloodless field [3].

Analysis of current best available evidence [4] from randomized controlled trials [6–28] indicates that OPCAB reduces the systemic inflammatory response but does not prevent it (grade A/level Ib). Use of OPCAB decreases concentrations of cytokines such as tumor necrosis factor (TNF)-α, interleukin (IL)-6, IL-8, IL-10, TNFsr1, and TNFsr2. It also attenuates the cellular inflammatory response, decreasing neutrophil and monocyte counts, neutrophil elastase, intracellular heat shock protein 70, and E-selectin concentrations. Indices of complement activation, such as C3a and C5a, are decreased. In addition, OPCAB attenuates other indices including platelet ß-thromboglobulin and procalcitonin. Finally, OPCAB decreases injury induced by reactive oxygen species (Table 27.3).

It would, however, be incorrect to expect that OPCAB will abolish the systemic inflammatory response completely. It is worth remembering that while performing OPCAB, the response to surgical trauma, manipulation of the heart, pericardial suction, heparin, protamine, other drugs, and anesthesia are still there, and all produce an increase in the markers of acute inflammation. Increasing acceptance to perform OPCAB in elderly patients and those with comorbid conditions is proof that this attenuated systemic inflammatory response reduces organ dysfunction [3].

Technical Strategies

Minimized Extracorporeal Circulation System

Recently, a minimized extracorporeal circulation (MECC) system has been developed based on the concept of a short closed total CPB circuit [29]. The basic elements are a centrifugal pump, a membrane oxygenator, and an arterial filter. The priming volume can be reduced to 500 ml or less, thus limiting hemodilution. The complete circuit is coated with heparin to maximize biocompatibility. The blood-air interface is eliminated, and suction of shed blood is carried out only through a cell-saving device. Thus, blood is washed before retransfusion into the patient. In a randomized controlled trial, Fromes and colleagues [29] showed that the MECC system initiated a milder inflammatory reaction than standard CPB: IL-6, TNF-α, and elastase release was significantly less in patients who were operated on with the MECC system. However, currently there is a paucity of randomized controlled trials highlighting long-term survival, clinical outcomes, and delayed complications in this area. Despite this, MECC remains a promising alternative to conventional extracorporeal circulation, especially in terms of its inflammatory results.

Heparin-Bonded Circuits

Coating the artificial surfaces of the CPB circuit with heparin was initially suggested in the late 1960s [30], predominantly because of its known antithrombotic property [31]. Since then, however, it has been proven to have many other biocompatibile properties, including inhibition of contact, activation of complement and neutrophil, reduction in the release of proinflammatory cytokines, and improvement of platelet function [32]. Furthermore, it adsorbs lipoproteins to create a surface that may simulate cell membranes [32].

The method by which the circuit is coated and the type of heparin used may have implications for its effects on the coagulation and complement systems. The Duraflo II HCC (Baxter Healthcare Corp., Irvine, CA), which uses ionically bonded unfractionated heparin, reduces kallikrein and com-

Table 27.3 Randomized controlled trials comparing impact of OPCAB and conventional CABG on systemic inflammatory response

Study	Level of evidence	Intervention (*n* per group)	Main result
Lin et al., 2010 [5]	Level Ib	CABG with CPB (25)[a] vs. OPCAB (20)	Elevated serum IL-8, IL-10, and IL-12 were found in all three groups. HSP70 expression within leukocytes was enhanced in CABG patients
Onorati et al., 2010 [6]	Level Ib	CABG with CPB (40)[b] vs. OPCAB (20)	OPCAB was associated with slight endothelial activation and cytokine response. Pulsatile cardiopulmonary bypass CABG significantly attenuates endothelial/cytokine leakage
Serrano et al., 2010 [7]	Level Ib	CABG with CPB (41) vs. OPCAB (40)	OPCAB better preserves the myocardium and attenuates inflammation compared to on-pump CABG
Rasmussen et al., 2007 [8]	Level Ib	CABG with CPB (17) vs. OPCAB (18)	Oxygenation was more affected by OPCAB. Only part of the systemic inflammatory response (IL-8 and IL-10) was attenuated by OPCAB
Parolari et al., 2007 [9]	Level Ib	CABG with CPB (16) vs. OPCAB (14)	The postoperative protracted activation of inflammation is not affected by surgical strategy (on-pump or off-pump)
Tatoulis et al., 2006 [10]	Level Ib	CABG with CPB (50) vs. OPCAB (50)	The incidence of low SVR and patterns of SVR changes were similar in both groups and were clinically unimportant as few patients required vasopressor support. Cardiac outputs and clinical outcomes were excellent in both groups
Cavalca et al., 2006 [11]	Level Ib	CABG with CPB (25) vs. OPCAB (25)	OPCAB revealed less perioperative oxidative stress, as reflected by lack of excretion of iPF2alpha-III in urine, by lack of increase of plasma free malondialdehyde, and by lower decreases in plasma total antioxidant status
Wehlin et al., 2005 [12]	Level Ib	CABG with CPB (9) vs. OPCAB (11)	Monocyte expression and in vitro mobilization of complement receptors, CD11b and CD35, were similar in both study groups during and after surgery, as was the expression of CD62L
Wan et al., 2004 [13]	Level Ib	CABG with CPB (19) vs. OPCAB (18)	IL-10, 1 L-6, 1 L-8, TNFα, and VCAM-1significantly higher in CABG+CPB group
Wehlin et al., 2004 [14]	Level Ib	CABG with CPB (16) vs. OPCAB (21)	Less complement activation in low- risk OPCAB patients
Dorman et al., 2004 [15]	Level Ib	CABG with CPB (25) vs. OPCAB (25)	Postoperative ET levels were higher in patients who underwent CPB for CABG
Al-Ruzzeh et al., 2004 [16]	Level Ib	CABG with CPB (10) vs. OPCAB (10)	Less activation of circulating neutrophils in OPCAB patients
Moller et al., 2003 [17]	Level Ib	CABG with CPB (15) vs. OPCAB (15)	Platelets after OPCAB are more easily activated in the early postoperative period. After CABG with CPB there is a temporary platelet dysfunction that improves within the first postoperative day
Jemielity et al., 2003 [18]	Level Ib	CABG with CPB (25) vs. OPCAB (25)	Peak IL-6 level significantly lower after OPCAB; CRP higher after CABG; AGP rise comparable
Okubo et al., 2003 [19]	Level 1b	CABG with CPB (10) vs. OPCAB (10)	Postoperative expression of m-RNA for IL-1, -8, and -10, TNF-alpha, HO-1, PECAM, and Mac-1 increased significantly in the on-pump group but not in the off-pump group ($p<0.05$)
Wildhirt et al., 2001 [20]	Level Ib	CABG with CPB (13) vs. OPCAB (13)	Significant reduction in systemic and cardiac adhesion molecular expression after OPCAB
Schulze et al., 2000 [21]	Level Ib	CABG with CPB (13) vs. OPCAB (13)	Significant increase in the TNF system and sIL-2r in CABG; no difference in IL-6 levels; CRP and total nitrate/nitrite levels significantly lower in OPCAB
Wildhirt et al., 2000 [22]	Level Ib	CABG with CPB (13) vs. OPCAB (13)	OPCAB reduces myocardial cell damage and lipid peroxidation and is also associated with a reduced activation of endothelin
Gulielmos et al., 2000 [23]	Level 1b	CABG with CPB (20)[c] vs. OPCAB (20)	The use of CPB was associated with higher levels of troponin-T and CK- MB as signs of myocardial damage. Surgical access was identified as a trigger of inflammatory response, as minithoracotomy was related to higher levels of IL-6
Czerny et al., 2000 [24]	Level Ib	CABG with CPB (16) vs. OPCAB (14)	Significantly lower IL-10, P-selectin, ICAM-1, myoglobin, CK-MB, and troponin I release after OPCAB
Ascione et al., 2000 [25]	Level Ib	CABG with CPB (30) vs. OPCAB (30)	Neutrophil elastase ($p<0.0001$), IL-8 levels ($p=0.01$), WBC counts ($p<0.01$) and incidence of postoperative infection ($p<0.0001$) higher in CABG

(continued)

Table 27.3 (continued)

Study	Level of evidence	Intervention (*n* per group)	Main result
Diegeler et al., 2000[d] [26]	Level Ib	Full sternotomy CABG with CPB (10), full sternotomy OPCAB (10), limited LAT OPCAB (10)	A significant increased release of C3d, C5a, IL-8 IL-10, TNF-α receptors p55 and p75 after CABG
Matata et al., 2000 [27]	Level Ib	CABG with CPB (10) vs. OPCAB (10)	Significant increase in lipid H_2O_2 (190 % at 4 h), protein carbonyls (250 % at 0.5 h), and nitrotyrosine (510 % at 0.5 h), IL-8, elastase, C3a and sE-selectin in CABG
Gu et al., 1998 [28]	Level Ib	CABG with CPB (31) vs. MIDCAB (31)	Leukocyte elastase, platelet beta- thromboglobulin, and C3a levels significantly increased in CABG

CABG coronary artery bypass grafting, *CPB* cardiopulmonary bypass, *OPCAB* off-pump coronary artery bypass surgery, *HSP70* heat shock protein 70, *IL* interleukin, *VCAM-1* vascular cell adhesion molecule-1, *ICAM-1* intercellular adhesion molecule-1, *TNF* tumor necrosis factor, *CRP* C reactive protein, *AGP* acid glycoprotein, *CK-MB* creatine kinase-MB, *LAT* left anterior thoracotomy, *MIDCAB* minimally invasive direct coronary artery bypass, *SVR* systemic vascular resistance, *HO-1* heme oxygenase-1, *PECAM* platelet endothelial cellular adhesion molecule, *ET* endothelin

[a]CABG on-pump with cardioplegic arrest = 12, CABG on-pump beating heart = 13

[b]CABG with pulsatile cardiopulmonary bypass = 20, CABG with linear cardiopulmonary bypass

[c]Four surgical techniques were compared: group 1, median sternotomy with CPB in ten patients (eight male, two female; aged 59.6 ± 11.0 years (mean ± SD); group 2, median sternotomy and off-pump in ten patients (seven male, three female; aged 65.1 ± 10.0 years); group 3, minithoracotomy with CPB in ten patients (seven male, three female, aged 61.2 ± 10.4 years); group 4, minithoracotomy and off-pump in ten patients (nine male, one female, aged 62.9 ± 9.8 years). All patients received a left internal mammary artery graft to the left anterior descending artery (LAD)

[d]The type of operative approach did not influence this immune response

plement activation but is less effective in attenuating coagulation or fibrinolysis [33, 34]. The Carmeda Bioactive Surface system (Medtronic, Inc., Minneapolis, MN) uses end-attached, covalently bonded heparin that has been fragmented by treatment with nitric acid. The Carmeda circuit seems superior to the Duraflo II in reducing complement and neutrophil activation and endothelin-1 concentrations [35, 36].

A significant amount of work has been performed to evaluate any potential benefit in using heparin-bonded circuits (HBCs), but controversy remains. HBCs have been shown to reduce transfusion requirements, lung injury, neurocognitive dysfunction, and markers of occult myocardial damage in patients undergoing CPB [32]. A large multicenter randomized trial investigating HBCs for high-risk patients undergoing CPB showed reduced hospital length of stay (LOS) and intensive care unit (ICU) LOS and reduced renal and pulmonary postoperative dysfunction [33]. However, other studies have reported no difference between HBCs and standard circuits when investigating a range of differing outcomes [37, 38].

A meta-analysis of 41 randomized trials including 3,434 patients found significant reductions in the duration of ventilation, the incidence of postoperative transfusion, resternotomy rates, ICU LOS, and hospital LOS [39]. This meta-analysis failed to show effect of HBCs on other adverse events evaluated. However, many of these positive effects were marginal and of moderate clinical significance.

Currently, the majority of trials performed in this area have been relatively underpowered to adequately explore key clinically relevant outcomes, have involved heterogeneous patient groups, and have studied a number of different HBCs [39]. Furthermore, the use of HBCs in clinical practice appears to vary among different centers and countries [40] with little up-to-date data available at present.

Hemofiltration

Hemofiltration is a process that uses ultrafiltration (convection or osmosis under a hydrostatic pressure gradient) to remove fluid and low-molecular-weight substances from plasma. Initially introduced to treat patients with renal failure and to correct accumulation of extravascular water following CPB, hemofiltration appears to exert beneficial antiinflammatory effects, particularly in pediatric patients (Table 27.4) [41–48].

The hemodilution associated with CPB is most marked in the pediatric population, and, as a result, modified ultrafiltration (MUF) has been studied more extensively and with more definitive outcomes within this population. Several pediatric studies have suggested that MUF may effectively remove some of the inflammatory mediators released during CPB, including complement, TNF-α, IL-6, IL-1, IL-8, and myeloperoxidase [41–48]. However, these findings have not always been replicated [49]. Clinical benefits also have been reported, including increased hematocrit, improved cardiovascular performance, and reduced postoperative chest tube drainage [41].

MUF is used less frequently in adult CPB patients, and any potential benefits remain controversial. There are a number of randomized controlled trials and case control studies that have reported positive clinical outcomes for adult

Table 27.4 Impact of modified ultrafiltration on systemic inflammatory response

Author	Study type (level of evidence)	No. of patients MUF	No. of patients Control	Key result
Hiramatsu et al. [42]	RCT (level 1b)	11[a]	11[b]	Significant increase in ET-1 levels in the control group
Chew et al. [43]	RCT[c] (level 1b)	10	8	No intergroup differences detectable for TNF-α, IL-1β, IL-1ra, C3d, and C4d
Pearl et al. [44]	Non-RCT (level 3)	22	12	MUF does not appear to have a significant effect on post-CPB levels of TXB2, ET-1, and LTB4
Portela et al. [45]	Single group (level 3)	22[d]	–	Significant decrease in levels of IL-6, ICAM-1, and VCAM-1 after MUF
Wang et al. [46]	RCT (level 1b)	20	20	Significant decrease in IL-8 and ET levels and no change in TNF-α levels after MUF
Journois et al. [47]	RCT (level 1b)	10	10	Significant decrease in TNF-α, IL-8, IL-1, IL-6, myeloper-oxidase, and C3a after MUF
Journois et al. [48]	RCT (level 1b)	16	16	Significant decrease in TNF-α, C3a, C5a, and IL-6 after MUF

RCT randomized controlled trial, *MUF* modified ultrafiltration, *ET-1* endothelin-1, *IL-8* interleukin-8, *TNF-α* tumor necrosis factor-alpha, *CPB* cardiopulmonary bypass, *TXB2* thromboxane B2, *LTB4* leukotriene B4, *IL-6* interleukin-6, *ICAM-1* intercellular adhesion molecule-1, *VCAM-1* vascular cell adhesion molecule-1, *IL-1ra* interleukin-1ra, *C3d & C4d* complement split products

[a]Combined dilutional and modified ultrafiltration group

[b]Control group had conventional ultrafiltration

[c]Methylprednisolone added to pump prime

[d]Combined conventional and modified ultrafiltration done

patients [32]. It is noteworthy that there is a significant variation in the techniques used to perform UF and that the technique has been studied in a variety of patient subgroups, including CABG surgery patients, high-risk patients, and patients on chronic renal dialysis [32]. UF does appear to improve post-CPB hematocrit and in some instances postoperative transfusion requirements [32]. Luciani et al. [50] have performed the largest randomized controlled trial in adults and showed a significant reduction in hospital morbidity and a statistically nonsignificant fall in mortality. The reduction of proinflammatory cytokines and adhesion molecules by UF during or after CPB has been shown in adults, but has not always been associated with clinical advantage in terms of postoperative complications or LOS [51]. Finally, a recent meta-analysis of randomized trials investigated the effect of UF on perioperative coagulopathy in adult cardiac surgery and found that UF does appear to reduce postoperative hemorrhage and transfusion requirements, although the extent of these reductions was of arguable clinical benefit according to the authors [52].

In both patient groups, uncertainty does remain concerning both the type and combination of UF strategies [32]. Work is ongoing to clarify this and the overall risk/benefit to the patient because not only do some benefits appear transitory, but also UF is not without risk; increased plasma heparin concentrations, entrainment of air through the aortic cannula, an increase in the duration of exposure of the patient's blood to nonendothelialized surfaces, hemodynamic instability, and human or equipment error all can occur [32, 53].

Leukocyte Depletion

Leukocytes play a central role in the inflammatory response to cardiac surgery. Leukocyte depletion during cardiac surgery, by means of leukocyte-specific filters, decreases circulating leukocyte and platelet concentrations and attenuates indices of inflammation and oxidative stress [54–58]. There is increasing evidence that leukocyte depletion may limit pulmonary and myocardial injury following CPB. Benefits appear to be the most consistent in patients with risk factors such as left ventricular dysfunction, urgent surgery, or long CPB time. Leukocyte depletion has been shown to improve postoperative respiratory function in CPB patients, particularly in those with a low preoperative oxygenation capacity or long CPB time [56, 57]. In addition, leukocyte depletion of the residual heart-lung machine blood, which contains large quantities of activated leukocytes, prior to re-transfusion improved lung function in patients undergoing elective CABG [54]. Leukocyte depletion during CPB, combined with leukocyte depletion of transfused blood, decreased indices of myocardial cell injury in patients undergoing urgent CABG for unstable angina [58]. Conversely, in low-risk patients, depletion of activated neutrophils during CPB did not confer a clinical benefit [59]. Limiting leukocyte depletion to the reperfusion phase of CPB (following aortic declamping) did not appear to provide any clinical benefit to CABG patients [60]. Leukocyte depletion of blood cardioplegia alone attenuated myocardial cell injury and improved early myocardial function in patients with left ventricular dysfunction undergoing CABG with CPB [61, 62].

Leukocyte depletion of terminal blood cardioplegia (blood cardioplegia administered for 10 min immediately prior to aortic declamping as an adjunct to crystalloid cardioplegia) decreased myocardial injury and improved cardiac function in patients with left ventricular hypertrophy undergoing valve surgery [63].

Despite the aforementioned benefits, currently, there is not enough high-quality or consistent evidence to advocate the routine use of leukofiltration as an anti-inflammatory strategy within routine CPB.

Centrifugal Pumps

Under physiologic conditions, blood flow occurs in a pulsatile manner, but during CPB this situation changes, a variation that may worsen the inflammatory response [1, 32]. A large number of studies have thus been conducted to investigate any possible benefits in using centrifugal pumps, originally developed for prolonged postoperative cardiac assist and for extracorporeal membrane oxygenation [32]. Centrifugal pumps have been reported to reduce platelet aggregation (and thus lower susceptibility to postoperative thrombotic phenomena) [64], decrease the incidence of neurologic and renal complications [65], decrease chest tube drainage, and reduce transfusion requirements [66]. However, other randomized controlled trials comparing the two pump types have failed to show improvements in blood transfusion rates, postoperative cardiac performance, duration of postoperative mechanical ventilation, ICU LOS, hospital LOS, and mortality [64]. More importantly, the impact of centrifugal pumps on inflammation is an underexplored area, and there is a paucity of evidence to validate their universal usage as a strategy to reduce SIRS.

Cardiopulmonary Bypass Temperature

The optimal temperature at which to conduct CPB remains a controversial area. The controversy is further compounded by the varying definitions of "normothermia" used by different investigators. Some groups refer to a temperature of 33–34 °C as normothermia, while others regard 36–37 °C as physiologic normothermia [32]. Significant reductions in the levels of inflammatory mediators (e.g., p-selectin, IL-1, IL-8, and elastase) have been shown when comparing hypothermic patients (28–30 °C) with patients at 34 °C [67]. However, although hypothermia appears to delay this reaction, it does not prevent it entirely, and other groups looking at similar molecular markers have found no difference among three differing temperatures [68]. The clinical outcome data are no more convincing. Some studies suggest that moderate hypothermia (32 °C) may reduce neuropsychologic injury, but benefits are best described as modest [69]. It can be said that although there is a significant level of evidence to suggest that hyperthermia must be avoided in patients on CPB [70], there is currently not enough evidence to clearly identify the optimal temperature at which CPB should be conducted.

Pharmacologic Strategies

Corticosteroids

Corticosteroid pretreatment may blunt the inflammatory response in humans by several distinct mechanisms. Administration of glucocorticoids prior to CPB may attenuate endotoxin release and complement activation [71, 72]. Methylprednisolone lowers post-CPB concentrations of the proinflammatory cytokines TNF-α, IL-6, and IL-8 and increases concentrations of the antiinflammatory cytokines IL-10 and IL-1ra, but not IL-4 [73]. Corticosteroids also attenuate post-CPB leukocyte activation, neutrophil adhesion molecule upregulation, and pulmonary neutrophil sequestration [2, 74]. Pre-bypass administration of methylprednisolone in aprotinin-treated patients improves early postoperative indices of pulmonary, cardiovascular, hemostatic, and renal function [75]. Glucocorticoid pretreatment may improve cardiac performance and reduce evidence of bronchial inflammation following CPB [76]. Low-dose methylprednisolone in the pump prime solution appears to attenuate myocardial cell damage [77]. However, the ability of corticosteroid pretreatment to attenuate post-CPB pulmonary inflammation, endotoxemia, and complement activation is disputed [2, 78]. The clinical implications of corticosteroid use are not yet fully elucidated, and clear benefit is not yet demonstrated. The dosage, formulation, and timing of administration of corticosteroids may be critical, and differences in dosage regimens may explain conflicting results. Preoperative combined with pre-bypass administration may be superior to pre-bypass administration alone [79]. It is premature to advocate the use of corticosteroids in the absence of proven outcome benefit, determination of optimal dosage regimens, and characterization of the harmful effects that may result from their use [2].

The Cochrane review regarding the use of prophylactic steroids in pediatric patients undergoing CPB reported that the existing evidence did not support this practice in this patient group [80]. Similarly, the Cochrane review for this practice in adults showed no beneficial effect of corticosteroid use on mortality or cardiac and pulmonary complications in cardiac surgery patients [81].

Finally, recent expert guidelines on CABG surgery from the American Heart Association and the American College of Cardiology state "corticosteroid administration is inexpensive and appears to reduce the risk of the systemic inflammatory response associated with CPB with little downside risk. Current understanding supports liberal prophylactic use in patients undergoing extracorporeal circulation" [82]. Hence, at present, evidence for the efficacy and safety of corticosteroids is controversial.

Serine Protease Inhibitors (Aprotinin)

Many effector proteins of the cytokine, complement, and hemostatic cascades are serine proteases; when activated, they catalyze the next step in the cascade by hydrolyzing and activating further proteins, a process termed "cascade amplification". Control processes that limit inflammation to the sites of injury and reduce systemic inflammation include serine protease inhibitors. Aprotinin is the best known and most studied of these inhibitors [2]. Aprotinin, a nonspecific serine protease inhibitor isolated from bovine lung tissue, was first used clinically in the 1960s to treat acute pancreatitis [83]. Knowing that it inhibited kallikrein, one of the key components of the contact system, led in the 1980s to it being tested as a potential antiinflammatory agent in CPB. However, the key findings of initial studies were that it significantly decreased the perioperative hemorrhage associated with cardiac surgery [84]. These findings led to the widespread adoption of aprotinin to reduce postoperative bleeding in cardiac surgery.

Subsequent studies confirmed that aprotinin possesses important antiinflammatory properties. It inhibits trypsin, chymotrypsin, plasmin, kallikrein, elastase, and thrombin [85]. By inhibiting kallikrein and plasmin, it reduces the levels of contact activation and limits fibrinolysis. It prevents proteolysis of the major thrombin receptor on platelets (protease activated receptor 1) [86], inhibiting platelet activation and suggesting simultaneous pro- and antithrombotic effects. Aprotinin reduces complement activation; the levels of circulating proinflammatory cytokines such as Il-6, IL-8, and TNF-α; and expression of leukocyte adhesion molecules (MAC-1) [87]. Aprotinin has been shown to reduce markers of myocardial injury (troponin T, CK-MB, and lactate dehydrogenase) in patients undergoing CABG surgery [88], and a meta-analysis suggested a decrease in all-cause mortality of almost twofold [89].

Despite the aforementioned benefits, aprotinin is no longer available for routine use. This restriction came into force following publication of the results of the studies by Mangano et al. [90], Karkouti et al. [91], and more importantly the Canadian BART (Blood Conservation using Antifibrinolytics) trial, which compared aprotinin to two lysine analogs (tranexamic acid and aminocaproic acid) in high-risk patients undergoing cardiac surgery [92]. The high-quality BART trial reported in late May 2008 and provided modest evidence that aprotinin was the more effective hemostatic agent because patients who received it had a reduced risk of massive postoperative bleeding and need for postsurgical administration of blood products [92]. Despite this, patients who received aprotinin had an increased risk of 30-day mortality of more than 50 % (relative risk, 1.53; 95 % confidence interval, 1.06–2.22), an outcome that led trial investigators to conclude that aprotinin should no longer be used in patients undergoing high-risk cardiac surgery [92]. Whether aprotinin now has a role in cardiac surgery appears doubtful; the conventional wisdom had always been that it was for patients at a high risk of bleeding who had the most to gain from aprotinin, but it was precisely this cohort whom BART was set up to investigate, and the study subsequently provided convincing evidence of the superiority of lysine analogs in this role. What is clear is that many lessons can be learned from the "aprotinin story" regarding the assessment of new pharmaceuticals as they enter clinical practice [32, 93].

Antioxidants

A key part of the cellular damage witnessed during the ischemia-reperfusion (I/R) injury that occurs during CPB is attributable to the reactive oxygen species (ROS, also known as oxygen-free radicals) released by activated neutrophils. This is compounded by CPB depleting the endogenous ROS scavengers, such as vitamins E and C. Experimental animal studies have investigated the efficacy of exogenous antioxidants, such as mannitol, allopurinol, and N-acetyl cysteine, in preventing or attenuating ROS-mediated damage [2, 32]. Encouraging results were seen using superoxide dismutase and catalase, both oxygen free radical scavengers, to reperfuse heart transplants in a rat model [94]. Reperfusion of human myocardium with blood cardioplegic solution instead of with crystalloid may reduce I/R injury because of the endogenous ROS scavengers present in erythrocytes [95]. Improved myocardial function and reduced perioperative morbidity have been found in patients undergoing CABG surgery who were administered preoperative oral vitamin E, a lipid-soluble chain-breaking antioxidant, both in isolation [96] and in combination with vitamin C and allopurinol [97]. Despite some of these promising results, most human studies have not shown any significant benefits, and, thus, antioxidant therapy cannot be recommended as a regular therapeutic option.

Complement Inhibitors

Therapies that utilize endogenous soluble complement inhibitors may be a suitable approach to reducing contact activation and thereby controlling the inflammatory response. A two-stage randomized clinical trial of a monoclonal antibody specific for human C5 demonstrated its efficacy and safety in patients undergoing CPB [98]. The generation of activated complement mediators and leukocyte adhesion molecule formation was inhibited in a dose-dependent manner. Furthermore, C5 inhibition resulted in a dose-dependent reduction in myocardial injury, postoperative cognitive deficits, and coagulation dysfunction. These data suggest that C5 inhibition may represent a promising therapeutic modality for preventing complement-mediated inflammation and tissue injury in patients undergoing CPB [98]. Compstatin, a recently discovered peptide inhibitor of complement, may have the potential to prevent complement activation during and after cardiac surgery. In preliminary primate studies, compstatin completely inhibited in vivo heparin-protamine-induced complement activation, without adverse effects [99]. Other promising strategies include the C1 inhibitor, recombinant soluble inhibitor-1, monoclonal antibodies to C3 and C5a, and strategies that attenuate complement receptor 3-mediated adhesion of inflammatory cells to the vascular endothelium. Utilization of membrane-bound complement regulators may also be feasible by means of transfection techniques [100]. Although not enough data currently exist to recommend routine incorporation into clinical practice, it would seem complement inhibitors have significant potential to play a future role [2].

Phosphodiesterase Inhibitors

Phosphodiesterase inhibitors increase intracellular cyclic adenosine monophosphate levels, thereby increasing myocardial inotropy and lowering systemic vascular resistance by causing peripheral vasodilatation. They also have been shown to exert an antiinflammatory effect, possibly through the same mechanism [2]. Immune cells contain type IV and type III phosphodiesterase, and phosphodiesterase inhibitors appear to directly limit inflammatory activation and organ dysfunction in sepsis models [101]. Milrinone attenuates the reduction in gastric intramucosal pH, reduces both venous and hepatic endotoxin concentrations, and may decrease postoperative IL-6 concentrations in healthy patients undergoing cardiac surgery, although this has been disputed [102, 103]. Dopexamine attenuates the postoperative increase in IL-6 concentrations and reduces gastrointestinal permeability, but does not improve splanchnic perfusion (as measured by intramucosal pH) or decrease plasma endotoxin concentrations following CPB [104, 105].

Cyclooxygenase Inhibitors

Aspirin, the prototype nonsteroidal antiinflammatory drug (NSAID), is widely used in cardiac surgical patients for the purposes of pain relief and antiplatelet activity. However, the potential for NSAIDs to attenuate the inflammatory response to cardiac surgery has not been widely evaluated in clinical trials. Traditional NSAIDs, such as indomethacin, inhibit both the constitutive cyclooxygenase 1 (COX-1) as well as COX-2, the inducible isoform activated by inflammatory stimuli [32]. Nonspecific COX inhibition attenuates the increase in pulmonary vascular resistance and acute lung injury and reverses pulmonary microvascular dysfunction in CPB models [106]. The only published clinical study of indomethacin demonstrated that it decreased the duration of postoperative fever, chest pain, malaise, and myalgias following CPB [107]. However, inhibition of COX-1 appears to increase free-radical-generated isoprostane formation, which aggravates postischemic myocardial dysfunction [108].

Specific COX-2 inhibitors exhibit considerable potential to attenuate the inflammatory response following cardiac surgery. COX-2 has been implicated in the pathogenesis of adverse events after cardiac surgery [109]. COX-2 is upregulated in multiple tissues following CPB, including the brain, while COX-2 products, particularly thromboxanes and vasoconstrictor prostaglandins, are increased [107, 110]. COX-2 upregulation following experimental CPB may contribute to postoperative coronary vasospasm and increased pulmonary vascular resistance [111]. In addition, myocardial COX-2 is upregulated during cardiac allograft rejection and myocardial infarction and contributes to endotoxin-induced myocardial depression [112]. Inhibition of COX-2 attenuates the myocardial inflammatory response during cardiac allograft rejection, reduces endothelial dysfunction following myocardial ischemia and reperfusion, and improves cardiac function in experimental myocardial infarction [112, 113]. In addition, COX-2 inhibition decreases endotoxin-induced myocardial depression and lung ischemia and reperfusion injury [114]. However, the clinical efficacy of specific COX-2 inhibitors in attenuating the inflammatory response to cardiac surgery remains to be determined.

Strategies to Reduce Endotoxemia

Antimediator and Antiendotoxin Therapies

Direct antimediator therapies that focus on the endotoxin molecule itself and the proinflammatory cytokine cascade following CPB offer new approaches. A recently published small randomized controlled trial of IgM-enriched intravenous immunoglobulin preparation showed it to be effective when used prophylactically in patients undergoing procedures with CPB [115]. However, the complex pathway observed in patients with SIRS does not appear to respond readily to antimediator therapy. Multicenter clinical trials blocking endotoxin and proinflammatory mediators such as IL-1 or TNF-α conducted in SIRS patients have shown no benefit in reducing mortality secondary to sepsis [116]. Reasons for the relative failure of immunomodulatory therapies to date may include the timing of intervention, the heterogeneous nature of the inflammatory response, and the reciprocating and redundant nature of the proinflammatory cascades. High circulating concentrations of antiinflammatory mediators, such as the cytokine antagonists IL-1ra, TNFsr1, and TNFsr2, may also limit the efficacy of therapies that aim to augment natural defenses against endotoxin or the proinflammatory cytokines [117].

Selective Digestive Decontamination

Selective digestive decontamination (SDD) is a technique to reduce the gut content of enterobacteria. This is achieved by preoperative administration of oral nonabsorbable antibiotics such as polymyxin E, tobramycin, and amphotericin B and has been demonstrated to reduce plasma concentrations of endotoxin, TNF-α, and IL-6 in patients undergoing CPB [118]. A recent meta-analysis of SDD suggests that it reduces rates of postoperative infection, but not mortality, in patients undergoing cardiac surgery [119]. Since mortality reduction with SDD in critically ill patients appears to be related to baseline mortality risk, trials of SDD in cardiac surgery thus far contain too many low-risk patients, resulting in inadequate study power. In high-risk cardiac surgical patients, SDD may prove worthwhile, but since its use raises both practical issues (notably the logistics of performing it) and theoretical concerns (changes in bacterial flora, emergence of resistance), its adoption is unlikely pending further studies [119].

Enteral Nutrition and Immunonutrition

Hypoalbuminemia and low body mass index independently predict increased morbidity and mortality after cardiac operations [120]. In an early study, well-nourished patients undergoing valve surgery had a much shorter hospital stay compared to those with preoperative malnutrition [121]. Laboratory evidence in animals suggests that protein-calorie malnutrition decreases left ventricular function, and that myocardial glycogen concentration correlates with left ventricular function following CPB [122]. The beneficial role of early institution of enteral nutrition, particularly immunonutrition that contains supplements such as arginine, purine nucleotides, and omega-3 fatty acids, which are considered to enhance immune function, has been established in other groups of postoperative and critically ill patients. In critically ill patients, immunonutrition reduced the duration of ICU and hospital stay, infectious complications, duration of SIRS, and mechanical ventilation compared to patients receiving conventional nutrition [123]. In patients scheduled for elective gastrointestinal surgery, preoperative and postoperative immunonutrition had beneficial effects on immune function, complication rates, and duration of hospital stay [124]. The use of glutamine supplementation may improve the survival of patients with organ failure who require parenteral nutrition [125]. There is no information available concerning the effect of nutritional support in patients undergoing cardiac surgery who have a complicated postoperative course.

Conclusion

The therapeutic potential of strategies to control the systemic inflammatory response after cardiac surgery is clear. However, the optimal therapeutic strategy (or strategies), as well as the optimal target subgroup of cardiac surgical patients, remains to be fully elucidated. Our goal must be to attenuate the deleterious effects of the systemic inflammatory response while preserving the ability of the patient to mount an appropriate defense to the physiologic trespasses of the perioperative period. Modulation of the stress response, rather than simple inhibition, is likely to confer substantial benefit. Furthermore, therapeutic strategies should be focused on the subset of cardiac surgical patients most likely to suffer deleterious consequences and hence most likely to experience benefit. This subgroup of high-risk patients is increasingly well characterized. Large-scale clinical trials of the more promising therapeutic strategies, restricted to the patient group at significant risk of perioperative morbidity, are urgently needed. Finally, many of these interventions have been studied in isolation, and it may be that, to be truly effective, methods of combining both pharmacologic and mechanical strategies are required to inhibit the differing pathways by which the inflammatory response is triggered and propagated.

References

1. Paparella D, Yau TM, Young E. Cardiopulmonary bypass induced inflammation: pathophysiology and treatment. An update. Eur J Cardiothorac Surg. 2002;21:232–44.
2. Raja SG, Dreyfus GD. Modulation of systemic inflammatory response after cardiac surgery. Asian Cardiovasc Thorac Ann. 2005;13:382–95.
3. Raja SG, Berg GA. Impact of off-pump coronary artery bypass surgery on systemic inflammation: current best available evidence. J Card Surg. 2007;22(5):445–55.
4. CEBM. Oxford centre for evidence based medicine. Available at http://www.cebm.net/index.aspx?o=1025. Accessed 7 Oct 2011.
5. Lin CY, Yang TL, Hong GJ, Li CY, Lin FY, Tsai CS. Enhanced intracellular heat shock protein 70 expression of leukocytes and serum interleukins release: comparison of on-pump and off-pump coronary artery surgery. World J Surg. 2010;34:675–81.
6. Onorati F, Rubino AS, Nucera S, Foti D, Sica V, Santini F, et al. Off-pump coronary artery bypass surgery versus standard linear or pulsatile cardiopulmonary bypass: endothelial activation and inflammatory response. Eur J Cardiothorac Surg. 2010;37:897–904.
7. Serrano Jr CV, Souza JA, Lopes NH, Fernandes JL, Nicolau JC, Blotta MH, et al. Reduced expression of systemic proinflammatory

and myocardial biomarkers after off-pump versus on-pump coronary artery bypass surgery: a prospective randomized study. J Crit Care. 2010;25:305–12.
8. Rasmussen BS, Laugesen H, Sollid J, Grønlund J, Rees SE, Toft E, et al. Oxygenation and release of inflammatory mediators after off-pump compared with after on-pump coronary artery bypass surgery. Acta Anaesthesiol Scand. 2007;51:1202–10.
9. Parolari A, Camera M, Alamanni F, Naliato M, Polvani GL, Agrifoglio M, et al. Systemic inflammation after on-pump and off-pump coronary bypass surgery: a one-month follow-up. Ann Thorac Surg. 2007;84:823–8.
10. Tatoulis J, Rice S, Davis P, Goldblatt JC, Marasco S. Patterns of postoperative systemic vascular resistance in a randomized trial of conventional on-pump versus off-pump coronary artery bypass graft surgery. Ann Thorac Surg. 2006;82:1436–44.
11. Cavalca V, Sisillo E, Veglia F, et al. Isoprostanes and oxidative stress in off-pump and on-pump coronary bypass surgery. Ann Thorac Surg. 2006;81:562–7.
12. Wehlin L, Vedin J, Vaage J, Lundahl J. Peripheral blood monocyte activation during coronary artery bypass grafting with or without cardiopulmonary bypass. Scand Cardiovasc J. 2005;39:78–86.
13. Wan IY, Arifi AA, Wan S, et al. Beating heart revascularization with or without cardiopulmonary bypass: evaluation of inflammatory response in a prospective randomized study. J Thorac Cardiovasc Surg. 2004;127:1624–31.
14. Wehlin L, Vedin J, Vaage J, Lundahl J. Activation of complement and leukocyte receptors during on- and off pump coronary artery bypass surgery. Eur J Cardiothorac Surg. 2004;25:35–42.
15. Dorman BH, Kratz JM, Multani MM, et al. A prospective, randomized study of endothelin and postoperative recovery in off-pump versus conventional coronary artery bypass surgery. J Cardiothorac Vasc Anesth. 2004;18:25–9.
16. Al-Ruzzeh S, Hoare G, Marczin N, et al. Off-pump coronary artery bypass surgery is associated with reduced neutrophil activation as measured by the expression of CD11b: a prospective randomized study. Heart Surg Forum. 2003;6:89–93.
17. Møller CH, Steinbrüchel DA. Platelet function after coronary artery bypass grafting: is there a procoagulant activity after off-pump compared with on-pump surgery? Scand Cardiovasc J. 2003;37:149–53.
18. Jemielity MM, Perek B, Buczkowski P, Lesniewska K, Wiktorowicz K, Dyszkiewicz W. Inflammatory response following off-pump and on-pump coronary artery bypass grafting. Heart Surg Forum. 2003;6 Suppl 1:S40–1.
19. Okubo N, Hatori N, Ochi M, Tanaka S. Comparison of m-RNA expression for inflammatory mediators in leukocytes between on-pump and off-pump coronary artery bypass grafting. Ann Thorac Cardiovasc Surg. 2003;9:43–9.
20. Wildhirt SM, Schulze C, Schulz C, et al. Reduction of systemic and cardiac adhesion molecule expression after off-pump versus conventional coronary artery bypass grafting. Shock. 2001;16 Suppl 1:55–9.
21. Schulze C, Conrad N, Schutz A, et al. Reduced expression of systemic proinflammatory cytokines after off-pump versus conventional coronary artery bypass grafting. Thorac Cardiovasc Surg. 2000;48:364–9.
22. Wildhirt SM, Schulze C, Conrad N, et al. Reduced myocardial cellular damage and lipid peroxidation in off-pump versus conventional coronary artery bypass grafting. Eur J Med Res. 2000;5:222–8.
23. Gulielmos V, Menschikowski M, Dill H, et al. Interleukin-1, interleukin-6 and myocardial enzyme response after coronary artery bypass grafting – a prospective randomized comparison of the conventional and three minimally invasive surgical techniques. Eur J Cardiothorac Surg. 2000;18:594–601.
24. Czerny M, Baumer H, Kilo J, et al. Inflammatory response and myocardial injury following coronary artery bypass grafting with or without cardiopulmonary bypass. Eur J Cardiothorac Surg. 2000;17:737–42.
25. Ascione R, Lloyd CT, Underwood MJ, Lotto AA, Pitsis AA, Angelini GD. Inflammatory response after coronary revascularization with or without cardiopulmonary bypass. Ann Thorac Surg. 2000;69:1198–204.
26. Diegeler A, Doll N, Rauch T. Humoral immune response during coronary artery bypass grafting: a comparison of limited approach, "off-pump" technique, and conventional cardiopulmonary bypass. Circulation. 2000;102(19 Suppl 3):III95–100.
27. Matata BM, Sosnowski AW, Galinanes M. Off-pump bypass graft operation significantly reduces oxidative stress and inflammation. Ann Thorac Surg. 2000;69:785–91.
28. Gu YJ, Mariani MA, van Oeveren W, Grandjean JG, Boonstra PW. Reduction of the inflammatory response in patients undergoing minimally invasive coronary artery bypass grafting. Ann Thorac Surg. 1998;65:420–4.
29. Fromes Y, Gaillard D, Ponzio O, et al. Reduction of the inflammatory response following coronary bypass grafting with total minimal extracorporeal circulation. Eur J Cardiothorac Surg. 2002;22:527–33.
30. Gott VL, Whiffen JD, Dutton RC. Heparin bonding on colloidal graphite surfaces. Science. 1963;142:1297–8.
31. Gott VL, Daggett RL. Serendipity and the development of heparin and carbon surfaces. Ann Thorac Surg. 1999;68(3 Suppl):S19–22.
32. Warren OJ, Watret AL, de Wit KL, et al. The inflammatory response to cardiopulmonary bypass: part 2-anti-inflammatory therapeutic strategies. J Cardiothorac Vasc Anesth. 2009;23:384–93.
33. Ranucci M, Mazzucco A, Pessotto R, et al. Heparin-coated circuits for high-risk patients: a multicenter, prospective, randomized trial. Ann Thorac Surg. 1999;67:994–1000.
34. te Velthuis H, Baufreton C, Jansen PG, et al. Heparin coating of extracorporeal circuits inhibits contact activation during cardiac operations. J Thorac Cardiovasc Surg. 1997;114:117–22.
35. Baufreton C, Moczar M, Intrator L, et al. Inflammatory response to cardiopulmonary bypass using two different types of heparin-coated extracorporeal circuits. Perfusion. 1998;13:419–27.
36. Lundblad R, Moen O, Fosse E. Endothelin-1 and neutrophil activation during heparin-coated cardiopulmonary bypass. Ann Thorac Surg. 1997;63:1361–7.
37. Fosse E, Thelin S, Svennevig JL, et al. Duraflo II coating of cardiopulmonary bypass circuits reduces complement activation, but does not affect the release of granulocyte enzymes: a European multicentre study. Eur J Cardiothorac Surg. 1997;11:320–7.
38. Boonstra PW, Gu YJ, Akkerman C, et al. Heparin coating of an extracorporeal circuit partly improves hemostasis after cardiopulmonary bypass. J Thorac Cardiovasc Surg. 1994;107:289–92.
39. Mangoush O, Purkayastha S, Haj-Yahia S, et al. Heparin-bonded circuits versus nonheparin-bonded circuits: an evaluation of their effect on clinical outcomes. Eur J Cardiothorac Surg. 2007;31:1058–69.
40. Baker RA, Willcox TW. Australian and New Zealand perfusion survey: equipment and monitoring. J Extra Corpor Technol. 2006;38:220–9.
41. Raja SG, Yousufuddin S, Rasool F, Nubi A, Danton M, Pollock J. Impact of modified ultrafiltration on morbidity after pediatric cardiac surgery. Impact of modified ultrafiltration on morbidity after pediatric cardiac surgery. Asian Cardiovasc Thorac Ann. 2006;14:341–50.
42. Hiramatsu T, Imai Y, Kurosawa H, et al. Effects of dilutional and modified ultrafiltration in plasma endothelin-1 and pulmonary vascular resistance after the Fontan procedure. Ann Thorac Surg. 2002;73:861–5.
43. Chew MS, Brix-Christensen V, Ravn HB, et al. Effect of modified ultrafiltration on the inflammatory response in paediatric open-heart surgery: a prospective, randomized study. Perfusion. 2002;17:327–33.

44. Pearl JM, Manning PB, McNamara JL, Saucier MM, Thomas DW. Effect of modified ultrafiltration on plasma thromboxane B2, leukotriene B4, and endothelin-1 in infants undergoing cardiopulmonary bypass. Ann Thorac Surg. 1999;68:1369–75.
45. Portela F, Espanol R, Quintans J. Combined perioperative ultrafiltration in pediatric cardiac surgery. The preliminary results. Rev Esp Cardiol. 1999;52:1075–82.
46. Wang W, Huang HM, Zhu DM, Chen H, Su ZK, Ding WX. Modified ultrafiltration in paediatric cardiopulmonary bypass. Perfusion. 1998;13:304–10.
47. Journois D, Israel-Biet D, Pouard P, et al. High-volume, zero-balanced hemofiltration to reduce delayed inflammatory response to cardiopulmonary bypass in children. Anesthesiology. 1996;85:965–76.
48. Journois D, Pouard P, Greeley WJ. Hemofiltration during cardiopulmonary bypass in pediatric cardiac surgery. Effects on hemostasis, cytokines, and complement components. Anesthesiology. 1994; 81:1181–9.
49. Saatvedt K, Lindberg H, Geiran OR, et al. Ultrafiltration after cardiopulmonary bypass in children: effects on hemodynamics, cytokines and complement. Cardiovasc Res. 1996;31:596–602.
50. Luciani GB, Menon T, Vecchi B, et al. Modified ultrafiltration reduces morbidity after adult cardiac operations: a prospective, randomized clinical trial. Circulation. 2001;104(12 Suppl 1): I253–9.
51. Grünenfelder J, Zünd G, Schoeberlein A, et al. Modified ultrafiltration lowers adhesion molecule and cytokine levels after cardiopulmonary bypass without clinical relevance in adults. Eur J Cardiothorac Surg. 2000;17:77–83.
52. Boodhwani M, Williams K, Babaev A, et al. Ultrafiltration reduces blood transfusions following cardiac surgery: a meta-analysis. Eur J Cardiothorac Surg. 2006;30:892–7.
53. Williams GD, Ramamoorthy C, Chu L, et al. Modified and conventional ultrafiltration during pediatric cardiac surgery: clinical outcomes compared. J Thorac Cardiovasc Surg. 2006;132:1291–8.
54. Gu YJ, de Vries AJ, Boonstra PW, van Oeveren W. Leukocyte depletion results in improved lung function and reduced inflammatory response after cardiac surgery. J Thorac Cardiovasc Surg. 1996;112:494–500.
55. Gu YJ, de Vries AJ, Vos P, Boonstra PW, van Oeveren W. Leukocyte depletion during cardiac operation: a new approach through the venous bypass circuit. Ann Thorac Surg. 1999;67:604–9.
56. Johnson D, Thomson D, Mycyk T, Burbridge B, Mayers I. Depletion of neutrophils by filter during aortocoronary bypass surgery transiently improves postoperative cardiorespiratory status. Chest. 1995;107:1253–9.
57. Morioka K, Muraoka R, Chiba Y, et al. Leukocyte and platelet depletion with a blood cell separator: effects on lung injury after cardiac surgery with cardiopulmonary bypass. J Thorac Cardiovasc Surg. 1996;111:45–54.
58. Di Salvo C, Louca LL, Pattichis K, Hooper J, Walesby RK. Does activated neutrophil depletion on bypass by leukocyte filtration reduce myocardial damage? A preliminary report. J Cardiovasc Surg (Torino). 1996;37(6 Suppl 1):93–100.
59. Hurst T, Johnson D, Cujec B, et al. Depletion of activated neutrophils by a filter during cardiac valve surgery. Can J Anaesth. 1997; 44:131–9.
60. Baksaas ST, Flom-Halvorsen HI, Ovrum E, et al. Leucocyte filtration during cardiopulmonary reperfusion in coronary artery bypass surgery. Perfusion. 1999;14:107–17.
61. Roth M, Kraus B, Scheffold T, et al. The effect of leukocyte-depleted blood cardioplegia in patients with severe left ventricular dysfunction: a randomized, double-blind study. J Thorac Cardiovasc Surg. 2000;120:642–50.
62. De Vecchi E, Paroni R, Pala MG, et al. Role of leucocytes in free radical production during myocardial revascularisation. Heart. 1997;77:449–55.
63. Sawa Y, Taniguchi K, Kadoba K, et al. Leukocyte depletion attenuates reperfusion injury in patients with left ventricular hypertrophy. Circulation. 1996;93:1640–6.
64. Andersen KS, Nygreen EL, Grong K, Leirvaag B, Holmsen H. Comparison of the centrifugal and roller pump in elective coronary artery bypass surgery – a prospective, randomized study with special emphasis upon platelet activation. Scand Cardiovasc J. 2003; 37:356–62.
65. Klein M, Dauben HP, Schulte HD, Gams E. Centrifugal pumping during routine open heart surgery improves clinical outcome. Artif Organs. 1998;22:326–36.
66. Klein M, Mahoney CB, Probst C, Schulte HD, Gams E. Blood product use during routine open heart surgery: the impact of the centrifugal pump. Artif Organs. 2001;25:300–5.
67. Menasché P, Peynet J, Haeffner-Cavaillon N. Influence of temperature on neutrophil trafficking during clinical cardiopulmonary bypass. Circulation. 1995;92(9 Suppl):II334–40.
68. Birdi I, Caputo M, Underwood M, Bryan AJ, Angelini GD. The effects of cardiopulmonary bypass temperature on inflammatory response following cardiopulmonary bypass. Eur J Cardiothorac Surg. 1999;16:540–5.
69. McLean RF, Wong BI. Normothermic versus hypothermic cardiopulmonary bypass: central nervous system outcomes. J Cardiothorac Vasc Anesth. 1996;10:45–52.
70. Shann KG, Likosky DS, Murkin JM, et al. An evidence-based review of the practice of cardiopulmonary bypass in adults: a focus on neurologic injury, glycemic control, hemodilution, and the inflammatory response. J Thorac Cardiovasc Surg. 2006;132:283–90.
71. Wan S, LeClerc JL, Huynh CH, et al. Does steroid pretreatment increase endotoxin release during clinical cardiopulmonary bypass? J Thorac Cardiovasc Surg. 1999;117:1004–8.
72. Dernek S, Tunerir B, Sevin B, et al. The effects of methylprednisolone on complement, immunoglobulins and pulmonary neutrophil sequestration during cardiopulmonary bypass. Cardiovasc Surg. 1999;7:414–8.
73. Kawamura T, Inada K, Nara N, Wakusawa R, Endo S. Influence of methylprednisolone on cytokine balance during cardiac surgery. Crit Care Med. 1999;27:545–8.
74. Jansen NJ, van Oeveren W, van Vliet M, et al. The role of different types of corticosteroids on the inflammatory mediators in cardiopulmonary bypass. Eur J Cardiothorac Surg. 1991;5:211–7.
75. Tassani P, Richter JA, Barankay A, et al. Does high-dose methylprednisolone in aprotinin-treated patients attenuate the systemic inflammatory response during coronary artery bypass grafting procedures? J Cardiothorac Vasc Anesth. 1999;13:165–72.
76. Kawamura T, Inada K, Okada H, Okada K, Wakusawa R. Methylprednisolone inhibits increase of interleukin 8 and 6 during open heart surgery. Can J Anaesth. 1995;42:399–403.
77. Yilmaz M, Ener S, Akalin H, Sagdic K, Serdar OA, Cengiz M. Effect of low-dose methyl prednisolone on serum cytokine levels following extracorporeal circulation. Perfusion. 1999;14: 201–6.
78. van Overveld FJ, De Jongh R, Jorens PG, et al. Pretreatment with methylprednisolone in coronary artery bypass grafting influences the levels of histamine and tryptase in serum but not in bronchoalveolar lavage fluid. Clin Sci (Lond). 1994;86:49–53.
79. Lodge AJ, Chai PJ, Daggett CW, Ungerleider RM, Jaggers J. Methylprednisolone reduces the inflammatory response to cardiopulmonary bypass in neonatal piglets: timing of dose is important. J Thorac Cardiovasc Surg. 1999;117:515–22.
80. Robertson-Malt S, Afrane B, El Barbary M. Prophylactic steroids for pediatric open heart surgery. Cochrane Database Syst Rev. 2007;(4):CD005550.
81. Dieleman JM, van Paassen J, van Dijk D, et al. Prophylactic corticosteroids for cardiopulmonary bypass in adults. Cochrane Database Syst Rev. 2011;(5):CD005566.

82. Eagle KA, Guyton RA, Davidoff R, American College of Cardiology; American Heart Association. ACC/AHA 2004 guideline update for coronary artery bypass graft surgery: a report of the American College of Cardiology/American Heart Association Task Force on Practice Guidelines (Committee to Update the 1999 Guidelines for Coronary Artery Bypass Graft Surgery). Circulation. 2004;110: e340–437.
83. Castiglioni GC, Lojacono L, Tamborini G. Effects of trypsin and kallikrein inhibition in acute pancreatitis. Arch Ital Chir. 1965; 91:365–76.
84. Royston D, Bidstrup BP, Taylor KM, Sapsford RN. Effect of aprotinin on need for blood transfusion after repeat open-heart surgery. Lancet. 1987;2:1289–91.
85. Poullis M, Manning R, Laffan M, et al. The antithrombotic effect of aprotinin: actions mediated via the proteaseactivated receptor 1. J Thorac Cardiovasc Surg. 2000;120:370–8.
86. Greilich PE, Brouse CF, Whitten CW, et al. Antifibrinolytic therapy during cardiopulmonary bypass reduces proinflammatory cytokine levels: a randomized, double-blind, placebo-controlled study of epsilon-aminocaproic acid and aprotinin. J Thorac Cardiovasc Surg. 2003;126:1498–503.
87. Hill GE, Pohorecki R, Alonso A, Rennard SI, Robbins RA. Aprotinin reduces interleukin-8 production and lung neutrophil accumulation after cardiopulmonary bypass. Anesth Analg. 1996; 83:696–700.
88. Wendel HP, Heller W, Michel J, et al. Lower cardiac troponin T levels in patients undergoing cardiopulmonary bypass and receiving high-dose aprotinin therapy indicate reduction of perioperative myocardial damage. J Thorac Cardiovasc Surg. 1995;109:1164–72.
89. Levi M, Cromheecke ME, de Jonge E, et al. Pharmacological strategies to decrease excessive blood loss in cardiac surgery: a meta-analysis of clinically relevant endpoints. Lancet. 1999;354: 1940–7.
90. Mangano DT, Tudor IC, Dietzel C, Multicenter Study of Perioperative Ischemia Research Group; Ischemia Research and Education Foundation. The risk associated with aprotinin in cardiac surgery. N Engl J Med. 2006;354:353–65.
91. Karkouti K, Beattie WS, Dattilo KM, et al. A propensity score case–control comparison of aprotinin and tranexamic acid in high-transfusion-risk cardiac surgery. Transfusion. 2006;46: 327–38.
92. Fergusson DA, Hébert PC, Mazer CD, BART Investigators. A comparison of aprotinin and lysine analogues in high-risk cardiac surgery. N Engl J Med. 2008;358:2319–31.
93. Ray WA, Stein CM. The aprotinin story – is BART the final chapter? N Engl J Med. 2008;358:2398–400.
94. Sun SC, Appleyard R, Masetti P, et al. Improved recovery of heart transplants by combined use of oxygen-derived free radical scavengers and energy enhancement. J Thorac Cardiovasc Surg. 1992; 104:830–7.
95. Julia PL, Buckberg GD, Acar C, Partington MT, Sherman MP. Studies of controlled reperfusion after ischemia. XXI. Reperfusate composition: superiority of blood cardioplegia over crystalloid cardioplegia in limiting reperfusion damage-importance of endogenous oxygen free radical scavengers in red blood cells. J Thorac Cardiovasc Surg. 1991;101:303–13.
96. Yau TM, Weisel RD, Mickle DA. Vitamin E for coronary bypass operations. A prospective, double-blind, randomized trial. J Thorac Cardiovasc Surg. 1994;108:302–10.
97. Sisto T, Paajanen H, Metsä-Ketelä T, et al. Pretreatment with antioxidants and allopurinol diminishes cardiac onset events in coronary artery bypass grafting. Ann Thorac Surg. 1995;59: 1519–23.
98. Fitch JC, Rollins S, Matis L, et al. Pharmacology and biological efficacy of a recombinant, humanized, single-chain antibody C5 complement inhibitor in patients undergoing coronary artery bypass graft surgery with cardiopulmonary bypass. Circulation. 1999;100:2499–506.
99. Soulika AM, Khan MM, Hattori T, et al. Inhibition of heparin/protamine complex-induced complement activation by Compstatin in baboons. Clin Immunol. 2000;96:212–21.
100. Kirschfink M. Controlling the complement system in inflammation. Immunopharmacology. 1997;38:51–62.
101. Takeuchi K, del Nido PJ, Ibrahim AE, et al. Vesnarinone and amrinone reduce the systemic inflammatory response syndrome. J Thorac Cardiovasc Surg. 1999;117:375–82.
102. Mollhoff T, Loick HM, Van Aken H, Schmidt C, Rolf N, Tjan TD, et al. Milrinone modulates endotoxemia, systemic inflammation, and subsequent acute phase response after cardiopulmonary bypass (CPB). Anesthesiology. 1999;90:72–80.
103. McNicol L, Andersen LW, Liu G, Doolan L, Baek L. Markers of splanchnic perfusion and intestinal translocation of endotoxins during cardiopulmonary bypass: effects of dopamine and milrinone. J Cardiothorac Vasc Anesth. 1999;13:292–8.
104. Berendes E, Mollhoff T, Van Aken H, et al. Effects of dopexamine on creatinine clearance, systemic inflammation, and splanchnic oxygenation in patients undergoing coronary artery bypass grafting. Anesth Analg. 1997;84:950–7.
105. Sinclair DG, Houldsworth PE, Keogh B, Pepper J, Evans TW. Gastrointestinal permeability following cardiopulmonary bypass: a randomised study comparing the effects of dopamine and dopexamine. Intensive Care Med. 1997;23:510–6.
106. Shafique T, Johnson RG, Dai HB, Weintraub RM, Sellke FW. Altered pulmonary microvascular reactivity after total cardiopulmonary bypass. J Thorac Cardiovasc Surg. 1993;106:479–86.
107. Livelli Jr FD, Johnson RA, McEnany MT. Unexplained in-hospital fever following cardiac surgery. Natural history, relationship to postpericardiotomy syndrome, and a prospective study of therapy with indomethacin versus placebo. Circulation. 1978;57: 968–75.
108. Mobert J, Becker BF. Cyclooxygenase inhibition aggravates ischemia-reperfusion injury in the perfused guinea pig heart: involvement of isoprostanes. J Am Coll Cardiol. 1998;31:1687–94.
109. Hindman BJ, Moore SA, Cutkomp J, et al. Brain expression of inducible cyclooxygenase 2 messenger RNA in rats undergoing cardiopulmonary bypass. Anesthesiology. 2001;95:1380–8.
110. Erez E, Erman A, Snir E, et al. Thromboxane production in human lung during cardiopulmonary bypass: beneficial effect of aspirin? Ann Thorac Surg. 1998;65:101–6.
111. Sato K, Li J, Metais C, Bianchi C, Sellke F. Increased pulmonary vascular contraction to serotonin after cardiopulmonary bypass: role of cyclooxygenase. J Surg Res. 2000;90:138–43.
112. Yang X, Ma N, Szabolcs MJ, Zhong J, Athan E, Sciacca RR, et al. Upregulation of COX-2 during cardiac allograft rejection. Circulation. 2000;101:430–8.
113. Bouchard JF, Lamontagne D. Mechanisms of protection afforded by cyclooxygenase inhibitors to endothelial function against ischemic injury in rat isolated hearts. J Cardiovasc Pharmacol. 1999; 34:755–63.
114. Grandel U, Fink L, Blum A, et al. Endotoxin-induced myocardial tumor necrosis factor-alpha synthesis depresses contractility of isolated rat hearts: evidence for a role of sphingosine and cyclooxygenase-2-derived thromboxane production. Circulation. 2000;102:2758–64.
115. Friedrich I, Silber RE, Baumann B, Fischer C, Holzheimer RG. IgM-enriched immunoglobulin preparation for immunoprophylaxis in cardiac surgery. Eur J Med Res. 2002;7:544–9.
116. Opal SM, Gluck T. Endotoxinas a drug target. Crit Care Med. 2003;31(1 Suppl):S57–64.
117. Goldie AS, Fearon KC, Ross JA. Natural cytokine antagonists and endogenous antiendotoxin core antibodies in sepsis syndrome. The Sepsis Intervention Group. JAMA. 1995;274:172–7.

118. Martinez-Pellus AE, Merino P, Bru M. Endogenous endotoxemia of intestinal origin during cardiopulmonary bypass. Role of type of flow and protective effect of selective digestive decontamination. Intensive Care Med. 1997;23:1251–7.
119. Nathens AB, Marshall JC. Selective decontamination of the digestive tract in surgical patients: a systematic review of the evidence. Arch Surg. 1999;134:170–6.
120. Engelman DT, Adams DH, Byrne JG, et al. Impact of body mass index and albumin on morbidity and mortality after cardiac surgery. J Thorac Cardiovasc Surg. 1999;118:866–73.
121. Walesby RK, Goode AW, Bentall HH. Nutritional status of patients undergoing valve replacement by open heart surgery. Lancet. 1978;1:76–7.
122. Abel RM, Grimes JB, Alonso D, Alonso M, Gay WA. Adverse hemodynamic and ultrastructural changes in dog hearts subjected to protein-calorie malnutrition. Am Heart J. 1979;97:733–44.
123. Gianotti L, Braga M, Vignali A, et al. Effect of route of delivery and formulation of postoperative nutritional support in patients undergoing major operations for malignant neoplasms. Arch Surg. 1997;132:1222–30.
124. Braga M, Gianotti L, Radaelli G, et al. Perioperative immunonutrition in patients undergoing cancer surgery: results of a randomized double-blind phase 3 trial. Arch Surg. 1999;134:428–33.
125. Griffiths RD. Outcome of critically ill patients after supplementation with glutamine. Nutrition. 1997;13:752–4.

The Systemic Inflammatory Response Syndrome Following Cardiopulmonary Bypass in Children

28

Harald L. Lindberg and Tom N. Hoel

To a large extent, reducing the effects of the surgical trauma itself is not possible. However, delicate tissue handling and a short operative time may reduce this factor and should be striven for, but not at the cost of the patient's safety or the quality of operative repair.

The effects of the cardiopulmonary bypass and blood exposure to a foreign surface can be modified by trying to make the artificial surfaces as biocompatible as possible. This can be done in different ways by coating the surfaces. Also, modification of the secondary effects of the activation of signal substances, such as complement factors and cytokines, has been attempted with pharmacological agents. Other measures, such as leukocyte filtration and ultrafiltration, have been in use to attenuate the SIRS. Generally, the most effective method for brain protection is the use of hypothermia during cardiopulmonary bypass. This chapter discusses these factors in detail.

The Endothelium

The endothelium fulfills the definition of an organ because of its physical size (5,000 m^2 surface area) and its ability to synthesize and release a large number of physiologically active products. It is a dynamic participant in cellular and organ function rather than a static barrier. It is intimately involved in a variety of physiologic and pathologic processes and has emerged as the central focus of many of the biologic events that affect the perioperative course of the patient.

The inflammatory response to cardiopulmonary bypass (CPB) is characterized by a state of widespread endothelial activation and diffuse endothelial dysfunction. Inflammatory mediators, including tumor necrosis factor alpha (TNF)-α and interleukin one (IL)-1, bind to specific receptors on the endothelium, initiating diverse signal transduction pathways, which in turn activate a specific set of genes within the nucleus of the endothelial cell, termed *activation genes*. Sheppard et al. [1] showed that transcription factor nuclear factor B plays a pivotal role in the signal transduction process. This process results in the translation of proteins, including adhesion molecules (e.g., E-selectin, intercellular adhesion molecule-1) and cytokines (e.g., IL-8) required for endothelial cell activation, a process that takes approximately 4 h and peaks at 8–24 h, depending on the gene.

The activated endothelial cell plays a major role in linking the inflammatory and coagulation systems by expressing proteins central to the activation of coagulation and inflammation [2, 3]. Endothelial cell adhesion molecule expression mediates the interaction between the neutrophil and the endothelial cell, resulting in neutrophil adhesion, activation, and degranulation. This further damages the endothelium, causing diffuse capillary leak and edema formation [2, 4]. Endothelial injury results in the expression of tissue factor, augmented by IL-1 and TNF-α, which activates the extrinsic pathway of coagulation as shown by Cicala and Cirino [3] and may result in disseminated intravascular coagulation [5]. In addition, protein C, a key inhibitory regulator of hemostasis, is antagonized in inflammatory states, most probably by TNF-α, further shifting the balance toward a procoagulant state [3].

Vascular endothelium plays a central role in the pathogenesis of microcirculatory derangement following CPB. Endothelial regulation of local vascular tone is mediated via a variety of endothelium-derived relaxing and contracting factors such as nitric oxide (NO), prostacyclin, endothelium-derived hyperpolarizing factor, endothelin, and thromboxane A2 [6]. The increase in pulmonary vascular resistance following CPB is attributed to reduced NO release from dysfunctional pulmonary endothelium and is reversed by NO supplementation [6].

H.L. Lindberg, MD, PhD (✉) • T.N. Hoel, MD, PhD
Department of Thoracic and Cardiovascular Surgery, University of Oslo, Rikshospitalet University Hospital, Oslo, Norway
e-mail: hlindber@ous-hf.no

E.A. Gabriel, S.A. Gabriel (eds.), *Inflammatory Response in Cardiovascular Surgery*,
DOI 10.1007/978-1-4471-4429-8_28, © Springer-Verlag London 2013

Biocompatible Surfaces

In order to attenuate the inflammatory response to CPB, tremendous efforts have been made to synthesize CPB surfaces that the body would recognize as non-self as little possible. Already in 1963, Gott et al. [7] described an attempt to intervene in the artificial surface-induced blood activation by coating surfaces with heparin. Later studies showed that such a surface modification of the CPB circuit reduced the activation of some of the cascade systems, both in vitro [8–10] and in vivo [11, 12]. The role of heparin in reducing the inflammatory response is still controversial despite reports on a favorable clinical outcome [13] and a reduced need for systemic anticoagulation [14]. In a meta-analysis of heparin-coated circuits, the authors concluded that heparin coating reduces postoperative bleeding as well as the need for reoperations [15].

Different coatings are available for clinical use, both heparin-based coatings and non-heparin coatings:

The Carmeda bioactive surface (CBAS) is composed of a layer of polyethyleneimine onto which the end point is attached and partially degraded heparin is covalently bound.

Duraflo II is based on an ionically bound heparin-benzalkonium-chloride complex, which enables a relatively firm connection with the foreign substance. This coating is somewhat unstable since approximately 10 % of the bound heparin leaks into the circulation [16].

The Trillium Bio-passive Surface is a water-soluble synthetic polymer. The polymer is covalently bound to a primer and is composed of sulfate and sulfonate groups, polyethylene oxide chains (PEO), and heparin. The hydrophilic PEO chains are thought to decrease protein adsorption and cell adhesion. Sulfonation is intended to mimic the functional groups responsible for heparin's anticoagulant effect. The Trillium coating also incorporates small amounts of covalently bound heparin.

BioLine coating brings high molecular weight heparin onto a base layer of immobilized polypeptides. This polypeptide adsorption can occur on hydrophilic as well as hydrophobic surfaces.

Phosphorylcholine inert surface (PHISIO) is a non-heparin coating. The idea is to produce a surface that largely mimics the main lipid head group component of the outer cell membrane. These neutral phospholipids do not activate the clotting system and are therefore thought to be non-thrombogenic [17].

Surface-modifying additive (SMA) is a non-heparin coating based on a mixture of two copolymers added to the resin polymer structure. During processing, these two amphipathic copolymers migrate and concentrate at the lumen surface, thus determining a mosaic structure with alternating hydrophilic and hydrophobic groups. This reduces fibrinogen adsorption and consequently platelet activation.

The Complement System and Inflammation

The complement system has the capability of initiating an inflammatory response whenever it comes into contact with foreign surfaces. It is one of the body's cascade systems that initiate an accurately tuned reaction, tightly controlled by several membrane-bound and fluid-phase inhibitors. Almost all mammalian cells express regulators of the complement system to protect against an autologous attack on the self [18]. There is considerable cross talk between the cascade systems in the body sharing some common regulatory proteins [19]. Complement components C3a, C4a, and C5a (anaphylotoxins) mediate many inflammatory effects, such as chemotaxis for human neutrophils and mast cells, smooth muscle cell contraction, increased permeability of the vessels, platelet aggregation and activation, and histamine release from mast cells. The complement system, a key factor in acute and chronic inflammatory response, is capable of promoting a powerful inflammatory response when the organism is exposed to "non-self" or "danger," subsequently adjusting the response in proportion to the intensity of the stimuli and finally terminating the response when the normal condition is restored.

Cytokines

Cytokines are mainly produced by monocytes, macrophages, lymphocytes, and endothelial cells and can be either protective or damaging depending on the concentration of each cytokine, the receptor, the cell types they are acting on, and the presence of other cytokines. Many of the cytokines are produced through stimulation of the transcription factor NF-kB [10]. The cytokines are produced locally, but in case of extensive stimulation there is a spillover to peripheral blood, and they have potential harmful effects on organ function [8] (partly through different cascades such as complement activation and the coagulation cascade) (Fig. 28.1). The cytokines interact in a complex network and exhibit pro- or antiinflammatory properties or both. The most important cytokines in relation to cardiac surgery are the proinflammatory cytokines TNF-a, IL-6, and IL-8 and the anti-inflammatory cytokines IL-10 and IL-1ra. They are mostly measured in blood samples or in bronchoalveolar lavage (BAL) fluid.

Proinflammatory Cytokines

TNF-a plays an important role for leukocyte-endothelium interaction and the release of oxygen radicals from adherent polymorphonuclear neutrophils (PMNs) [20]. Reports on the TNF-a response after CPB are conflicting. A significant increase in TNF-a was demonstrated after release of the aor-

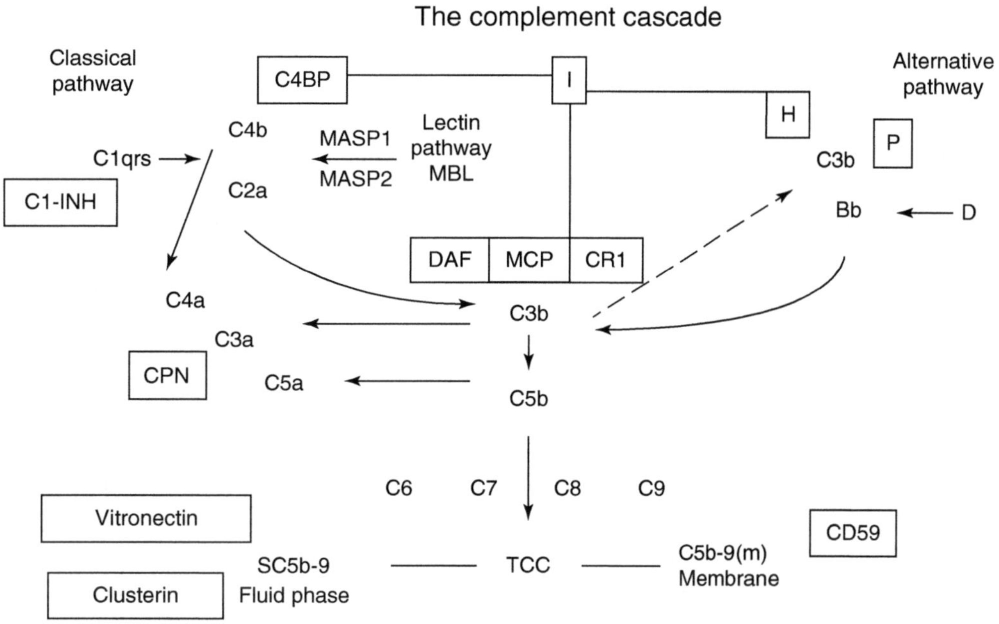

Fig. 28.1 Schematic illustration of the complement system and some of its inhibitors and activators. *C* complement, *MBL* mannose-binding lactin, *H and I* factors H and I, inhibitors of C3 formation in the fluid phase, *DAF* decay accelerating factor (CD 55), *MCP* membrane cofactor protein, *MASPI and MASP2* MBL-associated serine proteases, *CR1* complement receptor 1, *C4RP* C4 binding protein, *C1-INH* C1 inhibitor, *CPN* carboxypeptidase N, *CD59* protectin, *P* properdin, *TCC* terminal complement complex (By courtesy of Tom Eirik Mollnes)

tic cross clamp and termination of CPB in some studies [21], while others reported no detectable TNF-a [22]. In a few studies, TNF-a was detectable preoperatively but without further changes in the TNF-a plasma concentration during or after CPB. A similar inconsistency in TNF-a response was found in pigs subjected to CPB [23]. Animal studies have further revealed that administration of small amounts of TNF-a decrease myocardial performance, suggesting that even small TNF-a levels may also contribute to myocardial dysfunction in humans.

IL-6 is a good predictor of clinical outcome [24] and is thought to be related to the extent of tissue injury. Normally, IL-6 is undetectable in peripheral blood in healthy individuals, but has been found preoperatively in some children with congenital heart disease [25]. In general, IL-6 plasma levels increase during and after surgery and CPB and are related to the duration of aortic clamp time [26]. It is still not clear whether it is the CPB procedure, the surgery, or the combination that elicits the IL-6 response as no differences were found between pediatric patients subjected to surgery with or without CPB [27].

In children subjected to cardiac surgery during CPB, an early IL-8 response has been detected with increasing concentration in the following hours. The plasma levels were related to the duration of ischemia/reperfusion and total bypass time [21].

The proinflammatory cytokine response in children undergoing cardiac surgery with CPB shows a large variation in the release pattern and plasma concentrations. This is in contrast to the proinflammatory response in adults, which is well defined and temporary. It is still unknown whether the preoperative high cytokine levels in children are of clinical importance, but neonates with clinical signs of capillary leak syndrome after heart surgery showed signs of a preoperative inflammatory state measured as increased plasma levels of elastase and the complement split products C3d/ C3 [28].

Anti-inflammatory Cytokines

IL-10 and IL-1 receptor antagonists (IL-1ra) seem to be the most consistent antiinflammatory cytokines released during and after cardiac surgery with CPB, both in adults and children [28]. The antiinflammatory response is not caused by blood contact with the circuit because none of these cytokines were detectable when blood was drawn through an isolated pediatric CPB circuit [29]. However, when the CPB is connected to an animal, the stress from the CPB procedure itself elicits an IL-10 response when compared to sham-operated animals [23].

C-reactive protein (CRP*)* is an acute-phase protein with antiinflammatory properties as it downregulates PMN chemotaxis. Clinically, CRP is often used as an unspecific marker for infections, and its plasma concentration correlates to the extent of the surgical trauma. High CRP levels are unequivocally found in children after heart surgery during CPB with a peak on the first to third postoperative day, and the response is delayed compared with the IL-6 release [30]. It has been suggested that the stress of sternotomy is sufficient to elicit a CRP response as piglets subjected to anesthesia and sternotomy show the same CRP response as piglets exposed to the CPB procedure [23].

In conclusion, the antiinflammatory response in pediatric cardiac patients shows a more clear release pattern compared to the proinflammatory counterpart. Evidence has emerged that the balance between the pro- and antiinflammatory mediators is most important for the outcome of patients experiencing a systemic inflammatory response [19]. It is therefore irrelevant to follow changes in a single cytokine concentration in the patient at present. In general, the cytokine response is characterized by great variability and interindividual differences. In uncomplicated cases, the systemic response is temporary, balanced, and of a few days' duration in both pediatric and adult patients [31].

Steroid Pretreatment

Although steroids have been used for years to attenuate post-bypass inflammation, data to support this derive almost entirely from trials in adults with coronary artery disease. Even in adults, steroid use for cardiac surgery is controversial, and data in children are inconclusive.

The actions of steroids are protean with both immediate and delayed effects. The limitation of inflammatory capillary permeability by either by diminishing recruitment of activated white blood cells to vascular beds or inhibiting prostacyclin production and induction of nitric oxide synthase has been shown [32, 33]. Also, steroids appear to increase antiinflammatory and decrease proinflammatory cytokine levels [34]. Corticosteroids upregulate the production of b-adrenergic receptors and decrease reuptake, thus increasing the availability of these receptors to respond to endogenous or exogenous catecholamines. The availability of cytosolic calcium in myocardial and vascular smooth muscle cells, augmenting contractility, may be increased by physiologic doses of corticosteroids.

Methylprednisolone is able to reliably (and beneficially) alter the balance of proinflammatory and antiinflammatory mediators in the blood of patients subjected to CPB, indicating that the drug decreases the SIRS associated with CPB. Specific hemodynamic benefits (increased CI, decreased SVR) seem to be associated with use of the drug in this setting, yet these alterations may increase the need for postoperative IV hemodynamic agents (vasoconstrictors, etc.). Pulmonary compliance seems not to be influenced by steroids. Increased P(A-a)O_2 (perhaps by increasing pulmonary shunt) and early postoperative tracheal extubation may be hindered for undetermined reasons. Several studies have used different doses of MP and dexamethasone. There is no general agreement on the type of preparation and dose of the steroid. Most of the studies are concerned with adult patients. Varan et al. [35] demonstrated that the increase in cytokine levels and CRP was not significantly different between high and low doses. Niazi et al. [36] demonstrated an increase in the cardiac index during and after CPB in patients undergoing coronary artery bypass surgery that received 30 mg/kg of MP. In this study, after an initial increase in the cardiac index, it gradually decreased in the post-bypass period. Jansen et al. [37] reported normothermia, higher blood pressure levels without supportive treatment, and a shorter stay in the intensive care unit for dexamethasone-treated patients (receiving 1 mg/kg) compared to nontreated patients. Another study showed that two doses of 30 mg/kg MP before CPB and before declamping of the aorta suppressed the production of IL-8 and 6 [38]. The authors also found a higher post-surgical cardiac index in the MP-treated group. In the Varan study, the increase in IL-6 and 8 levels after surgery was not significantly different in low- and high-dose MP groups. The cumulative inotropic support required, the duration of mechanical ventilation, the stay in intensive care unit, urine volume, blood loss, and peak core temperature were not significantly different between the two groups. Several studies have demonstrated suppression of levels of interleukins. Jorens et al. [39] showed that MP pretreatment of 30 mg/kg failed to prevent IL-8-mediated pulmonary neutrophil infiltration after CPB, although an increase in serum IL-8 levels was less pronounced in MP-treated than in nonsteroid-treated patients. Butler et al. [40] investigated the levels of cytokines during cardiopulmonary bypass and the effects of intraoperative MP at a dose of 10 mg/kg versus no steroids in the pediatric age group. Clinical and hemodynamic consequences were not mentioned. The IL-6 level was elevated above baseline, peaking earlier in the nonsteroid group. Both IL-6 and CRP levels at 24 h postoperatively were higher in the nonsteroid group.

Cardiopulmonary bypass has also been shown to play a role in the development of pulmonary dysfunction after open-heart surgery. Increased protein leakage as early as 10 min after the onset of CPB in patients with clinical signs of capillary leak syndrome has also been demonstrated by Seghaye et al. [41]. Corticosteroids in several doses have been used with the hope of preventing pulmonary dysfunction after CPB surgery. Varan et al. [35] did not observe any difference in oxygenation parameters for any patients in the two groups, indicated by similar ratios of PaO_2/FiO_2 in the early postoperative period.

They concluded that CPB surgery initiates an SIR and high-dose MP is not superior to low-dose MP in suppressing this reaction. In this study, a low-dose treatment with MP (2 mg/kg) is preferable to a high-dose treatment considering the possible side effects, although none were observed. Children who received steroids prior to CPB had fewer febrile episodes, improved respiratory gas exchange, and better renal function, and they required less supplemental fluid postoperatively than did controls. As a result, the group given dexamethasone required fewer days of mechanical ventilatory support and was discharged from the ICU sooner.

Gessler et al. [42] evaluated the effects of steroids on SIRS by measuring, among other parameters, IL-8 and the total neutrophil count (TNC), as well as some clinical parameters. In this study, administration of steroids did not show a significant impact on the clinical outcome and the degree of the inflammatory response following cardiac surgery. They concluded that the lack of suppression of the inflammatory reaction may have been due to the dose and timing of steroid administration, the lower inflammatory reaction in patients with shorter time on CPB and less severe operative trauma, or an age older than 3 months at the time of surgery.

Although not measuring the amount of SIRS, some publications have shown beneficial effects of steroid administration by measuring other parameters. Checchia et al. [43] showed in 2003 that steroids reduced the postoperative troponin levels in a pediatric population, indicating better myocardial preservation. The Group from Toronto has shown clinically improved outcomes after the use of steroids in a study of high-risk pediatric cardiac surgery [44].

Additional well-designed (prospective, randomized, double-blind, placebo-controlled) clinical investigations (with large numbers of patients and tightly controlled perioperative management) involving corticosteroids and patients undergoing cardiac surgery with CPB need to be done. Whether or not suppression of the SIRS associated with CPB with corticosteroids (or any other drug/technique) is clinically desirable and beneficial remains to be determined.

Platelet Activation

Platelets are known to be activated during CPB because of contact with the foreign surfaces of the extra-corporeal circuit and also because of numerous other factors, such as hypothermia, shear forces, use of exogenous drugs, and release of endogenous chemicals [45]. Platelets are also activated by surgical trauma where the surgical incision, via activation of tissue factor and subsequently factor VII and factor X, may at least partly explain this process [46]. Activated platelets express reorganized surface molecules, such as glycoprotein IIb/IIIa, which forms a fibrinogen-binding complex. Simultaneously, there is a movement of cytoplasmic granules toward the cell surface. These granules fuse with the cell membrane and extrude their contents. This is the secretion method of platelet factor-4, β-TG, and von Willebrand factor. At the same time, those molecules that previously were an integral part of the granule membrane, such as P-selectin, now will be expressed on the surface of the activated platelets [45]. Extracorporeal circuits are manufactured from synthetic materials, and there is a material-derived platelet activation dependent on glycoprotein IIb/IIIa receptors [47]. P-selectin is upregulated by several mechanisms. One is through thrombin, which is redundant because of formation during CPB [48]; another is through newly generated cytokines that stimulate platelets [49]. Both the prothrombotic and the proinflammatory mechanisms occurring during CPB might be attributed to the release of soluble CD 40 ligand (sCD40L) by platelets [50]. Platelets activated during CPB form conjugates both between themselves and with leukocytes. P-selectin is expressed by activated platelets, which contribute to leukocyte conjugate formation by binding P-selectin glycoprotein. Activated platelets use this adhesion pathway to stimulate conjoined monocytes, thus leading to secretion of the proinflammatory cytokines IL-1β, IL-8, and MCP-1. P-selectin also induces tissue factor expression and fibrin deposition by monocytes, thus contributing to the evolution of thrombus. Endothelial cells express the adhesion molecule CD40 and activated platelets express the complementary CD40 ligand on their surface. CD40 ligand is structurally related to TNF-α and induces endothelium to secrete chemokines and express further adhesion molecules. Substantial secretion of IL-8 and MCP-1 was noted on platelets binding to endothelium [51].

Assessment of platelet activation can be done my means of flow cytometry and the analysis of granule proteins (such as β-TG) after degranulation. Thrombospondin, an extracellular matrix protein, has also been investigated, but β-TG seems superior to thrombospondin as a marker for platelet activation in vivo [52].

Temperature

Along with CPB came hypothermia, representing another milestone in the history of open-heart surgery. Hypothermia was used as a tool for lowering the metabolic needs of selected regional beds and/or the whole body. Although hypothermia was introduced in the 1950s by Dr. Wilfred Gordon Bigelow, allowing open-heart operations to be performed in a bloodless field after interruption of blood flow, it was not until the 1960s that hypothermia begun to be used in conjunction with CPB, ushering in the era of modern-day open-heart surgery.

There are a number of proposed clinical applications of hypothermia, including traumatic brain injury. During cardiac surgery with cardiopulmonary bypass (CPB), deep hypothermia is used to protect immature organs from ischemia when surgery requires complete arrest of the systemic circulation. CPB itself, because of the contact of blood with the large non-endothelial surfaces and air/blood interface, triggers the whole body inflammatory response. This often leads to capillary leakage, edema, organ dysfunction, and SIRS. This might explain why in this condition prolonged inflammation together with an acute systemic inflammatory response is one of the major correlates with the adverse clinical outcomes associated with CPB and a major cause of postoperative morbidity [31, 53, 54]. Hypothermia has been suggested to play a protective role in reducing the acute inflammation, but there are scant data demonstrating a beneficial effect of hypothermic CPB [55]. Data focusing on cellular and molecular effects of hypothermia are limited.

The inflammatory response that accompanies open-heart surgery is multifactorial, in both adults and children [56]. The mismatches between the foreign surfaces in the heart-lung machine and blood vessel surfaces are extreme in children. Therefore, specially designed heart-lung machines with small priming volumes and surfaces have been developed [57]. The surgical trauma, anesthesia, and deviation from normal organ perfusion are other important factors causing inflammatory activation [58]. It has also been suggested that the degree of hypothermia may influence the inflammatory response during CPB. Deep hypothermia and circulatory arrest have been shown to trigger less-pronounced inflammatory response than low-flow CPB in newborns, as assessed by measurements of IL-6, IL-8, and C3a [59]. This phenomenon may be the result of a shorter CPB time, but a protective effect of hypothermia per se may also be part of the explanation [60, 61]. However, in a randomized study [62], designed to further elucidate this issue, researchers did not find any significantly attenuated inflammatory response in the moderate hypothermia group. In fact, this group showed an enhanced IL-8 response and an attenuated IL-10 response during CPB, potentially suggesting an inflammatory net effect.

Diestel et al. [61] used endothelial cells as they play a pivotal role during activation of the inflammatory cascade by expression of cytokines. A special cell culture model was used to exclusively study the effects of hypothermia and drug treatment on the inflammatory response of endothelial cells. Using time-temperature settings analogous to clinical application during CPB in children, they measured the concentrations of IL-6, IL-8, and MCP-1. They concluded that hypothermia upregulated IL-6 and TNF-a and that MP-pretreatment attenuated this response.

Qing and colleagues [63] investigated the cell mechanisms by which hypothermia could ameliorate inflammation using a pig model of CPB and sham cardiac operation. In half of the animals ($n=6$), the core temperature was maintained at 28 °C during CPB and in the other half at 37 °C. Measurements made in liver samples obtained before CPB and 6 h after corroborated previous findings indicating that hypothermia increases intrahepatic concentrations of IL-10 while decreasing TNF-a. This effect was associated with less hepatic cell necrosis but without effects on apoptosis. They further documented increased activation of the signal transducer and activator of the transcription (STAT)-3 pathway and increased expression of the suppressor of cytokine signaling (SOCS)-3. These two signaling events are important because they have been associated with antiinflammatory effects in settings other than hypothermia [64]. Activation of STAT-3 is known to increase IL-10, and both IL-10 and activated STAT-3 can increase expression of SOCS-3 with subsequent decreases in TNF-a. These data demonstrate that moderate hypothermia during CPB is associated with activation of the Jak/STAT pathway, leading to the expression of IL-10, which in turn upregulates SOCS-3 and finally attenuates TNF-a production. This antiinflammatory shift in the cytokine balance is associated with liver protection.

Hypothermia has become the subject of scientific and clinical interest as growing evidence points to therapeutic effects not only during but also after an ischemic event. A widely publicized study has shown improved survival and neurologic recovery when hypothermia is instituted in patients who remain comatose after resuscitation from cardiac arrest [65]. Hypothermia also has been shown to be effective in selected subsets of patients presenting with stroke [66], head trauma [67], and myocardial infarction [68]. Thus, there is considerable interest in understanding the mechanisms by which hypothermia works and especially to determine whether benefits may involve mechanisms other than reduction in metabolic activity. Recent studies have in fact shown that hypothermia can activate cell- protecting pathways. For example, hypothermia can induce expression of heat shock protein 70 [69] and cause a shift in the inflammatory cascade during CPB, reducing proinflammatory mediators and increasing the antiinflammatory cytokine IL-10 [70].

A recent study by Stocker et al. [71] has addressed an important and previously unresolved clinical question regarding the most appropriate temperature during pediatric CPB. This study has shown that moderate hypothermia at 24 °C does not offer any advantages over mild hypothermia at 34 °C during pediatric CPB for repair of congenital heart disease in terms of the postoperative clinical course and severity of SIRS or markers of organ injury. Moreover, there was a tendency toward a shorter duration of mechanical ventilation with mild hypothermia. The depth of hypothermia during CPB did not influence the risk of postoperative bleeding, blood product transfusion requirements, or infection. As expected, there was a trend toward a shorter duration of CPB in the mildly hypothermic group, although this was related to the shorter duration of the rewarming period.

When considering the biochemical and cellular manifestations of inflammation, CPB resulted in a marked acute phase reaction in all children, but this was not influenced by temperature. In keeping with previous observations, CPB also resulted in activation of the receptor pathways and in deactivation of circulating monocytes. No influence by the temperature during CPB was noted. Of particular interest is the fact that TNF-a was not influenced by CPB in either group. In this study, no difference in any clinical or biochemical markers of end-organ injury between the two study groups was found. As would be expected, there was postoperative deterioration in lung and renal function, but again, the CPB temperature did not influence this. A transient microalbuminuria early after bypass indicated a significant capillary leak, although independent of bypass temperature.

Chemokines such as IL-8 and MCP-1 are, respectively, potent activators of neutrophils and monocytes [72]. Activation of neutrophils results in degranulation with increased release of myeloperoxidase (MPO) that together with increased production of reactive oxygen species may lead to tissue damage and are important contributors to inflammation. A long CPB time has previously been associated with increased levels of IL-8 and MPO, potentially reflecting enhanced activation of neutrophils [70]. The results in this study further support such a notion by showing raised IL-8 and MPO levels accompanied by increased leukocyte counts in patients with long CPB times. A similar pattern was observed in patients with long aortic cross-clamp times. Both long CPB time and long aortic cross-clamp time may induce enhanced oxidative stress, possibly contributing to the enhanced IL-8 and MCP-1. Eggum et al. [62] showed in a randomized study that duration of CPB will be longer in those with moderate compared with those with mild hypothermia in that it takes longer to cool and rewarm patients from 25 °C, rendering it difficult to evaluate the relative importance of each factor. Nevertheless, although those with moderate hypothermia showed some trends for a higher degree of inflammation than those with mild hypothermia during CPB, the differences were rather modest. In this study, the aortic cross-clamp time and time on CBP were associated with increased chemokine levels and leukocyte activation, underscoring that these procedures should be as short as possible to avoid an excessive inflammatory response and possible adverse clinical effects.

Caputo and colleagues [73] used biochemical and molecular markers of outcome and concluded that there was a need for a prospective trial with clinical end points.

Rasmussen and colleagues [74] studied the influence of CPB temperature only on markers of neuronal injury in 20 children, and in a recent comparison, Eggum and colleagues [62] investigated its effects on inflammatory mediators in 30 children. This study suggests that the temperature has little effect on nonclinical outcomes, as also suggested in previous studies. This conclusion is further supported by three large retrospective studies confirming the feasibility, safety, and potential clinical advantages of warmer CPB temperature when compared with cooler CPB temperature in pediatric cardiac surgery [75–77].

Hypothermia has been widely used in clinical practice to offer organ protection when perfusion may be jeopardized. Hypothermia has been applied during open surgery with the aim of providing organ protection for more than 50 years. Still, it remains debatable whether the increased safety concerning brain protection should be neglected for the benefits to the myocardium. In our opinion, we believe that normothermia can be used in straightforward cases without systemic to pulmonary collaterals and that some degree of hypothermia increases the safety in complex cases. However, there is still need for future research in this field on a molecular and cellular level, as well as clinical long-term follow-up studies.

References

1. Sheppard KA, Rose DW, Haque ZK, Kurokawa R, McInerney E, Westin S, et al. Transcriptional activation by NF-kappaB requires multiple coactivators. Mol Cell Biol. 1999;19(9):6367–78.
2. Boyle EM, Pohlman TH, Johnson MC, Verrier ED. Endothelial cell injury in cardiovascular surgery: the systemic inflammatory response. Ann Thorac Surg. 1997;63(1):277–84.
3. Cicala C, Cirino G. Linkage between inflammation and coagulation: an update on the molecular basis of the crosstalk. Life Sci. 1998;62(20):1817–24.
4. Elliott MJ, Finn AH. Interaction between neutrophils and endothelium. Ann Thorac Surg. 1993;56(6):1503–8.
5. Esmon CT, Fukudome K, Mather T, Bode W, Regan LM, Stearns-Kurosawa DJ, et al. Inflammation, sepsis, and coagulation. Haematologica. 1999;84(3):254–9.
6. Hill GE, Whitten CW. The role of the vascular endothelium in inflammatory syndromes, atherogenesis, and the propagation of disease. J Cardiothorac Vasc Anesth. 1997;11(3):316–21.
7. Gott VL, Whiffen JD, Dutton RC. Heparin bonding on colloidal graphite surfaces. Science. 1963;142(3597):1297–8.
8. Videm V, Mollnes TE, Garred P, Svennevig JL. Biocompatibility of extracorporeal circulation. In vitro comparison of heparin-coated and uncoated oxygenator circuits. J Thorac Cardiovasc Surg. 1991;101(4):654–60.
9. Baksaas ST, Videm V, Fosse E, Karlsen H, Pedersen T, Mollnes TE, et al. In vitro evaluation of new surface coatings for extracorporeal circulation. Perfusion. 1999;14(1):11–9.
10. Videm V, Fosse E, Mollnes TE, Garred P. Complement activation by extracorporeal circulation: effects of precoating a membrane oxygenator circuit with human whole blood. Scand J Thorac Cardiovasc Surg. 1988;22(3):251–6.
11. Fosse E, Moen O, Johnson E, Semb G, Brockmeier V, Mollnes TE, et al. Reduced complement and granulocyte activation with heparin-coated cardiopulmonary bypass. Ann Thorac Surg. 1994;58(2): 472–7.
12. Moen O, Fosse E, Dregelid E, Brockmeier V, Andersson C, Høgåsen K, et al. Centrifugal pump and heparin coating improves cardiopulmonary bypass biocompatibility. Ann Thorac Surg. 1996;62(4):1134–40.
13. Paparella D, Radi Al OO, Meng QH, Venner T, Teoh K, Young E. The effects of high-dose heparin on inflammatory and coagulation parameters following cardiopulmonary bypass. Blood Coagul Fibrinolysis. 2005;16(5):323–8.
14. Øvrum E, Tangen G, Tølløfsrud S, Ringdal MAL. Heparin-coated circuits and reduced systemic anticoagulation applied to 2500 consecutive first-time coronary artery bypass grafting procedures. Ann Thorac Surg. 2003;76(4):1144–8. discussion 1148.
15. Mangoush O, Purkayastha S, Haj-Yahia S, Kinross J, Hayward M, Bartolozzi F, et al. Heparin-bonded circuits versus nonheparin-bonded circuits: an evaluation of their effect on clinical outcomes. Eur J Cardiothorac Surg. 2007;31(6):1058–69.
16. Larm O, Larsson R, Olsson P. A new non-thrombogenic surface prepared by selective covalent binding of heparin via a modified reducing terminal residue. Biomater Med Devices Artif Organs. 1983;11(2–3):161–73.
17. De Somer F, François K, Van Oeveren W, Poelaert J, De Wolf D, Ebels T, et al. Phosphorylcholine coating of extracorporeal circuits provides natural protection against blood activation by the material surface. Eur J Cardiothorac Surg. 2000;18(5):602–6.
18. Liszewski MK, Post TW, Atkinson JP. Membrane cofactor protein (MCP or CD46): newest member of the regulators of complement activation gene cluster. Annu Rev Immunol. 1991;9:431–55.
19. Carroll MC. The complement system in regulation of adaptive immunity. Nat Immunol. 2004;5(10):981–6.
20. Christensen VB. The systemic inflammatory response after cardiac surgery with cardiopulmonary bypass in children. Acta Anaesthesiol Scand. 2001;45(6):671–9.

21. Ozawa T, Yoshihara K, Koyama N, Watanabe Y, Shiono N, Takanashi Y. Clinical efficacy of heparin-bonded bypass circuits related to cytokine responses in children. Ann Thorac Surg. 2000;69(2):584–90.
22. Finn A, Naik S, Klein N, Levinsky RJ, Strobel S, Elliott M. Interleukin-8 release and neutrophil degranulation after pediatric cardiopulmonary bypass. J Thorac Cardiovasc Surg. 1993;105(2):234–41.
23. Brix-Christensen V, Petersen TK, Ravn HB, Hjortdal VE, Andersen NT, Tønnesen E. Cardiopulmonary bypass elicits a pro- and anti-inflammatory cytokine response and impaired neutrophil chemotaxis in neonatal pigs. Acta Anaesthesiol Scand. 2001;45(4):407–13.
24. Hauser GJ, Ben-Ari J, Colvin MP, Dalton HJ, Hertzog JH, Bearb M, et al. Interleukin-6 levels in serum and lung lavage fluid of children undergoing open heart surgery correlate with postoperative morbidity. Intensive Care Med. 1998;24(5):481–6.
25. Duval EL, Kavelaars A, Veenhuizen L, van Vught AJ, van de Wal HJ, Heijnen CJ. Pro- and anti-inflammatory cytokine patterns during and after cardiac surgery in young children. Eur J Pediatr. 1999;158(5):387–93.
26. Eggum R, Ueland T, Mollnes TE, Videm V, Fiane AE, Aukrust P, et al. Perfusion temperature, thyroid hormones and inflammation during pediatric cardiac surgery. Interact Cardiovasc Thorac Surg. 2010;10(1):76–80.
27. Tárnok A, Hambsch J, Emmrich F, Sack U, van Son J, Bellinghausen W, et al. Complement activation, cytokines, and adhesion molecules in children undergoing cardiac surgery with or without cardiopulmonary bypass. Pediatr Cardiol. 1999;20(2):113–25.
28. Seghaye M, Duchateau J, Bruniaux J, Demontoux S, Bosson C, Serraf A, et al. Interleukin-10 release related to cardiopulmonary bypass in infants undergoing cardiac operations. J Thorac Cardiovasc Surg. 1996;111(3):545–53.
29. el Habbal MH, Carter H, Smith LJ, Elliott MJ, Strobel S. Neutrophil activation in paediatric extracorporeal circuits: effect of circulation and temperature variation. Cardiovasc Res. 1995;29(1):102–7.
30. Behr D, Hernvann A, POUARD P, Spizzi I, Leca F, VOUHE P. Interleukin-6 and C-reactive protein during pediatric cardiopulmonary bypass. Clin Chem. 1995;41(3):467–9.
31. Chew MS, Brandslund I, Brix-Christensen V, Ravn HB, Hjortdal VE, Pedersen J. Tissue injury and the inflammatory response to pediatric cardiac surgery with cardiopulmonary bypass: a descriptive study. Anesthesiology. 2001;94(5):745–53. discussion 5A.
32. Chaney MA, Durazo-Arvizu RA, Nikolov MP, Blakeman BP, Bakhos M. Methylprednisolone does not benefit patients undergoing coronary artery bypass grafting and early tracheal extubation. J Thorac Cardiovasc Surg. 2001;121(3):561–9.
33. Seri I, Tan R, Evans J. Cardiovascular effects of hydrocortisone in preterm infants with pressor-resistant hypotension. Pediatrics. 2001;107(5):1070–4.
34. Duffy JY, Nelson DP, Schwartz SM, Wagner CJ, Bauer SM, Lyons JM, et al. Glucocorticoids reduce cardiac dysfunction after cardiopulmonary bypass and circulatory arrest in neonatal piglets. Pediatr Crit Care Med. 2004;5(1):28–34.
35. Varan B, Tokel K, Mercan S, Dönmez A, Aslamaci S. Systemic inflammatory response related to cardiopulmonary bypass and its modification by methyl prednisolone: high dose versus low dose. Pediatr Cardiol. 2002;23(4):437–41.
36. Niazi Z, Flodin P, Joyce L, Smith J, Mauer H, Lillehei RC. Effects of glucocorticosteroids in patients undergoing coronary artery bypass surgery. Chest. 1979;76(3):262–8.
37. Jansen NJ, Van Oeveren W, van den Broek L, Oudemans-van Straaten HM, Stoutenbeek CP, Joen MC. Inhibition by dexamethasone of the reperfusion phenomena in cardiopulmonary bypass. J Thorac Cardiovasc Surg. 1991;102(4):515–25.
38. Kawamura T, Inada K, Okada H, Okada K, Wakusawa R. Methylprednisolone inhibits increase of interleukin 8 and 6 during open heart surgery. Can J Anaesth. 1995;42(5 Pt 1):399–403.
39. Jorens PG, De Jongh R, De Backer W, Van Damme J, Van Overveld F, Bossaert L. Interleukin-8 production in patients undergoing cardiopulmonary bypass. The influence of pretreatment with methylprednisolone. Am Rev Respir Dis. 1993;148(4 Pt 1):890–5.
40. Butler J, Pathi V, Paton R, Logan R. Acute-phase responses to cardiopulmonary bypass in children weighing less than 10 kilograms. Ann Thorac Surg. 1996;62(2):538–42.
41. Seghaye MC, Grabitz RG, Duchateau J, Busse S, Däbritz S, Koch D, et al. Inflammatory reaction and capillary leak syndrome related to cardiopulmonary bypass in neonates undergoing cardiac operations. J Thorac Cardiovasc Surg. 1996;112(3):687–97.
42. Gessler P, Hohl V, Carrel T, Pfenninger J, Schmid ER, Baenziger O. Administration of steroids in pediatric cardiac surgery: impact on clinical outcome and systemic inflammatory response. Pediatr Cardiol. 2005;26(5):595–600.
43. Checchia PA, Backer CL, Bronicki RA, Baden HP, Crawford SE, Green TP, et al. Dexamethasone reduces postoperative troponin levels in children undergoing cardiopulmonary bypass. Crit Care Med. 2003;31(6):1742–5.
44. Clarizia NA, Manlhiot C, Schwartz SM, Sivarajan VB, Maratta R, Holtby HM, et al. Improved outcomes associated with intraoperative steroid use in high-risk pediatric cardiac surgery. Ann Thorac Surg. 2011;91(4):1222–7.
45. Weerasinghe A, Taylor KM. The platelet in cardiopulmonary bypass. Ann Thorac Surg. 1998;66(6):2145.
46. Boisclair M, Lane D, Philippou H. Mechanisms of thrombin generation during surgery and cardiopulmonary bypass. Blood. 1993;82(11):3350–7.
47. Gluszko P, Rucinski B, Musial J. Fibrinogen receptors in platelet adhesion to surfaces of extracorporeal circuit. Am J Physiol. 1987;252(3 Pt 2):H615–21.
48. Dewanjee MK. Molecular biology of nitric oxide synthases. Reduction of complications of cardiopulmonary bypass from platelets and neutrophils by nitric oxide generation from L-arginine and nitric oxide donors. ASAIO J. 1997;43(3):151–9.
49. Lumadue JA, Lanzkron SM, Kennedy SD, Kuhl DT, Kickler TS. Cytokine induction of platelet activation. Am J Clin Pathol. 1996;106(6):795–8.
50. Nannizzi-Alaimo L, Rubenstein MH, Alves VL, Leong GY, Phillips DR, Gold HK. Cardiopulmonary bypass induces release of soluble CD40 ligand. Circulation. 2002;105(24):2849–54.
51. Day J. The systemic inflammatory response syndrome and cardiopulmonary bypass. Int J Surg. 2005;3(2):129–40.
52. Bergseth G, Lappegård KT, Videm V, Mollnes TE. A novel enzyme immunoassay for plasma thrombospondin. Comparison with beta-thromboglobulin as platelet activation marker in vitro and in vivo. Thromb Res. 2000;99(1):41–50.
53. Laffey JG, Boylan JF, Cheng DCH. The systemic inflammatory response to cardiac surgery: implications for the anesthesiologist. Anesthesiology. 2002;97(1):215–52.
54. Warltier DC, Laffey JG, Boylan JF, Cheng DCH. The systemic inflammatory response to cardiac surgery: implications for the anesthesiologist. Anesthesiology. 2002;97(1):215.
55. Menasché P, Peynet J, Haeffner-Cavaillon N, Carreno MP, de Chaumaray T, Dillisse V. Influence of temperature on neutrophil trafficking during clinical cardiopulmonary bypass. Circulation. 1995;92(9 Suppl):II334–40.
56. Alcaraz AJ, Manzano L, Sancho L, Vigil MD, Esquivel F, Maroto E. Different proinflammatory cytokine serum pattern in neonate patients undergoing open heart surgery. Relevance of IL-8. J Clin Immunol. 2005;25(3):238–45.
57. Hickey E, Karamlou T, You X, Komanapalli C, Person T, Wehrley K, et al. Seiler Resident Award paper. The use of a miniaturized circuit and bloodless prime to avoid cerebral no-reflow after neonatal cardiopulmonary bypass. Ann Thorac Surg. 2007;83(3):895–901.
58. Levy JH, Tanaka KA. Inflammatory response to cardiopulmonary bypass. Ann Thorac Surg. 2003;75(2):S715–20.

59. Tassani P, Barankay A, Haas F, Paek SU, Heilmaier M, Hess J, et al. Cardiac surgery with deep hypothermic circulatory arrest produces less systemic inflammatory response than low-flow cardiopulmonary bypass in newborns. J Thorac Cardiovasc Surg. 2002;123(4):648–54.
60. Diestel A, Roessler J, Berger F, Schmitt KRL. Hypothermia downregulates inflammation but enhances IL-6 secretion by stimulated endothelial cells. Cryobiology. 2008;57(3):216–22.
61. Diestel A, Roessler J, Pohl-Schickinger A, Koster A, Drescher C, Berger F, et al. Specific p38 inhibition in stimulated endothelial cells: a possible new anti-inflammatory strategy after hypothermia and rewarming. Vascul Pharmacol. 2009;51(4):246–52.
62. Eggum R, Ueland T, Mollnes TE, Videm V, Aukrust P, Fiane AE, et al. Effect of perfusion temperature on the inflammatory response during pediatric cardiac surgery. Ann Thorac Surg. 2008;85(2):611–7.
63. Qing M, Nimmesgern A, Heinrich PC, Schumacher K, Vazquez-Jimenez JF, Hess J, et al. Intrahepatic synthesis of tumor necrosis factor-alpha related to cardiac surgery is inhibited by interleukin-10 via the Janus kinase (Jak)/signal transducers and activator of transcription (STAT) pathway. Crit Care Med. 2003;31(12):2769–75.
64. Hennein HA, Ebba H, Rodriguez JL, Merrick SH, Keith FM, Bronstein MH, et al. Relationship of the proinflammatory cytokines to myocardial ischemia and dysfunction after uncomplicated coronary revascularization. J Thorac Cardiovasc Surg. 1994;108(4):626–35.
65. Bernard SA, Gray TW, Buist MD, Jones BM, Silvester W, Gutteridge G. Treatment of comatose survivors of out-of-hospital cardiac arrest with induced hypothermia. N Engl J Med. 2002;346(8):557–63.
66. Feigin VL, Anderson CS, Rodgers A, Anderson NE, Gunn AJ. The emerging role of induced hypothermia in the management of acute stroke. J Clin Neurosci. 2002;9(5):502–7.
67. Zhi D, Zhang S, Lin X. Study on therapeutic mechanism and clinical effect of mild hypothermia in patients with severe head injury. Surg Neurol. 2003;59(5):381–5.
68. Dixon SR, Whitbourn RJ, Dae MW, Grube E, Sherman W, Schaer GL. Induction of mild systemic hypothermia with endovascular cooling during primary percutaneous coronary intervention for acute myocardial infarction. J Am Coll Cardiol. 2002;40(11):1928–34.
69. Bes S, Roussel P, Laubriet A, Vandroux D, Tissier C, Rochette L, et al. Influence of deep hypothermia on the tolerance of the isolated cardiomyocyte to ischemia-reperfusion. J Mol Cell Cardiol. 2001;33(11):1973–88.
70. Qing M, Vazquez-Jimenez JF, Klosterhalfen B, Sigler M, Schumacher K, Duchateau J, et al. Influence of temperature during cardiopulmonary bypass on leukocyte activation, cytokine balance, and post-operative organ damage. Shock. 2001;15(5):372–7.
71. Stocker CF, Shekerdemian LS, Horton SB, Lee KJ, Eyres R, D'Udekem Y, et al. The influence of bypass temperature on the systemic inflammatory response and organ injury after pediatric open surgery: a randomized trial. J Thorac Cardiovasc Surg. 2011; 142(1):174–80.
72. Rot A, von Andrian UH. Chemokines in innate and adaptive host defense: basic chemokinese grammar for immune cells. Annu Rev Immunol. 2004;22:891–928.
73. Caputo M, Bays S, Rogers C, Pawade A. Randomized comparison between normothermic and hypothermic cardiopulmonary bypass in pediatric open-heart surgery. Ann Thorac Surg. 2005;80:982–8.
74. Rasmussen L, Sztuk F, Christiansen M. Normothermic versus hypothermic cardiopulmonary bypass during repair of congenital heart disease. J Cardiothorac Vasc Anesth. 2001;15(5):563–6.
75. Walther T, Rastan A, Dähnert I, Jacobs S, Scheer K, Wild F, et al. Moderate versus deep hypothermia for arterial switch operation. Thorac Cardiovasc Surg. 2006;54(4):255–8.
76. Pouard P, Pouard P, Mauriat P, Mauriat P, Ek F, Ek F, et al. Normothermic cardiopulmonary bypass and myocardial cardioplegic protection for neonatal arterial switch operation. Eur J Cardiothorac Surg. 2006;30(5):695–9.
77. Durandy Y, Hulin S, Lecompte Y. Normothermic cardiopulmonary bypass in pediatric surgery. J Thorac Cardiovasc Surg. 2002; 123(1):194.

Vacuum-Assisted Venous Drainage in Cardiac Surgery

29

Wakako Fukuda, Takeshi Goto, and Ikuo Fukuda

In 1937, the first heart-lung machine was built by John Heysham Gibbon, who also performed the first human open-heart operation [2]. Around 1954, the SigmaMotor pump, a multiple finger pump, was produced, and it became extremely popular. The multiple finger pump or the roller pump was used for years in the cardiopulmonary bypass circuit for venous drainage by surgeons and perfusionists. However, because they were difficult to control, these were discarded in favor of the more simple and effective gravity siphon method [3]. Gravity siphon drainage, which has been employed as the standard for venous return during CPB for many years, is accomplished with a pressure gradient of approximately 40 mmHg, attributable to the height difference between the patient and the venous reservoir [4].

With the advent of minimally invasive cardiac surgery and the progression of congenital heart surgery, there is a desire to reduce the diameter of the venous cannula to improve surgical access, decrease pump priming volumes, and enable cannulation of vessels remote from the heart [5]. Unfortunately, decreasing cannula diameter increases resistance; thus, blood drainage is limited. Gravity siphon or passive venous drainage may provide insufficient blood return for adequate tissue perfusion [6]. This drawback has led to the development of assisted venous drainage (AVD), which can increase venous return to more acceptable levels of perfusion.

AVD is generally divided into kinetic-assisted venous drainage (KAVD) and vacuum-assisted venous drainage (VAVD) (Fig. 29.1). KAVD uses a centrifugal pump placed in the venous line to generate negative pressure and consequently increase venous return. This technique has been shown to guarantee adequate global tissue perfusion for use in minimally invasive CPB procedures [6]. VAVD involves a constant vacuum pressure onto an airtight venous reservoir, allowing more blood to be drained from the patient via the venous line [6]. Murai et al. [7] suggested the indications for use of VAVD were insufficient venous return by siphon drainage alone, persistent elevation of the central venous pressure and insufficient venous drainage in the operative field.

Advantages of Vacuum-Assisted Venous Drainage

The Use of Smaller Cannulae and Shorter Tubing

In several situations, such as minimally invasive surgery, repeat-cardiovascular operation, pediatric cardiac surgery, and emergency cardiac resuscitation, peripheral venous cannulae are needed. Smaller venous cannulae facilitate venous cannulation.

Vacuum-assisted venous drainage (VAVD) does not rely on the height differential between the patient's heart and the venous reservoir, unlike conventional gravity siphon venous drainage. It is possible to raise the height of the venous reservoir, shorten the venous and arterial lines, and decrease the tubing diameter. This allows remodeling of the pump console and circuit. With smaller cannulae and shorter tubing, VAVD could dramatically reduce priming volumes, maximally decrease tubing dead space, and lower patient hemodilution [8]. VAVD is becoming especially advantageous in the neonate and pediatric populations for reducing circuit size and thereby decreasing priming volume [3].

Banbury et al. [9] reported that a VAVD resulted in a smaller CPB volume (1.4 ± 0.4 l with VAVD vs. 2.0 ± 0.4 l with gravity siphon, $p < 0.0001$) in valve operations. In neonates and infants, with use of 3/16-in. venous and arterial tubing, no arterial line filter, no prime in the venous line,

W. Fukuda, MD • I. Fukuda, MD, PhD (✉)
Department of Thoracic and Cardiovascular Surgery, Hirosaki University Graduate School of Medicine, 5 Zaifu-cho, Hirosaki, Aomori 036-8562, Japan
e-mail: ikuofuku@cc.hirosaki-u.ac.jp

T. Goto, ME
Department of Clinical Engineering, Hirosaki University School of Medicine and Hospital, Aomori, Japan

E.A. Gabriel, S.A. Gabriel (eds.), *Inflammatory Response in Cardiovascular Surgery*, DOI 10.1007/978-1-4471-4429-8_29, © Springer-Verlag London 2013

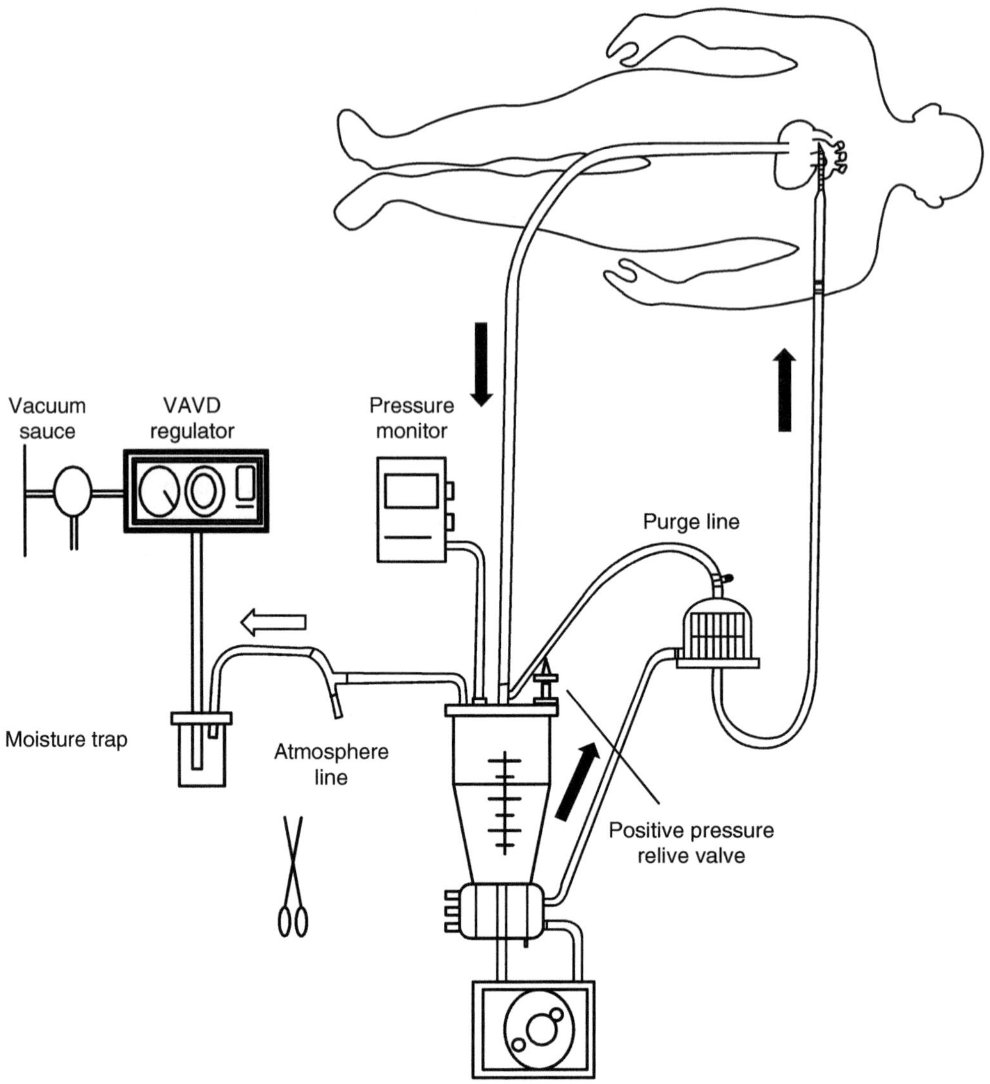

Fig. 29.1 Vacuum-assisted venous drainage

and the use of VAVD, the prime volume for a neonatal circuit reportedly is as low as 200 ml [10].

Improved venous drainage reduces the fluid overload of patients. Less interstitial edema should result in better organ function and faster recovery. Reduced flow through the right atrium and less blood in the heart should reduce rewarming of the heart and contribute to improved myocardial protection [11]. It may ameliorate the inflammatory reaction caused by contact activation of neutrophils on the CPB circuit.

Provide an Unobstructed Surgical Field

VAVD can provide total cardiopulmonary support with adequate cardiac decompression and reduce blood exposure to the damaging effects of pump suction and basket suction salvage. At the same time, VAVD can maintain higher arterial perfusion flow and higher blood levels in the venous reservoir, resulting in a drier, "bloodless" surgical field while also minimizing blood cell trauma [9].

Shin et al. [12] reported a case in which the huge right atrial malignant lymphoma was successfully resected using VAVD without snaring the inferior vena cava. Fukuda et al. [13] described a case of re-tricuspid valve replacement with VAVD. CPB with VAVD established before median sternotomy facilitated surgery by decompressing the heart and allowed safe reentry to the mediastinum [13]. Aklog et al. [14] performed bicaval orthotopic heart transplantation in ten patients using an open IVC anastomosis with VAVD, and they have reported good results. They stated the visualization during performance of IVC anastomosis was improved [14].

Increases Venous Drainage and Eliminates the Risk of Air Blocks in the Venous Line

In VAVD, additional negative pressure in the venous line will augment venous blood return. An in vitro study conducted by Fiorucci et al. [15] found that the VAVD can increase venous drainage by as much as 50 %. Munster et al. [11] showed positive relationships between vacuum pressure and venous drainage and between blood temperature and venous drainage.

According to LaPietra et al. [16], negative pressure easily handled the macrobubbles and eliminated the risk of air blocks in the venous line in the event that gross air entered the venous line. VAVD permits the use of smaller caliber venous cannulae and allows the right heart chambers to be opened without the threat of venous air block.

Disadvantages and Pitfalls of VAVD

Possibility of Transmission of Gaseous Microemboli from the Venous Line to the Arterial Side of the Circuit

Cardiac surgery and the use of CPB are associated with damage to end organs [5]. Roach et al. [17], in the largest prospective study on cerebral outcome after coronary artery bypass surgery, found that 6.1 % of the 2,108 patients developed serious neurological complications ranging from stroke to seizures and to deterioration of intellectual function after surgery. There is substantive evidence particularly with regard to brain injury implicating emboli as a cause of organ damage during CPB. Emboli may be gaseous, liquid, or particulate, and they may originate in the circulation or be introduced into the circulation [5].

VAVD is based on the application of a vacuum to a hard-shell venous reservoir, and it facilitates the pull of air into the venous line from around the venous cannula. Gaseous micro-emboli (GME) that pass through the oxygenator and arterial filter could enter the patient's body and be responsible for neurocognitive impairment after CPB [18]. Wilcox [19] have shown that VAVD can increase entrainment of venous air with vacuum-assisted drainage and have raised safety issues concerning the system. In their study, arterial line emboli increased eight- to tenfold after the introduction of air into the venous line of a salvaged clinical adult circuit. Wang et al. [18] demonstrated that, when a fixed volume air was introduced into the venous line of a simulated neonatal CPB circuit, VAVD with higher negative pressures, increased flow rates, and pulsatile flow delivered more gaseous microemboli at the post-pump site.

Carrier et al. [20] compared the incidence of neurological complications in patient who underwent valvular surgery with and without VAVD added to standard CPB system, and they concluded that the use of VAVD during CPB in patients undergoing valve replacements does not increase the risk of significant neurological injuries. Jegger et al. [6] analyzed the vacuum pressure required to produce bubble transgression using an in vitro circuit successively including a closed reservoir, a pump (centrifugal or roller), and an oxygenator, and they stated that VAVD is a safe technique as long as the perfusionist stops the vacuum when the arterial pump is no longer in use. Wilcox [19] suggests the development of novel de-airing devices that can be incorporated safely into the perfusion circuit.

Overpressurization of the Sealed Venous Reservoir Induces Blood Trauma

During CPB, red blood cells are damaged mainly by shear stresses, and this damage results in either immediate hemolysis, with release of free hemoglobin, or a shortened red cell life span with delayed hemolysis. This damage may potentially be increased by VAVD because of the negative pressure within the circuit and because of the turbulence generated at the tip of the smaller venous cannulae, especially when they lie in the vena cava [21].

In *in vitro* and in vivo studies, investigators have reported that VAVD does not increase trauma to blood cells and hemolysis caused by VAVD is not a clinical problem [11, 12, 21]. However, the safe range of VAVD is unknown [7].

VAVD Makes the CPB Circuit More Complicated

VAVD equipment attaches to the venous reservoir and changes an open system to a closed system. Using a closed system is different from using routine gravity venous drainage and requires additional training of perfusionists to ensure functional understanding of the principles underlying VAVD [8].

VAVD Reduces Pump Flow Rate

When using higher negative pressure, VAVD reduces the pump flow rate. Fiorucci et al. [15] investigated the efficiency of the VAVD and the VAVD+gravitational drainage in increasing the venous return and quantified the relationship between the negative pressure applied to the reservoir and the resultant flow delivered by the pump. Their study showed that VAVD with a negative pressure >50 mmHg could reduce the flow delivered by the roller pump. Increased negative pressure at the inlet of the raceway tubing reduces its re-expansion, resulting in a net reduction in the stroke volume.

VAVD May Lead to Serious Accidents

There are reports on accidents. Davila et al. [22] reported a complication of VAVD by inadvertent positive pressurization of a venous circuit resulting in a paradoxic air embolus across a patent arterial septal defect. Jahangiri et al. [23] reported a cerebrovascular accident after VAVD in a Fontan patient. Cautious use of VAVD and real-time monitoring of microemboli during CPB with VAVD are important [8]. Errors can be moderated by training the perfusionists and following the appropriate procedures.

Applying VAVD allows for reduced circuit size and prime volume. It also improves venous drainage and flow rates through the smaller cannulae used in neonates and in peripheral cannulation for minimally invasive cardiac surgery. VAVD is a useful adjunct to modern CPB systems and offers a number of potential benefits to CPB.

References

1. Murphy GS, Hessel II EA, Groom RC. Optimal perfusion during cardiopulmonary bypass: an evidence-based approach. Anesth Analg. 2009;108:1394–417.
2. Gibbon Jr JH. Artificial maintenance of circulation during experimental occlusion of pulmonary artery. Arch Surg. 1937;34(6):1105–31.
3. Gravlee GP. Cardiopulmonary bypass: principles and practice. 2nd ed. Philadelphia: Lippincott Williams & Wilkins; 2007. p. 69.
4. Humphries K, Sistino J. Laboratory evaluation of the pressure flow characteristics of venous cannulas during vacuum-assisted venous drainage. J Extra Corpor Technol. 2002;34:111–4.
5. Jones TJ, Deal DD, Vernon JC, Blackburn N, Stump DA. Does vacuum-assisted venous drainage increase gaseous microemboli during cardiopulmonary bypass? Ann Thorac Surg. 2002;74:2132–7.
6. Jegger D, Tevaearai HT, Mueller XM, Horisberger J, von Segesser LK. Limitations using the vacuum-assist venous drainage technique during cardiopulmonary bypass procedures. J Extra Corpor Technol. 2003;35:207–11.
7. Murai N, Cho M, Okada S, Chiba T, Saito M, Shioguchi S, et al. Venous drainage method for cardiopulmonary bypass in single-access minimally invasive cardiac surgery: siphon and vacuum-assisted drainage. J Artif Organs. 2005;8:91–4.
8. Wang S, Üudar A. Vacuum-assisted venous drainage and gaseous microemboli in cardiopulmonary bypass. J Extra Corpor Technol. 2008;40:249–56.
9. Banbury MK, White JA, Blackstone EH, Cosgrove DM. Vacuum-assisted venous return reduces blood usage. J Thorac Cardiovasc Surg. 2003;126:680–7.
10. Lake CL, Booker PD. Pediatric cardiac anesthesia. 4th ed. Philadelphia: Lippincott Williams & Wilkins; 2004. p. 230.
11. Münster K, Anderson U, Mikkelsen J, Pettersson G. Vacuum assisted venous drainage (VAVD). Perfusion. 1999;14:419–23.
12. Shin H, Mori M, Matayoshi T, Suzuki R, Yozu R. Resection of giant right atrial lymphoma using vacuum-assisted cardiopulmonary bypass without snaring the inferior vena cava. Ann Thorac Cardiovasc Surg. 2004;10(4):249–51.
13. Fukuda W, Aoki C, Daitoku K, Fukuda I. Vacuum-assisted venous drainage in tricuspid valve re-replacement. Interact Cardiovasc Thorac Surg. 2011;13(1):101–3.
14. Aklog L, Sepic J, Filsoufi F, Bryne JG, Adams DH. Open inferior vena caval anastomosis during bicaval heart transplantation. Ann Thorac Surg. 2002;73(2):671–2.
15. Fiorucci A, Gerometta PS, DeVecchi M, Guzman C, Costantino ML, Arena V. In vitro assessment of the vacuum-assisted venous drainage (VAVD) system: risks and benefits. Perfusion. 2004;19(2):113–7.
16. LaPietra A, Grossi EA, Pua BB, Esposito RA, Galloway AC, Derivaux CC, et al. Assisted venous drainage presents the risk of undetected air microembolism. J Thorac Cardiovasc Surg. 2000;120:856–63.
17. Roach GW, Kanchuger M, Mangano CM, Multicenter Study of Perioperative Ischemia Research Group and the Ischemia Research and Education Foundation Investigators. Adverse cerebral outcomes after coronary bypass surgery. N Engl J Med. 1996;335:1857–63.
18. Wang S, Baer L, Kunselman AR, Myers JL, Üudar A. Delivery of gaseous microemboli with vacuum-assisted venous drainage during pulsatile and nonpulsatile perfusion in a simulated neonatal cardiopulmonary bypass model. ASAIO J. 2008;54:416–22.
19. Willcox TW. Vacuum-assisted venous drainage: to air or no to air, that is the question. Has the bubble burst? J Extra Corpor Technol. 2002;34:24–8.
20. Carrier M, Cyr A, Voisine P, Pellerin M, Perrault LP, Cartier R, et al. Vacuum-assisted venous drainage does not increase the neurological risk. Heart Surg Forum. 2001;5(3):285–8.
21. Mueller XM, Tevaearai HT, Horisberger J, Augstburger M, Burki M, Von Segesser LK. Vacuum assisted venous drainage does not increase trauma to blood cells. ASAIO J. 2001;47:651–4.
22. Davila RM, Rawles T, Mack MJ. Venoarterial air embolus: a complication of vacuum-assisted venous drainage. Ann Thorac Surg. 2001;71:1369–71.
23. Jahangiri M, Rayner A, Keogh B, Lincoln C. Cerebrovascular accident after vacuum-assisted venous drainage in a fontan patient: a cautionary tale. Ann Thorac Surg. 2001;72:1727–8.

30 Miniaturize CPB Versus Off-Pump Surgery

Francesco Formica

Introduction

Off-pump coronary artery bypass grafting (OPCABG) surgery has been accepted since the early 1990s when it was recognized that conventional extracorporeal circulation (cECC) is associated with a systemic inflammatory response syndrome (SIRS). SIRS is implicated in myocardial, renal, pulmonary, and neurologic dysfunction. For these reasons, the OPCABG technique is widely applied as the first choice in patients affected by acute or chronic renal dysfunction, obstructive pulmonary disease, cerebrovascular disease, and peripheral obstructive arteriopathy [1]. However, although the effects of cECC are often subclinical, in some situations they can be responsible for worse outcomes in the early postoperative period. OPCABG has produced very encouraging results, and this technique has seen wide popularity during the last decade, with many cardiac centers performing OPCABG in more than 80 % of coronary patients [2]. However, the OPCABG technique presents some drawbacks, such as the significant learning curve for the surgeon, the high rate of incomplete revascularization in dilated and hypokinetic hearts due to the very difficult exposure of obtuse coronary marginal branches, and the lesser quality of the coronary anastomosis with an increased graft restenosis identified [3, 4]. Over the past 10 years, miniaturized extracorporeal circulation (MECC) has been developed with the aim of reducing the side effects of cECC, strengthening the advantages of cECC, and eliminating the drawbacks of OPCABG [5, 6]. Utilizing a shorter circuit without the interposition of a venous reservoir may offer several benefits, such as a reduction in hemodilution, coagulopathy, and SIRS. In other words, MECC should combine the best of cECC with the best of "off-pump" surgery. However, it is not yet clear whether the combination of these advantages is superior in MECC compared to OPCABG in terms of mortality and morbidity because multicenter randomized studies currently are lacking.

F. Formica, MD
Cardiac Surgery Clinic, Department of Surgical Science, University of Milano-Bicocca, San Gerardo Hospital, Via Pergolesi 33, 20900 Monza, Italy
email: francesco_formica@fastwebnet.it

Anatomy of the Miniaturized Extracorporeal Circulation System

Different types of MECC circuits are available on the market, and although they can have some differences in terms of characteristics of the blood pump, oxygenator membrane, length of tubing, and arterial and venous filters, the main concept is substantially the same for each system: a closed circuit without a venous cardiotomy reservoir that strongly reduces the blood-air interfaces. Several other key components forming the structure of MECC are the following:

(a) *Circuit coating*. All components of the MECC circuit are coated with heparin, phosphorylcholine, or polymer according to the different techniques available on the market. The heparin pre-treatment of the circuit minimizes the systemic heparinization dose requirements (usually a half dose of the conventional ECC: 150 IU/kg instead of 300 IU/kg) [7–10] and provides biocompatibility for blood cells [5, 6, 11, 12].

(b) *Tubing length*. The MECC circuit is usually shorter than that of the conventional ECC. Tubing length of about 100 cm is frequently reported as well as a smaller tubing section than in conventional ECC tubing (3/8″ size instead of 1/2″ size) [8, 13]. These characteristics are reflected in a lower prime volume ranging between 200 and 650 ml for the MECC compared to 1,200–1,600 ml for the standard ECC [8, 12, 14]. The combination of short length tubing, heparin pre-treatment, small size tubing, and absence of a venous reservoir leads to a significant reduction of hemodilution, clotting factor consumption, and triggering of SIRS [5, 15, 16].

E.A. Gabriel, S.A. Gabriel (eds.), *Inflammatory Response in Cardiovascular Surgery*,
DOI 10.1007/978-1-4471-4429-8_30, © Springer-Verlag London 2013

(c) *Centrifugal pump.* The blood pump included in the circuit is a centrifugal pump, which is very versatile, reducing the cell trauma in the erythrocytes and platelets with possible lower effects on hemolysis.
(d) *Oxygenator.* The oxygenator of the MECC is one of the most important components of the circuit itself. Oxygenators have an oxygenation membrane of either microporous polypropylene [16, 17] or polymethylpentene [8, 12, 18, 19]. In the latter case, the membrane is considered a diffusion membrane. Usually the oxygenator has an integrated heat exchanger and one of the largest gas exchange surface areas, reaching about 2.4 m^2. In this way, the oxygenator can give full oxygenation also with a high-blood-flow pump up to 7 l/min.
(e) *Arterial and venous filters.* Many MECC circuits include an arterial filter between the oxygenator and the aortic cannula and a venous bubble trap between the venous cannula and the centrifugal pump. The arterial filter has a prime volume ranging between 150–200 ml and strongly reduces the risk of cerebral and systemic embolization. The venous bubble trap reduces large air entrainment in the circuit, which could be one of the causes of accidental blockage of the MECC circuit. Aortic and atrial cannulation is equal to that in conventional ECC. Usually an aortic vent catheter is positioned in the ascending aorta, and a further vent is inserted in the pulmonary main trunk during aortic valve surgery.
(f) *Cell-saver device.* This can be associated with the MECC with the aim of removing all the pericardial bloodshed. This can then be washed and transfused during the surgery by means a soft reservoir bag or in the immediate postoperative period via an intravenous cannula.

The major difference between the MECC and cECC is the absence of a venous reservoir; also, the capillary vascular bed of the patient works as a *biological human venous reservoir*. The direct collaboration among the cardiac surgeon, the anesthesiologist, and the perfusionist is extremely important to guarantee the best outcome. Use of vasodilator and vasoconstrictor drugs, Trendelenburg or anti-Trendelenburg position of the patient, and reducing or increasing the centrifugal pump flow are all fundamental keys to handling an MECC system with the aim of avoiding malperfusion syndrome, systemic embolization, failure of MECC, and rapid conversion to cECC.

Table 30.1 shows the different types of MECC systems currently available.

Systemic Inflammatory Response Syndrome (SIRS)

Recent publications have described the association of the MECC with minimal activation of inflammation and coagulopathy, less hemodilution with low blood transfusion, and a low incidence of cerebral stroke [8, 20, 21]. The SIRS is a complex multifactorial syndrome that is known to be associated with ECC. The SIRS to ECC is initiated by many aggressive factors, including surgical trauma, blood contact with nonendothelial surfaces, cardioplegia, and ischemia-reperfusion injury [22–24]. Several blood elements, such as neutrophils, monocytes, endothelial cells, platelets, and complement proteins, are involved in the SIRS. When activated, these blood components release cytotoxic and vasoactive substances, produce inflammatory and inhibitory cytokines, and express cell receptors interacting with specific cellular substance [24]. Therefore, when the SIRS has been initiated, several inflammatory mediators, including anti- and proinflammatory cytokines, could be associated with a worse postoperative course.

Cytokines are small proinflammatory peptides strongly involved in the myocardial stunning process and in multiorgan failure syndrome [23]. Important cytokines involved in the SIRS are interleukin 1β (IL-1β), interleukin 6 (IL-6), tumor necrosis factor α (TNF-α), and soluble CD 40 ligand (sCD40L).

IL-1β is produced mainly by monocytes. This cytokine derives from IL-1 by the action of the IL-1β-converting enzyme. An increase of IL-1β was found after ECC with a peak concentration after 24 h [5].

IL-6 is produced and released by the monocytes and endothelial cells following a stimulus by IL-1 and TNF-α. IL-6 has its peak concentration a few hours after the end of ECC and gradually decreases within the following 24 h [5, 10, 16]. The IL-6 concentration also increases after major noncardiac operations, and the peak concentration occurs 6–24 h after the end of the operation.

TNF-α is a cytokine produced by neutrophils and monocytes. A significant increase of TNF-α was shown after removal of the cross clamp, and a peak concentration is reached 24 h after the end of ECC. TNF-α has a negative inotropic effect, and the myocardium is a major source after ischemic reperfusion injury.

sCD40L is produced by activated platelets and upregulates the expression of inflammatory adhesion receptors including E-selectin, VCAM-1, tissue factor, and matrix metalloproteinases [25]. Furthermore, sCD40L has been described as a major mediator of vascular inflammation [26]. Plasma levels of CD40L increased within 1 h on ECC and increased by fourfold after 2 h [25]. A high preoperative level of CD40L was associated with a high risk of postoperative atrial fibrillation in patients who underwent off-pump myocardial revascularization [27].

Miniaturized Extracorporeal Circulation Compared to Off-Pump Surgery

At this time, there are not many publications comparing MECC to off-pump surgery, and obviously many further randomized studies are needed to verify the superiority of

Table 30.1 Different types of MECC systemc currently available

	Resting Heart (Medtronic)	MECC (Maquet)	ECC.O (Sorin)	ROCSafe (Terumo)	CORx (CardioVention)
Circuit coating	Carmeda bioactive surface (with heparin)	Bioline (with heparin)	Prosphorylcoline	Xcoating, biopassive polymer coating	Not coated
Centrifugal pump	Affinity (prime volume 40 ml)	Rotaflow (prime volume 32 ml)	Revolution Impeller type integrated with oxygenator	Sarns (prime volume 48 ml)	Impeller, integrated with oxygenator
Oxigenator	Affinity (hollow fibers)	QuadroxD (polymethilpentene diffusion membrane)	Hollow fiber	Capiox (microporous polypropylene)	Hollow fiber polypropylene
Filters	Arterial and venous: Affinity (38 μm pore size)	Arterial (40 μm pore size) and venous bubble trap (175 μm pore size)	Arterial filter (40 μm pore size). Venous bubble trap	Arterial filter (37 μm pore size). Venous bubble trap (170 μm pore size)	Integrated (defoamer)
Total prime volume (ml)	1,000	800–900	400	665	820

one technique over the other. The few studies available did not identify significant differences between the two techniques in terms of hospital mortality, neurocognitive disturbance, triggering of SIRS, blood loss and transfusion requirements, and rate of postoperative atrial fibrillation.

In-hospital mortality did not differ among the different studies. Puehler et al. [9] did not find significant in-hospital mortality in patients undergoing CABG with MECC or cECC or off-pump surgery. Each group had 558 patients, and overall in-hospital mortality in the MECC group was 3.22 % compared to the off-pump group, which was 3.76 %. However, in a subgroup of an emergent population, the in-hospital mortality of the MECC group was significantly lower than that of the off-pump group (5.6 and 10.7 %, respectively). However the in-hospital mortality ranged between 0 and 5.4 % in the different studies [8, 16, 19, 28].

SIRS, hemolysis, and coagulopathy are among the most studied events in the studies comparing MECC to off-pump surgery. Wippermann et al. [16] reported no significant changes in prothrombin fragment 1.2 levels, interleukin 6 releases, and plasmin-antiplasmin complex levels between the MECC and off-pump groups over the immediate postoperative course. Instead, they found a significant difference when these two groups were compared to cECC patients. Van Boven et al. [29] reported no differences in serum concentrations of malondialdehyde, allantoin/urate ratios, and lung epithelium-specific proteins (CC16) in MECC compared to off-pump patients. The release of these biomarkers was higher in cECC patients, and they speculated that the oxidative stress parameters showed a tendency toward improved global organ protection in MECC and off-pump patients compared to cECC patients.

Mazzei et al. [13] compared interleukin 6 and serum S-100 protein levels between MECC and off-pump surgery in a prospective randomized trial. No differences were reported in terms of release of these biomarkers over a 24 h period, and this evidence suggests that off-pump surgery and MECC with cardioplegic arrest should be considered equivalent tools.

Recently, Formica et al. [8] in a prospective randomized study evaluated the release of tumor necrosis factor-α and interleukin 6 in a group of patients operated on with MECC compared to off-pump surgery. They observed a higher release of interleukin 6 in off-pump surgery than in MECC surgery 24 h after the operation, whereas levels of tumor necrosis factor-α were not different in the two groups. Moreover, the authors observed no difference in the cardiac release of these cytokines in the two groups. The authors suggested that, according to their findings, MECC can be used extensively in all patients with multivessel disease in whom off-pump surgery could have more operative risks.

Neurocognitive disturbance and cerebrovascular events such as stroke/transient ischemic attack can seriously complicated the postoperative course of patients undergoing coronary surgery. It has been recognized that off-pump surgery is associated with a lower incidence of cerebral stroke when compared to CABG with ECC, above all in patients who have undergone off-pump surgery with the no-touch aorta technique. At this time, no reports exist showing evidence of an increased rate of neurological sequelae in MECC patients. However, neurological complications are always caused by multifactorial events such as micro- and macroembolizations, cerebral hypoperfusion, cerebrovasculopathy, and carotid disease, and for this reason, it is not possible to find a direct correlation between MECC and postoperative neurological outcome.

At the present time, few studies study have primarily investigated the incidence of postoperative atrial fibrillation (AF) in MECC compared to off-pump surgery. In their study, Panday et al. [30] reported a lower incidence of postoperative AF in the MECC and off-pump groups (25 and 21.7 %, respectively) compared to the cECC group (35.6 %). Other authors reported a very low incidence of postoperative atrial fibrillation without differences in the MECC, off-pump, and cEE groups (3.6, 3.9, and 5.4 %, respectively) [9].

Formica et al. [8] reported no significant difference in the incidence of AF, but the rate of AF in the MECC group was higher than in the off-pump group (40 and 23.3 %, respectively; $p = 0.9$). Postoperative AF is considered a multifactorial complication in which hypoglycemia due to hemodilution, release of proinflammatory cytokines, need for blood, and advanced age can be associated with the development of this event.

Completeness of revascularization, reoperation for graft failure, and composite outcome at midterm are considered some of the main weaknesses of off-pump surgery. Some recent large trials compared off-pump surgery to cECC and reported survival of less than 10 years for off-pump surgery [31], more early reinterventions after the off-pump procedure [32], fewer grafts performed, poorer long-term graft patency, and increased incidence of composite outcome (death and major cardiac events) in off-pump surgery [3]. These results have led to less acceptance of off-pump surgery worldwide. Formica et al. [8] reported fewer grafts performed and less use of bilateral internal arteries in off-pump surgery compared to MECC. Other authors reported similar findings [13, 19, 33]. With MECC surgery, the incidence of complete revascularization and total arterial myocardial revascularization is higher because, like with cECC, the handling of the heart during coronary anastomosis is safer with the MECC even in unstable patients with a dilated and dysfunctional left heart. Currently, only one randomized trial has focused on 1-year follow-up in MECC and off-pump patients. In this trial, the authors reported no difference in the incidence of death and recurrence of angina in both groups, and the incidence of both events was low [13].

Perioperative blood transfusions are one of the most common events that physicians encounter clinically. Among the factors that increase the incidence of the red cell requirement, the most reported include advancing age, redo surgery, the preoperative use of anti-platelet agents, preoperative hemodilution, and other non-cardiac causes such as renal dysfunction and lessr impairment [34, 35]. Off-pump CABG has been reported to significantly reduce the mean blood loss and transfusion requirement when compared to cECC [36]. One of the aims of the MECC circuit is to reduce hemodilution and thereby to reduce the need for transfusions. Analysis of the data presently available has shown no significant difference in the mean blood loss or number of patients transfused when MECC is compared to OPCAB [8, 9, 36]. Interestingly, Gerritsen et al. [37] reported a significantly lower blood loss with MECC compared to off-pump surgery. This is most likely because of the different antiplatelets/anticoagulation therapy strategies applied in cardiac units, the variation in anticoagulation strategies employed by the different units, and the more aggressive approach to anticoagulation that is applied by this group.

In conclusion, data comparing MECC to off-pump surgery for CABG are limited by the small number of comparative studies currently available and by the lack of large randomized controlled trials. However, current data suggest that MECC is comparable to OPCAB, with no significant difference in mortality, morbidity, length of stay, neurological outcomes, blood transfusions, or blood loss. Further to this, both techniques have shown several advantages when compared to conventional techniques of cardiopulmonary bypass in terms of less SIRS, less morbidity, reduced blood loss, and fewer blood transfusions. Further randomized trials are needed focusing not only on the short-term endpoints, but also the long-term outcomes and differences between these techniques, including angina recurrence, the need for repeat revascularization, and mortality and morbidity.

References

1. Kuss O, von Salviati B, Borgermann J. Off-pump versus on-pump coronary artery bypass grafting: a systematic review and meta-analysis of propensity score analyses. J Thorac Cardiovasc Surg. 2010;140:829–35.
2. Lytle BW, Sabik JF. On-pump and off-pump bypass surgery: tools for revascularization. Circulation. 2004;109:810–2.
3. Shroyer AL, Grover FL, Hattler B, et al. On-pump versus off-pump coronary-artery bypass surgery. N Engl J Med. 2009;361:1827–37.
4. Hueb W, Lopes NH, Pereira AC, et al. Five-year follow-up of a randomized comparison between off-pump and on-pump stable multivessel coronary artery bypass grafting. The MASS III Trial. Circulation. 2010;122 suppl 1:S48–52.
5. Fromes Y, Gaillarda D, Ponzio O, et al. Reduction of the inflammatory response following coronary bypass grafting with total minimal extracorporeal circulation. Eur J Cardiothorac Surg. 2002;22:527–33.
6. Remadi JP, Marticho P, Butoi I, et al. Clinical experience with the mini-extracorporeal circulation system: an evolution or a revolution? Ann Thorac Surg. 2004;77:2172–6.
7. Curtis N, Vohra HA, Ohri SK. Mini extracorporeal circuit cardiopulmonary bypass system: a review. Perfusion. 2010;25:115–24.
8. Formica F, Broccolo F, Martino A, et al. Myocardial revascularization with miniaturized extracorporeal circulation versus off pump: evaluation of systemic and myocardial inflammatory response in a prospective randomized study. J Thorac Cardiovasc Surg. 2009;137:1206–12.
9. Puehler T, Haneya A, Philipp A, et al. Minimal extracorporeal circulation: an alternative for on-pump and off-pump coronary revascularization. Ann Thorac Surg. 2009;87:766–72.
10. Beghi C, Nicolini F, Agostinelli A, et al. Mini-cardiopulmonary bypass system: results of a prospective randomised study. Ann Thorac Surg. 2006;81:1396–400.
11. Koivisto SP, Wistbacka JO, Rimpiläinen R, et al. Miniaturized versus conventional cardiopulmonary bypass in high-risk patients undergoing coronary artery bypass surgery. Perfusion. 2010;25:65–70.
12. Remadi JP, Rakotoarivelo Z, Marticho P, Benamar A. Prospective randomized study comparing coronary artery bypass grafting with the new mini-extracorporeal circulation Jostra System or with a standard cardiopulmonary bypass. Am Heart J. 2006;151:198e1–7.
13. Mazzei V, Nasso G, Salamone G, Castorino F, Tommasini A, Anselmi A. Prospective randomized comparison of coronary bypass grafting with minimal extracorporeal circulation system (MECC) versus off-pump coronary surgery. Circulation. 2007;116:1761–7.

14. Stalder M, Gygax E, Immer FF, et al. Minimized cardiopulmonary bypass combined with a smart suction device: the future of cardiopulmonary bypass? Heart Surg Forum. 2007;3:E235–8.
15. Ohata T, Mitsuno M, Yamamura M, et al. Minimal cardiopulmonary bypass attenuates neutrophil activation and cytokine release in coronary artery bypass grafting. J Artif Organs. 2007;10:92–5.
16. Wippermann J, Albes JM, Hartrumpf M, et al. Comparison of minimally invasive closed circuit extracorporeal circulation with conventional cardiopulmonary bypass and with off-pump technique in CABG patients: selected parameters of coagulation and inflammatory system. Eur J Cardiothorac Surg. 2005;28:127–32.
17. El-Essawi A, Hajek T, Skorpil J, et al. A prospective randomised multicentre clinical comparison of a minimised perfusion circuit versus conventional cardiopulmonary bypass. Eur J Cardiothorac Surg. 2010;38:91–7.
18. Anastasiadis K, Chalvatzoulis O, Antonitsis P, et al. Neurocognitive outcome after coronary artery bypass surgery using minimal versus conventional extracorporeal circulation: a randomised controlled pilot study. Heart. 2011;97:1082–8.
19. Puehler T, Haneya A, Philipp A, et al. Minimized extracorporeal circulation system in coronary artery bypass surgery: a 10-year single-center experience with 2243 patients. Eur J Cardiothorac Surg. 2011;39:459–64.
20. Rimpilainen R, Biancari F, Wistbacka JO, et al. Outcome after coronary artery bypass surgery with miniaturized versus conventional cardiopulmonary bypass. Perfusion. 2008;23:361–7.
21. Zangrillo A, Garozzo FA, Biondi-Zoccai G, et al. Miniaturized cardiopulmonary bypass improves short-term outcome in cardiac surgery: a meta-analysis of randomized controlled studies. J Thorac Cardiovasc Surg. 2010;139:1162–9.
22. Raja SG, Berg GA. Impact of off-pump coronary artery bypass surgery on systemic inflammation: current best available evidence. J Card Surg. 2007;5:445–55.
23. Larmann J, Theilmeier G. Inflammatory response to cardiac surgery: cardiopulmonary bypass versus non-cardiopulmonary bypass surgery. Best Pract Res Clin Anaesthesiol. 2004;18:425–38.
24. Royston D. The inflammatory response and extracorporeal circulation. J Cardiothorac Vasc Anesth. 1997;11:341–54.
25. Nannizzi-Alaimo L, Rubenstein MH, Alves VL, et al. Cardiopulmonary bypass induces release of soluble CD40 ligand. Circulation. 2002;105:2849–54.
26. Antoniades C, Bakogiannis C, Tousoulis D, et al. The CD40/CD40 ligand system. Linking inflammation with atherothrombosis. J Am Coll Cardiol. 2009;54:669–77.
27. Antoniades C, Van-Assche T, Shirodaria C, et al. Preoperative sCD40L levels predict risk of atrial fibrillation after off-pump coronary artery bypass graft surgery. Circulation. 2009;120:S170–6.
28. Munos E, Calderon J, Pillois X, et al. Beating-heart coronary artery bypass surgery with the help of mini extracorporeal circulation for very high-risk patients. Perfusion. 2011;2:123–31.
29. van Boven WJ, Gerritsen WB, Waanders FG, et al. Mini extracorporeal circuit for coronary artery bypass grafting: initial clinical and biochemical results: a comparison with conventional and off-pump coronary artery bypass grafts concerning global oxidative stress and alveolar function. Perfusion. 2004;19:239–46.
30. Panday GF, Fischer S, Bauer A, et al. Minimal extracorporeal circulation and off-pump compared to conventional cardio- pulmonary bypass in coronary surgery. Interact Cardiovasc Thorac Surg. 2009; 9:832–6.
31. Filardo G, Grayburn PA, Hamilton C, et al. Comparing long-term survival between patients undergoing off-pump and on-pump coronary artery bypass graft operations. Ann Thorac Surg. 2011;92: 571–7.
32. Ben-Gal Y, Stone GW, Smith CR, et al. On-pump versus off-pump surgical revascularization in patients with acute coronary syndromes: analysis from the acute catheterization and urgent intervention triage strategy trial. J Thorac Cardiovasc Surg. 2011;142:e33–9.
33. Reber D, Brouwer R, Buchwald D, et al. Beating-heart coronary artery bypass grafting with miniaturized cardiopulmonary bypass results in a more complete revascularization when compared to off-pump grafting. Artif Organs. 2010;34:179–84.
34. Ferraris VA, Ferraris SP, Saha SP, et al. Perioperative blood transfusion and blood conservation in cardiac surgery: the Society of Thoracic Surgeons and the Society of Cardiovascular Anesthesiologists clinical practice guideline. Ann Thorac Surg. 2007;83:S27–86.
35. Whitson BA, Huddleston SJ, Savik K, Shumway SJ. Risk of adverse outcomes associated with blood transfusion after cardiac surgery depends on the amount of transfusion. J Surg Res. 2010; 158(1):20–7.
36. Puskas JD, Thourani VH, Marshall JJ, et al. Clinical outcomes, angiographic patency, and resource utilization in 200 consecutive off-pump coronary bypass patients. Ann Thorac Surg. 2001;71: 1477–83.
37. Gerritsen WB, van Boven WJ, Wesselink RM, et al. Significant reduction in blood loss in patients undergoing minimal extracorporeal circulation. Transfus Med. 2006;16:329–34.

31 Thyroid Hormones and Cardiovascular Surgery

Edmo Atique Gabriel and Sthefano Atique Gabriel

At some point, it seems to be incompatible to correlate thyroid hormones with cardiovascular surgery. Furthermore, it is unusual to think about thyroid function when surgeons are performing any kind of cardiovascular surgery [1, 2].

However, from now on, we postulate that cardiopulmonary bypass and its complex inflammatory universe can interfere with thyroid hormone levels in such a way that postoperative heart function may become considerably depressed. This is possible because thyroid hormones play a cardiotonic and inotropic role. Some authors have correlated modifications of thyroid hormone levels with higher incidence of atrial fibrillation postoperatively. Some controversial hypotheses try to elucidate the real causes for depressed heart function in great detail. One of them considers irregular thyroid perfusion during cardiopulmonary bypass as a not entirely physiological state [3, 4].

Euthyroid sick syndrome encompasses a group of modifications in thyroid hormones levels that can be detected following heart surgery that requires cardiopulmonary bypass. The main features of this syndrome are depressed total and free triiodothyronine (T3) levels, whereas thyroid-stimulating hormone (TSH) and total and free thyroxine (T4) hormone concentrations tend to remain stable [5, 6].

Gabriel et al. [7] designed clinical research focusing on the profile of thyroid hormone variation over the early postoperative period following on-pump coronary artery bypass. In addition to some thyroid hormones, inflammatory and biochemical parameters were addressed over the same time point. These authors found out that on-pump coronary artery bypass can induce a significant reduction in some cellular, protein, and thyroid hormone concentrations at the end of bypass surgery. Moreover, they postulated that recovery of these parameters tends to occur by 24 h postoperatively (Tables 31.1, 31.2, 31.3, and 31.4; Figs. 31.1, 31.2, 31.3, 31.4, 31.5, 31.6, 31.7, 31.8 and 31.9) [7].

Many authors have assumed that decreased thyroid hormones levels occurring during cardiopulmonary bypass should be preoperatively balanced by T4 or T3 supplementation. The rationale for this undertaking is prevention of negative effects from depressed cardiac output, perfusion pressure, stroke volume, and contractility intra- and postoperatively [8, 9].

Nonetheless, as pointed out previously, this matter is so intriguing that some authors, such as Velissaris et al. [10], have advocated that a reduction in thyroid hormone levels might consist of an organic adaptive process of reduced catabolism rather than a true hypothyroid state. The basis for this theory was the association between low free T3 levels and high global oxygen consumption (Fig. 31.10) [10].

Anyway, turning our attention to the role of thyroid hormones during cardiovascular surgery is somehow wise, particularly in case of heart surgery requiring cardiopulmonary bypass. Furthermore, in the context of on-pump heart surgery, it is important to add some comments on the impact of ultrafiltration on thyroid hormone levels to such an interesting discussion [11].

The thyroid hormone concentration in the ultrafiltrate can be positively correlated with prolonged recovery in patients who have undergone heart surgery. Velissaris et al. [10] and Bartkowski et al. [12] demonstrated this trend in a clinical study encompassing infants who had undergone heart surgery with cardiopulmonary bypass and ultrafiltration. These authors noticed remarkable relationships between decreased thyroidhormone levels and eventful recovery postoperatively (Table 31.5; Fig. 31.11) [10, 12].

E.A. Gabriel, MD, PhD (✉)
Department of Cardiovascular Surgery, University Nove de Julho, São Paulo, Brazil
e-mail: edag@uol.com.br

S.A. Gabriel, MD
Department of Vascular Surgery, Pontifical Catholic University of Campinas,
São Paulo, Brazil

Department of Vascular Surgery, Celso Pierro Hospital and Maternity, Campinas São Paulo, Brazil
e-mail: sthefanogabriel@yahoo.com.br

E.A. Gabriel, S.A. Gabriel (eds.), *Inflammatory Response in Cardiovascular Surgery*,
DOI 10.1007/978-1-4471-4429-8_31, © Springer-Verlag London 2013

Table 31.1 Comparison among the time points of simultaneous observation for total leukocytes, neutrophils, and platelets

Block of variables	n	Average	SD	Minimum	Maximum	25th Quartile	Median	75th Quartile	Calculated significance (P)
Total leukocytes pre	18	7,369.44	2,629.74	2,090.00	12,450.00	5,980.00	7,180.00	9,190.00	
Total leukocyte intra	18	11,507.22	5,950.92	2,930.00	21,100.00	6,940.00	9,255.00	18,002.50	
Total leukocytes 24 h	18	13,738.33	3,763.50	7,990.00	23,980.00	10,655.00	13,680.00	15,275.00	<0.001
Total leukocytes 48 h	18	12,966.67	3,933.52	8,060.00	23,320.00	10,290.00	12,410.00	13,825.00	
Total neutrophils pre	18	7,927.22	13,646.36	690,00	62,000.00	3,920.00	4,670.00	6,520.00	
Total neutrophils intra	18	9,342.78	5,258.52	1,140.00	19,620.00	5,240.00	8,225.00	13,897.50	
Total neutrophils 24 h	18	11,646.67	3,926.20	6,310.00	23,260.00	8,920.00	11,480.00	12,807.50	<0.001
Total neutrophils 48 h	18	10,607.11	4,655.99	858.00	20,990.00	8,145.00	9,515.00	12,522.50	
Total platelet pre	18	244,444.44	76,814.69	130,000.00	385,000.00	177,750.00	247,000.00	307,750.00	
Total platelet intra	18	166,277.78	62,520.40	85,000.00	311,000.00	117,000.00	160,000.00	201,500.00	<0.001
Total Platelet 24	18	160,994.44	59,754.86	73,000.00	305,000.00	122,250.00	142,500.00	209,750.00	
Total platelet 48 h	18	160,994.44	63,178.99	83,000.00	306,000.00	129,250.00	147,500.00	223,500.00	

Table 31.2 Comparison between the time points of simultaneous observation for total protein and albumin

Block of variables	*n*	Average	SD	Minimum	Maximum	25th Quartile	Median	75th Quartile	Calculated significance (*P*)
Total protein pre	18	6.78	0.88	5.00	7.90	6.03	7.00	7.50	
Total protein intra	18	4.70	0.90	2.80	6.20	4.30	4.85	5.33	
Total protein 24	18	4.85	0.58	3.20	5.70	4.58	5.00	5.13	<0.001
Total protein 48 h	18	5.11	0.68	3.20	6.40	4.88	5.10	5.40	
Total albumins pre	18	4.05	0.56	2.80	4.90	3.73	4.10	4.40	
Total albumins intra	18	2.72	0.53	1.70	3.60	2.33	2.75	3.20	
Total albumins 24 h	18	2.86	0.39	2.00	3.50	2.68	2.90	3.03	<0.001
Total albumins 48 h	18	2.94	0.37	1.80	3.50	2.80	3.00	3.13	

Table 31.3 Comparison between the time points of simultaneous observation for total T3 and free T3

Block of Variables	*n*	Average	SD	Minimum	Maximum	25th Quartile	Median	75th Quartile	Calculated significance (*P*)
T3 pre	18	134.46	32.31	61.70	190.30	113.33	130.85	161.18	
T3 intra	18	103.81	37.18	51.90	187.30	79.68	101.10	122.10	
T3 24	18	84.77	19.57	56.70	124.30	73.05	79.95	91.78	<0.001
T3 48 h	18	138.60	191.35	53.80	899.00	78.00	89.60	127.25	
Free T3 pre	18	2.54	0.67	1.40	4.30	2.30	2.60	2.90	
Free T3 intra	18	2.14	0.82	0.50	4.10	1.60	2.35	2.60	
Free T3 24	18	1.72	0.65	0.60	2.80	1.30	1.75	2.15	<0.001
Free T3 48 h	18	1.73	0.76	0.50	3.10	1.10	1.90	2.15	

Table 31.4 Comparison among the time points of simultaneous observation for total T4, free T4, and TSH

Block of variables	*n*	Average	SD	Minimum	Maximum	25th Quartile	Median	75th Quartile	Calculated significance (*P*)
T4 pre	18	9.96	3.23	6.00	20.25	8.08	9.45	10.90	
T4 intra	18	8.27	2.20	4.70	13.00	6.58	8.30	10.00	
T4 24	18	7.80	2.11	4.90	12.10	6.00	7.55	9.40	< 0.001
T4 48 h	18	8.35	2.11	5.00	13.90	7.08	8.25	9.70	
Free T4 pre	18	1.36	0.29	0.90	1.80	1.10	1.30	1.70	
Free T4 intra	18	1.44	0.37	1.00	2.30	1.18	1.40	1.53	
Free T4 24 h	18	1.14	0.23	0.80	1.70	0.98	1.10	1.25	<0.002
Free T4 48 h	18	1.24	0.23	1.00	1.70	1.08	1.20	1.40	
TSH pre	18	3.04	2.00	0.20	7.90	1.40	2.75	4.55	
TSH intra	18	2.85	2.06	0.30	6.90	1.25	2.50	3.83	
TSH 24	18	1.69	1.90	0.30	8.60	0.68	1.25	1.95	<0.157
HRT 48 h	18	2.30	1.87	0.10	8.90	1.45	2.00	2.75	

Fig. 31.1 Comparison between time points regarding number of total leukocytes

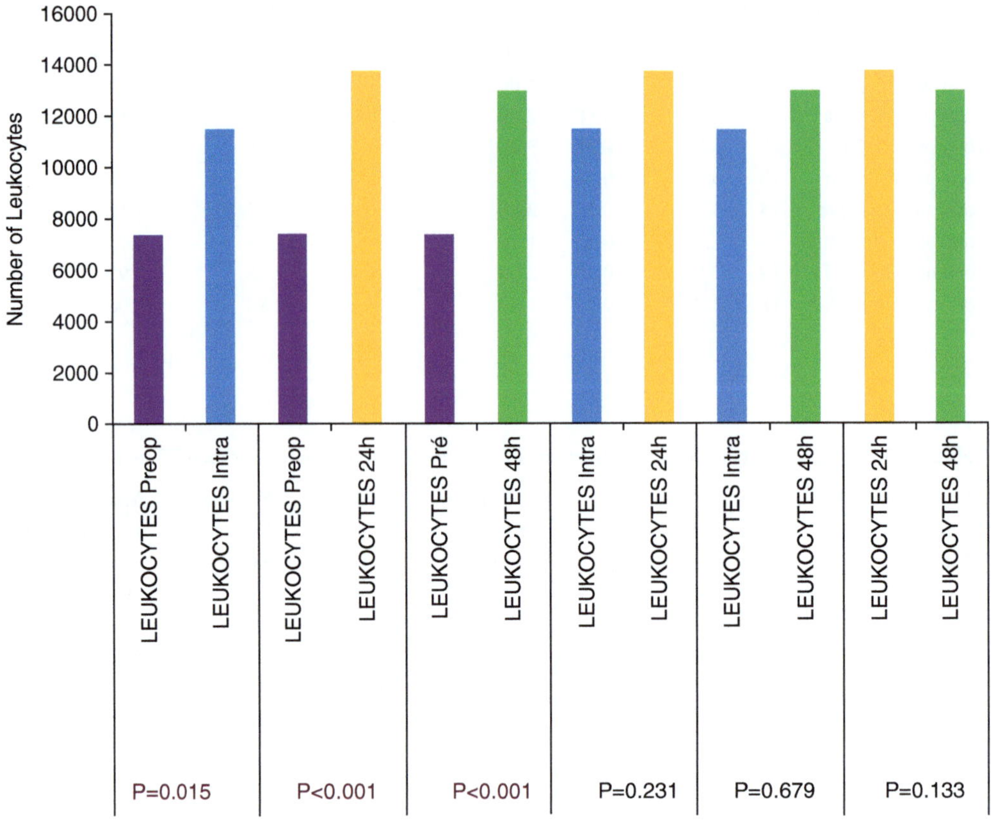

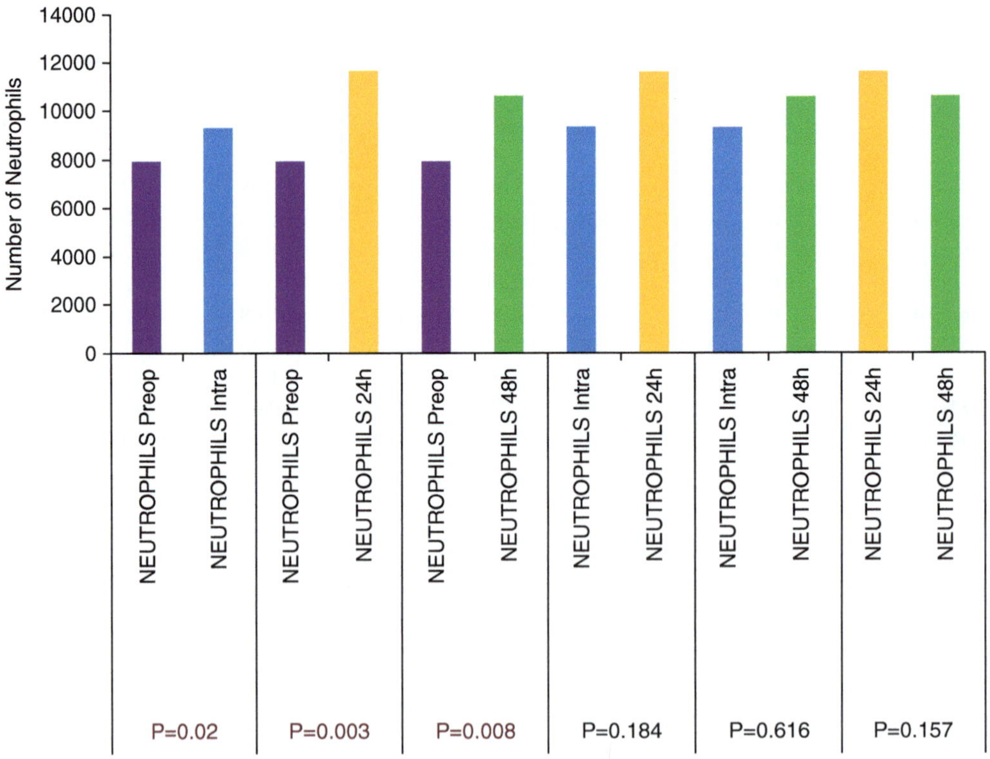

Fig. 31.2 Comparison between time points regarding number of neutrophils

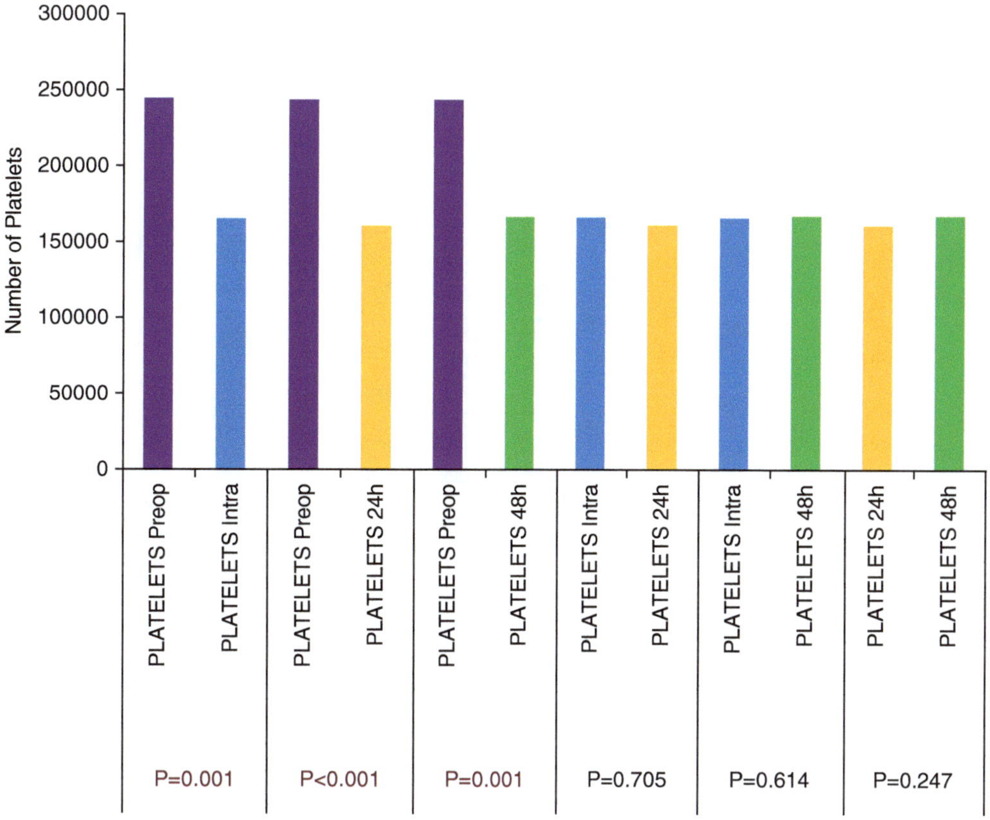

Fig. 31.3 Comparison between time points regarding number of platelets

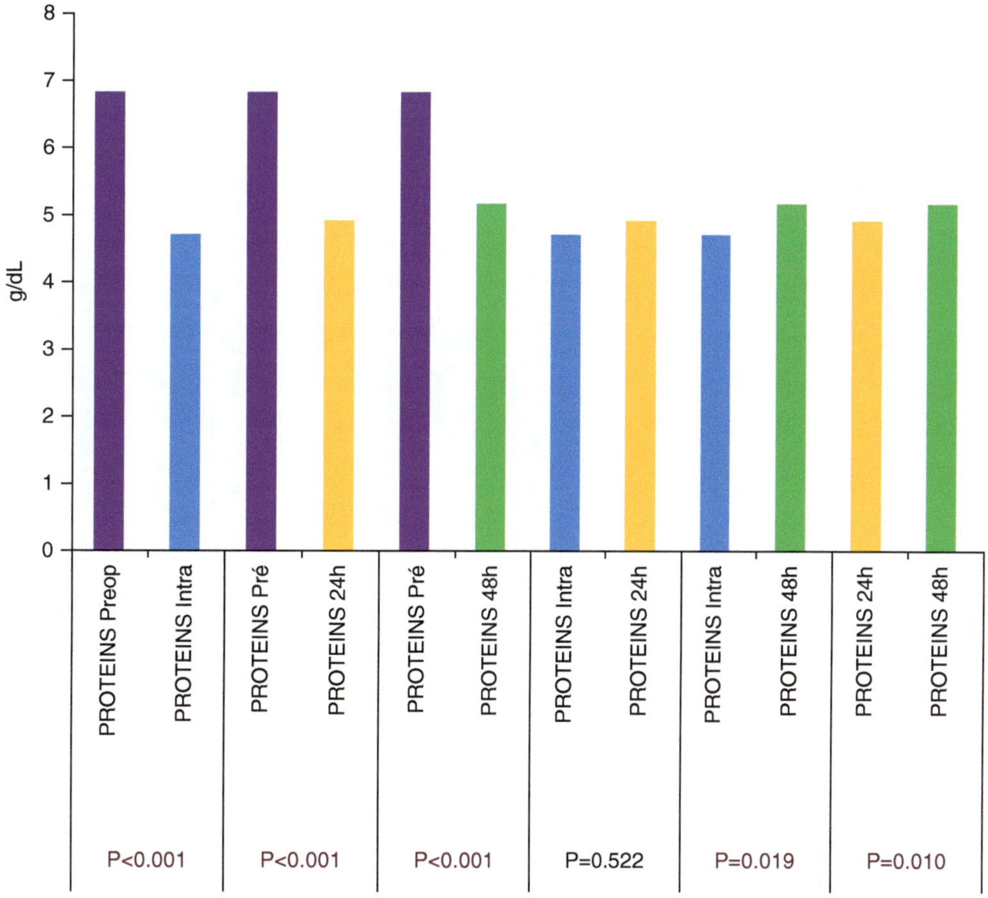

Fig. 31.4 Comparison between time points regarding levels of total proteins

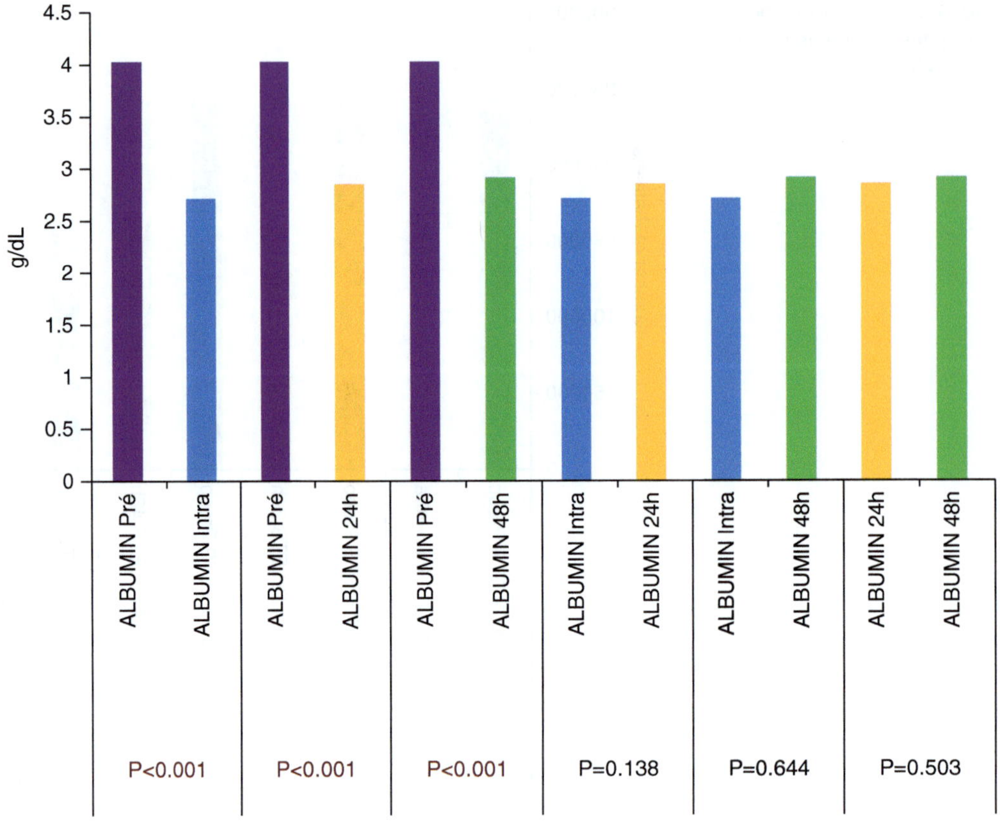

Fig. 31.5 Comparison between time points regarding levels of albumin

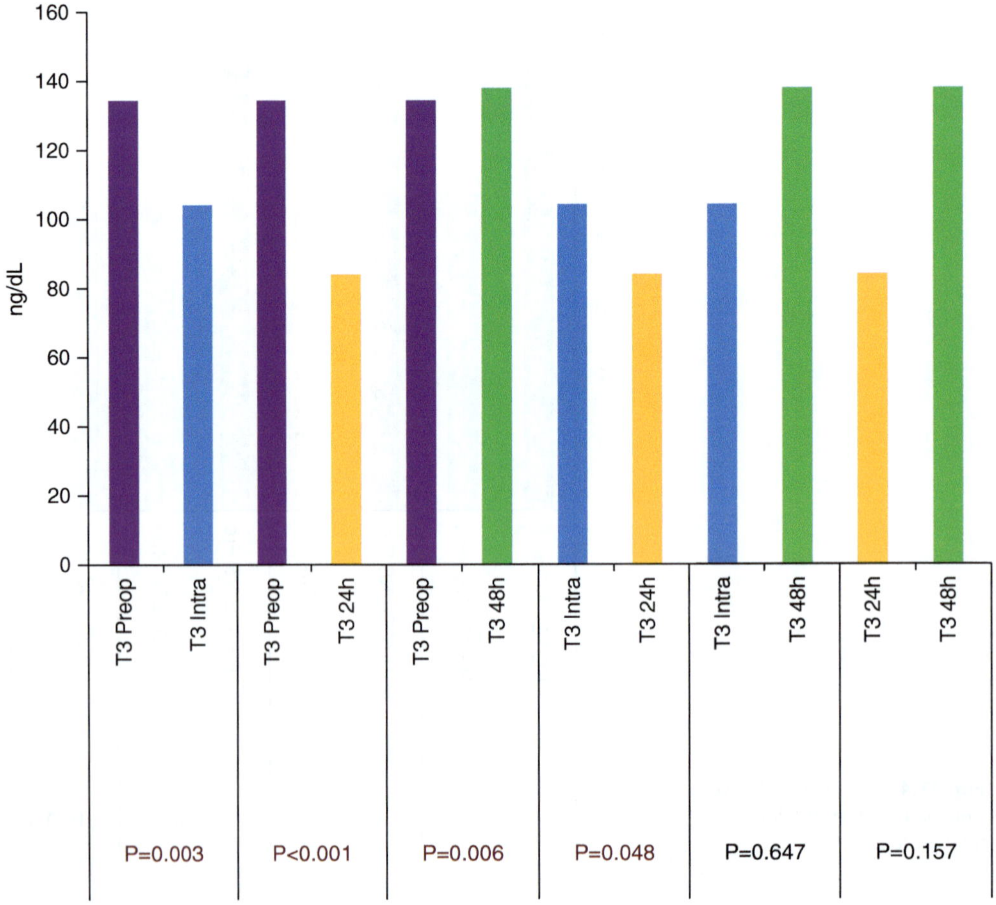

Fig. 31.6 Comparison between time points regarding levels of total T3

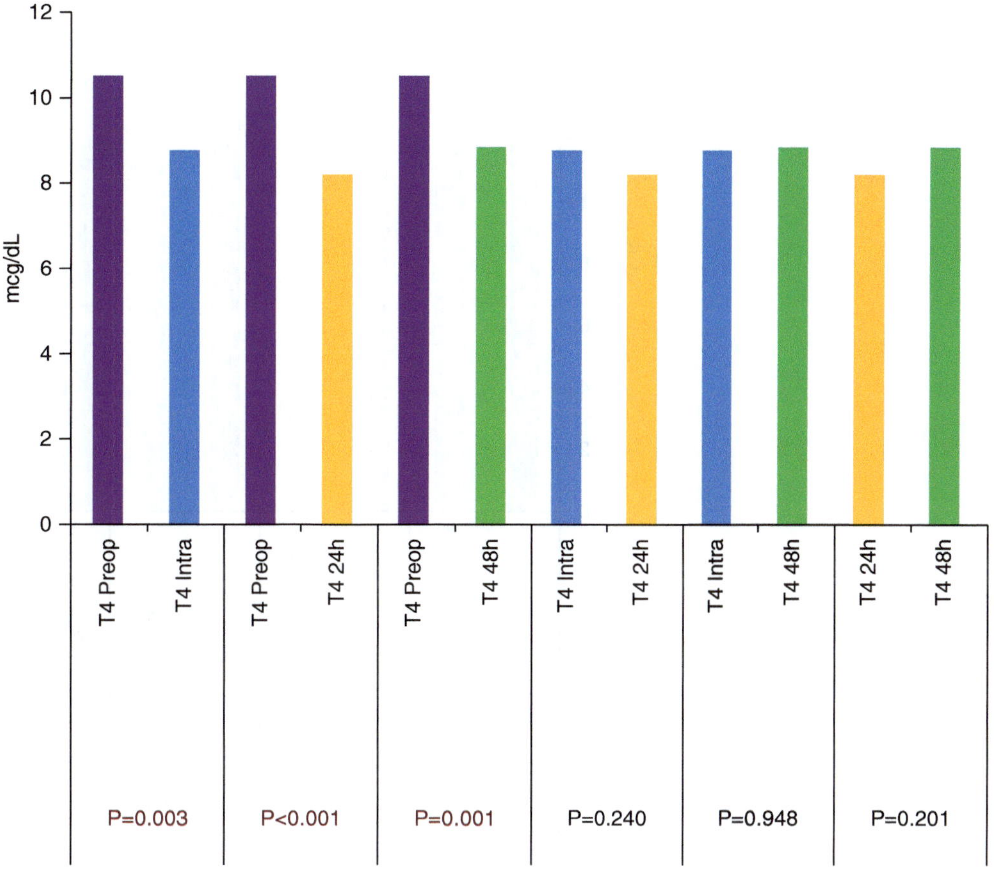

Fig. 31.7 Comparison between time points regarding levels of total T4

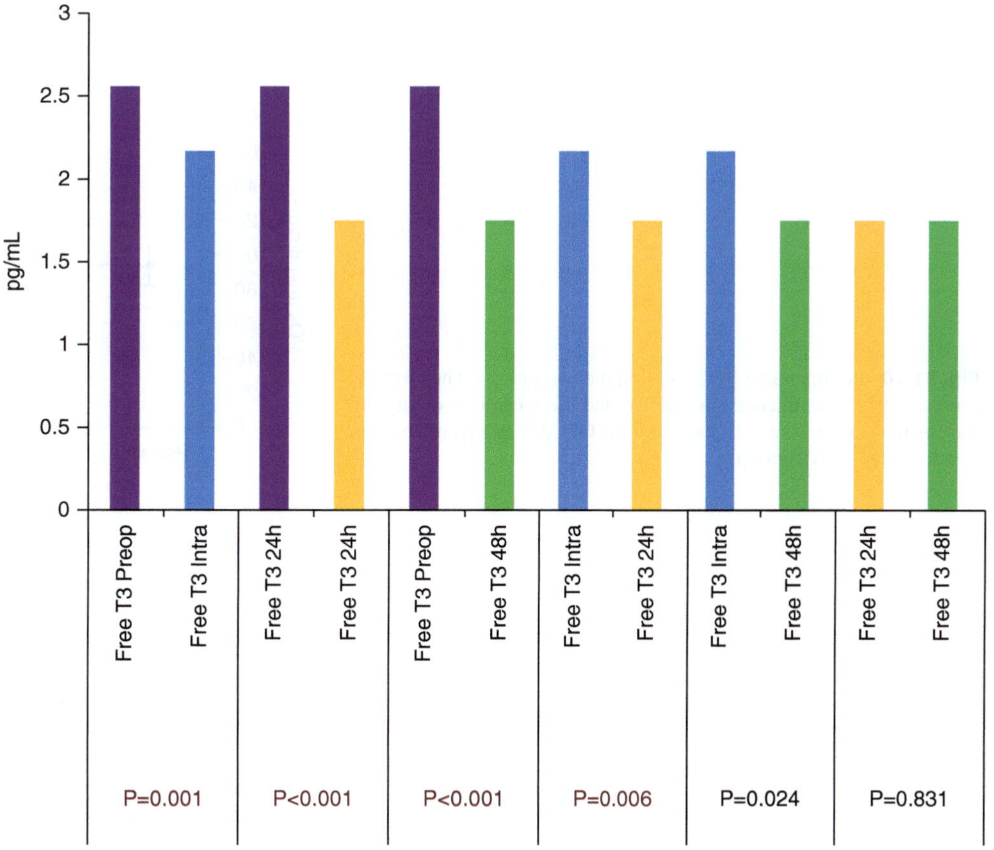

Fig. 31.8 Comparison between time points regarding levels of free T3

Fig. 31.9 Comparison between time points regarding levels of free T4

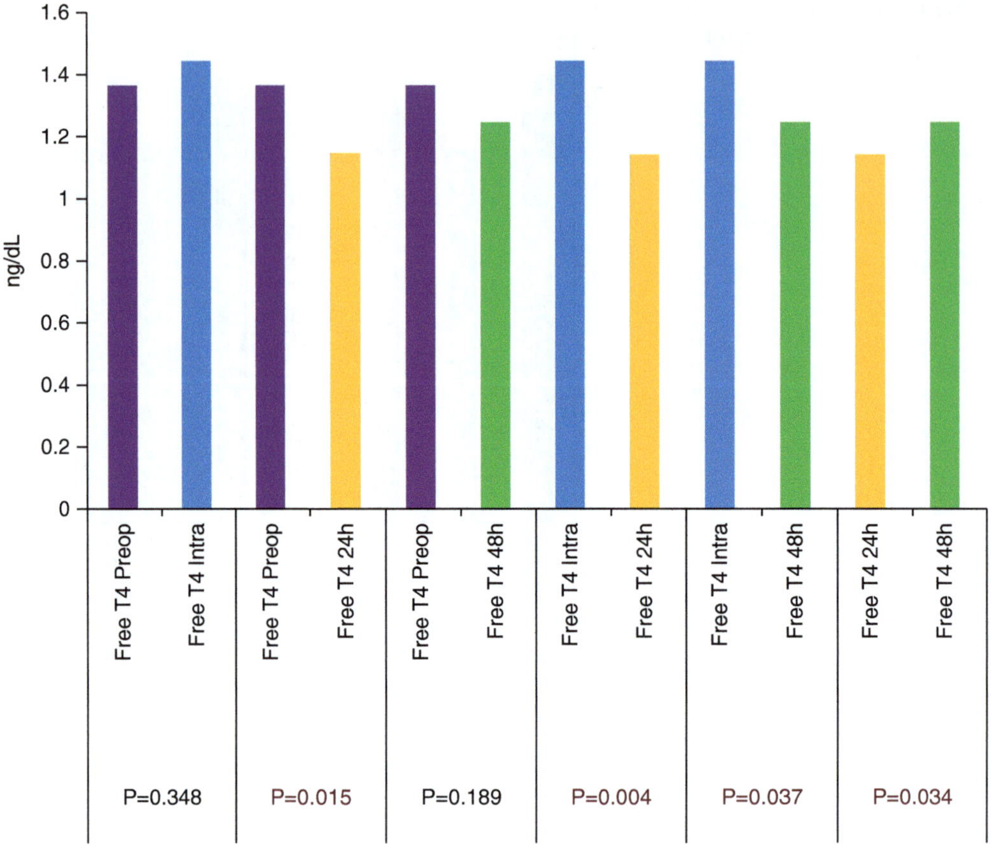

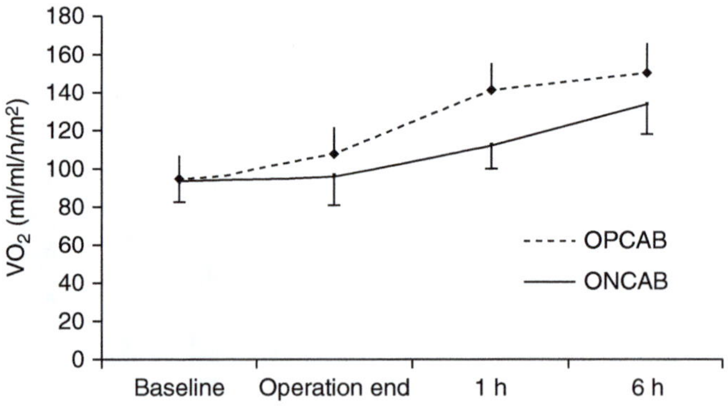

Fig. 31.10 Perioperative VO2 levels in the two groups. The error bars represent 95 % confidence intervals around the mean (for clarity only the positive error bars are displayed for the OPCAB group and the negative for the ONCAB group)

Table 31.5 Perioperative thyroid hormone levels in the two groups

Variable	Preop	Operation end	1 h	6 h	24 h
TSH (mU/l)					
ONCAB	2.16±2.45	2.11±2.31	1.60±1.37	1.01±0.77	1.89±1.36
OPCAB	2.74±1.57	1.94±1.17	1.49±0.98	1.01±0.59	2.07±1.70
fT4 (pmol/l)					
ONCAB	16.40±2.45	16.8±2.57	15.64±2.43	13.84±1.99	14.42±2.55
OPCAB	15.88±2.28	18.50±3.55	16.04±2.78	12.94±2.01	13.83±1.86
fT3 (pmol/l)					
ONCAB	5.12±0.41	4.62±0.43	4.56±0.47	3.68±0.63	3.31±0.69[a]
OPCAB	5.04±046	4.88±0.71	4.67±0.57	3.57±0.59	3.34±0.52[a]

Data are presented as mean±standard deviation. Reference ranges, fT4: 8.0–22.0 pmol/l, fT3: 3.5–7.0 pmol/l, TSH: 0.5–5.5 mU/l
TSH thyroid-stimulating hormone, *fT4* free thyroxine, *fT3* free triiodothyronine
[a]$p<0.001$ compared to preoperative value

Fig. 31.11 The average amount of triiodothyronine in the ultrafiltrate (in patients with or without intensive care treatment)

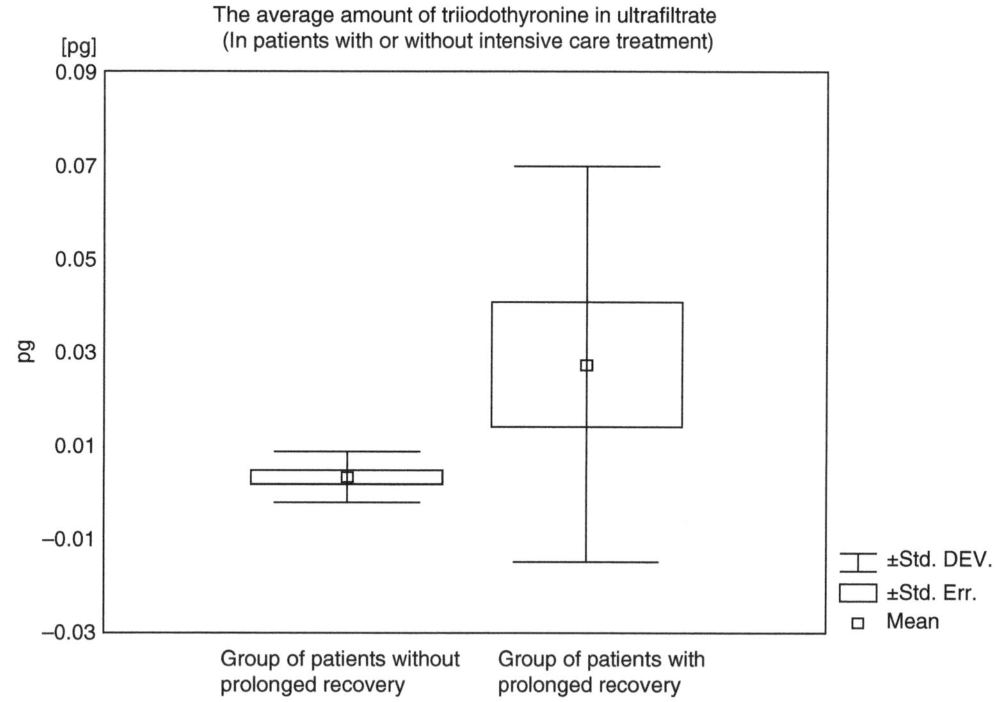

References

1. Murzi B, Iervasi G, Masini S, Moschetti R, Vanini V, Zucchelli G, et al. Thyroid hormones homeostasis in pediatric patients during and after cardiopulmonary bypass. Ann Thorac Surg. 1995;59:481–5.
2. Jones TH, Hunter SM, Price A, Angelini GD. Should thyroid function be assessed before cardiopulmonary bypass operations? Ann Thorac Surg. 1994;58:434–6.
3. Park YJ, Yoon JW, Kim KI, Lee YJ, Kim KW, Choi SH, et al. Subclinical hypothyroidism might increase the risk of transient atrial fibrillation after coronary artery bypass grafting. Ann Thorac Surg. 2009;87:1846–52.
4. Cerillo AG, Storti S, Clerico A, Iervasi G. Thyroid function and cardiac surgery: what should we measure, and when? Ann Thorac Surg. 2010;89:1010–1.
5. Portman MA, Fearneyhough C, Ning XH, Duncan BW, Rosenthal GL, Lupinetti FM. Triiodothyronine repletion in infants during cardiopulmonary bypass for congenital heart disease. J Thorac Cardiovasc Surg. 2000;120:604–8.
6. Wieselthaler GM, Riedl M, Schima H, Wagner O, Waldhäusl W, Wolner E, et al. Endocrine function is not impaired in patients with a continuous MicroMed–DeBakey axial flow pump. J Thorac Cardiovasc Surg. 2007;133:2–6.
7. Gabriel EA, Locali RF, Matsuoka PK, Cherbo T, Buffolo E. On-pump coronary artery bypass graft surgery:biochemical, hormonal and cellular features. Rev Bras Cir Cardiovasc. 2011;26(4):525–31.
8. Pearce EN, Yang Q, Benjamin EJ, Aragam J, Vasan RS. Thyroid function and left ventricular structure and function in the Framingham Heart Study. Thyroid. 2010;20(4):369–73.
9. Virtanen VK, Saha HH, Groundstroem KW, Salmi J, Pasternack AI. Thyroid hormone substitution therapy rapidly enhances

left-ventricular diastolic function in hypothyroid patients. Cardiology. 2001;96(2):59–64.
10. Velissaris T, Tang AT, Wood PJ, Hett DA, Ohri SK. Thyroid function during coronary surgery with and without cardiopulmonary bypass. Eur J Cardiothorac Surg. 2009;36(1):148–54.
11. Reinhardt W, Mocker V, Jockenhövel F, Olbricht T, Reinwein D, Mann K, et al. Influence of coronary artery bypass surgery on thyroid hormone parameters. Horm Res. 1997;47(1):1–8.
12. Bartkowski R, Wojtalik M, Korman E, Sharma G, Henschke J, Mrówczyński W. Thyroid hormones levels in infants during and after cardiopulmonary bypass with ultrafiltration. Eur J Cardiothorac Surg. 2002;22(6):879–84.

32 Inflammatory Response in Cardiovascular Surgery

Kaan Kaya

CPB, first performed by John H. Gibbon in 1953, is still a standard method to operate on most patients undergoing cardiac surgery. There are many studies in the literature of its use and complications, and systemic inflammatory response has been largely documented. Currently, the systemic inflammatory response to CPB is well diagnosed, but it is not clearly understood. Both the cellular and humoral complexes are activated during CPB, but their effects and interactions remain poorly defined. Recently, many surgeons tried to perform off-pump cardiac surgery to prevent systemic inflammation caused by CPB, but they did not succeed in preventing inflammation caused by the surgery itself. This chapter describes the etiopathogenesis and mechanisms of the development of the inflammatory response as well as its prevention in cardiac surgery.

Etiology and Pathogenesis

The inflammatory response can be caused by burns, chemical irritations, trauma, and infections. Inflammation can be classified into two categories: acute and chronic inflammation. Chronic inflammation can be observed during rheumatoid arthritis, systemic lupus erythematosus, atherosclerosis, and inflammatory bowel disease. In these diseases, inflammation may last several weeks or months. But during cardiac surgery, the extracorporeal circulation plays the major role, and the inflammatory response is acute.

Nonspecific activators of the stress response include surgical trauma, blood loss and transfusion, hypothermia, or hyperthermia. The extracorporeal circulation may activate the inflammatory response via at least three distinct mechanisms integrated with each other (Fig. 32.1). The major mechanism is exposure of blood to cardiopulmonary bypass (CPB) circuits. The second is ischemia-reperfusion injury of vital organs during CPB. The third mechanism is systemic endotoxemia from the gut following splanchnic hypoperfusion. Inflammatory mediators can be classified as humoral and cellular factors. These factors are shown in Table 32.1.

K. Kaya, MD
Division of Cardiovascular Surgery,
Kavaklidere Umut Hospital, Ankara, Turkey
e-mail: drkaankaya@yahoo.com

Humoral Response

The initial response is probably the humoral response, and it is initiated by the blood coming in contact with the foreign surfaces (the extracorporeal circuit). The greatest stimulus is the oxygenator as gas exchange requires a large surface area. Although the patient is heparinized, many cascades including coagulation, complement, kallikrein and fibrinolysis responds immediately. It has been shown that many split products resulting from all the cascades can be found in the circulation during and after CPB. Hageman factor (factor XII) activation has an important initial role in activation of these cascades. Activated products have strong physiologic effects. For example, by activation of the complement cascade powerful anaphylatoxins are produced (C3a and C5a), and they increase vascular permeability and leukocyte chemotaxis.

Complement System

The complement system includes a large number of plasma proteins, and it is activated by the classic and the alternative pathways during CPB. The exposure of blood to extracorporeal circuits activates the alternative pathway, which leads to the formation of C3a and C5a, and reversal of heparin with protamine activates the classical pathway that produces C4 and C2. Thus, C4 and C2 activation does not occur in patients

E.A. Gabriel, S.A. Gabriel (eds.), *Inflammatory Response in Cardiovascular Surgery*,
DOI 10.1007/978-1-4471-4429-8_32, © Springer-Verlag London 2013

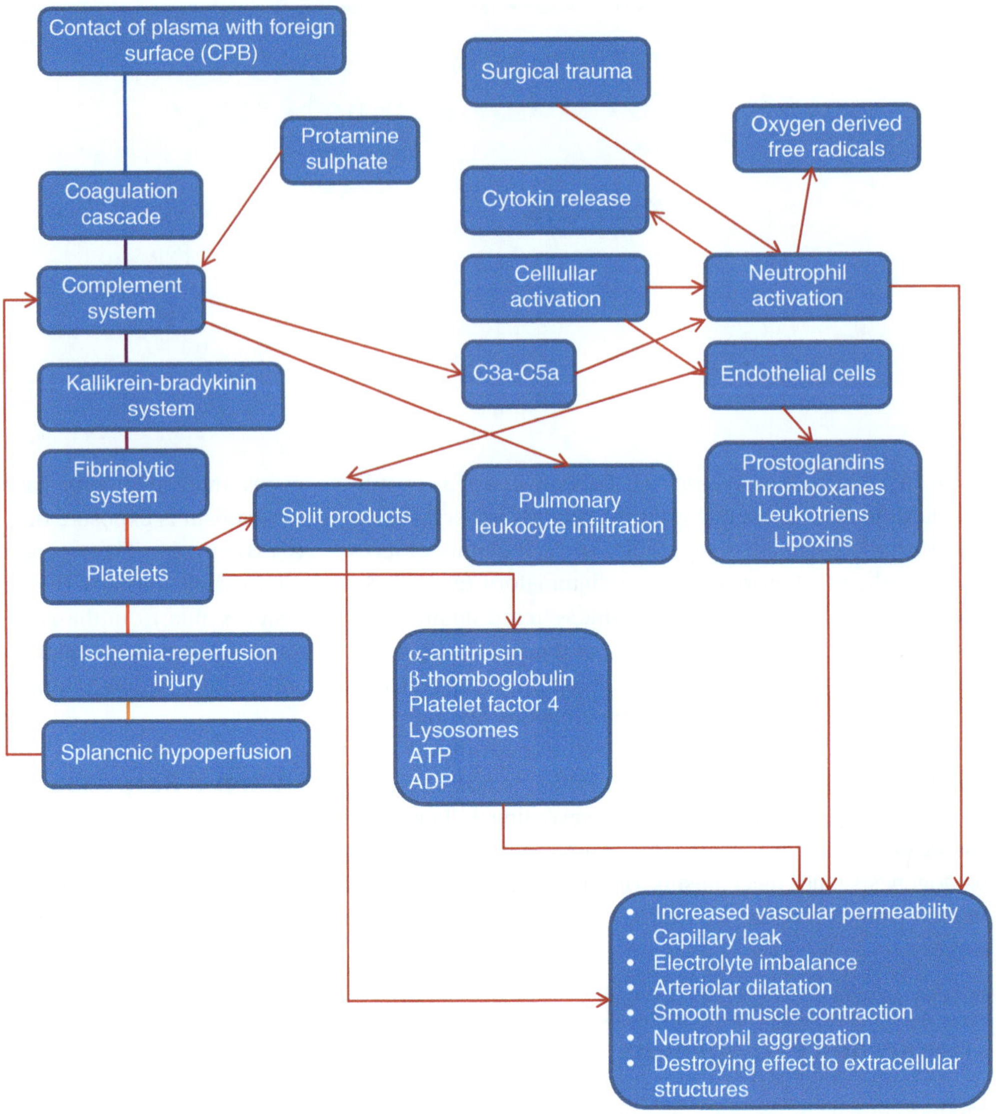

Fig. 32.1 Complexity of the inflammatory response in cardiac surgery

Table 32.1 Humoral and cellular factors of the inflammatory response

Humoral factors	Cellular factors
Contact activation products	Neutrophils
Factor XIIa	Endothelial cells
Thrombin	
Kallikrein	
Fibrinogen degradation products	
Complement system	
Cytokines	
Tumor necrosis factor	
Interleukin	
Leukotriene	

undergoing off-pump surgery without protamine administration. By activation of the complement system, a number of active products increase the vascular permeability, mast cells and basophils release histamine, and white blood cells release free oxygen radicals and lysosomal enzymes. The complement system can be activated by contact of blood with extravascular surfaces, probably by way of the Hageman factor. Complement activation has also been shown during hemodialysis during exposure of blood to the dialysis membrane.

The extent of complement activation during CPB correlates with the severity of the operation and the development of complications. However, most clinical problems do not occur until the first or second postoperative days. CRP, one of the acute-phase proteins, has strong potency to activate complement. But it is not clear whether CRP contributes to complement activation during or after CPB. The duration of the CPB does not affect the final C3a level, but protamine administration has a strong effect. Pretreatment of the patient with steroids may decrease complement activation but does not prevent it completely.

Pulmonary sequestration of the polymorphonuclear leukocytes and neutropenia during CPB has been shown to be related to complement system activation. Thus, activation of the complement system is involved in production of pulmonary edema. Once the complement system has been activated, pulmonary neutrophil migration occurs, neutrophil-mediated pulmonary endothelial injury begins, pulmonary vascular permeability increases, and reactive oxygen radicals may contribute to the adverse effects of CPB on pulmonary function.

Cytokines

Cytokines are a kind of protein produced by immune system cells. Myocardium, lungs and kidneys play a role in sequestrating proinflammatory cytokines. These cytokines may damage them in the presence of hypoperfusion [1]. They include interleukins (IL), tumor necrosis factor-α (TNFα), and transforming growth factor-β. They need to bind specific receptors to activate cells, and they can affect autocrine (effective in its own cell), paracrine (effective in the neighboring cells), and endocrine (effective in the remote cells). Proinflammatory cytokines are increased in pulmonary venous blood [2].

Interleukin-1: Its main role is a mediator in the inflammatory response. It has a chemotactic effect for macrophages and neutrophils. It also causes fever via central nervous system effects.

Interleukin-2: Mainly, this is produced from T-helper cells. Its most important role is proliferation of T-cells.

Interleukin-6: This is produced by macrophages, monocytes, fibroblasts, and endothelial cells. IL-6 is a proinflammatory cytokine. It has effects on proliferation of B-cells. Its most important effect is the coordination of the generalized systemic inflammatory response, and it is one of the acute phase reactants [3]. IL-6 has been accepted as the best proinflammatory cytokine predictor of LV systolic dysfunction and myocardial ischemia [4]. IL-6 levels rise in cardiac surgery with extracorporeal circulation [5].

Interleukin-8: This is produced by macrophages, monocytes, fibroblasts, and endothelial cells. It is an activator of neutrophils, and it has a chemotactic effect on neutrophils. IL-8 levels rise in cardiac operations with using CPB [5].

Tumor necrosis-alpha (*TNF-α*): This is mainly produced by activated macrophages. It is produced by activated monocytes and plays a very significant role in inflammation [6]. During CPB, its plasma levels have been shown to rise [7]. It is a powerful activator of neutrophils and phagocytes. It causes fever, hypoglycemia, and vasodilatation, and it stimulates the coagulation cascade. TNF-α can directly cause hypotension, coagulopathy, and renal dysfunction [8].

Platelet-activating factor (*PAF*): This is a phospholipid released from endothelial cells. It has strong vasoactive effects And causes the release of cytokines.

Leukotriene: This causes endothelial cell contraction and increases capillary leakage.

Thromboxane A_2: This is derived from macrophages and platelets. It has forcing effects on platelet aggregation and causes vasoconstriction and thrombosis.

Free Oxygen Radicals

These products increase permeability via its effect on membrane lipids, and they cause organ dysfunction. Hyperoxic CPB is widely used during cardiac operations, but it induces oxygen-derived free radicals. These products represent a potential risk for the myocardium and lungs [9, 10].

Endotoxins

Endotoxins have very strong effects on the inflammatory cascade during cardiac surgery. It has been shown that there is a significant increase of endotoxin levels during CPB. Extracorporeal circulation, pulmonary arterial catheters, intravenous fluid administration, and blood transfusions are believed to be responsible for endotoxemia. The presence of circulating endotoxins is a major stimulus for producing TNF-α. In addition, endotoxins activate the complement system and cause the release of some cytokines. During CPB, splanchnic hypoperfusion can result in increased permeability of the gut mucosal barrier and consequently endotoxemia. Endotoxemia causes the release of inflammatory and antiinflammatory mediators [11].

Kallikrein-Bradykinin System

Many investigations have shown that the amount of bradykinin increases during CPB. Because the lungs play a primary role in the elimination of bradykinin, reduced pulmonary circulation causes reduced bradykinin elimination during CPB. Bradykinin is a powerful vasodilator, and this effect has great importance in the body's inflammatory response to CPB.

Coagulation System

Exposure of blood to the extracorporeal circuit activates the contact system because the CPB circuit lacks endothelial cells. Although coagulation is largely inhibited by administering heparin during CPB, its activation cannot be completely prevented. Due to incomplete inhibition of the coagulation cascade by heparin, small amounts of fibrin are present during routine CPB. Because of this process, some of the coagulation factor levels are reduced by the end of CPB.

The coagulation system has two pathways: intrinsic (contact activation) and extrinsic. The intrinsic pathway is activated by the Hageman factor, and at the end of this pathway, thrombin is produced. The intrinsic pathway is mostly activated by tissue damage. The extrinsic pathway is activated by infection and systemic inflammation. Activation of the coagulation system is not only important for cloth formation, it is also important for the proinflammatory response.

Fibrinolytic Cascade

The fibrinolytic cascade may be initiated by activation of the Hageman factor during CPB. Kallikrein is produced by activation of the Hageman factor, and it facilitates the conversion of plasminogen to plasmin.

Arachidonic Acid Cascade

During CPB, the lungs are the major site of synthesis, release, and degradation of the eicosanoids (products of the arachidonic acid cascade). Prostacyclin and prostaglandin E_2 production appears to be increased during CPB, and they can cause pulmonary vasodilation, while leukotriene-C4 and thromboxane tend to cause vasoconstriction. It is believed that thromboxane-A_2 is mostly produced by platelets, but its release occurs in the lungs. Platelet-activating factor (PAF) is another factor in the arachidonic acid cascade, and it is an important mediator of the inflammatory response. Leukotriene-B_4 is another product of this cascade and promotes plasma leakage and leukocyte adhesion; it is also increased after CPB.

Cellular Response

Whole blood cells (platelets, neutrophils, etc.), endothelial cells, and lymphocytes participate in the cellular inflammatory response. Polymorphonuclear leukocytes play a major role in the response to CPB. Neutrophils are activated by complement and other mediators. Once they are activated, they become more adhesive, and they secrete cytotoxic substances, such as oxygen-derived free radicals. Platelets are strongly affected during CPB. They can be activated by direct surface contact, abnormal shear stress, and mechanical injury. Endothelial cells are also activated by shear stress, localized ischemia, and increased concentrations of abnormal mediators and split products.

Neutrophil Activation

During CPB, an initial leukopenia occurs, but it returns to baseline levels soon. At the end of CPB, leukocytosis is present. Pulmonary sequestration of neutrophils develops during CPB. Activation of complement system produces C3a and C5a complement fragments, and these products activate neutrophils to liberate oxygen-derived free radicals. This is associated with the damaging effects of CPB.

In healthy persons, neutrophils are resting cells. However, when stimulated, they aggregate and cluster with each other and the other cell types. This process is rapid, and it is a critical step in the development of inflammatory and immune responses.

Platelet Response

During extracorporeal circulation, the platelet count decreases significantly. Membrane oxygenators tend to reduce more than bubble oxygenators. The number of platelets in circulating blood after CPB is decreased to about 60 % of the pre-bypass value, but it doesn't correlate with the duration of CPB.

Erythrocytes

Shear stress results in injury of the erythrocyte membrane during CPB. This causes the release of free hemoglobin into the circulating blood. Viscosity and oncotic pressure are increased, and tissue perfusion is decreased. After autooxidation of hemoglobin, cytotoxic free oxygen radicals are released.

Metabolic Response

During CPB, because of the acute elevation of catecholamine levels, a strong metabolic response to stress may develop. Its magnitude is directly correlated with catecholamine levels in the circulating blood.

Anti-inflammatory Strategies

Many investigations have been performed to prevent the systemic antiinflammatory response, and some drugs (corticosteroids, sodium nitroprusside, etc.) or some manipulations (off-pump cardiac surgery, minimal invasive surgery, normothermic approaches, etc.) have been used. However, it should not be forgotten that the antiinflammatory response is a kind of defense mechanism, and we do not know if it is stopped completely.

Corticosteroids

Commonly used corticosteroids in the prevention of the systemic inflammatory response during cardiac surgery are methyl-prednisolone and dexamethasone. They inhibit phospholipase activity and protect myocardial cells. These effects reduce damage in the myocardium and lungs. Steroids cannot prevent endotoxemia during CPB but prevent activation of complement and reduce the release of proinflammatory cytokines. Bronicki et al. [12] demonstrated that preoperative administration of 1 mg/kg dexamethasone decreases the inflammatory response.

Aprotinin

This is a protease inhibitor derived from bovine lungs. It has antagonist effects on proteolytic enzymes such as kallikrein and plasmin. It inhibits complement activation and production of TNF-α and IL-6. Aprotinin also reduces neutrophil migration to the lungs and IL-8 production.

Adenosine

Adenosine can block oxygen-derived free radical production from neutrophils.

Sodium Nitroprusside

Nitric oxide decreases ischemia-reperfusion injury. Nitric oxide also has cardiac protective effects. Sodium nitroprusside is a nitric oxide donor. It inhibits complement activation.

Heparin-Coated Circulation

During cardiopulmonary bypass, blood exposure to the extracorporeal circulation circuit is the most important factor causing systemic inflammatory reactions. It has been thought that heparin-coated extracorporeal circuit lines can prevent thrombosis. Many studies have shown that heparin-coated circuits decrease leukocyte activation and repair platelet functions [13]. Levels of TNF-α, IL-6, IL-8, and thrombin-antithrombin complex were significantly reduced with the use of heparin-coated circuits [14, 15].

Leukocyte Filters

Inflammation has been reported to be reduced by implanting a leukocyte filter in the arterial line, but there have been many contrasting investigations. Some clinics use leukocyte filters routinely, but others do not believe that they have beneficial effects. Using leukocyte filtering during CPB may limit the postoperative inflammatory response as measured by reduced IL-8 production [16]. Some of the investigators have reported leukocyte filtering did not improve pulmonary hemodynamics [16], but others have reported better lung functions [17, 18].

Off-Pump Beating Heart Technique

Perhaps the most effective prevention method against the inflammatory response is using the off-pump cardiac surgery technique. This technique involves some technical difficulties and cannot be used for all types of cardiac surgery (valve surgery, etc.). The perioperative release of inflammatory response markers IL-6 and TNF-α was found to be significantly lower after off-pump cardiac surgery. It has also been shown that the number of circulating monocytes and polymorphonuclear cells was significantly lower following off-pump cardiac surgery [19]. Gu et al. reported that C3a, β-thromboglobulin, and leukocyte elastase levels are lower than in patients who undergo on-pump cardiac surgery [20]. This result shows that CPB is the major factor in activating the complement system. It is also reported that higher TNF-α levels are observed in patients undergoing on-pump surgery [21]. However, there is no difference in IL-6 levels between the patients who were operated on off-pump and on-pump with median sternotomy [22] (Table 32.2).

Table 32.2 Inflammatory mediators during cardiac surgery

	Off-pump	On-pump
Complement activation [11]	↓	↑
TNF-α level [11]	↓	↑
IL-6 level [2, 12]	↔	↔
IL-8 level [8]	↓	↑
IL-10 level [2]	↓	↑
Neutrophil elastase level [11, 15]	↓	↑
Leukocyte activation [12]	↔	↔
C-reactive protein	↔	↔
C3a and C5a levels [11]	↓	↑

↔ no difference, ↓ significantly lower, ↑ significantly higher

References

1. Ng CSH, Wan S, Yim APC, Arifi AA. Pulmonary dysfunction after cardiac surgery. Chest. 2002;121:1269–77.
2. Massoudy P, Zahler S, Becker BF, Braun SL, Barankay A, Meisner H. Evidence for inflammatory response of the lungs during coronary artery bypass grafting with cardiopulmonary bypass. Chest. 2001;119:31–6.
3. Cassey WF, Hauser GJ, Hannalah RS, Midgley FM, Khan W. Circulating endotoxin and tumour necrosis factor during paediatric cardiac surgery. Crit Care Med. 1992;20:1090–6.
4. Fortenberry JD, Bhardwaj V, Niemer P, et al. Neutrophil and cytokine activation with neonatal extracorporeal membrane oxygenation. J Pediatr. 1996;128:670–8.
5. Gessler P, Pfenninger J, Pfammatter JP, Carrel T, Baenziger O, Dahinden C. Plasma levels of interleukin-8 and expression of interleukin-8 receptors on circulating neutrophils and monocytes after cardiopulmonary bypass in children. J Thorac Cardiovasc Surg. 2003;126:718–25.
6. Jansen NJ, van Oeveren W, van der Brock L, et al. Inhibition by dexamethasone of the reperfusion phenomenon in cardiopulmonary bypass. J Thorac Cardiovasc Surg. 1991;102:515–25.
7. Sun D, Xu C, Li J, Jiao X, Chen Y. Changes of inflammatory factors in patients with coronary artery disease during perioperation. Zhonghua Wai Ke Za Zhi. 2002;40:571–3.
8. Khabar KS, elBarbary MA, Khouqeer F, et al. Circulating endotoxins and cytokines after cardiopulmonary bypass: differential correlation with duration of bypass and systemic inflammatory response/multiple organ dysfunction syndromes. Clin Immunol Immunopathol. 1997;85:97–103.
9. Clermont G, Vergely C, de Girard C, Rochette L. Cellular injury associated with extracorporeal circulation. Ann Cardiol Angeiol. 2002;51:38–43.
10. Ulus AT, Aksoyek A, Ozkan M, Katircioglu SF, Basu S. Cardiopulmonary bypass as a cause of free radical-induced oxidative stress and enhanced blood-borne isoprostanes in humans. Free Radic Biol Med. 2003;34:911–7.
11. Kirklin JK, Westaby S, Blackstone EH, et al. Complement and the damaging effects of cardiopulmonary bypass. J Thorac Cardiovasc Surg. 1983;86:845–57.
12. Bronicki RA, Backer CL, Baden HP, Mavroudis C, Crawford SE, Gren TP. Dexamethasone reduces the inflammatory response to cardiopulmonary bypass in children. Ann Thorac Surg. 2000;69:1490–5.
13. Matheve C. Clinical evidence of improved biocompatibility using heparin-coated surfaces. Perfusion. 1996;11:264–9.
14. Moen O, Hogasen K, Fosse E, et al. Attenuation of changes in leukocyte surface markers and complement activation with heparin-coated cardiopulmonary bypass. Ann Thorac Surg. 1997;63:105–11.
15. Hamulu A, Discigil B, OZbaran M, et al. Complement consumption during cardiopulmonary bypass: comparison of Duraflo II heparin-coated and uncoated circuits in fully heparinized patients. Perfusion. 1996;11:333–7.
16. Gu YJ, de Vries AJ, Vos P, et al. Leukocyte depletion during cardiac operation. A new approach through the venous bypass circuit. Ann Thorac Surg. 1999;67:604–9.
17. Olivencia-Yurvatti AH, Ferrara CA, Tierney N, Wallace N, MAllet RT. Strategic leukocyte depletion reduces pulmonary microvascular pressure and improves pulmonary status post-cardiopulmonary bypass. Perfusion. 2003;18 suppl 1:23–31.
18. Morioka K, Muraoka R, Chiba Y, et al. Leukocyte and platelet depletion with the blood cell separator: effects on lung injury after cardiac surgery with cardiopulmonary bypass. J Thorac Cardiovasc Surg. 1996;111:45–54.
19. Ascione R, Lloyd CT, Underwood MJ, et al. Inflammatory response after coronary revascularization with or without cardiopulmonary bypass. Ann Thorac Surg. 2000;69:1198–204.
20. Gu YJ, MAriani MA, van Oeveren W, et al. Reduction of the inflammatory response in patients undergoing minimally invasive coronary artery bypass grafting. Ann Thorac Surg. 1998;65:420–4.
21. Brasil LA, Gomes WJ, Salomao R, et al. Inflammatory response after myocardial revascularization with or without cardiopulmonary bypass. Ann Thorac Surg. 1998;66:56–9.
22. Wan S, LeClere JL, Vincent JL. Inflammatory response to cardiopulmonary bypass. Chest. 1997;112:676–92.

33 Lung Protection in Cardiovascular Surgery

Edmo Atique Gabriel and Sthefano Atique Gabriel

Lung protection is a cutting-edge topic for cardiovascular surgeons; for several decades the main concern has been just to protect the heart by preventing ischemia-reperfusion injury [1].

Nonetheless, in recent years, some heart teams have turned their attention to the importance of the lungs throughout and following cardiovascular surgery. The lungs have lagged behind everything considering that the heart-lung machine has an unmatchable ability to carry out pulmonary function without metabolic, biochemical, or structural modifications [2, 3].

The concept of lung protection has evolved so far that many cardiovascular surgeons worldwide have published numerous papers consistently advocating this idea and carrying it out during heart operations. Furthermore, one of the greatest breakthroughs on this topic was proving that bronchial arterial circulation alone is not enough to provide blood flow to the lungs, and thus one could conclude that bronchial circulation will not protect the lungs from ischemia-reperfusion injury. Even when the heart is placed on a bypass machine and kept beating during surgery, lung protection is inadequate because the flow provided by conventional cardiopulmonary bypass is low and not pulsatile [4–6].

Many steps should be taken to obtain optimal results after cardiovascular surgery in terms of adequate lung protection. First, heart teams must be aware of the importance of lung circulation for the postoperative quality of the procedure. In addition, they must be concerned about managing inflammatory factors, which can considerably impair surgical outcomes, and bear in mind that coronary perfusion is as relevant as lung perfusion. Perhaps we still need to devote major effort to convincing heart teams to add lung protection to their operative checklist [7, 8]. Implementation of lung protection can be carried out by employing some of the strategies depicted in Table 33.1 [9].

The role of two substances in lung protection – protein C and adenosine – has been extensively addressed in recent papers worldwide. Thus, understanding their mechanism of action and the effective impact on pulmonary function will allow heart surgeons to attenuate the inflammatory response and ischemia-reperfusion injury during heart surgery [10].

Protein C has an activated form – activated protein C; this is a natural anticoagulant generated by the thrombin-thrombomodulin complex on endothelial cells. In addition to the anticoagulant role, this activated protein has antiinflammatory properties as it downregulates proinflammatory cytokines and regulates cardiopulmonary bypass-induced neutrophil activation [10, 11].

Yamakazi et al. [12] designed intriguing experimental research depicting the inflammatory and functional benefits of using activated protein C in heart surgery requiring

Table 33.1 Strategies for lung protection in heart surgery

Utilization of heparin-coated circuits
Utilization of synthetic co-polymer(methacrylate)-coated circuits
Utilization of phosphorylcholine-coated circuits
Use of ultrafiltration techniques
Use of leukocytes filters
Use of the Drew-Anderson technique[a]
Lung perfusion with controlled perfusion pressure
Lung perfusion with antibiotics and antiinflammatory solutions
Lung perfusion with pulsatile flow
Lung perfusion with low-volume ventilation
Inhalation of NO
Inhalation of CO
Miniaturized cardiopulmonary circuit
Management of hemodilution
Monoclonal anticytokine antibodies

[a]Technique designed to keep lungs ventilating in such a way that lungs are natural oxygenators.

E.A. Gabriel, MD, PhD (✉)
Department of Cardiovascular Surgery,
University Nove de Julho, São Paulo, Brazil
e-mail: edag@uol.com.br

S.A. Gabriel, MD
Department of Vascular Surgery,
Pontifical Catholic University of Campinas,
São Paulo, Brazil

Department of Vascular Surgery,
Celso Pierro Hospital and Maternity,
Campinas, São Paulo, Brazil
e-mail: sthefanogabriel@yahoo.com.br

E.A. Gabriel, S.A. Gabriel (eds.), *Inflammatory Response in Cardiovascular Surgery*,
DOI 10.1007/978-1-4471-4429-8_33, © Springer-Verlag London 2013

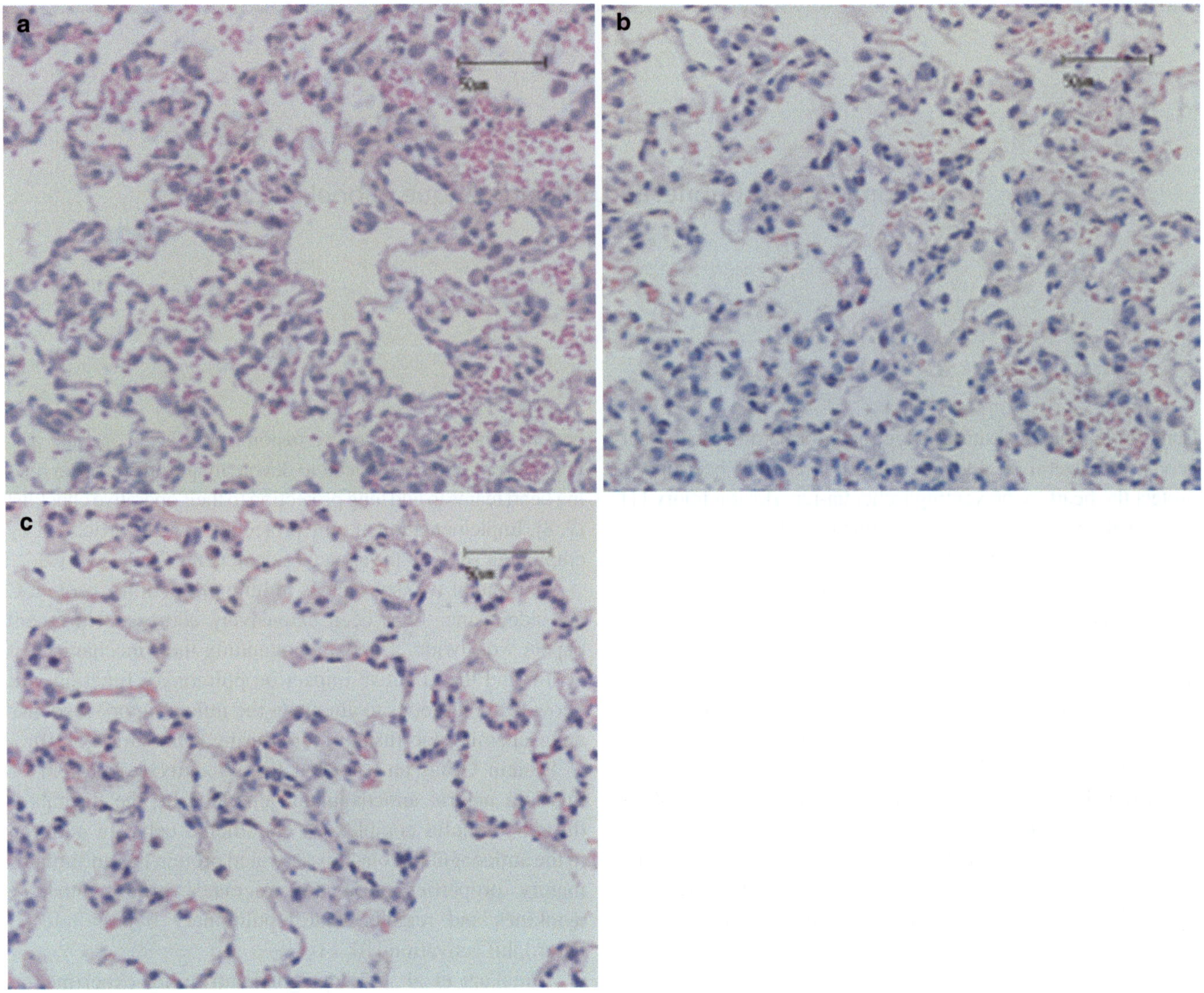

Fig. 33.1 Microphotograph of the left lung. The left lung section in each group was stained with hematoxylin & eosin. Lungs in the control and DIP groups show interstitial edema, alveolar hemorrhage, and severe neutrophil accumulation. Inflammatory change in the APC group lung is minimized. Original magnification: x200. *Black bar* = 50 μm. Control (**a**), DIP (**b**), and APC (**c**) groups

cardiopulmonary bypass. These authors defined three groups as follows: control, DIP (intravenous inactive derivative of activated protein C), and APC (intravenous activated protein C). Histological analysis, arterial oxygen pressure, proinflammatory marker concentration, and CD11b expression are shown in Figs. 33.1, 33.2, 33.3, and 33.4. These figures allow us to suggest that, in terms of pulmonary function, activated protein C can play a protective role, minimizing inflammatory injury and providing functional balance [12].

Adenosine is a useful substance for lung protection that can be employed either during heart-lung procedures or during ex vivo lung perfusion. Thus, it is evident that adenosine plays a remarkable role in conventional heart-lung operations and some particular operations, such as heart-lung transplantation/lung transplantation [13].

Taking into consideration that adenosine has many relevant benefits for lung protection, a feasible strategy would be to use adenosine agonists in an attempt to improve lung function. Based on this concept, Emaminia et al. [14] just published an experimental study in which two groups were assigned according to the strategy of ex vivo lung perfusion. The control group (EVLP) underwent 14 h of ischemia, and subsequently the lungs were perfused with a protective solution for 5 h. The treatment group (EVLP+ adenosine agonist) underwent the same procedure, but the lungs were perfused with the same protective solution plus a selective adenosine agonist.

Some results obtained by Emaminia et al. [14] corroborate the protective effects of adenosine as well as adenosine agonists in lung function (Figs. 33.5 and 33.6). Its benefits are seen in terms of less mean airway pressure and less expression of inflammatory markers.

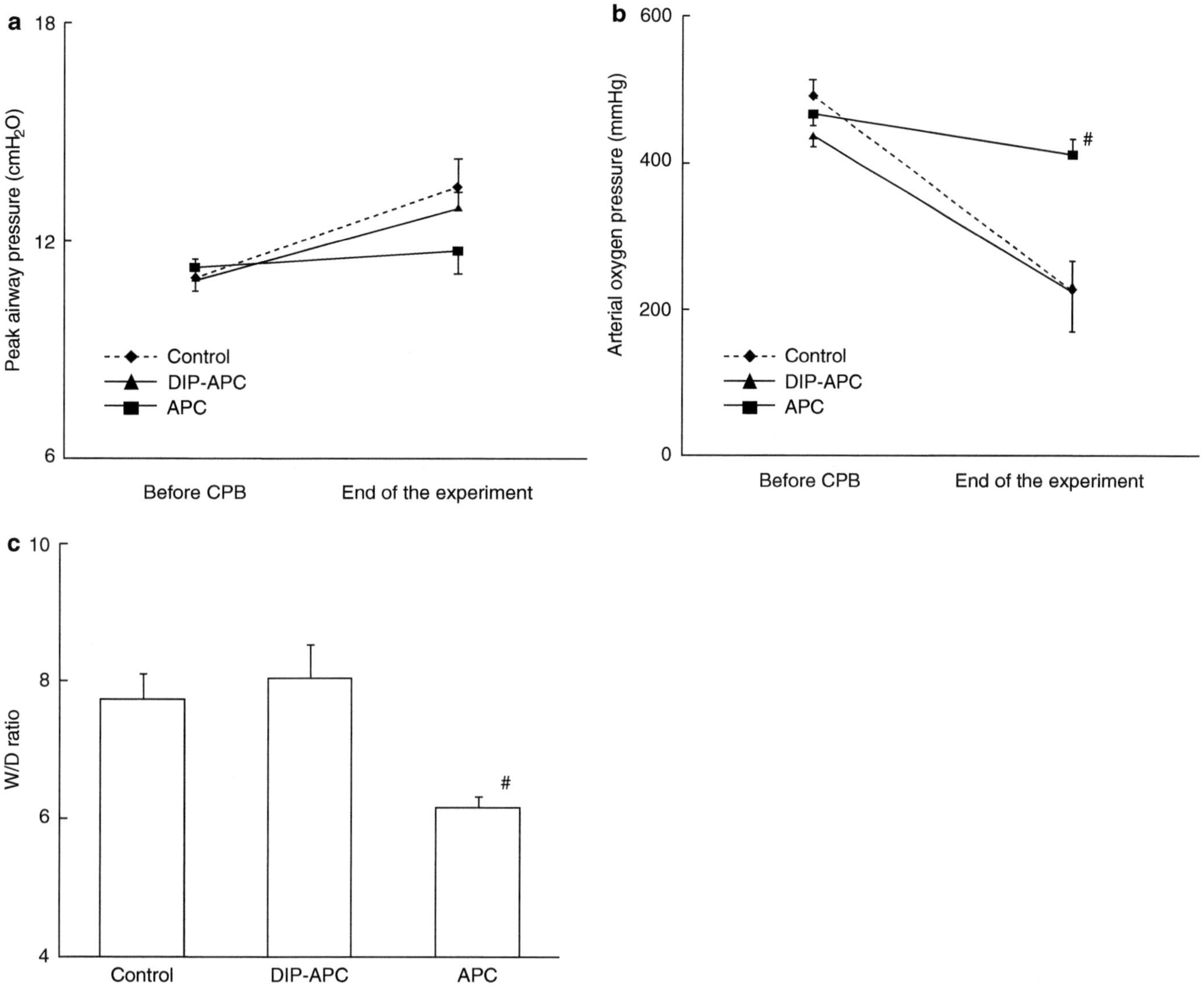

Fig. 33.2 (**a**) Peak airway pressure before CPB and at the end of the experiment. The APC group shows a relatively lower value than the other groups at the end of the experiment, although there are no significant differences among the groups. Results are expressed as mean ± standard error of the mean (SEM). (**b**) Arterial oxygen pressure before CPB and at the end of the experiment. The APC group shows a significantly higher value than the other groups at the end of the experiment. Results are expressed as mean ± SEM. #$P<0.01$ versus the control or DIP group. (**c**) W/D weight ratio of the left lung. The APC group shows a significantly lower value than the other groups. Results are expressed as mean ± SEM. #$P<0.01$ versus the control or DIP group. *APC* activated protein C, *CPB* cardiopulmonary bypass, *DIP* diisopropyl fluorophosphate, *W/D* wet to dry

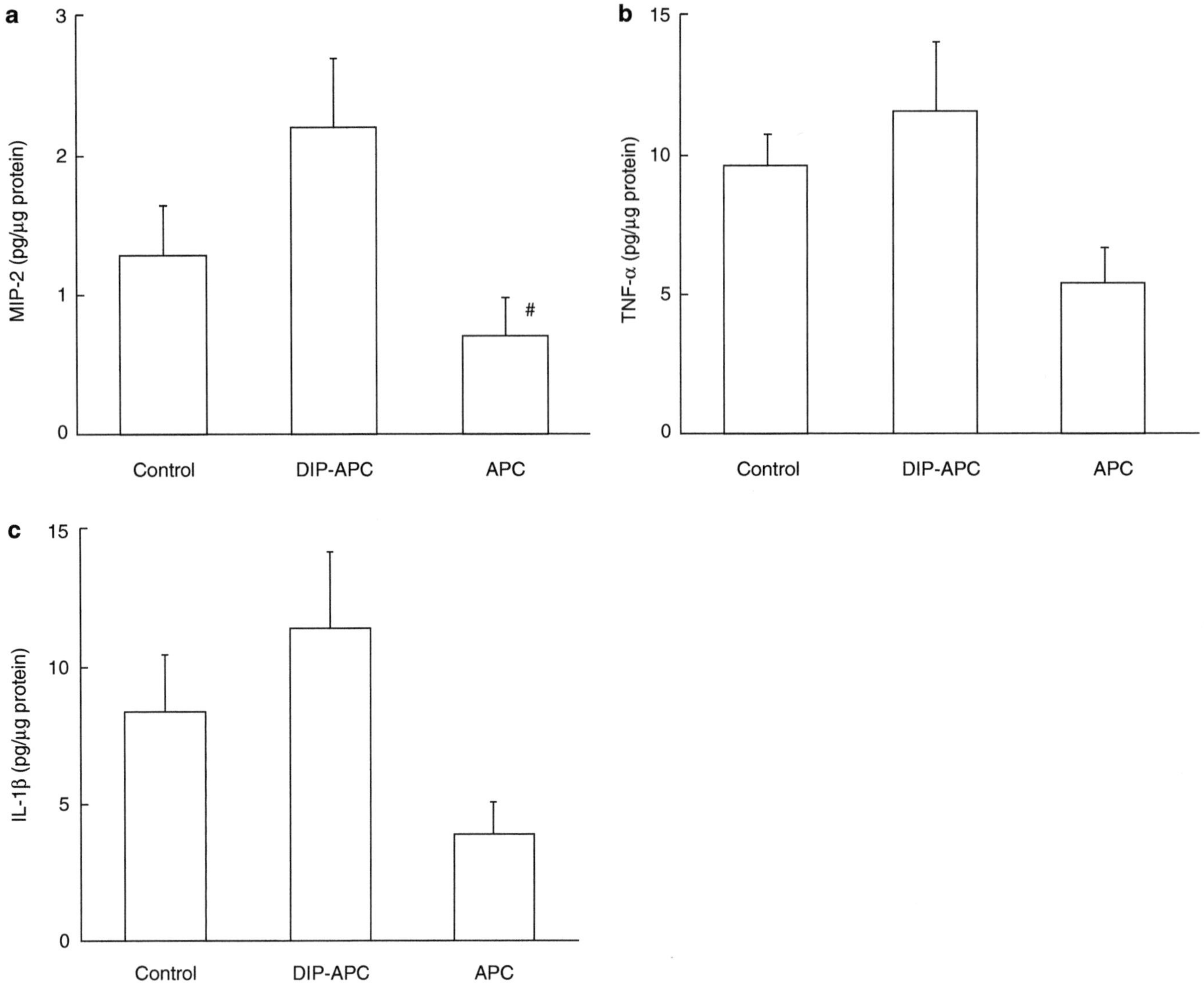

Fig. 33.3 (**a**) Tissue MIP-2 concentration in the left lung. The APC group shows a relatively lower value than the control group and a significantly lower value than the DIP group. Results are expressed as mean ± SEM. #$P<0.01$ versus the DIP group. (**b**) Tissue TNF-a concentration in the left lung. The APC group shows a relatively lower value than the other groups, although there are no significant differences among the groups. Results are expressed as mean ± SEM. (**c**) Tissue IL-1b concentration in the left lung. The APC group shows a relatively lower value than the other groups, although there are no significant differences among the groups. Results are expressed as mean ± SEM. *DIP* diisopropyl fluorophosphate, *APC* activated protein C, *TNF* tumor necrosis factor, *MIP* macrophage inflammatory protein, *IL* interleukin

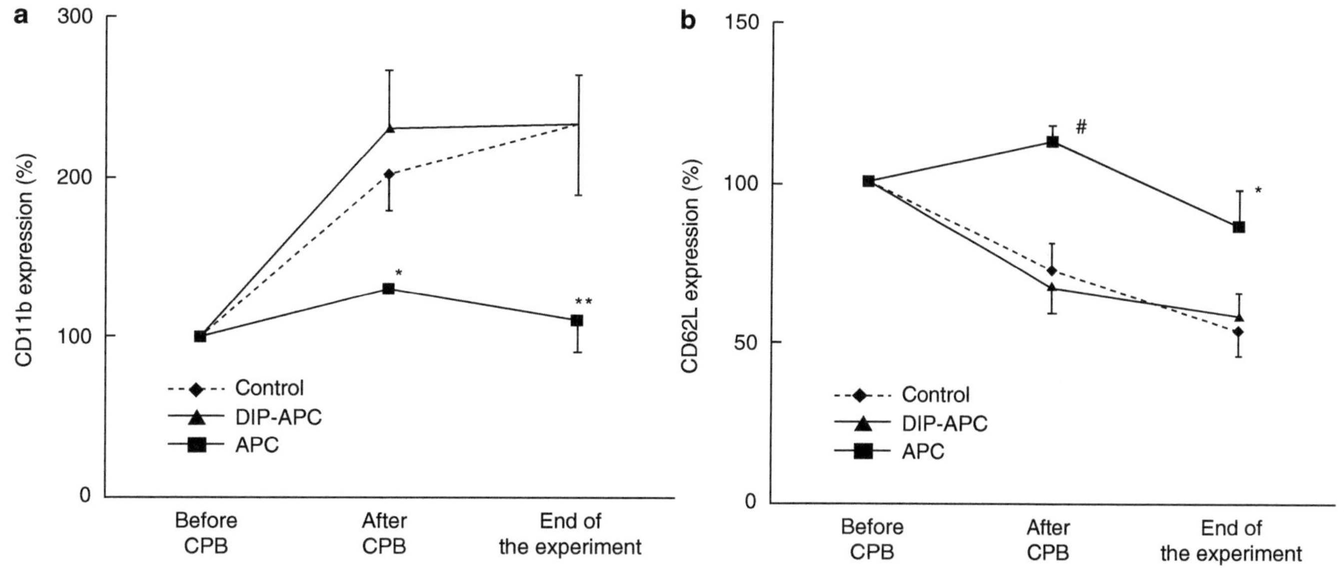

Fig. 33.4 (**a**) CD11b expression in circulating neutrophils. Percentage change in geometric mean from the value before CPB was calculated. The APC group maintains level CD11b expression at all of the time points, whereas expression in the control and DIP groups approximately doubles at 60 and 120 min after the initiation of CPB. Results are expressed as mean ± SEM. *$P<0.05$ versus the DIP group. **$P<0.05$ versus the control or DIP group. (**b**) CD62L expression on circulating neutrophils. Percentage change in geometric mean from the value before CPB was calculated. CD62L expression remains level in the APC throughout the experiment, whereas expression in the control and DIP groups gradually decreases to approximately 50 % at 120 min after the initiation of CPB. Results are expressed as mean ± SEM. #$P<0.01$ versus the control or DIP group. *$P<0.05$ versus the DIP group. *CPB* cardiopulmonary bypass, *DIP* diisopropyl fluorophosphate, *APC* activated protein C

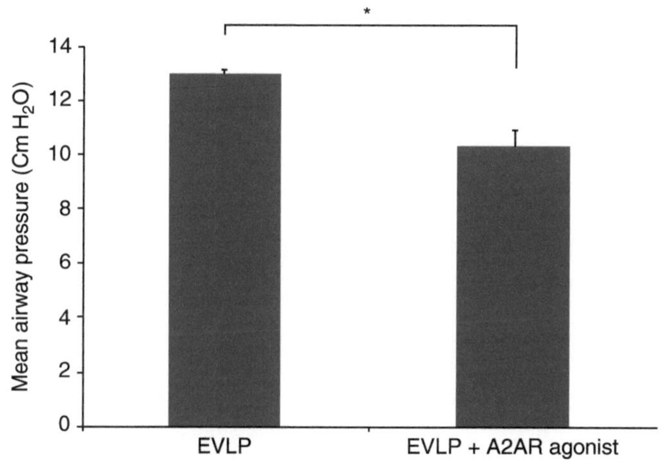

Fig. 33.5 Comparison of the wet-dry (W/D) weight ratio between the treatment and control groups. Low edema formation rates were observed in lungs exposed to the A2A agonist; *$P = 0.03$. *EVLP* ex vivo lung perfusion, *A2AR* A2A receptor

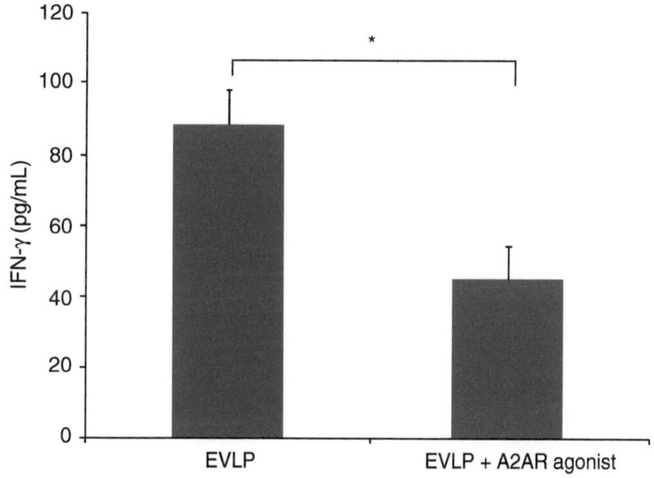

Fig. 33.6 Tissue level of interferon gamma (IFNγ) was significantly lower in treatment lungs after 5 h of ex vivo lung perfusion (*EVLP*) and exposure to adenosine A2A agonist; *$P = 0.05$. *A2AR* A2A receptor

References

1. Sievers HH, Freund-Kaas C, Eleftheriadis S, Fischer T, Kuppe T, Kraatz EG, et al. Lung protection during total cardiopulmonary bypass by isolated lung perfusion: preliminary results of a novel perfusion strategy. Ann Thorac Surg. 2002;74:1167–72.
2. Farivar AS, Delgado MF, McCourtie AS, Barnes AD, Verrier ED, Mulligan MS. Crosstalk between thrombosis and inflammation in lung reperfusion injury. Ann Thorac Surg. 2006;81:1061–7.
3. Zhang L, Kumar S, Kaminski A, Kasch C, Sponholz C, Stamm C, et al. Importance of endothelial nitric oxide synthase for the hypothermic protection of lungs against ischemia-reperfusion injury. J Thorac Cardiovasc Surg. 2006;131:969–74.
4. Iglesias M, Jungebluth P, Petit C, Matute MP, Rovira I, Martínez E, et al. Extracorporeal lung membrane provides better lung protection than conventional treatment for severe postpneumonectomy noncardiogenic acute respiratory distress syndrome. J Thorac Cardiovasc Surg. 2008;135:1362–71.
5. Gazoni LM, Walters DM, Unger EB, Linden J, Kron IL, Laubach VE. Activation of A1, A2A, or A3 adenosine receptors attenuates lungischemia-reperfusion injury. J Thorac Cardiovasc Surg. 2010;140:440–6.
6. Krishnadasan B, Naidu BV, Byrne K, Fraga C, Verrier ED, Mulligan MS. The role of proinflammatory cytokines in lung ischemia-reperfusion injury. J Thorac Cardiovasc Surg. 2003;125:261–72.
7. Naidu BV, Woolley SM, Farivar AS, Thomas R, Fraga CH, Goss CH, et al. Early tumor necrosis factor-α release from the pulmonary macrophage in lung ischemia-reperfusion injury. J Thorac Cardiovasc Surg. 2004;127:1502–8.
8. Anvari F, Sharma AK, Fernandez LG, Hranjec T, Ravid K, Kron IL, et al. Tissue-derived proinflammatory effect of adenosine A_{2B} receptor inlung ischemia – reperfusion injury. J Thorac Cardiovasc Surg. 2010;140:871–7.
9. Carvalho EMF, Gabriel EA, Salerno TA. Pulmonary protection during cardiac surgery: systematic literature review. Asian Cardiovasc Thorac Ann. 2008;16:503–7.
10. Murakami K, Okajima K, Uchiba M, Johno M, Nakagaki T, Okabe H, et al. Activated protein C prevents LPS-induced pulmonary vascular injury by inhibiting cytokine production. Am J Physiol. 1997;272:L197–202.
11. Lisle TC, Gazoni LM, Fernandez LG, Sharma AK, Bellizzi AM, Schifflett GD, et al. Inflammatory lung injury after cardiopulmonary bypass is attenuated by adenosine A_{2A} receptor activation. J Thorac Cardiovasc Surg. 2008;136:1280–8.
12. Yamazaki S, Inamori S, Nakatani T, Suga M. Activated protein C attenuates cardiopulmonary bypass-induced acutelung injury through the regulation of neutrophil activation. J Thorac Cardiovasc Surg. 2011;141:1246–52.
13. Link AA, Kino T, Worth JA, McGuire JL, Crane ML, Chrousos GP, et al. Ligand-activation of the adenosine A2a receptors inhibits IL-12 production by human monocytes. J Immunol. 2000;164:436–42.
14. Emaminia A, LaPar DJ, Zhao Y, Steidle JF, Harris DA, Laubach VE, et al. Adenosine A_{2A} agonist improves lung function during ex vivo lung perfusion. Ann Thorac Surg. 2011;92:1840–6.

Part X

Coronary Artery Disease

Fifteen Years of 'No-Touch' Saphenous Vein Harvesting in Patients Undergoing Coronary Artery Bypass Surgery: What Have We Learned?

34

Michael R. Dashwood and Domingos S.R. Souza

Introduction

Coronary artery disease (CAD) is the major cause of mortality in the Western world. Methods for restoring blood supply to the heart have changed over the years and include percutaneous transluminal coronary angioplasty (PTCA), bare metal or drug-eluting stents, with more recent attempts using techniques such as gene targeting and stem cell therapy. Once these techniques have failed, the remaining method for revascularization of the myocardium is coronary artery bypass surgery (CABG) using autologous blood vessel grafts as 'conduits,' restoring blood supply to diseased heart muscle. The main vessels used include the internal thoracic artery (ITA), radial artery (RA), and saphenous vein (SV). The success of CABG relies on the long-term patency of the conduit used for revascularization. Originally, SV grafts were used, but the ITA has subsequently become the first conduit of choice since it has superior patency compared with SV grafts [1, 2]. The poor long-term results with SV grafts and the encouraging results with ITA have led to a search for other arterial conduits for CABG. Among arterial grafts, the radial artery (RA) has gained the widest popularity as in many studies it has shown an excellent long-term patency [3] compared to SV grafts. However, recent studies have shown no difference between RA and SV grafts regarding their clinical outcome [4] or patency [5]. There is no doubt that the SV remains an important and the most widely used complementary conduit for patients undergoing CABG, and improvement of its long-term patency has been a major goal.

M.R. Dashwood, PhD (✉)
Department of Clinical Biochemistry,
Royal Free and University College Medical School,
London NW3 2QG, UK
e-mail: m.dashwood@ucl.ac.uk

D.S.R. Souza, MD, PhD
Department of Cardiovascular Surgery
and Anesthesiology, Örebro University Hospital,
Örebro, Sweden
e-mail: domingos.souza.orebro@gmail.com

Saphenous Vein: Structure

As with most blood vessels, the SV is characterized by three main layers (Fig. 34.1):

1. The innermost layer, the intima, consisting of little more than a thin basement membrane and its endothelial lining.
2. The middle layer, the media, consisting mainly of vascular smooth muscle cells (VSMCs) separated by collagen in which the vasa vasorum is located.
3. The outermost layer, the adventitia, is the thickest layer and is composed of collagen fibers and fibroblasts that merge with the surrounding connective tissue and fat. Also, within the adventitia are embedded the vascular (autonomic) nerves and vasa vasorum. Surrounding the adventitia is a pronounced cushion of perivascular fat (PVF).

The inner border of the media and intima is divided by the internal elastic lamina. In medium-sized veins, such as the SV, the intima is thrown into folds, and there may be signs of thickening due to the presence of smooth muscle cells and collagen within regions of neointimal hyperplasia. These features are only seen in 'normal,' non-distended/immersion-fixed sections and often not represented by published examples that have been perfusion fixed at ~100 mmHg compared with the vein's normal ~10 mmHg basal pressure. The media and adventitia are divided by the external elastic lamina, which is less distinct in veins than arteries. The vascular nerves are located in the adventitia, and also within this layer is a microvessel network, the vasa vasorum, which penetrates the media and may extend into the vessel lumen. During conventional vein harvesting, all vessel layers are damaged to varying degrees.

Intima and Endothelium

The single layer of cells lining the vein lumen, the endothelium, is affected during harvesting. There may be some 'mechanical' detachment of endothelial cells caused during removal and handling during surgery. The most striking

E.A. Gabriel, S.A. Gabriel (eds.), *Inflammatory Response in Cardiovascular Surgery*,
DOI 10.1007/978-1-4471-4429-8_34, © Springer-Verlag London 2013

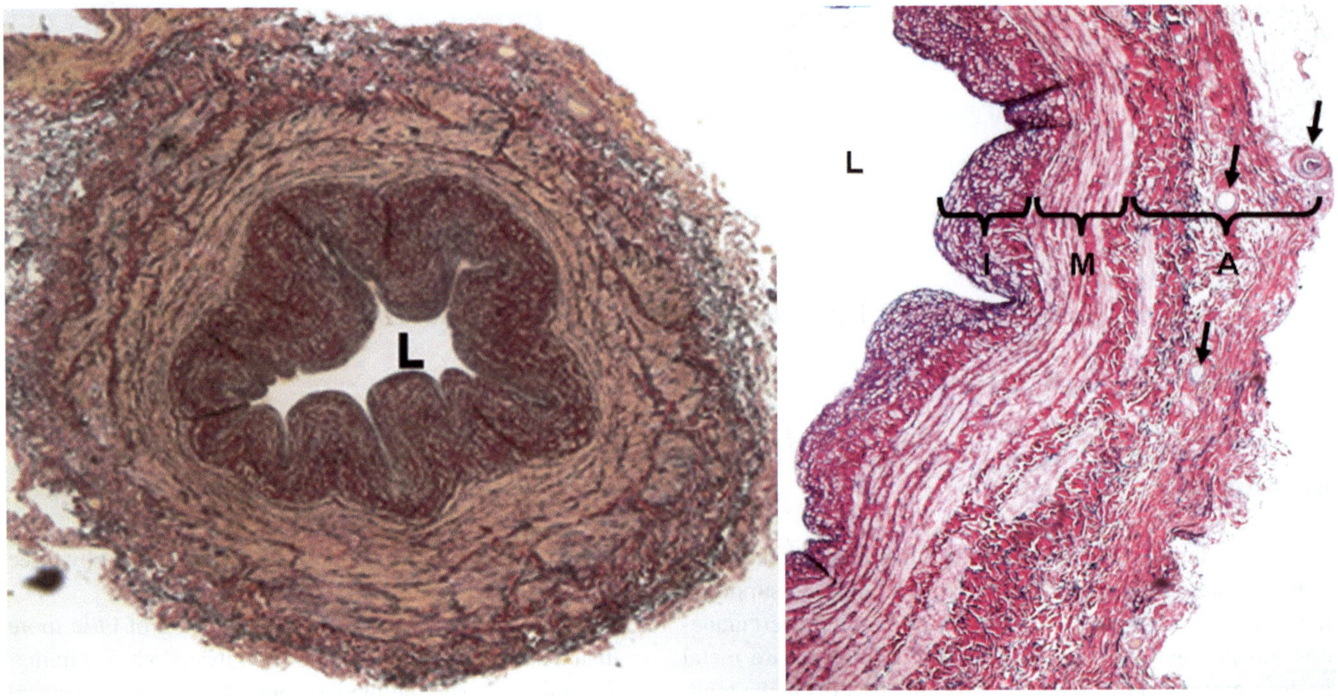

Fig. 34.1 Structure of human saphenous vein. (*Left*) Whole transverse section of non-distended human saphenous vein (*SV*) where the intima, surrounding the lumen (*L*) is thrown into folds. (*Right*) High magnification of the wall of the SV showing the three distinct layers (*I* intima, *M* media, *A* adventitia). The *arrows* indicate the vasa vasorum

effect is the dramatic endothelial denudation caused by distension at pressures of up to or over 700 mmHg [6]. While these effects are apparent by light microscopy [7], further shape changes and cell detachment are revealed using electron microscopy [8, 9] (Fig. 34.2). Apart from the striking effects observed on the endothelium, distension-induced 'smoothing' of the intima has been described where the folds that are evident in non-distended vein segments are absent in veins that have been subjected to high-pressure intraluminal distension [10] (Fig. 34.3). There may also be evidence of damage to cells within the intima as well as rupture of the internal elastic lamina.

Media

While the VSMCs that predominate within the media control venous tone, they may also alter their phenotype from contractile to synthetic. In this state these cells migrate and proliferate and are associated with the medial and intimal thickening observed in occluded vein grafts. Although there may be some damage to the media caused by manipulation by surgical instruments, the most pronounced effect is due to high-pressure distension during harvesting. This additional insult causes considerable thinning of the vessel wall [10] (Fig. 34.3), presumably because of overstretching of smooth muscle cells exposed to high/raised circumferential pressures. Again, dramatic cellular changes have been reported within the media, with striking shape changes to VSMCs as well as intracellular effects, including increased signs of nuclear division [8]. In addition to the effects on medial VSMCs, there are signs of damage to the vasa vasorum, where many of these microvessels appear collapsed and their endothelial cells misshapen and/or occluded by erythrocytes [8].

Adventitia

It is the adventitia, the outermost layer of the SV, that is generally removed or severely damaged during conventional harvesting but spared when using Souza's 'no-touch' technique [11] (Figs. 34.3 and 34.4). First, along with its adjacent connective tissue and cushion of surrounding fat, the adventitia constitutes a robust perivascular structure that protects the vein against the effects of altered hemodynamics once implanted into the coronary arterial system. In addition to this mechanical role, the adventitia contains the major proportion of autonomic nerves innervating the vessel, as well the vasa vasorum, microvessels responsible for the exchange of gases and nutrient supply to the vessel wall. Although the excised vein is essentially denervated, removal of the adventitia will further reduce the perivascular nerves, although these have been shown to proliferate in experimental porcine grafts [12, 13].

Perhaps the most serious consequence of removing the adventitia is the damage caused to the vasa vasorum (Fig. 34.5). There is convincing evidence from experimental

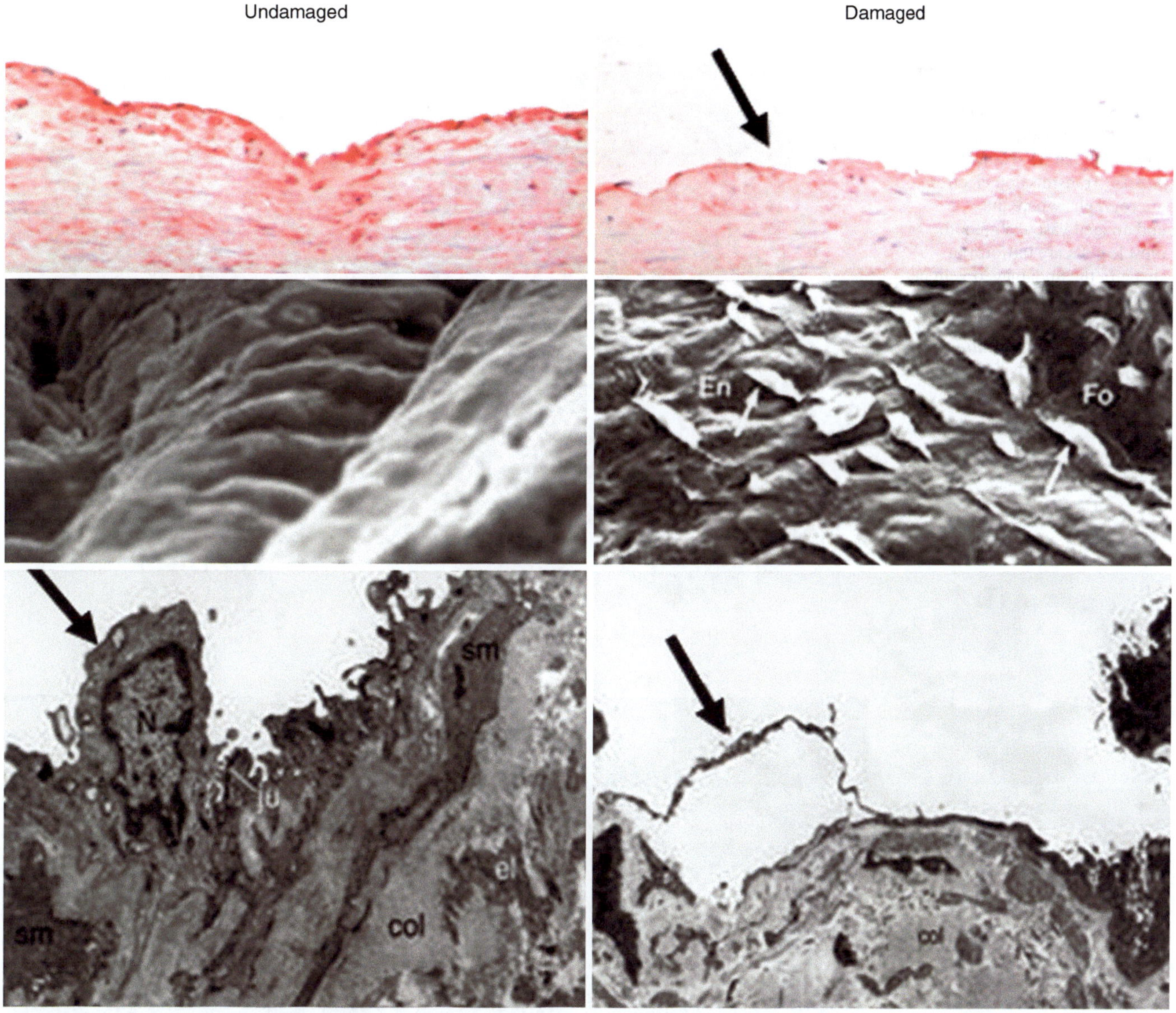

Fig. 34.2 Endothelium of undamaged and damaged human saphenous vein. The panels on the *left* are representative examples from undamaged (no-touch) veins and on the *right* are damaged (conventional) veins. The *top panels* show immunohistochemical localization of luminal endothelium (identified using CD31: *red stain*), which is continuous in the undamaged vein. In the damaged (conventional) vein, there are large areas of endothelial denudation (*arrow*). The *middle panels* show examples of scanning electron micrographs of en face preparations of human SV where there is a smooth, intact endothelium lining of undamaged veins but denudation and shape change of endothelial cells of the damaged vein. The *lower panels* show examples of transmission electron micrographs of luminal endothelial cells. There is a marked alteration in endothelial cells (*En*, *arrows*) in damaged versus undamaged veins. *sm* smooth muscle, *col* collagen, *N* nucleus, *Fo* luminal fold, *ju* junction, *el* elastin (Modified from Refs. [8, 9])

animal models that occlusion of the vasa vasorum by a close-fitting external collar [14] or adventitial removal [15] leads to neointimal hyperplasia and atherosclerosis, both features associated with vein graft failure. It has been suggested that these effects are mainly due to ischemia of the vessel's media, and this is supported by studies showing that reduced transmural oxygen levels are detected in occluded femoral arteries in an experimental model of atherosclerosis [14]. Interestingly, it has been shown that the vasa vasorum is affected by application of both dilator and constrictor compounds, suggesting that they play a role in the regulation of the tone of the vasa vasorum, implicating this microvessel network in conduit vessel physiology [16].

Perivascular Fat

Using the no-touch harvesting technique, the SV is removed with minimal surgical damage and complete with its pronounced cushion of perivascular fat (PVF) (Fig. 34.4). In this

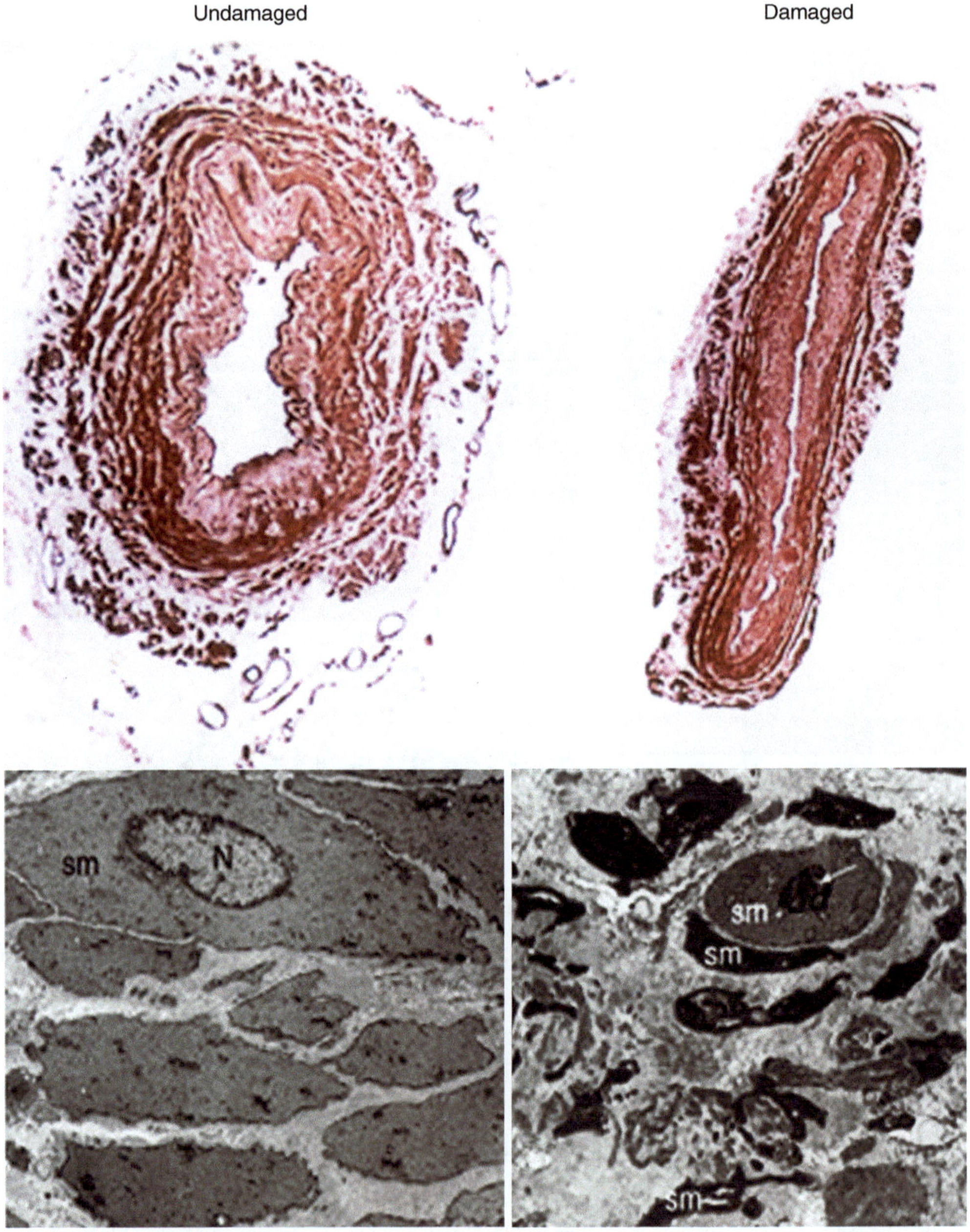

Fig. 34.3 Media and vascular smooth muscle of undamaged and damaged human saphenous vein. (*Top panels*) Representative transverse sections of undamaged vein (*left*) and damaged (*right*) human SV. (*Lower panels*) Transmission electron micrographs where the undamaged vascular smooth muscle cells are uniform in shape in the undamaged vein but exhibit dramatic shape changes in the damaged cells. *sm* smooth muscle, *N* nucleus, *small white arrow* nuclear division (Modified from Ref. [8])

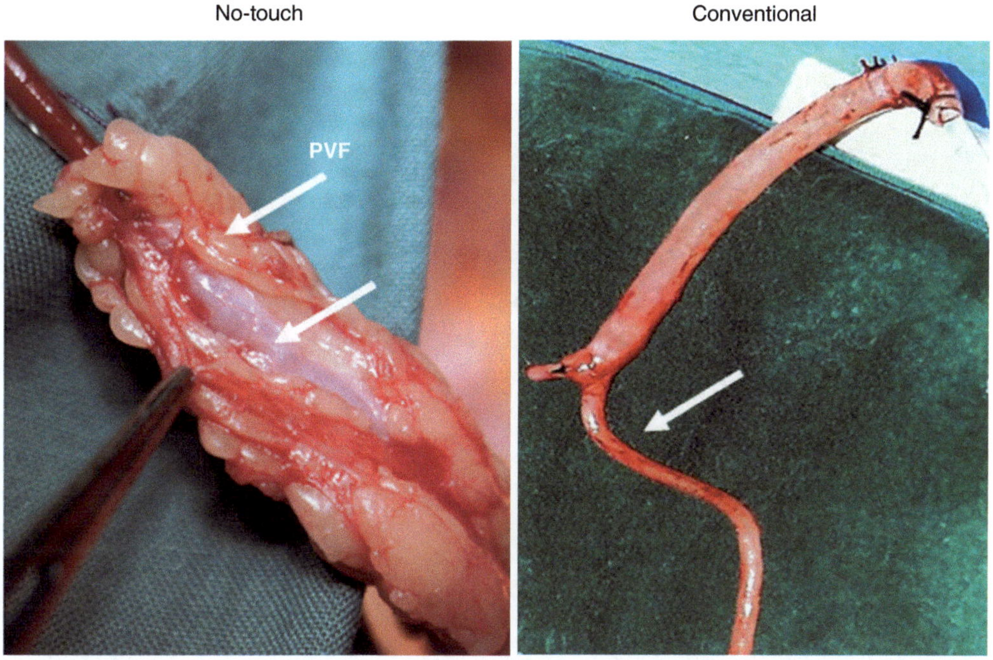

Fig. 34.4 No-touch and conventional saphenous vein used as bypass grafts in CABG. (*Left*) The no-touch vein is removed complete with its cushion of surrounding perivascular fat (*PVF*). Handling the vein via this cushion prevents the vein from going into spasm (*lower arrow*). (*Right*) Conventionally harvested vein is stripped of surrounding tissue causing spasm (*arrow*) that is overcome using high-pressure saline distension (shown at upper segment of the vein). To the *left* is a tied off side branch

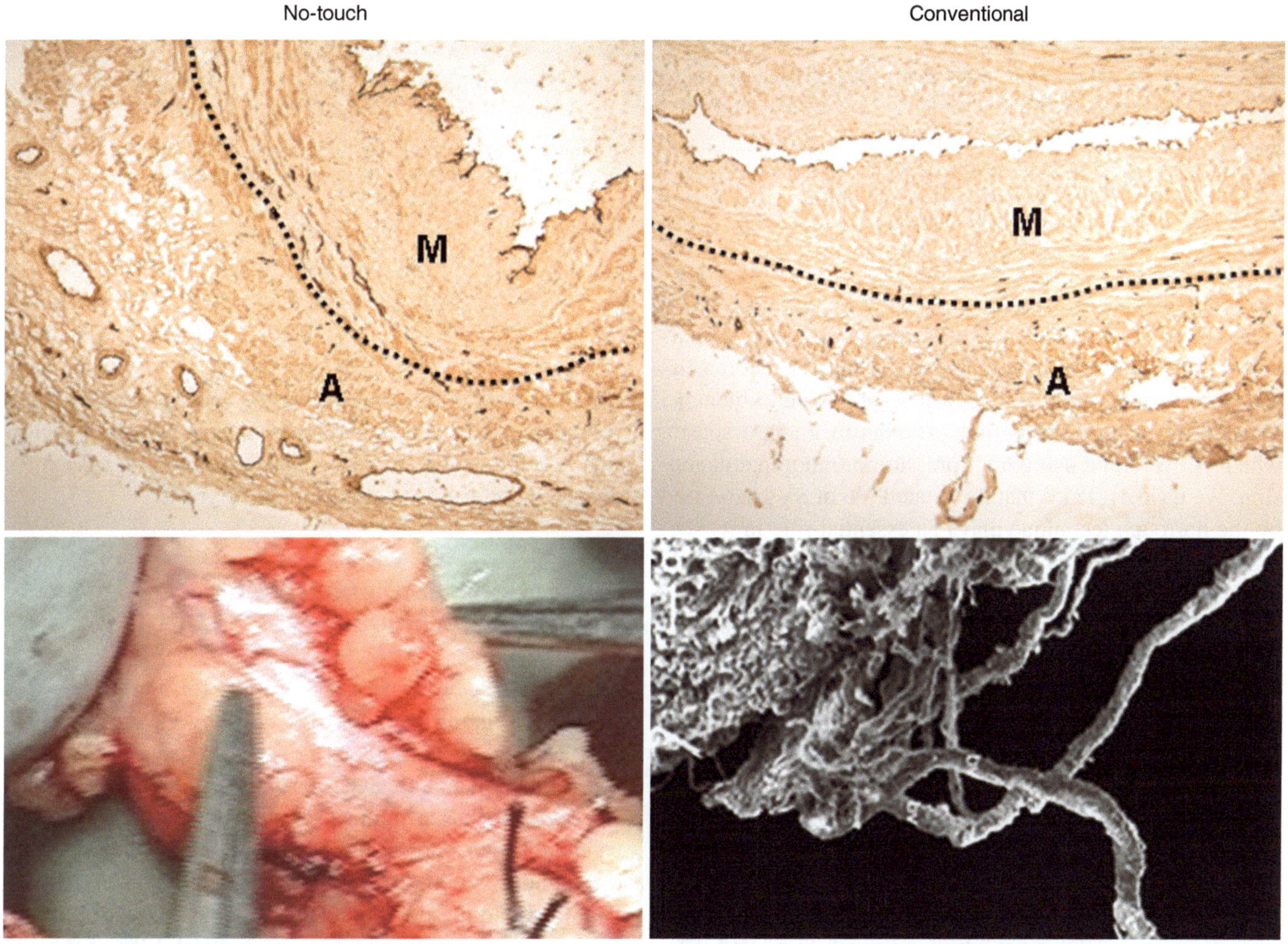

Fig. 34.5 Vasa vasorum of no-touch and conventionally harvested saphenous vein. *Left panels* show representative examples of a no-touch vein with adventitia intact. The *lower panel* shows retrograde blood flow through the adventitial vasa vasorum on release of vascular clamps at completion of graft insertion – evidence of luminal termination. *Right panels* show examples of conventionally harvested veins with much of the adventitia removed (*top panel*) with the *lower panel* showing a scanning electron micrograph of the damage to the adventitial vasa vasorum. The endothelial cells lining both the lumen and vasa vasorum in the *top panels* are identified using CD31 (dark immunostaining). The *dotted line* shows the external elastic lamina that separates the media (*M*) and adventitia (*A*)

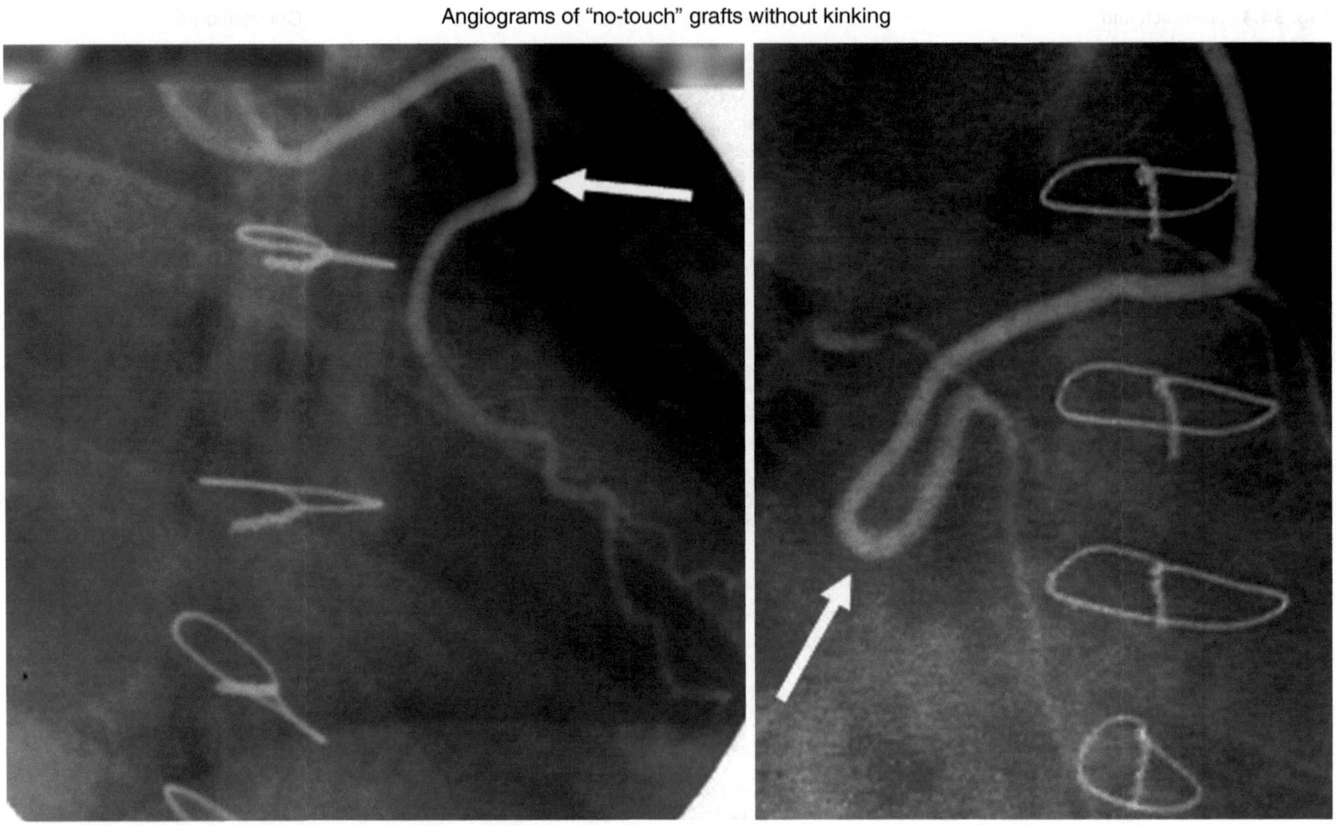

Fig. 34.6 Angiographic examples of no-touch saphenous vein grafts. Two examples of angiograms of no-touch saphenous vein grafts in CABG patients where the surrounding cushion of tissue prevents kinking (*arrows*), maintaining blood flow in excessively long grafts

way, the vein retains its normal architecture, providing superior graft patency when compared with veins prepared by conventional methods. When performing conventional harvesting, the vein is stripped of much of its surrounding tissue, a procedure that inflicts considerable vascular damage. In addition, a high proportion of veins to go into spasm, which is overcome using high-pressure intraluminal distension. We have evidence that the intact PVF of SVs harvested by the no-touch technique plays an essential role in its success. Since the vein is handled during surgery by the PVF, direct contact by surgical instruments and consequent spasm are avoided, distension is unnecessary, and the luminal endothelium remains intact. In addition, the vasa vasorum is preserved and the supply of oxygen and nutrients to the graft wall maintained. The PVF also provides mechanical support to the vein once implanted into the coronary arterial circulation where it acts as a buffer, protecting the graft against arterial hemodynamics as well as preventing kinking of excessively long grafts (Fig. 34.6). Finally, the surrounding cushion of fat is a source of adipocyte-derived relaxing factors (ADRFs) [17–19], many of which are vasculoprotective. For example, PVF surrounding no-touch-harvested SVs obtained from patients undergoing CABG is a potential source of NO, a vasorelaxant factor with antithrombotic, anti-inflammatory, and antiproliferative properties [20, 21]. We have also identified leptin in extracts of PVF from human SV [22]. Positive immunostaining for leptin is associated with adipocytes of the PVF surrounding the SV, and, as an adipokine with both vasorelaxant and angiogenic properties, we hypothesize that this, and other adipocyte-derived factors such as adiponectin [23], may play an important role in the improved performance of no-touch SV grafts.

Conventional Saphenous Vein Harvesting Technique

The SV has been the vessel of choice for autologous vein grafts since its introduction for CABG by Favarolo in 1969 [24]. The use of autologous grafts eliminates problems of tissue rejection and the need for tissue typing and matching. The SV also has a number of practical advantages: it is expendable, since lower limb drainage can rely solely on the deep venous system; its long length allows its use for multiple grafts, and its superficial position renders it easily accessible, facilitating its exposure at harvest [25]. Since its introduction as a graft, the SV has become the most commonly used conduit in patients undergoing CABG. However, the patency rate of this vessel is poor, with 15–25 % grafts occluding within 1 year and over 50 % patients requiring redo surgery within 10 years [26].

Although there may be minor modifications made by cardiac surgeons, during conventional harvesting, the SV is either harvested endoscopically or exposed by a longitudinal leg incision, where the surrounding connective tissue, including the adventitia, is stripped off and its side branches ligated. Generally, veins are then distended with saline to check for leakage, often at high pressure to overcome the spasm that occurs because of surgical trauma [25]. Rather than preserving their normal architecture, SV grafts are frequently prepared in such a way that they merely serve as channels (hence the general term "conduit") for redirecting blood flow past occluded regions of the coronary vasculature in order to maintain or restore myocardial perfusion. For example, the original paper describing the use of the SV as a bypass graft for CABG states that, "Care must be taken to dissect only the vein, avoiding as much as possible the adventitia that surrounds it" [24]. These instructions have been taken by many cardiac surgeons to indicate that the vein should be stripped of surrounding tissue at harvesting. Consequently, a high proportion of SVs go into spasm, with the high pressure saline distension employed causing further damage to the vein [22, 25]. The potential effect of vascular damage on graft patency has been recognized for some time, and various atraumatic dissecting techniques have been introduced in an attempt to improve vein graft performance [11, 27, 28].

No-Touch Saphenous Vein Harvesting

The particular 'no-touch' technique that is the focus of this chapter was described by Souza in1996 [11]. Various minor modifications have been made subsequently, with details of the technique, including video footage, available online (http://mmcts.ctsnetjournals.org/cgi/content/full/2009/0731/mmcts.2008.003624) [29]. Briefly, the day before the operation, a Duplex examination of the SV should be performed in order to mark the course of the vein on the skin. This allows an incision to be made precisely over the vein to avoid creating a flap of subcutaneous tissue, thus reducing the risk of complications such as hematomas, seromas, or infection. Also, on the day of CABG, the SV is located and harvested with minimal delay. It is imperative to follow the surgical technique in all details from harvesting to implantation. A longitudinal incision is made over the skin and the required length of vein exposed, keeping its perivascular tissue in place (Fig. 34.4). After exposure, a margin of about 0.5 cm is created around the vein to include the fat pedicle using electrocautery, and all visible side braches are ligated and divided at the same level (0.5 cm from the vein). The SV, together with its cushion of surrounding tissue, is then separated from its bed using scissors and electrocautery. The vein should be left in situ and covered with a moistened compress at least until a few minutes after heparinization. This allows continuous heparinized blood perfusion to be carried out and obviates the need for rinsing or flushing the vein with saline solution. After removal, the vein is stored in heparinized blood obtained from the aortic cannula. While performing the anastomosis, the vein is handled via the surrounding cushion, thereby avoiding direct contact between the vein and instruments. This prevents spasm from occurring. After each completed distal anastomosis, the vein graft is briefly connected to the arterial cannula of the cardiopulmonary bypass system using a three-way stopcock to check for any leakage from the anastomosis or side branches. Manual distension using a syringe should be avoided, as this procedure damages the endothelial lining of the lumen [3, 7, 10]. After removal of the aortic cross-clamp, and before suturing the proximal anastomoses, the grafts are once again connected to the arterial line. This procedure assists in determining the graft length and maintains the vein in a dilated condition. Accordingly, this is a true "no-touch" technique as the SV is not handled with instruments nor is it distended or flushed during the whole procedure. SVs prepared by this no-touch technique exhibit an improved early graft performance [30, 31] with patency at 18 months for no-touch SV grafts of 95 % versus 89 % for conventional grafts and similar to the ITA. A long-term (mean 8.5 years) follow-up study described a no-touch SV graft patency that was comparable to the ITA (both 90 %) and superior to conventional SV grafts (76 %) [32].

Vein Harvesting and Vascular Damage

Clearly, damage to the proximal and distal segments of the SV to be grafted is inevitable since the vessel is 'disconnected' from the remainder of the native vein during harvesting. There seems no basis for the additional damage caused when 'clearing' the vein of surrounding tissue apart from identifying leaks and ligating side branches. Otherwise, stripping the vein of adherent tissue appears to be only for 'aesthetic' purposes. In isolating the vein from its outer cushion, we believe that subsequent graft occlusion is associated with a number of factors ranging from endothelial disruption to medial ischemia and altered vascular smooth muscle compliance and deformation resulting from the removal of the mechanical influences of the vein's outer layer and surrounding cushion of tissue. When using conventional harvesting procedures the luminal endothelium is denuded mainly because of the high pressure distension used to overcome spasm [7–9, 33] (Fig. 34.2), ultrastructural changes occur to the VSMCs in the media [8] (Fig. 34.3), and the damage to the adventitia when removing the SV causes severing of the vasa vasorum [10, 34] (Fig. 34.5) and sectioning of the perivascular nerves [35, 36]. A clinical study demonstrated that, by avoiding this vascular damage, more patients receiving no-touch-harvested SV grafts were free from angina with fewer patients with cardiac death or myocardial infarction than with conventionally harvested grafts [37]. A study employing angiography and intravascular ultrasound showed that, at a mean time of 8.3 years, no-touch SV grafts had a lower intimal thickness, fewer multiple/advanced plaques and less plaque thickness, as well as a lower progression of atherosclerosis than conventional SV grafts [38].

Vascular Damage and Vein Graft Performance

When using the SV as a graft, this vessel, which is normally subjected to low pressures (~5–8 mmHg), non-pulsatile flow, and a shear stress of ~0.2 dyn/cm^2, is grafted into the coronary arterial system where it is subjected to high pressures (~60–140 mmHg), pulsatile flow, and a shear stress of ~3–6 dyn/cm^2 [39]. These conditions lead to the 'remodeling' or 'arterialization' that contributes to graft failure when the SV is used in revascularization procedures. The combined effects of altered hemodynamics, shear stress, and increased pulsatile flow stimulates the release of a number of endothelium-derived factors [40] and causes a proportion of the VSMCs to undergo a phenotypic change from the contractile to synthetic, factors associated with vein graft occlusion [41]. Furthermore, although the role of the vasa vasorum in supplying the vessel wall with oxygen and nutrients has been recognized for some time [42], the importance of this microvessel network in maintaining 'healthy vessels' is frequently ignored, and it is severely damaged when using most conventional harvesting techniques. This interruption of transmural flow renders the vessel wall ischemic, a condition triggering many of the processes involved in vein graft failure [14, 15].

Endovascular Vein Harvesting (EVH)

In recent years, endoscopic vein harvesting (EVH) has become popular, particularly in the USA. Apart from reducing the incidence of wound infection associated with conventional 'open' surgery, a major attraction of this method is the cosmetic outcome. Although the patency rates of conventionally harvested SVs and those prepared by EVH are similar, an early review discusses the need to consider the cost implications of prolonged operating time and disposable instruments when converting from conventional harvesting to EVH [43]. Results from early multicentre studies describe the potential benefits of EVH, in particular the reduced wound-healing problems and shortening recuperation period when compared with conventional harvesting procedures [44].

There can be no doubt that EVH inevitably causes a degree of vascular damage, in particular to the outer layers of the vein. While a number of studies suggest that SV prepared by EVH, using the Mayo extraluminal dissector, preserves endothelial function [45] as well as endothelial integrity and eNOS content [46], our data suggest that any damage to, or removal of, the adventitia (as occurs using EVH) is likely to have a detrimental effect on the SV when used as a graft in CABG [7, 25], in particular through adverse effects on vascular tissue sources of nitric oxide [7, 20]. A recent study comparing the patency of 'open harvested' grafts versus those prepared by EVH showed that endoscopic harvesting resulted in increased vein graft failure and adverse clinical outcomes [47], supporting our suggestion that no-touch harvesting would result in superior SV grafts to those prepared endoscopically [48].

Concluding Remarks

The no-touch technique outlined in this chapter was introduced in 1996, a major aim being to reduce surgical trauma at harvesting and to preserve the vessel's normal architecture. Subsequent early and long-term follow-up studies showed that no-touch-harvested SVs have a dramatically improved patency rate, comparable to the ITA. Laboratory-based research techniques into mechanisms underlying the improved performance of no-touch SV grafts have revealed various potential processes, many of which were unexpected. With such promising follow-up results and supporting laboratory-based research data, it is disappointing that so many cardiac surgeons are not prepared to adopt this technique, particularly considering the profound benefits to patients undergoing CABG.

References

1. Lytle BW, Loop FD, Cosgrove DM, Ratliff NB, Easley K, Taylor PC. Long-term (5 to 12 years) serial studies of internal mammary artery and saphenous vein coronary bypass grafts. J Thorac Cardiovasc Surg. 1985;89:248–58.
2. Cameron A, Davis KB, Green G, Schaff HV. Coronary bypass surgery with internal-thoracic-artery grafts – effects on survival over a 15-year period. N Engl J Med. 1996;334:216–20.
3. Achouh P, Boutekadjirt R, Toledano D, et al. Long-term (5- to 20-year) patency of the radial artery for coronary bypass grafting. J Thorac Cardiovasc Surg. 2010;140:73–79.e2.
4. Acar C, Jebara VA, Portoghese M, et al. Revival of the radial artery for coronary artery bypass grafting. Ann Thorac Surg. 1992;54:652–9.
5. Tatoulis J, Royse AG, Buxton BF, et al. The radial artery in coronary surgery: a 5-year experience–clinical and angiographic results. Ann Thorac Surg. 2002;73:143–8.
6. Rosenfeldt FL, He GW, Buxton BF, Angus JA. Pharmacology of coronary artery bypass grafts. Ann Thorac Surg. 1999;67(3):878–88.
7. Tsui JC, Souza DS, Filbey D, Bomfim V, Dashwood MR. Preserved endothelial integrity and nitric oxide synthase in saphenous vein

grafts harvested by a 'no-touch' technique. Br J Surg. 2001;88: 1209–15.
8. Ahmed SR, Johansson BL, Karlsson MG, Souza DS, Dashwood MR, Loesch A. Human saphenous vein and coronary bypass surgery: ultrastructural aspects of conventional and "no-touch" vein graft preparations. Histol Histopathol. 2004;19(2):421–33.
9. Vasilakis V, Dashwood MR, Souza DS, Loesch A. Human saphenous vein and coronary bypass surgery: scanning electron microscopy of conventional and "no-touch" vein grafts. Vasc Dis Prev. 2004;1:133–9.
10. Dashwood MR, Savage K, Tsui JC, Dooley A, Shaw SG, Fernández Alfonso MS, et al. Retaining perivascular tissue of human saphenous vein grafts protects against surgical and distension-induced damage and preserves endothelial nitric oxide synthase and nitric oxide synthase activity. J Thorac Cardiovasc Surg. 2009;138(2): 334–40.
11. Souza D. A new "no-touch" preparation technique. Scand J Thorac Cardiovasc Surg. 1996;30:41–4.
12. Dashwood MR, Gibbins R, Mehta D, Bashar Izzat M, Angelini GD, Jeremy JY. Neural reorganisation in porcine vein grafts: a potential role for endothelin-1. Atherosclerosis. 2000;150(1):43–53.
13. Dashwood MR, Angelini GD, Wan S, Yim A, Mehta D, Izzat MB, et al. Does external stenting reduce porcine vein-graft occlusion via an action on vascular nerves? J Card Surg. 2002;17(6): 556–60.
14. Barker SG, Talbert A, Cottam S, Baskerville PA, Martin JF. Arterial intimal hyperplasia after occlusion of the adventitial vasa vasorum in the pig. Arterioscler Thromb. 1993;13:70–7.
15. Barker SG, Tilling LC, Miller GC, Beesley JE, Fleetwood G, Stavri GT, et al. The adventitia and atherogenesis: removal initiates intimal proliferation in the rabbit which regresses on generation of a 'neoadventitia'. Atherosclerosis. 1994;105:131–44.
16. Scotland RS, Vallance PJ, Ahluwalia A. Endogenous factors involved in regulation of tone of arterial vasa vasorum: implications for conduit vessel physiology. Cardiovasc Res. 2000;46(3): 403–11.
17. Gollasch M, Dubrovska G. Paracrine role for periadventitial adipose tissue in the regulation of arterial tone. Trends Pharmacol Sci. 2004;25(12):647–53.
18. Maenhaut N, Van de Voorde J. Regulation of vascular tone by adipocytes. BMC Med. 2011;9:25.
19. Gollasch M. Vasodilator signals from perivascular adipose tissue. Br J Pharmacol. 2012;165(3):633–42.
20. Dashwood MR, Dooley A, Shi-Wen X, Abraham DJ, Souza DS. Does periadventitial fat-derived nitric oxide play a role in improved saphenous vein graft patency in patients undergoing coronary artery bypass surgery? J Vasc Res. 2007;44(3):175–81.
21. Malinowski M, Deja MA, Gołba KS, Roleder T, Biernat J, Woś S. Perivascular tissue of internal thoracic artery releases potent nitric oxide and prostacyclin-independent anticontractile factor. Eur J Cardiothorac Surg. 2008;33(2):225–31.
22. Dashwood MR, Dooley A, Shi-Wen X, Abraham DJ, Dreifaldt M, Souza DS. Perivascular fat-derived leptin: a potential role in improved vein graft performance in coronary artery bypass surgery. Interact Cardiovasc Thorac Surg. 2011;12(2):170–3.
23. Fésüs G, Dubrovska G, Gorzelniak K, Kluge R, Huang Y, Luft FC, et al. Adiponectin is a novel humoral vasodilator. Cardiovasc Res. 2007;75(4):719–27.
24. Favaloro RG. Saphenous vein graft in the surgical treatment of coronary artery disease. Operative technique. J Thorac Cardiovasc Surg. 1969;58:178–85.
25. Tsui JC, Dashwood MR. Recent strategies to reduce vein graft occlusion: a need to limit the effect of vascular damage. Eur J Vasc Endovasc Surg. 2002;23(3):202–8.
26. Mehta D, Izzat MB, Bryan AJ, Angelini GD. Towards the prevention of vein graft failure. Int J Cardiol. 1997;62 Suppl 1:S55–63.
27. Gottlob R. The preservation of the venous endothelium by <<dissection without touching>> and by an atraumatic technique of vascular anastomosis. Minerva Chir. 1977;32:693–700.
28. Angelini GD, Bryan AJ, Hunter S, Newby AC. A surgical technique that preserves human saphenous vein functional integrity. Ann Thorac Surg. 1992;53(5):871–4.
29. Souza DSR, Arbeus M, Botelho Pinheiro B, Filbey D. The no-touch technique of harvesting the saphenous vein for coronary artery bypass grafting surgery. http://mmcts.ctsnetjournals.org/cgi/content/full/2009/0731/mmcts.2008.003624. Accessed on Jan 1, 2009.
30. Souza DS, Bomfim V, Skoglund H, Dashwood MR, Borowiec JW, Bodin L, et al. High early patency of saphenous vein graft for coronary artery bypass harvested with surrounding tissue. Ann Thorac Surg. 2001;71(3):797–800.
31. Souza DS, Dashwood MR, Tsui JC, Filbey D, Bodin L, Johansson B, et al. Improved patency in vein grafts harvested with surrounding tissue: results of a randomized study using three harvesting techniques. Ann Thorac Surg. 2002;73(4):1189–95.
32. Souza DS, Johansson B, Bojö L, Karlsson R, Geijer H, Filbey D, et al. Harvesting the saphenous vein with surrounding tissue for CABG provides long-term graft patency comparable to the left internal thoracic artery: results of a randomized longitudinal trial. J Thorac Cardiovasc Surg. 2006;132(2):373–8.
33. Souza DS, Christofferson RH, Bomfim V, Filbey D. "No-touch" technique using saphenous vein harvested with its surrounding tissue for coronary artery bypass grafting maintains an intact endothelium. Scand Cardiovasc J. 1999;33(6):323–9.
34. Dreifaldt M, Souza DS, Loesch A, Muddle JR, Karlsson MG, Filbey D, et al. The "no-touch" harvesting technique for vein grafts in coronary artery bypass surgery preserves an intact vasa vasorum. J Thorac Cardiovasc Surg. 2011;141(1):145–50.
35. Dashwood MR, Loesch A. The saphenous vein as a bypass conduit: the potential role of vascular nerves in graft performance. Curr Vasc Pharmacol. 2009;7(1):47–57.
36. Loesch A, Dashwood MR. On the sympathetic innervation of the human greater saphenous vein: relevance to clinical practice. Curr Vasc Pharmacol. 2009;7(1):58–67.
37. Johansson BL, Souza DS, Bodin L, Filbey D, Bojö L. No touch vein harvesting technique for CABG improves the long-term clinical outcome. Scand Cardiovasc J. 2009;43(1):63–8.
38. Johansson BL, Souza DS, Bodin L, Filbey D, Loesch A, Geijer H, et al. Slower progression of atherosclerosis in vein grafts harvested with 'no touch' technique compared with conventional harvesting technique in coronary artery bypass grafting: an angiographic and intravascular ultrasound study. Eur J Cardiothorac Surg. 2010;38(4): 414–9.
39. Lemson MS, Tordoir JH, Daemen MJ, Kitslaar PJ. Intimal hyperplasia in vascular grafts. Eur J Var Endovasc Surg. 2000;19: 336–50.
40. Vanhoutte PM. Endothelium and control of vascular function. State of the art lecture. Hypertension. 1989;13(6 Pt 2):658–67.
41. Dashwood MR, Mehta D, Izzat MB, Timm M, Bryan AJ, Angelini GD, et al. Distribution of endothelin-1 (ET) receptors (ET(A) and ET(B)) and immunoreactive ET-1 in porcine saphenous vein-carotid artery interposition grafts. Atherosclerosis. 1998;137(2):233–42.
42. Heistad DD, Marcus ML. Role of vasa vasorum in nourishment of the aorta. Blood Vessels. 1979;16(5):225–38.
43. Iafrati MM. Less-invasive saphenous harvest. Surg Clin North Am. 1999;79(3):623–44.
44. Rosenthal D, Arous EJ, Friedman SG, Ingegno MD, Johnson BL, Kraiss LW, et al. Endovascular-assisted versus conventional in situ saphenous vein bypass grafting: cumulative patency, limb salvage, and cost results in a 39-month multicenter study. J Vasc Surg. 2000;31(1 Pt 1):60–8.
45. Narayan P, Yeatman M, Caputo M, Capoun R, Ciulli F, Jeremy JY, et al. Saphenous vein harvest with the Mayo extraluminal dissector:

is endothelial function preserved? J Thorac Cardiovasc Surg. 2009;138(2):508–10.

46. Nowicki M, Buczkowski P, Miskowiak B, Konwerska A, Ostalska-Nowicka D, Dyszkiewicz W. Immunocytochemical study on endothelial integrity of saphenous vein grafts harvested by minimally invasive surgery with the use of vascular Mayo strippers. A randomized controlled trial. Eur J Vasc Endovasc Surg. 2004;27(3):244–50.
47. Lopes RD, Hafley GE, Allen KB, Ferguson TB, Peterson ED, Harrington RA, et al. Endoscopic versus open vein-graft harvesting in coronary-artery bypass surgery. N Engl J Med. 2009;361(3): 235–44.
48. Dashwood MR, Fremes S, Souza DS. Saphenous vein harvest with the Mayo extraluminal dissector: is endothelial function preserved? J Thorac Cardiovasc Surg. 2010;139(1):239–41.

35 Platelets and Coronary Artery Disease

Meinrad Gawaz, Harald Langer, and Tobias Geisler

Introduction

Platelets play a critical role in thrombosis and hemostasis [1, 2]. Beyond that, platelets have been recognized to act as an interface between thrombosis and inflammation [3]. Previous research has shown that inflammation plays a key role in the development of coronary artery disease (CAD) and other manifestations of atherosclerosis [4]. Recently, platelets have been recognized to trigger atherosclerotic lesion formation, to favor plaque instability, and to form thrombosis at areas of vulnerable plaques, resulting in myocardial infarction and tissue ischemia. During atherogenesis platelets interact with a variety of vascular and blood-borne cells (e.g., endothelial cells and leukocytes) and regulate chemotaxis, migration, and cytokine/chemokine release, which further propagate inflammation within vascular lesions [3, 5]. Understanding the role of platelets in atherogenesis will allow developing new strategies in the treatment of coronary artery disease.

Platelets Interact with Endothelium and Propagate Inflammation

In the past, numerous studies have shown that platelets can adhere to the intact endothelial monolayer and substantially modulate endothelial cell function [6–8]. Thus, under certain pathophysiological circumstances, endothelial denudation and exposure of the subendothelial matrix are not required for platelet adhesion to the vascular wall. Adherent platelets release a variety of proinflammatory mediators and growth hormones and have the potential to modify signaling cascades in vascular cells, inducing the expression of endothelial adhesion receptors and the release of endothelial chemoattractants [3]. In this manner, they might regulate the adhesion and infiltration of leukocytes, in particular of monocytes, into the vascular wall, a process, that is thought to play a key role in acute and chronic inflammation. Normal "resting" endothelium represents a non-adhesive and non-thrombogenic surface that prevents extravasation of circulating blood cells. In contrast, activated endothelial cells are pro-adhesive and promote the adhesion of circulating blood platelets. Adhesion of platelets to the intact but activated endothelium in the absence of previous endothelial denudation involves a surface receptor-dependent process that allows "capturing" of circulating platelets toward the vessel wall even under high shear stress. Similar to the recruitment of leukocytes [5], the adhesion of platelets to the vascular endothelial surface is a multistep process in which platelets are tethered to the vascular wall followed by platelet rolling and subsequent firm adhesion. Whereas the adhesion receptors involved in platelet attachment to the subendothelial matrix, e.g., following rupture of an atherosclerotic plaque, have been well defined during the past decade, few studies have focused on the molecular determinants that promote the interaction between platelets and the intact vascular endothelium.

During the adhesion process, platelets are activated and release an arsenal of potent proinflammatory and promitogenic substances into the local microenvironment, thereby altering chemotactic, adhesive, and proteolytic properties of endothelial cells (Fig. 35.1). These platelet-induced alterations of the endothelial phenotype support chemotaxis, adhesion, and transmigration of monocytes to the site of inflammation. Among the various platelet-derived proinflammatory proteins, IL-1β has been identified as a major mediator of platelet-induced activation of endothelial cells. The IL-1β activity expressed by platelets appears to be associated with the platelet surface [9], and co-incubation of endothelial cells with thrombin-activated platelets induces IL-1β-dependent secretion of IL-6 and IL-8 from endothelial cells. Furthermore, incubation of cultured endothelial cells with thrombin-stimulated platelets significantly enhances the secretion of endothelial monocyte chemoattractant protein-1 (MCP-1) in an IL-1β-dependent manner [10, 11].

M. Gawaz, MD (✉) • H. Langer, MD • T. Geisler, MD
Department of Cardiology, University of Tübingen, Tübingen, Germany
e-mail: meinrad.gawaz@med.uni-tuebingen.de

E.A. Gabriel, S.A. Gabriel (eds.), *Inflammatory Response in Cardiovascular Surgery*,
DOI 10.1007/978-1-4471-4429-8_35, © Springer-Verlag London 2013

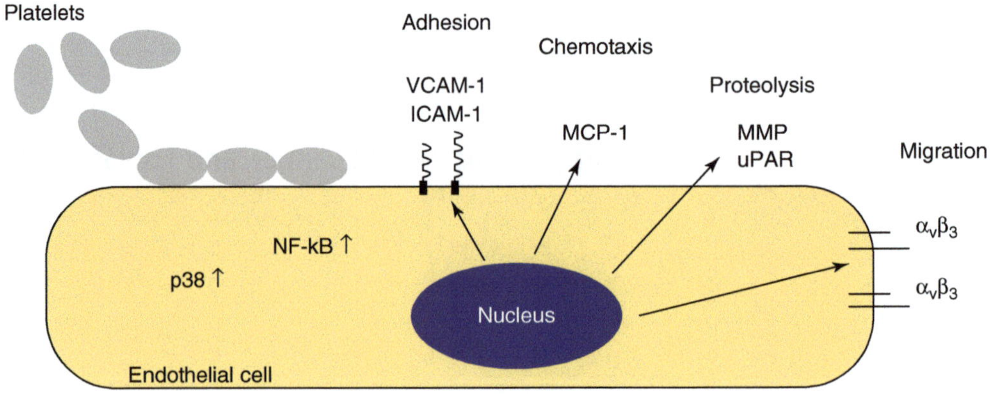

Fig. 35.1 Platelets induce chemotactic, adhesive, and proteolytic properties of endothelial cells

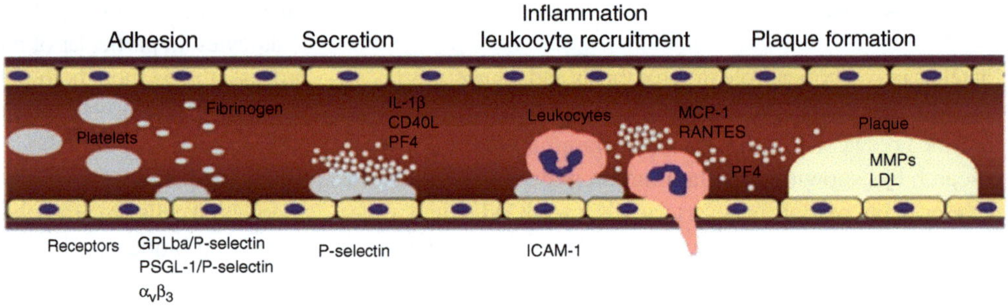

Fig. 35.2 Platelets activate the endothelial monolayer of arteries and induce monocyte chemotaxis and migration, thus propagating atherosclerotic lesion formation

However, platelet IL-1β not only modifies endothelial release of chemotactic proteins, but it also has the potential to increase endothelial expression of adhesion molecules. Surface expression of ICAM-1 and $\alpha_v\beta_3$ on endothelial cells is significantly enhanced by activated platelets via IL-1β [10, 12]. Both enhanced chemokine release and upregulation of endothelial adhesion molecules through platelet-derived IL-1β act in concert and promote neutrophil and monocyte adhesion to the endothelium. IL-1β-dependent expression of early inflammatory genes, such as MCP-1 or ICAM-1, involves the activation of the transcription factor nuclear factor kappa B (NF-κB). Transient adhesion of platelets to the endothelium initiates degradation of IκB and supports activation of NF-κB in endothelial cells, thereby inducing NF-κB-dependent chemokine gene transcription [11]. Parallel to this finding, transfection of "decoy" κB oligonucleotides or a dominant negative IKK mutant attenuates platelet-induced nuclear translocation of NF-κB and MCP-1 secretion in endothelial cells [10]. Likewise, platelet-induced NF-κB-activation was largely reduced by IL-1β antagonists, supporting the notion that platelet IL-1β is the molecular determinant of platelet-dependent activation of the transcription factor. Taken together, platelet-derived IL-1β initiates NF-κB-dependent expression of chemotactic and adhesive proteins in endothelial cells. In this manner, platelets promote the recruitment of both neutrophils and monocytes to the endothelial cell surface, thus inducing inflammation.

Another platelet-derived chemokine is RANTES, which has been identified to trigger monocyte arrest on inflamed and atherosclerotic endothelium [13]. Deposition of platelet RANTES induces monocyte recruitment mediated by P-selectin. Furthermore, release of platelet-derived CD40 ligand induces inflammatory responses in endothelium. CD154 (CD40L), a 30–33 kDa protein, belongs to the TNF family of cytokines, which includes TNF-α and Fas ligand. CD40L was originally thought to be restricted to $CD4^+$ T-lymphocytes, mast cells, and basophils. Henn et al. [14] showed that platelets store CD40L in high amounts and release CD40L within seconds following activation in vitro and in vivo. Ligation of CD40 on endothelial cells by CD40L expressed on the surface of activated platelets increased the release of IL-8 and MCP-1, the principal chemoattractants for neutrophils and monocytes. In addition, platelet CD40L enhanced the expression of endothelial adhesion receptors including E-selectin, VCAM-1, and ICAM-1, all molecules that mediate the attachment of neutrophils, monocytes, and lymphocytes to the inflamed vessel wall (Fig. 35.2). Hence, like IL-1β, CD40L expressed on platelets induces endothelial cells to release chemokines and to express adhesion molecules, thereby generating signals for the recruitment of leukocytes in the process of inflammation. CD40 ligation on endothelial cells, smooth muscle cells, and macrophages initiates the expression and release of matrix degrading enzymes, the matrix metalloproteinases (MMPs). These enzymes, which degrade extracellular matrix proteins, significantly contribute to destruction and remodeling of inflamed tissue. Adhesion of activated platelets to endothelial cells results in generation and secretion of MMP-9 and of the protease receptor uPAR on cultured endothelium [15]. The endothelial release of MMP-9 was dependent on both the fibrinogen receptor GPIIb–IIIa and CD40L because inhibition of either mechanism resulted in reduction of platelet-induced matrix degradation activity of endothelial cells. Moreover, GPIIb–IIIa ligation resulted in substantial release of CD40L in the absence of any further platelet agonist. These results propose that the release of platelet-derived proinflammatory mediators such as CD40L is dependent on GPIIb–IIIa-mediated adhesion. This mechanism may be pathophysiologically important to localize platelet-induced inflammation of the endothelium at a site of platelet-endothelium adhesion.

Platelets Interact with Leukocytes

Platelet adhesion to the endothelium or the subendothelial matrix induces platelet activation and the release of substances that are able to cause chemotaxis and migration of circulating leukocytes toward the site of platelet accumulation. Similar to platelet adhesion to the vessel wall, leukocyte recruitment to vascular endothelium requires multistep adhesive and signaling events, including selectin-mediated rolling, leukocyte activation, and integrin-mediated firm adhesion and diapedesis [5]. On leukocytes, members of the β_2-integrin family, LFA-1, MAC-1, and p150.95, as well as β_1-integrins interact with endothelial counterligands such as ICAM-1, surface-associated fibrinogen [16], or vascular cell adhesion molecule-1 (VCAM-1) to mediate the described heterotypic cell interaction. At sites of platelet adhesion to the endothelium or subendothelium, leukocyte infiltration can occur through interactions with platelets and fibrin [5]. Similar to the leukocyte-endothelium adhesion, a sequential adhesion process of leukocytes to adherent platelets has been proposed. Leukocyte adhesion to platelets involves surface expression of P-selectin on activated platelets and binding to PSGL-1, the counterreceptor present on neutrophils and monocytes [17]. Diacovo et al. [18, 19] have previously demonstrated that leukocytes tether, roll, and subsequently rest on activated platelet monolayers via sequential action of platelet P-selectin and ICAM-2 binding to their leukocyte counterreceptors PSGL-1 and CD11b/CD18, respectively. This suggests that platelets attached to the vessel wall may recruit leukocytes. In addition, P-selectin/PSGL-1-dependent platelet-leukocyte interaction brings platelets into close vicinity with neutrophils and may facilitate leukocyte activation by platelet proinflammatory mediators. Earlier studies indicated that GPIbα and JAM-3 on platelets are potential counterreceptors for MAC-1 [20] and that they mediate mechanism of platelet-leukocyte adhesion. Furthermore, ICAM-2 and $\alpha_{IIb}\beta_3$-associated fibrinogen have also been proposed to mediate MAC-1-dependent platelet-leukocyte adhesion. Thus, platelets either immobilized on a surface or activated in suspension express a complete machinery to recruit leukocytes: (1) platelet P-selectin is a mediator of the first contact (tethering), (2) interaction of platelet P-selectin with its counterreceptor PSGL-1 on leukocytes induces signaling events relevant for MAC-1 activation, and (3) the activated β_2-integrin (MAC-1) on leukocytes allows and reinforces firm platelet-leukocyte adhesion through binding to counterreceptors (ICAM-2, fibrinogen bound to GPIIb–IIIa, GPIbα, JAM-3) present on the platelet surface.

Platelets Interact with Circulating Progenitor Cells

There is increasing evidence showing that circulating progenitor cells contribute to vascular repair mechanisms and limit atheroprogression. Impairment of progenitor-dependent vascular repair due to either low numbers of circulating progenitor cells or dysfunctional progenitor cells leads to inadequate vascular healing and atheroprogression. Recently, the role of platelets for recruitment and subsequent differentiation of progenitor cells has been recognized [21–23]. Adherent platelets recruit circulating progenitor cells and induce differentiation of the latter into endothelial cells or macrophages and foam cells [21–23]. Further, the combination of platelets and fibrin promoted $CD34^+$ cell migration even to a greater extent than vascular endothelial growth factor in vitro [24]. Moreover, the chemokine stromal cell-derived factor-1 (SDF-1) was found to be secreted by activated platelets, which supports chemotaxis and primary recruitment of progenitor cells on the surface of arterial thrombi in vivo [22, 23]. Moreover, cytokine-mediated deployment of SDF-1 coming from activated platelets induces revascularization through mobilization of CXCR4 hemangiocytes [25].

Adhesion of human $CD34^+$ cells to immobilized platelets is significantly attenuated in the presence of blocking mAbs anti-CD162 or anti-CD62P, indicating that the platelet P-selectin interacts with the endothelial progenitor cells (EPCs) through interaction with P-selectin glycoprotein ligand-1 [24, 26, 27]. Thus, platelets act as an intermediate mediator to tether progenitor cells, indicating that platelets are a prerequisite for the initial step of the homing process of CD34+ cells to vascular injury.

Platelets play a critical part not only in the capture, but also in the subsequent differentiation of murine EPCs, inducing the differentiation of the latter into spindle-shaped cells that are positive for vWF [21]. Furthermore, human CD34 progenitor cells can form colonies on immobilized platelets similar to immobilized fibronectin and further differentiate into mature endothelial cells [23]. Under distinct circumstances, however, in vitro co-culture experiments between platelets and human CD34+ cells induce distinct morphological changes of the latter and differentiation into macrophages at an early phase and later on into foam cells [26].

Inhibition of Platelet Adhesion Attenuates Atheroprogression

Enhanced chronic interaction of platelets with the arterial wall results in endothelial inflammation and atheroprogression [3]. The platelet von Willebrand receptor GPIbα and the collagen receptor GPVI have been demonstrated to largely contribute to endothelial platelet adhesion in vivo in *ApoE*$^{-/-}$ mice [28], making them good candidates for inhibition. Inhibition of GP1b prevented adhesion of circulating platelets to endothelial cells at the carotid artery of *ApoE*$^{-/-}$ mice. Inhibition of platelet adhesion by blocking monoclonal anti-GPIb antibodies substantially attenuated atheroprogression in *ApoE*$^{-/-}$ mice [28]. Next, we studied the role of GPVI-mediated platelet adhesion for atheroprogression. Prolonged administration of the soluble form of GPVI [28] substantially reduced atheroprogression in ApoE-deficient mice. Further, gene transfer of GPVI-Fc to the carotid vascular wall significantly attenuated atheroprogression and endothelial dysfunction in atherosclerotic rabbits in vivo [29]. In addition, administration of soluble GPVI-Fc preferentially bound to sites of vascular injury and was able to inhibit neointimal formation after wire-induced vascular injury in *ApoE*$^{-/-}$ mice [30] (Fig. 35.3). Thus, inhibition of platelet adhesion via GPIb- or GPVI-blockers might be a promising strategy to attenuate lesion progression [31].

Conclusion

Platelets are central players in thrombosis and inflammation and contribute significantly to development of coronary artery disease. Understanding the molecular mechanisms of platelet-mediated inflammatory reactions within the vessel wall discloses important aspects of the pathophysiology of coronary artery disease. Platelet-mediated vascular inflammation is an attractive therapeutic strategy to limit atheroprogression.

Acknowledgement The authors were supported in part by the Deutsche Forschungsgemeinschaft and the Klinische Forschergruppe KFO-274 "*Platelets-Molecular Mechanisms and Translational Implications*".

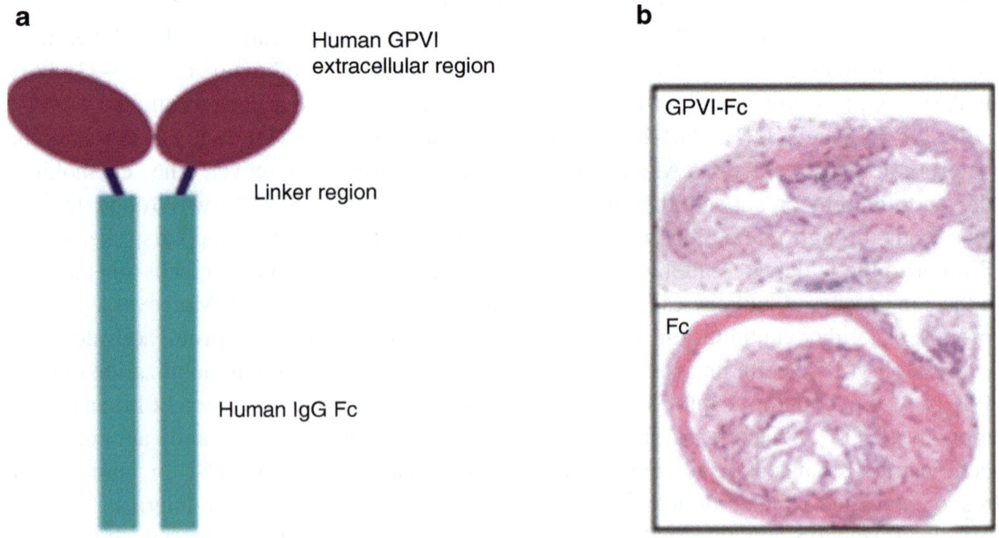

Fig. 35.3 Glycoprotein VI binds to vascular lesions and reduces atherosclerotic lesion formation. Glycoprotein VI binds to vascular lesions and reduces atherosclerotic lesion formation. (**a**) Schematic of the recombinant GPVI-Fc. (**b**) Reduced neointimal formation in GPVI-Fc-treated *ApoE*$^{-/-}$ mice after wire-induced injury of the carotid artery (H&E staining, *bar* 100 μm) [30]. (**c**) Binding of radiolabeled GPVI-Fc to injured carotid artery shown by PET/CT (*left*) and autoradiography (*right*) [30]

Fig. 35.3 (continued)

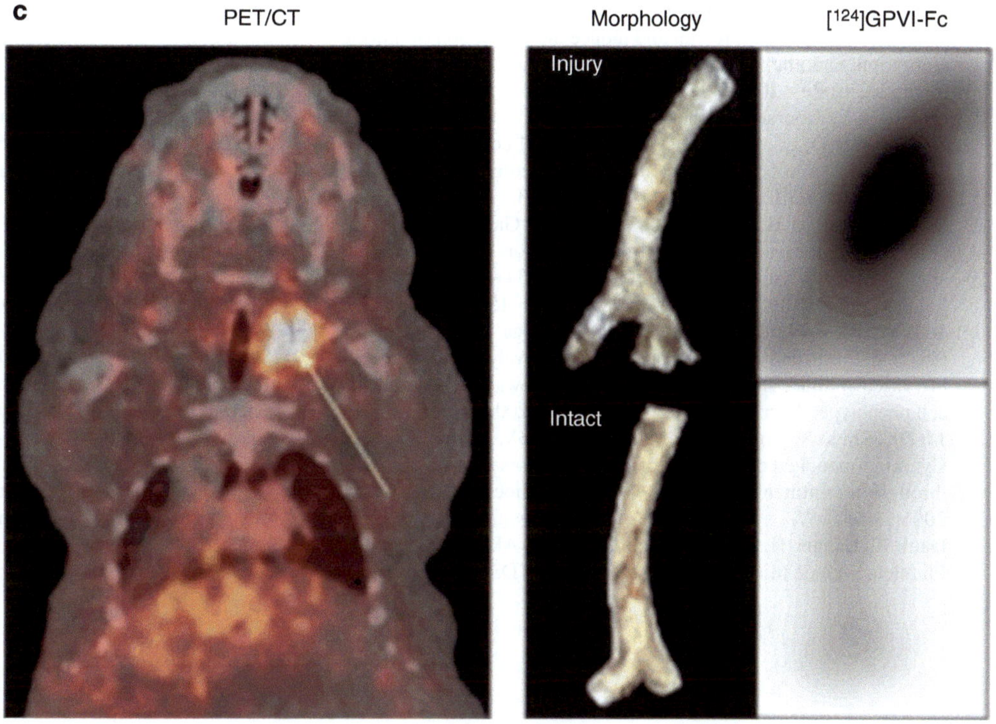

References

1. Davi G, Patrono C. Platelet activation and atherothrombosis. N Engl J Med. 2007;357:2482–94.
2. Ruggeri ZM. Platelets in atherothrombosis. Nat Med. 2002;8: 1227–34.
3. Gawaz M, Langer H, May AE. Platelets in inflammation and atherogenesis. J Clin Invest. 2005;115:3378–84.
4. Hansson GK. Inflammation, atherosclerosis, and coronary artery disease. N Engl J Med. 2005;352:1685–95.
5. May AE, Seizer P, Gawaz M. Platelets: inflammatory firebugs of vascular walls. Arterioscler Thromb Vasc Biol. 2008;28:S5–10.
6. Bombeli T, Schwartz BR, Harlan JM. Adhesion of activated platelets to endothelial cells: evidence for a GPIIbIIIa-dependent bridging mechanism and novel roles for endothelial intercellular adhesion molecule 1 (ICAM-1), alphavbeta3 integrin, and GPIbalpha. J Exp Med. 1998;187:329–39.
7. Gawaz M, Neumann FJ, Dickfeld T, Reininger A, Adelsberger H, Gebhardt A, et al. Vitronectin receptor (alpha(v)beta3) mediates platelet adhesion to the luminal aspect of endothelial cells: implications for reperfusion in acute myocardial infarction. Circulation. 1997;96:1809–18.
8. Gawaz M. Role of platelets in coronary thrombosis and reperfusion of ischemic myocardium. Cardiovasc Res. 2004;61:498–511.
9. Hawrylowicz CM, Howells GL, Feldmann M. Platelet-derived interleukin 1 induces human endothelial adhesion molecule expression and cytokine production. J Exp Med. 1991;174:785–90.
10. Gawaz M, Neumann FJ, Dickfeld T, Koch W, Laugwitz KL, Adelsberger H, et al. Activated platelets induce monocyte chemotactic protein-1 secretion and surface expression of intercellular adhesion molecule-1 on endothelial cells. Circulation. 1998;98:1164–71.
11. Gawaz M, Page S, Massberg S, Nothdurfter C, Weber M, Fisher C, et al. Transient platelet interaction induces MCP-1 production by endothelial cells via I kappa B kinase complex activation. Thromb Haemost. 2002;88:307–14.
12. Gawaz M, Brand K, Dickfeld T, Pogatsa-Murray G, Page S, Bogner C, et al. Platelets induce alterations of chemotactic and adhesive properties of endothelial cells mediated through an interleukin-1-dependent mechanism. Implications for atherogenesis. Atherosclerosis. 2000;148:75–85.
13. von Hundelshausen P, Weber KS, Huo Y, Proudfoot AE, Nelson PJ, Ley K, et al. RANTES deposition by platelets triggers monocyte arrest on inflamed and atherosclerotic endothelium. Circulation. 2001;103:1772–7.
14. Henn V, Slupsky JR, Grafe M, Anagnostopoulos I, Forster R, Muller-Berghaus G, et al. CD40 ligand on activated platelets triggers an inflammatory reaction of endothelial cells. Nature. 1998;391: 591–4.
15. May AE, Kalsch T, Massberg S, Herouy Y, Schmidt R, Gawaz M. Engagement of glycoprotein IIb/IIIa (alpha(IIb)beta3) on platelets upregulates CD40L and triggers CD40L-dependent matrix degradation by endothelial cells. Circulation. 2002;106:2111–7.
16. Springer TA. Traffic signals for lymphocyte recirculation and leukocyte emigration: the multistep paradigm. Cell. 1994;76: 301–14.
17. Gardiner EE, De Luca M, McNally T, Michelson AD, Andrews RK, Berndt MC. Regulation of P-selectin binding to the neutrophil P-selectin counter-receptor P-selectin glycoprotein ligand-1 by neutrophil elastase and cathepsin G. Blood. 2001;98:1440–7.
18. Diacovo TG, DeFougerolles AR, Bainton DF, Springer TA. A functional integrin ligand on the surface of platelets: intercellular adhesion molecule-2. J Clin Invest. 1994;94:1243–51.
19. Diacovo TG, Roth SJ, Buccola JM, Bainton DF, Springer TA. Neutrophil rolling, arrest, and transmigration across activated, surface-adherent platelets via sequential action of P-selectin and the beta 2-integrin CD11b/CD18. Blood. 1996;88:146–57.
20. Santoso S, Sachs UJ, Kroll H, Linder M, Ruf A, Preissner KT, et al. The junctional adhesion molecule 3 (JAM-3) on human platelets is a counterreceptor for the leukocyte integrin Mac-1. J Exp Med. 2002;196:679–91.

21. Langer H, May AE, Daub K, Heinzmann U, Lang P, Schumm M, et al. Adherent platelets recruit and induce differentiation of murine embryonic endothelial progenitor cells to mature endothelial cells in vitro. Circ Res. 2006;98:E2–10.
22. Massberg S, Konrad I, Schurzinger K, Lorenz M, Schneider S, Zohlnhoefer D, et al. Platelets secrete stromal cell-derived factor 1alpha and recruit bone marrow-derived progenitor cells to arterial thrombi in vivo. J Exp Med. 2006;203:1221–33.
23. Stellos K, Langer H, Daub K, Schoenberger T, Gauss A, Geisler T, et al. Platelet-derived stromal cell-derived factor-1 regulates adhesion and promotes differentiation of human CD34+ cells to endothelial progenitor cells. Circulation. 2008;117:206–15.
24. de Boer HC, Verseyden C, Ulfman LH, Zwaginga JJ, Bot I, Biessen EA, et al. Fibrin and activated platelets cooperatively guide stem cells to a vascular injury and promote differentiation towards an endothelial cell phenotype. Arterioscler Thromb Vasc Biol. 2006;26:1653–9.
25. Jin DK, Shido K, Kopp HG, Petit I, Shmelkov SV, Young LM, et al. Cytokine-mediated deployment of SDF-1 induces revascularization through recruitment of CXCR4(+) hemangiocytes. Nat Med. 2006;12:557–67.
26. Daub K, Langer H, Seizer P, Stellos K, May AE, Goyal P, et al. Platelets induce differentiation of human CD34(+) progenitor cells into foam cells and endothelial cells. FASEB J. 2006; 20:2559.
27. Lev EI, Patel R, Karim A, Kleiman A, Badimon JJ, Kleiman NS. Anti-thrombotic effect of bivalirudin compared with eptifibatide and unfractionated heparin in diabetic patients: an ex vivo human study. Thromb Haemost. 2006;95:441–6.
28. Massberg S, Brand K, Gruner S, Page S, Muller E, Muller I, et al. A critical role of platelet adhesion in the initiation of atherosclerotic lesion formation. J Exp Med. 2002;196:887–96.
29. Bultmann A, Li ZM, Wagner S, Peluso M, Schonberger T, Weis C, et al. Impact of glycoprotein VI and platelet adhesion on atherosclerosis-A possible role of fibronectin. J Mol Cell Cardiol. 2010;49: 532–42.
30. Schonberger T, Siegel-Axel D, Bussl R, Richter S, Judenhofer MS, Haubner R, et al. The immunoadhesin glycoprotein VI-Fc regulates arterial remodelling after mechanical injury in ApoE–/– mice. Cardiovasc Res. 2008;80:131–7.
31. Ungerer M, Rosport K, Bultmann A, Piechatzek R, Uhland K, Schlieper P, et al. Novel antiplatelet drug revacept (Dimeric Glycoprotein VI-Fc) specifically and efficiently inhibited collagen-induced platelet aggregation without affecting general hemostasis in humans. Circulation. 2011;123:1891–9.

Part XI

Heart Valve Diseases

Role of Bone Morphogenetic Proteins in Valvulogenesis

36

Russell A. Gould and Jonathan T. Butcher

Valvular Morphogenesis

Initiation of Valvular Morphogenesis

Valvulogenesis is a complex process involving the formation and morphogenesis of both the atrioventricular and semilunar valves. The early embryonic heart is a single myocardial tube lined with endocardial cells. During the looping process, simultaneous valve formation initiates by deposition of hyaluronan-rich gelatinous matrix, called cardiac jelly, forming swellings that project into the lumen. At the onset of Hamburger and Hamilton (HH14⁻, E9.0 in mouse), a process called EMT (epithelial-mesenchymal transition) takes place in which the lining of endocardial cell swellings differentiated from an EMT phenotype. This process is associated with downregulation of cell-cell contacts, such as E-cadherin and PECAM1, the acquisition of cell-matrix adhesions, and cytoskeleton rearrangement [1]. Loss of tight junctions in EMT is concomitant with the acquisition of a spindle-shaped morphology and migratory/invasive phenotype. The invasiveness of the mesenchymal phenotype is critical, as these cells dive into the hyaluronan-rich cardiac jelly, degrade the underlying matrix, and deposit newly synthesized collagen I, II, III, versican, and other proteoglycans [2]. These newly populated mesenchymal swellings are called "cushions" because of their soft visual appearance while stitched to the myocardial wall. Cushions are formed in pairs that oppose each other during the cardiac cycle to act as primitive valves by maintaining unidirectional blood flow [3]. One pair of cushions develops in the atrioventricular (AV) canal, and two (proximal and distal) develop in the outflow tract (OFT). The processes by which the AV and outflow cushions remodel into thin fibrous leaflets are discussed below.

R.A. Gould, BS
Department of Biomedical Engineering,
Cornell University, Ithaca, NY 14850, USA

J.T. Butcher, PhD (✉)
Department of Biomedical Engineering,
Cornell University, 304 Weill Hall,
Ithaca, NY 14853, USA
e-mail: jtb47@cornell.edu

Atrioventricular Valve Remodeling

By HH26 (E12.5 in mouse), the AV cushions fuse together at the midline along a superior/inferior axis, dividing the canal into the right and left conduits. Even before fusing, the expansion of the cushions creates a "dog-bone" shape of the ventricular inlet that begins to divert blood flow around the cushions, potentially contributing to their eventual fusion [4]. From the left and right lateral aspects of this fused central cushion mass evolves the septal leaflets of the left and right AV valves. At about the same time as central cushion fusion, new cushions begin to form from the left and right lateral walls, which will eventually form the mural AV leaflets. The process by which the AV leaflets form is thought to involve a process of proliferation, extension, condensation, and delamination [5]. Briefly, a subendocardial portion of the AV cushion expands and extends along the myocardial substrate, which is mediated in part by a fibroblast growth factor 4 (FGF4) section by the endocardium [6]. These cells form a progressive-like zone and begin to differentiate further toward a fibroblastic phenotype. This zone of differentiated cells condenses the cushion matrix into a thinner and more fibrous tissue consisting of a subendocardial surface, which is largely positive for laminin, while the ventricular side is predominately collagen III. Furthermore, fenestrations between the myocardial wall and valve tissue begin to form, possibly because of expansion of the ventricular cavities or changes in hemodynamic loading [7]. Upon further delamination, residual contacts between the valve tissue and myocardium form the site of newly developing papillary muscles. This creates mesenchymal tissue strands that develop into the tendinous chords of the AV valves. By HH36, full delamination from the myocardial wall occurs

E.A. Gabriel, S.A. Gabriel (eds.), *Inflammatory Response in Cardiovascular Surgery*,
DOI 10.1007/978-1-4471-4429-8_36, © Springer-Verlag London 2013

and the distinct tri-layer structure (atrialis/spongiosa, fibrosa, and ventricularis) with a largely organized lamellar network of elastin and newly formed collagen (I, II, III, V, VI) [8].

Semilunar Valve Morphogenesis

Similar to AV valves in terms of mesenchymal transformation and formation of the tri-layered valve structure, semilunar valves become excavated from the aortic side inward. Between HH17 and HH26 (E10–E12), the conal and truncal cushion pairs of the outflow tract become invaded and populated by activated endocardially derived cells. The aorticopulmonary (AP) septum spirals through the outflow tract lumen with a counterclockwise rotation so that the right portion of the semilunar ring is derived from the original left side of the primitive outflow tract [9, 10]. The splitting of the parietal and septal distal truncal cushions by the AP septum, combined with the intercalated cushions of the distal outflow tract creates the six cushions required for the formation of the semilunar valves, which is completed by HH34 (E14.5). The tissue on the arterial side becomes a more condensed fibrous matrix, as the small depression continues to deepen, sculpting the leaflet cusps. By HH39–40, the leaflets begin to appear trilaminar in nature, with an elastin–collagen lamellar structure forming at the ventricular surface. By HH45, fibrous tissue is seen radiating from the attachment of the valve cusps into the aortic wall from the base to the level of the commissures, creating an anchoring ring of fibro-cartilaginous tissue around the sinuses [11].

BMP Signaling

Canonical Smad Signaling

Bone morphogenetic proteins (BMP) are a subset within the cytokine superfamily transforming growth factor beta (TGFβ). They are multipotential proteins that regulate a wide variety of cellular functions during development. All BMP signaling occurs through a family of homodimeric proteins that interact with BMP type I and type II receptors. Thus far, three out of seven type I and three out of five type II receptors have been identified to transduce the BMP signal into the cell. Unlike the other TGFβ family members, BMP has a higher affinity for the type I than the type II receptors. The type I receptors are ACVR1 (Alk2), BMPRIA (Alk3), and BMPR1B (Alk6), and the type II are BMPR2 (BMPRII), ACVR2A (ActRIIA), and ACVR2B (ActRIIIB). BMP ligands (BMP2, 4, 5, 6, 7) directly bind to the type II receptors, which form heterodimers with type I receptors. This activates the receptors serine/threonine kinase activity to phosphorylate and activate the receptor Smads 1/5/8 [12]. Other ligands, e.g., NOG (Noggin), can directly bind BMP, inhibiting their interaction with the receptors. Phosphorylated Smads 1/5 (pSmad1/5) form heterodimers with partner Smad4 and translocate to the nucleus. During translocation to the nucleus, pSmad complexes can join with other co-activators to form a unique transcription factor complex capable of regulating specific genes. Intracellular BMP signal transduction can be negatively influenced by modulating Smad phosphorylation and transport into the nucleus, e.g., SMURF or Smad6 [13]. Also cross-talk with other signaling pathways has been observed to affect the phosphorylation status of the Smads and nuclear accumulation such as ERK modulation. Although Smad-mediated signaling is the most extensively studied, BMP signaling can also be mediated by MAP3K7/MAP3K7IP1 (Tak1/Tab1) leading to the activation of MAPK14 (p38 MAPK), as well as of PI3K (PI3 kinase), RAS, MAPK1 (ERK), and MAPK8 (JNK) (Fig. 36.1) [14, 15].

Spatial and Temporal Localization of BMP Signaling in Valve Development

BMPs are uniquely expressed during cushion formation and valve maturation in both the OFT and AV canal (AVC). BMP2 and BMP4 have been widely studied because of their localization within the myocardium along the cushion-forming regions. BMP2 and BMP4 are expressed within the myocardium of the AVC and OFT and thought to be a strong inducers of EMT and cushion formation. In mice, BMP2 expression dissipates in the OFT by E10.5 while continuing to persist throughout the AVC myocardium. On the other hand, BMP4 expression dissipates in the AVC by E10.5 while continuing to persist throughout the OFT myocardium. BMP5 is expressed in the myocardium before and during cardiac cushion EMT (at E8.5) [16]. However, it is later downregulated, and its role in cushion formation or maturation is thought to be minimal. BMP6 is found within the endocardium of the OFT at E8.5 and E9.5 [17], OFT myocardium at E10.5, and in the mesenchyme of the cushions of the AVC at E10.5 [18]. At later stages, however, it has been described in the cushion mesenchyme of the OFT. BMP7 is widely expressed throughout the myocardium with modest expression in AV valve mesenchyme [19, 20].

Traditional mouse knockout models used to define the role of BMP in valve morphogenesis has been challenging. Both BMP2 and BMP4 null mutant mice have early precardiac embryonic lethality [21, 22]. Interestingly, BMP5, BMP6, and BMP7 alone do not produce cardiac defects. However, combinations of BMP knockout mice models have proven to affect valve formation. Within the BMP5/BMP7 double–knockout mouse, cardiac cushions do not form, but the precise role is difficult to determine because of the global disruption in development [16]. BMP6/BMP7 double-knockout mice show a marked delay in the formation of outflow tract cushions because of reduced cell proliferation. Compared

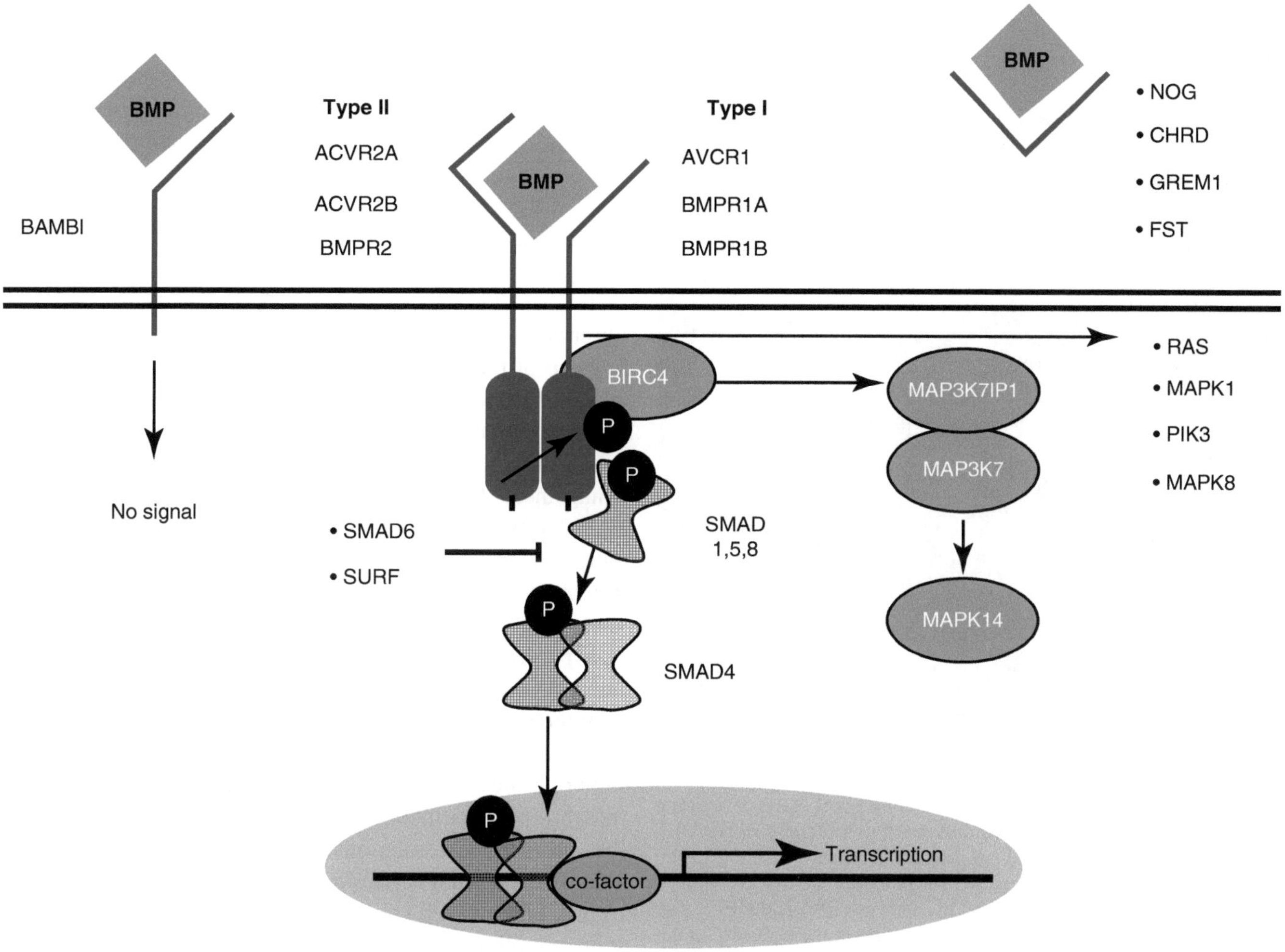

Fig. 36.1 Canonical BMP signaling pathways. BMP form a heteromeric complex with type I and type II BMP receptors. Subsequent to this complex formation, the type II receptor phosphorylates the type I receptor, through which the Smad1, Smad5, or Smad8 is phosphorylated. Phosphorylated Smad forms a complex with the common Smad4 and is transported into the nucleus. Besides signaling via Smads, the BMP signal can also be transduced via MAP3K7(Tak1)/MAP3K7IP1 (Tab1), RAS, MAPK1 (ERK), or PI3 kinase. Extracellularly, BMPs can be inhibited by secreted inhibitors, such as NOG, CHRD (chordin), GREM1 (Gremlin), and FST (follistatin), or by the decoy receptor BAMBI, which lacks the intracellular domain for signal propagation. BMP signal transduction is intracellularly inhibited by Smad6 or SMURF (van Wijk et al. [15])

with the outflow tract cushions, AV canal cushions are generally less compromised by the loss of BMP6 and BMP7 [17]. This suggests that the combinations of these growth factors are critical for valve morphogenesis.

Analysis of BMP receptor expression patterns and conditional mutations have provided additional insight into the role of BMP in valve formation and remodeling because of their reduced lethality. However, extracting mechanistic understanding is challenging because of their promiscuity. Of the type I receptors, Alk6 (BMPRIB) is not expressed, and Alk3 (BMPRIA) is ubiquitously expressed, while Alk2 (ACVR1) can transduce both BMP and TGFβ signals, is expressed in the heart rather widely [23, 24]. Two type II receptors have been described as being able to transduce a BMP signal. ActRII, originally described as a type II receptor for activins, can also transduce a BMP signal [25], although its pattern of expression in the heart has not been described in detail. The main type II BMP receptor, BMPRII (which mainly binds with Alk3), is ubiquitously expressed in the heart, and all tissues during development [20] (Fig. 36.2).

Mice lacking type II or type IA BMP receptors die at gastrulation and cannot be used to assess potential later roles in valvular morphogenesis. However, Cre/Lox-targeted deletion of Alk3 in cardiac myocytes revealed an unexpected role for this receptor in the formation of the AVC cushions. EMT in both AVC and OFT regions is normal, suggesting these BMP receptors were either not required or more likely redundant. However, during the remodeling process, cushions were found smaller in size and cushion fusion does not occur. Elimination of Alk3 was also found to diminish TGFβ2 expression in the AVC, which further supports the notion that BMP is an important contributor to the TGFβ paracrine

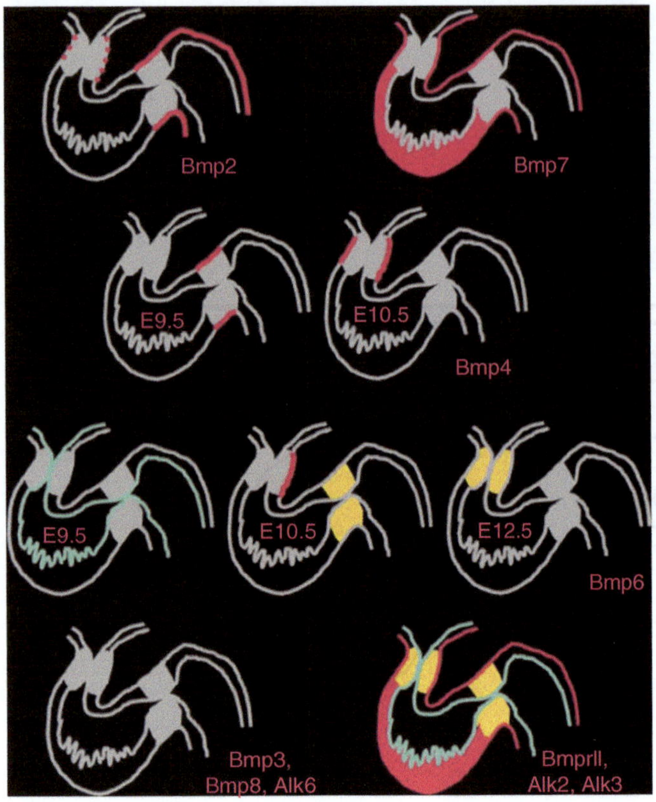

Fig. 36.2 Expression patterns of BMP family genes in the developing mouse heart. BMP2 is expressed only briefly and faintly in the OFT myocardium, but strongly and persistently in the myocardium of the AVC (and atria). BMP4 expression switches from the myocardium of the AVC to the myocardium of the OFT between E9.5 and E10.5. The very dynamic expression of BMP6 is seen first in the endocardium at E9.5, then in the mesenchyme of the AVC cushions and in the myocardium of the left OFT at E10.5, and finally becomes restricted to the mesenchyme of the OFT at E12.5. BMP7 is expressed strongly in all the myocardium at all stages described. BMP3, BMP8, and receptor Alk6 are not expressed in the developing heart, while Alk2, Alk3, and BMPRII are ubiquitous (Delot [20])

response [26]. Likewise, mice with a hypomorphic BMP receptor II allele (BMPR2) die before birth as a result of cardiovascular abnormalities. Similar to the Alk3 mutant mice, EMT is initiated in both the AV and OFT endocardial cushions. However, OFT cushions failed to develop past the initial EMT events, suggesting that BMPR2 is required for subsequent growth and maintenance of the conotruncal cushions [27].

Growth Factor Regulation of Valve Formation by BMP

Initiation of EMT

Efforts to investigate the mechanisms of EMT and cushion formation have been greatly facilitated by the use of a three-dimensional collagen gel explants. In this system, AV canals (chick or mouse embryos) are isolated and then explanted onto the collagen gel surface. The endocardium of the AV canal adheres to the surface, from which a subset of these cells undergoes the mesenchymal transformation and invades the underlying matrix. Interestingly, EMT does not take place if the myocardium is removed directly after the endocardium has been attached to the collagen gel surface. This suggests that the AV myocardium has a unique capacity to secrete specific signals for EMT [28]. After these landmark observational studies, the focus shifted to understand the makeup of the myocardial inductive signal for EMT in AV canal endocardial cells. Through segmental patterning, it was found that myocardial cells express BMP2 in a manner consistent with the segmental pattern of cushion formation. Using these AV explants in mice, Sugi et al. showed that BMP2 was sufficient to induce EMT in mouse AV canal cultures in the absence of AV myocardium [29]. Furthermore, treatment of AV cultures with Noggin, a BMP inhibitor, prevented mesenchymal cell formation in untreated cultures and also prevented BMP2 induced EMT in AV cultures with intact AV myocardium.

Interestingly, BMP2 treatments of AV explants resulted in increased TGFβ2 protein levels [29]. This is particularly important because antagonists to TGFβ2 and TGFβ3 show that they play distinct but complementary roles in regulating the initial transformation events in chick. Endocardial TGFβ2 expression is required for cell separation and hypertrophy, while TGFβ3 signaling is required for mesenchymal transformation and migration [30]. TGFβ3 induces expression of MMP-2 and MT-MMP, which digest the collagen IV endocardial matrix permitting invasion [31]. At the onset of EMT in chick cardiogenesis, TGFβ3 is expressed in transforming endothelial and invading mesenchymal cells, while BMP2 is expressed in the subjacent myocardium. To restrict this entire process to the cushion forming region in the lumen, endocardial Notch1 signals repress myocardial BMP2 through the Hey1 transcription factor [20]. Furthermore, chick AV explants experiments have investigated the combinatory role of both TGFβ3 and BMP2. In summary, it was found that (1) myocardially derived inductive signals upregulate the expression of AV endothelial TGFβ3 at the onset of EMT, (2) TGFβ3 needs to be expressed by these endothelial cells to trigger the initial phenotypic changes of EMT, and (3) myocardial BMP2 acts synergistically with TGFβ3 in the initiation of EMT [32].

Cushion Maturation

During cushion formation, type I BMP receptors, BMPR1A (Alk3), BMPR1B (Alk6), and Alk2, have all been localized in AV cushion mesenchyme in stage-24 chick embryos. AV

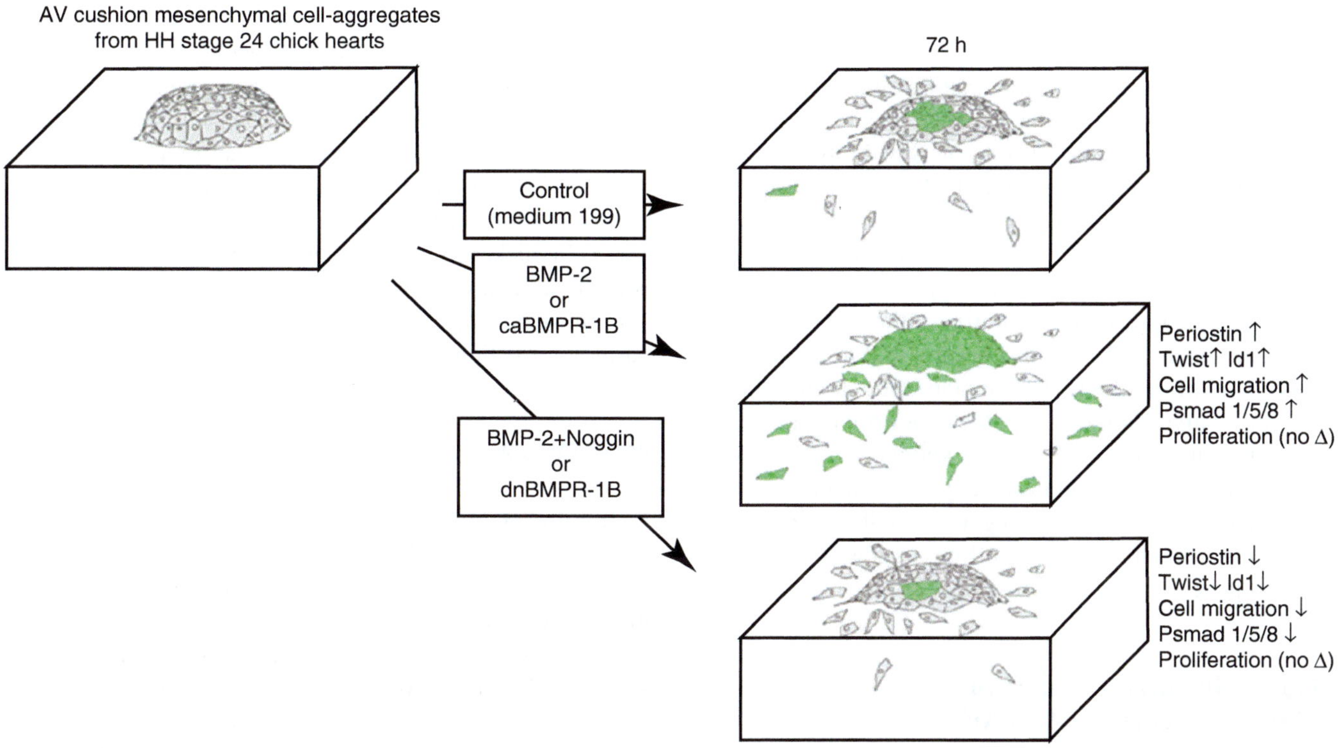

Fig. 36.3 Summary diagram illustrating the results from bioassays to assess the role of BMP2 and BMP signaling using AV cushion mesenchymal cell aggregates cultured on 3D-collagen gels. Exogenous BMP2 or caBMPR1B treatments induced mesenchymal cell migration and expression of periostin, Twist and Id1. In contrast, Noggin or dnBMPR1B treatment inhibited BMP2 promoted cell migration and expression of periostin, Twist, and Id1. Phospho-Smad 1/5/8 expression was induced by BMP2 or caBMPR1B treatments but reduced by Noggin or dnBMPR1B treatments (Inai et al. [33])

explant experiments applying exogenous BMP2 or caBMPR1B (Alk6) treatments significantly promoted expression of an extracellular matrix (ECM) protein periostin, a known valvulogenic matrix maturation mediator whereas periostin expression was repressed by adding Noggin or dnBMPR1B (Alk6)-virus to the culture [33]. Moreover, transcripts of Twist and Id1, were induced by BMP2 but repressed by Noggin in cushion mesenchymal cell cultures. This data provides evidence that BMP2 signaling induces biological processes involved in early AV valvulogenesis, i.e., mesenchymal cell migration and expression of periostin, indicating critical roles for BMP signaling in post-EMT AV cushion tissue maturation and differentiation (Fig. 36.3).

BMP2-induced periostin expression plays an important role in the developing cushion and maturation of valves. As a secreted fasciclin domain-ECM protein that associates with areas of fibrosis, periostin can directly interact with other ECM proteins, such as fibronectin, tenascin-C, collagen I, collagen V, and heparin sulfate proteoglycans. Periostin serves as a ligand for select integrins, such as αvβ3, αvβ5, and α4β6, where it can affect the ability of cells (fibroblasts or cancer cells) to migrate and/or undergo mesenchymal transformation in select tissues [34]. Using the aforementioned in vitro assays, Butcher et al. found that upon periostin overexpression, mesenchyme invasion was enhanced in a dose-dependent manner through 3D collagen gels and increased matrix compaction. It was also found that this invasion was dependent on αvβ3 more than β1 integrin signaling and was mediated differentially by Rho kinase and PI3 kinase [35].

BMP4 signaling is thought to be involved in both cardiac cushion EMT and later stage valve remodeling. By combining the use of a hypomorphic BMP4 allele with conditional gene inactivation, BMP4 was found to signal from the myocardium and directly mediate atrioventricular septation. Likewise, more pronounced reductions in myocardial BMP4 expression results in a complete atrioventricular septal defect (AVSD). The AVSDs in these mouse models appear to result from decreased cell proliferation within the AV cardiac cushions [36]. Furthermore, the anterior heart field (AHF)–derived myocardium, another essential source of BMP4, is required for normal endocardial cushion expansion and remodeling. Loss of BMP4 from the AHF in mice results in an insufficient number of cells in the developing OFT endocardial cushions, defective cushion remodeling, ventricular septal defects, persistent truncus arteriosus, and abnormal semilunar valve formation [37].

Downstream signaling through Smad phosphorylation is dependent upon the formation of the Smad1-Smad4 and/or Smad5-Smad4 transcription factor complexes. Smad6 is an important Smad protein capable of attenuating BMP signaling through competition of Smad4 binding [38]. Smad6 is expressed in the AV and OFT regions of the heart during development. Smad6 homozygous knockout mice displayed hypercellular AV and OFT cardiac cushions. The hypercellular cushion phenotype in Smad6 null mice is consistent with BMP mediating either EMT or subsequent mesenchymal cell proliferation within cardiac cushions. In addition, the role of Smad6 in the homeostasis of the adult valves is indicated by the development of bone-related ossification upon Smad6 knockout [39]. It would seem that BMP-induced mesenchyme formation or proliferation is controlled by a negative feedback mechanism involving Smad6 and controlling expression of bone-related genes in adult homeostasis [2].

Transcriptional Regulation of Valve Formation by BMP

The role of BMP directing the differentiation of mesenchymal valve progenitor cells is becoming more understood at the transcriptional level. Recent work by Chakraborty et al. conducted gene expression profiling analysis of murine E12.5 AV endocardial cushions compared with E17.5. They hypothesized the existence of shared regulatory pathways active in developing AV valves and bone progenitor cells. Overall, MC3T3 cells (pre-osteoblasts) were significantly more similar to E17.5 valves than to E12.5 cushions, supporting the hypothesis that valve maturation involves the expression of many genes also expressed in osteoblasts. Several transcription factors characteristic of mesenchymal and osteoblast precursor cells, including Twist1, Sox9, Tbx20, and Msx1/Msx2, are predominant in E12.5 cushion [40]. We will now discuss these transcription factors with regards to valve formation below.

Sox9

Sox9 is thought to be a master regulator required for endocardial cushion cell lineage expansion, as well as differentiation associated with cartilage progenitor cells [41, 42]. In both chick and mouse, Sox9 is expressed within the endocardial cushions and remodeling leaflets. BMP2 activates expression of Sox9 and the cartilage differentiation marker Col2a1, which has been observed in cultured avian endocardial cushion cells [43]. Upon gene knockout of Sox9 in mice, embryonic lethality occurs between E11.5 and E12.5 with hypoplastic endocardial cushions. It is thought that loss of Sox9 inhibits EMT after delamination and initial migration, but before definitive mesenchymal transformation [44]. During targeted loss of Sox9 with Col2a1Cre in the remodeling valve, decreased expression of cartilage-associated proteins Col2a1 occurs. In adult mice, heterozygous loss of Sox9 in Col2a1Cre results in thickened valve leaflets and calcification characteristic of valve disease [42]. This suggests that that a relationship between BMP and Sox9 has a critical role in endocardial cushion formation and valve remodeling.

Msx1/Msx2

Expression of the Msx1 and Msx2 homeobox genes has been shown to be co-coordinately regulated with the BMP2 and BMP4 ligands in a variety of developing tissues. It known that that both Msx1 and Msx2 are crucial downstream effectors of BMP signaling in endocardial cushion. Upon mouse knockout, Msx1 and Msx2 single homozygous mutant mice exhibited normal valve formation, while hypoplastic AV cushions and malformed AV valves were evident in the double Msx1 and Msx2 homozygous mutant mouse. These results support redundant functions for Msx1 and Msx2 during AV valve morphogenesis. In the Msx1/2 mutant embryos, endocardial expression of Notch1, BMP2/4, and NFATc1 is reduced, and patterning of the AVC myocardium is also abnormal, leading to compromised EMT [45]. In addition, loss of both Msx1 and Msx2 were also found to affect secondary heart field and neural crest anomalies related to defects in cell proliferation and migration [46]. Taken together, combined Msx1 and Msx2 mutations lead to a spectrum of cardiac malformations including double outlet right ventricle (DORV), a pulmonary stenosis, atrial and ventricular septal defects, and hypoplastic ventricle [47].

Twist1

Endocardial cushion expression of Twist1 is induced by BMP2 in both chicken and mouse embryos. During valve morphogenesis, Twist1 is expressed throughout the endocardial cushions of the AVC and OFT, and expression is downregulated in the remodeling valves [48]. Shelton et al. performed gain and loss of function studies in avian endocardial cushion cell cultures to demonstrate that Twist1 promotes cell proliferation and migration, while increasing the expression of periostin and MMP-2 [49]. Twist1 activity was examined in transgenic mice with persistent expression in the developing valves. Persistent expression leads to increased valve cell proliferation, increased expression of Tbx20, and increased ECM gene expression, characteristic of early valve progenitors. Among the ECM genes predominant in the endocardial cushions, Col2a1 was identified as a direct transcriptional target of Twist1. Increased expression also leads to dysregulation of fibrillar collagen and periostin expression, as well as enlarged hypercellular valve leaflets prior to birth [50].

Tbx20

Tbx20 is thought to maintain BMP2 expression localized to the AVC region. Tbx20 is strongly expressed in the myocardium of the AVC in both mouse and chick [51, 52]. Mice lacking Tbx20 in the AVC myocardium fail to form the AVC constriction, and EMT is severely perturbed. Furthermore, downstream genes, such as Twist1, Sox9, and Msx1 involved in the EMT initiation were found nearly absent. During re-expression of BMP2 in the AVC myocardium, BMP2 substantially rescues the EMT defects resulting from the lack of Tbx20, suggesting BMP2 is one of the key downstream targets of Tbx20 in AVC development [53]. Furthermore, Tbx20 gain and loss of function studies performed in chicken AVC explants were found to increase cell proliferation and migration while repressing ECM maturation. Tbx20 promotes expression of the ECM remodeling enzymes, MMP9 and MMP13, while repressing expression of the chondroitin sulfate proteoglycans, aggrecan, and versican [54]. Overall, Tbx20 has essential roles in regulating AVC development that coordinate early cushion formation.

BMP and Post-natal Valve Dysfunction

Degenerative valve calcification in cardiac valves has been associated with the expression of BMP [55]. However, their precise role in this process remains largely unknown. In human aortic leaflets, both BMP2 and BMP4 expression has been upregulated in calcific stenotic valves [56]. Interestingly, downstream signaling of BMP has been shown preferentially activated in a side-specific manner. Smad-1/5/8 was preferentially activated in the calcified fibrosa endothelium of human aortic valves and correlates with low expression of BMP antagonists and inhibitory Smad6. These results suggest a dominant role of BMP antagonists in the side-dependent calcification of human aortic valves [57]. Further in-vitro experiments with human valve interstitial cells have shown that exogenous addition of BMP2 and BMP4 induces a significant increase in the activity and expression of alkaline phosphatase, RUNX2, osteocalcin, and osteopontin [58]. Changes in RUNX2 and osteopontin expression levels are thought to be preceded by phosphorylation of Smad1 and extracellular signal-regulated kinase 1/2 but not p38 MAPK [59]. It is also important to note that elevated stretch may cause valve calcification via a BMP-dependent mechanism. For example, cyclic stretch of porcine aortic valve leaflets, pathological magnitudes elicited a stronger calcification response compared with physiological magnitudes in a fully osteogenic medium. BMP2, BMP4, and RUNX2 expression was also found upregulated on the fibrosa surface of the valve cusp in a stretch dependent manner after 3 days. Tissue calcium content and alkaline phosphatase activity were similarly stretch dependent and significantly reduced by Noggin in a dose-dependent manner. These results underline the potential role of BMP in valve calcification because of altered stretch [60]. Taken together, these findings suggest that excessive BMP signaling within the human aortic valves contribute to the calcification process in a side-specific manner.

Conclusion

Valvulogenesis is an extremely complex process by which a fragile gelatinous matrix is populated and remodeled during embryonic development into thin fibrous leaflets capable of maintaining unidirectional flow over a lifetime. Studies from transgenic knockout mice and in-vitro explant studies have shown that BMP are critical contributors to this process, regulating both the initiation of cushion formation and later stages of leaflet maturation. Understanding the role of BMP in this complex process is not only important for determining the origins of congenital defects, but may also provide insight into potential regenerative and/or therapeutic strategies to combat valvular dysfunction. Recently, Sox9 expression was found to have a protective role on calcific valve phenotypes in vivo, completely reversing the effects of mineralization, and activation of inflammatory and matrix remodeling processes [61]. This is a remarkable finding since BMP-induced Sox9 has been suggested as a master regulator of valve progenitor differentiation for proper valve maturation. Taken together, the orchestration of BMP signaling during valvulogenesis is critical. By exploiting these controlled embryonic derived paradigms, re-expression of BMP-associated factors may potentially be used to combat pathological stimuli within the clinic.

References

1. Nakajima Y et al. Expression of smooth muscle alpha-actin in mesenchymal cells during formation of avian endocardial cushion tissue: a role for transforming growth factor beta3. Dev Dyn. 1997;209(3):296–309.

2. Person AD, Klewer SE, Runyan RB. Cell biology of cardiac cushion development. Int Rev Cytol. 2005;243:287–335.
3. Moorman AF, Christoffels VM. Cardiac chamber formation: development, genes, and evolution. Physiol Rev. 2003;83(4):1223–67.
4. Yalcin HC et al. Hemodynamic patterning of the avian atrioventricular valve. Dev Dyn. 2011;240(1):23–35.
5. Butcher JT, Markwald RR. Valvulogenesis: the moving target. Philos Trans R Soc Lond B Biol Sci. 2007;362(1484):1489–503.
6. Sugi Y et al. Fibroblast growth factor (FGF)-4 can induce proliferation of cardiac cushion mesenchymal cells during early valve leaflet formation. Dev Biol. 2003;258(2):252–63.
7. Combs MD, Yutzey KE. Heart valve development: regulatory networks in development and disease. Circ Res. 2009;105(5):408–21.
8. Hurle JM et al. Elastic extracellular matrix of the embryonic chick heart: an immunohistological study using laser confocal microscopy. Dev Dyn. 1994;200(4):321–32.
9. Bajolle F et al. Rotation of the myocardial wall of the outflow tract is implicated in the normal positioning of the great arteries. Circ Res. 2006;98(3):421–8.
10. Thompson RP, Abercrombie V, Wong M. Morphogenesis of the truncus arteriosus of the chick embryo heart: movements of autoradiographic tattoos during septation. Anat Rec. 1987;218(4):434–40, 394–5.
11. Garcia-Martinez V, Sanchez-Quintana D, Hurle JM. Histochemical and ultrastructural changes in the extracellular matrix of the developing chick semilunar heart valves. Acta Anat (Basel). 1991; 142(1):87–96.
12. Massague J, Seoane J, Wotton D. Smad transcription factors. Genes Dev. 2005;19(23):2783–810.
13. Massague J, Wotton D. Transcriptional control by the TGF-beta/Smad signaling system. EMBO J. 2000;19(8):1745–54.
14. Nohe A et al. Signal transduction of bone morphogenetic protein receptors. Cell Signal. 2004;16(3):291–9.
15. van Wijk B, Moorman AF, van den Hoff MJ. Role of bone morphogenetic proteins in cardiac differentiation. Cardiovasc Res. 2007; 74(2):244–55.
16. Solloway MJ, Robertson EJ. Early embryonic lethality in Bmp5; Bmp7 double mutant mice suggests functional redundancy within the 60A subgroup. Development. 1999;126(8):1753–68.
17. Kim RY, Robertson EJ, Solloway MJ. Bmp6 and Bmp7 are required for cushion formation and septation in the developing mouse heart. Dev Biol. 2001;235(2):449–66.
18. Yamagishi T et al. Expression of bone morphogenetic protein-5 gene during chick heart development: possible roles in valvuloseptal endocardial cushion formation. Anat Rec. 2001;264(4):313–6.
19. Dudley AT, Robertson EJ. Overlapping expression domains of bone morphogenetic protein family members potentially account for limited tissue defects in BMP7 deficient embryos. Dev Dyn. 1997;208(3): 349–62.
20. Delot EC. Control of endocardial cushion and cardiac valve maturation by BMP signaling pathways. Mol Genet Metab. 2003;80(1–2): 27–35.
21. Zhang H, Bradley A. Mice deficient for BMP2 are nonviable and have defects in amnion/chorion and cardiac development. Development. 1996;122(10):2977–86.
22. Winnier G et al. Bone morphogenetic protein-4 is required for mesoderm formation and patterning in the mouse. Genes Dev. 1995;9(17):2105–16.
23. Dewulf N et al. Distinct spatial and temporal expression patterns of two type I receptors for bone morphogenetic proteins during mouse embryogenesis. Endocrinology. 1995;136(6):2652–63.
24. Verschueren K et al. Expression of type I and type IB receptors for activin in midgestation mouse embryos suggests distinct functions in organogenesis. Mech Dev. 1995;52(1):109–23.
25. Yamashita H et al. Osteogenic protein-1 binds to activin type II receptors and induces certain activin-like effects. J Cell Biol. 1995;130(1):217–26.
26. Gaussin V et al. Endocardial cushion and myocardial defects after cardiac myocyte-specific conditional deletion of the bone morphogenetic protein receptor ALK3. Proc Natl Acad Sci USA. 2002; 99(5):2878–83.
27. Delot EC et al. BMP signaling is required for septation of the outflow tract of the mammalian heart. Development. 2003;130(1): 209–20.
28. Krug EL, Mjaatvedt CH, Markwald RR. Extracellular matrix from embryonic myocardium elicits an early morphogenetic event in cardiac endothelial differentiation. Dev Biol. 1987;120(2):348–55.
29. Sugi Y et al. Bone morphogenetic protein-2 can mediate myocardial regulation of atrioventricular cushion mesenchymal cell formation in mice. Dev Biol. 2004;269(2):505–18.
30. Boyer AS et al. TGFβeta2 and TGFβeta3 have separate and sequential activities during epithelial-mesenchymal cell transformation in the embryonic heart. Dev Biol. 1999;208(2):530–45.
31. Song W, Jackson K, McGuire PG. Degradation of type IV collagen by matrix metalloproteinases is an important step in the epithelial-mesenchymal transformation of the endocardial cushions. Dev Biol. 2000;227(2):606–17.
32. Nakajima Y et al. Mechanisms involved in valvuloseptal endocardial cushion formation in early cardiogenesis: roles of transforming growth factor (TGF)-beta and bone morphogenetic protein (BMP). Anat Rec. 2000;258(2):119–27.
33. Inai K et al. BMP-2 induces cell migration and periostin expression during atrioventricular valvulogenesis. Dev Biol. 2008;315(2):383–96.
34. Conway SJ, Doetschman T, Azhar M. The inter-relationship of periostin, TGF beta, and BMP in heart valve development and valvular heart diseases. ScientificWorldJournal. 2011;11:1509–24.
35. Butcher JT et al. Periostin promotes atrioventricular mesenchyme matrix invasion and remodeling mediated by integrin signaling through Rho/PI 3-kinase. Dev Biol. 2007;302(1):256–66.
36. Jiao K et al. An essential role of Bmp4 in the atrioventricular septation of the mouse heart. Genes Dev. 2003;17(19):2362–7.
37. McCulley DJ et al. BMP4 is required in the anterior heart field and its derivatives for endocardial cushion remodeling, outflow tract septation, and semilunar valve development. Dev Dyn. 2008;237(11): 3200–9.
38. Hata A et al. Smad6 inhibits BMP/Smad1 signaling by specifically competing with the Smad4 tumor suppressor. Genes Dev. 1998; 12(2):186–97.
39. Galvin KM et al. A role for smad6 in development and homeostasis of the cardiovascular system. Nat Genet. 2000;24(2):171–4.
40. Chakraborty S et al. Shared gene expression profiles in developing heart valves and osteoblast progenitor cells. Physiol Genomics. 2008;35(1):75–85.
41. Wehrli BM et al. Sox9, a master regulator of chondrogenesis, distinguishes mesenchymal chondrosarcoma from other small blue round cell tumors. Hum Pathol. 2003;34(3):263–9.
42. Lincoln J et al. Sox9 is required for precursor cell expansion and extracellular matrix organization during mouse heart valve development. Dev Biol. 2007;305(1):120–32.
43. Lincoln J, Alfieri CM, Yutzey KE. BMP and FGF regulatory pathways control cell lineage diversification of heart valve precursor cells. Dev Biol. 2006;292(2):292–302.
44. Akiyama H et al. Essential role of Sox9 in the pathway that controls formation of cardiac valves and septa. Proc Natl Acad Sci USA. 2004;101(17):6502–7.
45. Chen YH et al. Msx1 and Msx2 are required for endothelial-mesenchymal transformation of the atrioventricular cushions and patterning of the atrioventricular myocardium. BMC Dev Biol. 2008;8:75.
46. Chen YH et al. Msx1 and Msx2 regulate survival of secondary heart field precursors and post-migratory proliferation of cardiac neural crest in the outflow tract. Dev Biol. 2007;308(2):421–37.
47. Chakraborty S, Combs MD, Yutzey KE. Transcriptional regulation of heart valve progenitor cells. Pediatr Cardiol. 2010;31(3):414–21.

48. Ma L et al. Bmp2 is essential for cardiac cushion epithelial-mesenchymal transition and myocardial patterning. Development. 2005;132(24):5601–11.
49. Shelton EL, Yutzey KE. Twist1 function in endocardial cushion cell proliferation, migration, and differentiation during heart valve development. Dev Biol. 2008;317(1):282–95.
50. Chakraborty S et al. Twist1 promotes heart valve cell proliferation and extracellular matrix gene expression during development in vivo and is expressed in human diseased aortic valves. Dev Biol. 2010;347(1):167–79.
51. Stennard FA et al. Cardiac T-box factor Tbx20 directly interacts with Nkx2-5, GATA4, and GATA5 in regulation of gene expression in the developing heart. Dev Biol. 2003;262(2):206–24.
52. Plageman Jr TF, Yutzey KE. T-box genes and heart development: putting the "T" in heart. Dev Dyn. 2005;232(1):11–20.
53. Cai X et al. Myocardial Tbx20 regulates early atrioventricular canal formation and endocardial epithelial-mesenchymal transition via Bmp2. Dev Biol. 2011;360(2):381–90.
54. Shelton EL, Yutzey KE. Tbx20 regulation of endocardial cushion cell proliferation and extracellular matrix gene expression. Dev Biol. 2007;302(2):376–88.
55. Mohler 3rd ER et al. Bone formation and inflammation in cardiac valves. Circulation. 2001;103(11):1522–8.
56. Kaden JJ et al. Expression of bone sialoprotein and bone morphogenetic protein-2 in calcific aortic stenosis. J Heart Valve Dis. 2004;13(4):560–6.
57. Ankeny RF et al. Preferential activation of SMAD1/5/8 on the fibrosa endothelium in calcified human aortic valves–association with low BMP antagonists and SMAD6. PLoS One. 2011;6(6): e20969.
58. Osman L et al. Role of human valve interstitial cells in valve calcification and their response to atorvastatin. Circulation. 2006; 114(1 Suppl):I547–52.
59. Yang X et al. Bone morphogenic protein 2 induces Runx2 and osteopontin expression in human aortic valve interstitial cells: role of Smad1 and extracellular signal-regulated kinase 1/2. J Thorac Cardiovasc Surg. 2009;138(4):1008–15.
60. Balachandran K et al. Elevated cyclic stretch induces aortic valve calcification in a bone morphogenic protein-dependent manner. Am J Pathol. 2010;177(1):49–57.
61. Peacock JD et al. Reduced sox9 function promotes heart valve calcification phenotypes in vivo. Circ Res. 2010;106(4):712–9.

Dysfunctional Mechanisms of Anti-inflammation in Aortic Stenosis

37

David A. Fullerton and Xianzhong Meng

Aortic valve disease is the third most common cardiovascular disease in the United States, exceeded only by hypertension and coronary artery disease. Approximately 2–7 % of the population older than 65 years has aortic stenosis [1], and calcific aortic stenosis is the most common indication for valve replacement. Despite its prevalence, the pathogenesis of calcific aortic stenosis is not well understood. In particular, the cellular mechanisms by which the aortic valve leaflets become calcified are unclear.

Calcific aortic stenosis has traditionally been considered a "degenerative" process with passive accumulation of calcium on the aortic valve leaflets. Recently, however, separate lines of investigation have begun to coalesce, suggesting that the pathogenesis of calcific aortic stenosis may be an active biologic process.

One such line of investigation includes epidemiologic studies that have identified several clinical risk factors for the development of aortic stenosis, including hypertension, hyperlipidemia, and diabetes mellitus [1–3]. Importantly, these same clinical risk factors are also associated with atherosclerosis. It is now appreciated that inflammatory mechanisms initiate and perpetuate atherosclerosis on a cellular level [4]. Hence, it is logical to postulate that given the similarity of clinical risk factors for the development of aortic stenosis and atherosclerosis, the cellular mechanisms of the two disease states may have common features as well (i.e., mechanisms of inflammation). It is therefore noteworthy that patients with aortic stenosis have circulating evidence of systemic inflammation such as elevated C-reactive protein and elevated levels of circulating soluble adhesion molecules [5–11].

Such clinical investigations are supported by studies in which histological evidence of inflammation has been found in calcified aortic valve leaflets removed at the time of aortic valve replacement. Early aortic valvular lesions demonstrate lipid accumulation as well as an infiltrate of chronic inflammatory cells such as macrophages, mast cells, and T lymphocytes [12, 13]. Histological data such as these provide circumstantial evidence that mechanisms of inflammation may play an important role in the pathogenesis of aortic stenosis.

In another line of investigation, histological evidence of active bone formation has been found in aortic valves removed at the time of aortic valve replacement. The calcified aortic leaflets have features that resemble the osteogenic bone formation found in skeletal bone [14]. Skeletal bone formation is dependent upon osteoblasts, which create a mineralized extracellular matrix [15]. Osteoblast cells are phenotypically characterized by several proteins associated with bone formation, including osteopontin, osteocalcin, and bone sialoprotein. Using RT-PCR, increased mRNA levels for all of these have been found in calcified aortic valves [14]. Such data indicate that bone-forming cells (osteoblasts or osteoblast-like cells) are present in calcified aortic valve leaflets and in fact are responsible for the calcification. The origin of the bone-forming cells is not known. It is noteworthy, however, that bone formation has been reported in cultured myofibroblasts from aortic valves [16], suggesting the possibility that aortic valve myofibroblasts may differentiate into bone-forming cells.

Taken together, these background studies strongly suggest that calcific aortic stenosis is (1) an inflammatory disease and (2) the process of calcification results from active bone-like formation.

The fact that calcified aortic valve leaflets have a histological appearance consistent with bone formation suggests that calcific aortic stenosis is a process of active bone formation rather that a passive degenerative process. This implies that bone-forming cells (osteoblasts or osteoblast-like cells) may be responsible for the calcification and that some cells within the valve may have the potential to become osteoblast-like. However, the origin of such cells is unknown.

D.A. Fullerton, MD (✉) • X. Meng, MD, PhD
Division of Cardiothoracic Surgery,
The University of Colorado School of Medicine,
12631 E. 17th Avenue, Room 6602, MS-C310,
Aurora, CO 80045, USA
e-mail: david.fullerton@ucdenver.edu

E.A. Gabriel, S.A. Gabriel (eds.), *Inflammatory Response in Cardiovascular Surgery*,
DOI 10.1007/978-1-4471-4429-8_37, © Springer-Verlag London 2013

The normal human aortic valve leaflet is a gossamer structure. It is primarily comprised of a single layer of endothelial cells on both the aortic surface and the ventricular surface overlying a very thin matrix of collagen and elastin fibrils. Interspersed among the collagen and elastin fibrils are cells. Some of these cells are fibroblasts, but the predominant cell type has a phenotype with features of both myoblasts and fibroblasts, hence it is called a myofibroblast. These myofibroblasts are referred to as aortic valve interstitial cells (AVICs).

The AVIC is a biologically active cell and has been implicated in the pathogenesis of aortic stenosis [14]. These cells have been shown to express Toll-like receptors (TLRs) 2 and 4 [17]. Toll-like receptors are phylogenetically preserved components of the innate immune system and mediate many mechanisms of inflammation; the central role of TLRs, specifically TLR2 and TLR4, in the mediation of inflammatory stimuli is well recognized. Toll-like receptor signaling induces gene transcription, and its downstream effects, which include cytokine, chemokine, and adhesion molecule production, are mediated through NF-kB. While the role of TLRs in atherosclerotic mineralization has been investigated, insight into the inflammatory TLR signaling in heart valves has only recently emerged.

It is important to note that NF-kB also has a central role in controlling the expression of genes associated with bone mineralization. An important effector protein for mineralization is Runx-2, which is held in check by the transcription factors Hes and Hey. The net effect of NF-kB activation is to inhibit Hes and Hey gene expression, thereby increasing Runx-2 expression. In turn, this has been shown to lead to mineralization.

In response to proinflammatory stimulation via TLRs 2 and 4, the phenotype of human AVICs changes from that of a myofibroblast to that of a bone-forming-like cell [17]. Characteristics of this osteogenic phenotype include an increased expression of the potent bone forming protein, bone morphogenetic protein 2 (BMP-2), the osteogenic transcription factor, Runx2, and expression and activity of alkaline phosphatase.

Such pro-osteogenic factors have important roles in bone formation. Bone morphogenetic proteins are osteogenic growth factors and are the principal inducers of osteoblast differentiation and bone formation. BMP-2 is the most extensively characterized osteogenic growth factor and the most widely studied to stimulate osteoblastic differentiation [15]. Runx2 is a transcription factor expressed in mineralized tissues or their precursors [16]. It directly stimulates transcription of osteoblast-related genes and is necessary for osteoblast differentiation and bone formation.

Stimulation of TLR-2 and 4 on AVICs also produces a profound proinflammatory response. Stimulation of both of these receptors causes a significant increase in the expression of genes for powerful proinflammatory cytokines such as interleukin (IL)-8, IL-6, and IL-1β. In addition, their stimulation leads to significantly increased expression of proinflammatory adhesion molecules, such as intercellular adhesion molecule 1 (ICAM1) and vascular cell adhesion molecule 1 (VCAM1). Further, such increased genetic expression is translated into significantly increased production of the respective proinflammatory cytokines and adhesion molecules [18]. Of great interest is the observation that once the human AVIC is stimulated by proinflammatory stimuli, it responds with an augmented inflammatory response and an osteogenic response [19, 20].

Hence, not only does evidence suggest that calcific aortic stenosis may be an inflammatory disease, but that the human AVIC may play a very important role in the pathogenesis of calcific stenosis. In response to inflammatory stimuli, the human AVIC produces proinflammatory cytokines, chemokines, and adhesion molecules. In turn, these proinflammatory factors act in a paracrine and autocrine fashion to act upon the AVIC and to perpetuate the proinflammatory response and to stimulate the cells to assume an osteogenic phenotype. In other words, the inflammatory stimulation of the AVIC produces an inflammo-ostiogenic response.

The net inflammatory state of any tissue is determined by the relative balance of proinflammatory and anti-inflammatory mechanisms. In response to proinflammatory stimulation, a deficiency of anti-inflammatory mechanisms will lead to unopposed actions of proinflammatory mechanisms. Such an imbalance of pro- and anti-inflammatory mechanisms has been implicated in the pathogenesis of many inflammatory diseases. Specifically, increased tissue levels of interleukin-one beta (IL-1β) relative to its anti-inflammatory antagonist, interleukin-one receptor antagnosist (IL-1RA), have been implicated in the pathogenesis of rheumatoid arthritis, inflammatory bowel disease, atherosclerosis, and other inflammatory diseases [21].

Interleukin-one beta (IL-1β) has been implicated in the pathogenesis of aortic stenosis as well [22]. Produced by circulating mononuclear cells, the proinflammatory actions of IL-1β are mediated by the membrane-bound IL-1 receptor (IL-1R). Once stimulated, the IL-1R induces the AVIC to assume an osteogenic phenotype marked by the production of BMP-2 and alkaline phosphatase. The specific antagonist of IL-1β is the anti-inflammatory cytokine, IL-1RA, which blocks the actions of its receptor. The balance between IL-1β and IL-1RA in a given tissue may determine the development of inflammatory disease. In fact, a deficiency of IL-1RA relative to IL-1β leads to inflammation and tissue destruction.

This important defense mechanism of anti-inflammation is dysfunctional in aortic stenosis. Normal aortic valve leaflets have been shown to have an abundance of IL-1RA. However, it is virtually absent in stenotic aortic valves. Further, AVICs have been shown to be an important source of IL-1RA in normal valve leaflets. In normal valve leaflets, AVICs respond to proinflammatory stimulation by significantly increased production of IL-1RA, an important defense mechanism. Conversely, human AVICs from stenotic valve leaflets contain anti-inflammatory IL-1RA in nearly undetectable levels. And in response to proinflammatory stimulation, AVICs from stenotic valves produce significantly less IL-1RA than do normal AVICs. Therefore, impaired mechanisms of anti-inflammation, specifically a deficiency of IL-1RA, are associated with the pathogenesis of calcific aortic stenosis [21]. It is unknown, however, whether this dysfunctional mechanism of anti-inflammation is a primary deficiency or is somehow lost somewhere as the disease of aortic stenosis progresses.

In summary, the pathogenesis of aortic stenosis is one in which mechanisms of inflammation play an important role. However, dysfunction of mechanisms may likewise be equally important and offer insight into the mechanisms of the disease.

References

1. Mohler ER, Gannon F, Reynolds C, et al. Bone formation and inflammation in cardiac valves. Circulation. 2001;103:1522–8.
2. O'Brien KD, Knusisto J, Reichenbach DD, et al. Osteopontin is expressed in human aortic valvular lesions. Circulation. 1995;92: 2163–8.
3. Srivatsa SS, Harrity PJ, Maercklein PB, et al. Increased cellular expression of matrix proteins that regulate mineralization is associated with calcification of native human and porcine xenograft bioprosthetic heart valves. J Clin Invest. 1997;99:996–1009.
4. Shao J-S, Cai J, Towler DA. Molecular mechanisms of vascular calcification. Lessons learned from the aorta. Arterioscler Thromb Vasc Biol. 2006;26:1423–30.
5. Kaden JJ, Bickelhaupt S, Grobholz R, et al. Expression of bone sialoprotein and bone morphogenetic protein-2 in calcific aortic stenosis. J Heart Valve Dis. 2004;13:560–6.
6. Osman L, Yacoub MH, Latif N, Amrani M, Chester AH. Role of human valve interstitial cells in valve calcification and their response to atorvastatin. Circulation. 2006;114(Suppl I):I-547–52.
7. Olsson M, Dalsgaard CJ, Haegerstrand A, Rosenqvist M, Ryden L, Nilsson J. Accumulation of T lymphocytes and expression of interleukin-2 receptors in nonrheumatic stenotic aortic valves. J Am Coll Cardiol. 1994;23:1162–70.
8. Rajamannan NM, Gersh B, Bonow RO. Calcific aortic stenosis: from bench to the bedside-emerging clinical and cellular concepts. Heart. 2003;89:801–5.
9. Galante A. C-reactive protein is increased in patients with degenerative aortic valvular stenosis. J Am Coll Cardiol. 2001;38:1078–82.
10. Sanchez PL, Mazzone AM. C-reactive protein in aortic valve disease. Cardiovasc Ultrasound. 2006;4:37–40.
11. Shahi CN. Elevated levels of circulating soluble adhesion molecules in patients with nonrheumatic aortic stenosis. Am J Cardiol. 1997; 79:980–2.
12. Karsenty G, Ducy P, Starbuck M, et al. Cbfa1 as a regulator of osteoblast differentiation and function. Bone. 1999;25:107–8.
13. Aubin JE, Liu F, Malaval L, et al. Osteoblast and chondroblast differentiation. Bone. 1995;17:77S–83.
14. Rajamannan NM, Subramanian M, Rickard D, et al. Human aortic valve calcification is associated with an osteoblast phenotype. Circulation. 2003;107:2181–4.
15. Mohler ER, Chawla MK, Chang AW, et al. Identification and characterization of calcifying valve cells from human and canine aortic valves. J Heart Valve Dis. 1999;8:254–60.
16. Lane JM. Bone morphogenic protein science and studies. J Orthop Trauma. 2005;19:S17–22.
17. Meng X, Banerjee A, Cleveland JC, Weyant MJ, Dinarello CA, Babu A, et al. Expression of functional Toll-like receptors 2 and 4 in human aortic valve interstitial cells: potential roles in aortic valve inflammation and stenosis. Am J Physiol Cell Physiol. 2008;294:C29–35.
18. Babu A, Meng X, Zou N, Yang X, Wang M, Song Y, et al. LPS stimulation of human aortic valve interstitial cells activates inflammation and osteogenesis. Ann Thorac Surg. 2008;86:71–6.
19. Yang X, Fullerton DA, Su X, Al L, Meng X. Pro-osteogenic phenotype of human aortic valve interstitial cells is associated with higher levels of Toll-like receptors 2 and 4 and enhanced expression of bone morphogenic proteins. J Am Coll Cardiol. 2009;53:491–500.
20. Yang X, Meng X, Su X, Mauchley DC, Ao L, Cleveland JC, et al. Bone morphogenic protein 2 induces Runx2 and osteopontin expression in human aortic valve interstitial cells: role of Smad1 and extracellular signal related kinase 1/2. J Thorac Cardiovasc Surg. 2009;138:1008–15.
21. Lee J, Meng X, Weyant MJ, Reece JB, Cleveland Jr JC, Fullerton DA. Stenotic aortic valves have dysfunctional mechanisms of anti-inflammation: implications for aortic stenosis. J Thorac Cardiovasc Surg. 2011;141:481–6.
22. Kaden JJ, Dempfle CE, Grobholz R, et al. Interleukin-1 beta promotes matrix metalloproteinase expression and cell proliferation in calcific aortic valve stenosis. Atherosclerosis. 2003;170:205–11.

Heart Valve Surgery and the Antiphospholipid Syndrome

38

Carlos A. Mestres, Cecilia Marcacci, Gerard Espinosa, Jose L Pomar, Andrea Colli, and Ricard Cervera

Antiphospholipid syndrome – Lupus eritematosus – Cardiac surgery – Valve replacement device

Introduction

For more than 5 decades, cardiac surgery has developed at a fast and steady pace. Since the early days of complex and cumbersome procedures initially developed at targeting the correction in congenital intracardiac defects [1, 2], all types of intra- and extracardiac procedures have been performed worldwide on a routine basis at all institutions that meet the minimum requirements for intrathoracic surgery according to international standards [3]. The lack of appropriate diagnostic tools and advanced equipment for intracardiac surgery is a stimulus for progression. The initial era of cardiac surgery was defined by the development of basic technology for diagnosis and treatment and marked by the enormous progression in clinical experience.

Currently, cardiac surgery is a fully standardized specialty covering all aspects of congenital and acquired cardiovascular diseases. Up-to-date technological development combined with massive accumulation of clinical work and knowledge on intra- and postoperative management has led to an increase in the complexity and condition of the patients submitted for surgical correction of cardiac defects [4].

Antiphospholipid syndome (APS), an autoimmune disorder characterized by venous and arterial thrombosis, fetal loss, and thrombocytopenia, in the presence of antiphospholipid antibodies (aPL), namely lupus anticoagulant (LA), anticardiolipin antibodies (aCL), or anti-β2 glycoprotein-I (β2GPI) antibodies [5], is an uncommon disease bringing difficulties in establishing an appropriate diagnosis and effective treatment.

APS belongs to a formally unclassified group of uncommon or infrequent diseases such as infective endocarditis (IE). As such, a number of cases might go underdiagnosed, and, because of the specific pathophysiology, it might also pose a number of problems at the time of the management. Considering the specific impact of APS on thrombosis and hemostasis, APS is an example of a challenging disease when cardiovascular complications develop and surgical treatment is indicated.

APS has been called to clinicians' attention in recent years as patients are increasingly being diagnosed at specifically dedicated units [6] focusing on autoimmune disorders.

The Antiphospholipid Syndrome

Antiphospholipid syndrome (APS) is defined by the occurrence of venous and arterial thrombosis, often multiple, and recurrent fetal loss, frequently accompanied by a moderate thrombocytopenia, in the presence of antiphospholipid antibodies (aPL), namely lupus anticoagulant (LA), anticardiolipin antibodies (aCL), or anti-β_2 glycoprotein I (β_2GPI) antibodies. Chronic biological false-positive serological tests for syphilis (BFP-STS) may be present in some of these patients, because these tests also detect the presence of aPL. Other autoantibodies have also been found in many patients with an APS, such as antimitochondrial (M5 type), antiendothelial cell, antiplatelet, antierythrocyte, and antinuclear antibodies.

C.A. Mestres, MD, PhD, FETCS (✉) • C. Marcacci, MD
J.L. Pomar, MD, PhD, FETCS
Department of Cardiovascular Surgery,
Hospital Clinico, University of Barcelona,
Villarroel 170, Barcelona 08036, Spain
e-mail: cmestres@clinic.ub.es

G. Espinosa, MD, PhD • R. Cervera, MD, PhD, FRCP
Department of Autoimmune Diseases,
Hospital Clinico, University of Barcelona,
Barcelona, Spain

A. Colli, MD, PhD
Department of Cardiovascular Surgery,
Cardiac Surgery Unit, University of Padova,
Padova, Italy

E.A. Gabriel, S.A. Gabriel (eds.), *Inflammatory Response in Cardiovascular Surgery*,
DOI 10.1007/978-1-4471-4429-8_38, © Springer-Verlag London 2013

Box 38.1 Revised Classification Criteria for APS (Sydney Criteria)

Clinical criteria

1. Vascular thrombosis:
   One or more clinical episodes of arterial, venous, or small vessel thrombosis, in any tissue or organ. Thrombosis must be confirmed by objective validated criteria (i.e., unequivocal findings of appropriate imaging studies or histopathology). For histopathological confirmation, thrombosis should be present without significant evidence of inflammation in the vessel wall.
2. Pregnancy morbidity:
   (a) One or more unexplained deaths of a morphologically normal fetus at or beyond the tenth week of gestation, with normal fetal morphology documented by ultrasound or by direct examination of the fetus, or
   (b) One or more premature births of a morphologically normal baby before the 34th weeks of gestation because of: (i) eclampsia or severe preeclampsia defined according to standard definitions or (ii) recognized features of placental failure, or
   (c) Three or more unexplained consecutive spontaneous abortions before the 10th week of gestation, with maternal anatomic or hormonal abnormalities and paternal and maternal chromosomal causes excluded.

Laboratory criteria

1. LA present in plasma on two or more occasions at least 12 weeks apart, detected according to the guidelines of the International Society on Thrombosis and Hemostasis
2. aCL antibody of IgG and/or IgM isotype in serum or plasma, present in medium or high titers (i.e. >40 GPL or MPL, or > the 99th percentile), on two or more occasions, at least 12 weeks apart, measured by a standardized ELISA
3. Anti-β2 glycoprotein-I antibody of IgG and/or IgM isotype in serum or plasma (in titers > the 99th percentile), present on two or more occasions, at least 12 weeks apart, measured by a standardized ELISA, according to recommended procedures

APS is present if at least one of the clinical criteria and one of the laboratory criteria are met.

APS can be found in patients having neither clinical nor laboratory evidence of another definable condition (primary APS) or it may be associated with other diseases. APS is the disorder with which systemic lupus erythematosus (SLE) is most commonly associated. Less frequently, aPL and, rarely, APS may also be encountered in other groups of patients, including those with malignancies [5].

The clinical picture of the APS is characterized by venous and arterial thrombosis, fetal loss, and thrombocytopenia. According to the largest survey of APS patients – the Europhospholipid project [6] – deep vein thrombosis, sometimes accompanied by pulmonary embolism, is the most frequently reported manifestation in this syndrome (38.9 %). Conversely, cerebrovascular accidents – either stroke (19.8 %) or transient ischemic attacks (11.1 %) – are the most common arterial thrombotic manifestations. Early fetal loss (35.4 %), late fetal loss (16.9 %), premature births (10.6 %), and pre-eclampsia (9.5 %) are the most frequent fetal and obstetric manifestations. Additionally, several other clinical features are relatively common in these patients, i.e., thrombocytopenia (29.6 %), livedo reticularis (24.1 %), heart valve lesions (11.6 %), hemolytic anemia (9.7 %), epilepsy (7 %), myocardial infarction (5.5 %), leg ulcers (5.5 %), and amaurosis fugax (5.4 %). However, a large variety of other clinical manifestations have been less frequently described in patients with the APS, with prevalences lower than 5 %.

Some patients have a catastrophic variant of the APS, and they have in common: (1) clinical evidence of multiple organ involvement developing over a very short period of time; (2) histopathological evidence of multiple small vessel occlusions, and (3) laboratory confirmation of the presence of aPL, usually at high titers. Furthermore, more than half of the catastrophic episodes are preceded by a precipitating event, mainly infections [7, 8]. Although patients with catastrophic APS represent less than 1 % of all patients with APS [6], they are usually in a life-threatening situation with a nearly 50 % mortality rate [8]. In order to correlate all the published case reports as well as newly diagnosed cases from all over the world, an international registry of patients with catastrophic APS (CAPS Registry) was created in 2000 by the European Forum on aPL. Currently, it documents the entire clinical, laboratory, and therapeutic data of more than 400 patients whose data have been fully registered (www.med.ub.es/MIMMUN/FORUM/CAPS.HTM). The analysis of this registry has allowed the characterization of the clinical and laboratory features of catastrophic APS as well as the establishment of preliminary criteria for its classification and guidelines for its management [9, 10].

In order to facilitate studies of treatment and causation, preliminary classification criteria for APS were formulated in 1998 in Sapporo [11] and revised in 2006 in Sydney [12] (Box 38.1). Classification criteria for catastrophic APS were published in 2003 and are depicted in Box 38.2 [9].

Heart Valve Lesions in the Antiphospholipid Syndrome

The heart is one of the major target organs in APS, and cardiac valve disease is the most common cardiac manifestation [13]. In the largest series, with 1,000 APS patients, the Europhospholipid cohort, valvular thickening and/or dysfunction

Box 38.2 Preliminary Criteria for the Classification of Catastrophic APS

1. Evidence of involvement of three or more organs, systems, and/or tissues[a]
2. Development of manifestations simultaneously or in less than a week
3. Confirmation by histopathology of small vessel occlusion in at least one organ or tissue[b]
4. Laboratory confirmation of the presence of antiphospholipid antibodies (lupus anticoagulant and/or anticardiolipin antibodies)[c]

[a]Usually, clinical evidence of vessel occlusions, confirmed by imaging techniques when appropriate. Renal involvement is defined by a 50 % rise in serum creatinine, severe systemic hypertension (>180/100 mmHg), and/or proteinuria (>500 mg/24 h)

[b]For histopathological confirmation, significant evidence of thrombosis must be present, although vasculitis may coexist occasionally

[c]If the patient had not been previously diagnosed as having an APS, the laboratory confirmation requires that the presence of antiphospholipid antibodies must be detected on two or more occasions at least 12 weeks apart (not necessarily at the time of the event), according to the revised criteria for the classification of definite APS

Definite catastrophic APS:

- All 4 criteria

Probable catastrophic APS:

- All 4 criteria, except for only two organs, systems, and/or tissues involvement
- All 4 criteria, except for the absence of laboratory confirmation at least 12 weeks apart because of the early death of a patient never previously tested for aPL prior to the catastrophic APS event
- 1, 2, and 4
- 1, 3, and 4 and the development of a third event in more than a week but less than a month, despite anticoagulation

appeared as a cumulative manifestation in 11.6 % of the patients, followed by vegetations in 2.7 % [6]. In the 5-year follow-up of this cohort, 1.7 % of patients developed new valvular thickening and/or dysfunction and 1.4 % valvular vegetations [14].

An international consensus statement published in 2006 provided relevant definitions of heart valve lesions in APS [12]. According to this consensus, valve lesions, as assessed by echocardiography, include valve thickness of more han 3 mm, localized thickening involving the leaflet's proximal or middle portion, and irregular nodules on the atrial face of the edge of the mitral valve or on the vascular face of the aortic valve. However, the differential diagnosis from infective endocarditis and rheumatic fever valve lesions remains difficult and will require clinical and microbiological assessment in addition to the echocardiographic findings.

There are discrepancies in the prevalence of valvular disease in SLE patients with or without aPL as well as in primary APS patients [15]. One of the reasons for this variability may be the different techniques [transthoracic (TTE) or transesophageal (TEE) echocardiography] used to detect valve lesions. In particular, TTE is less sensitive, and TEE may detect minor non-specific valvular thickening compared with TTE. In this regard, TEE has a higher sensitivity to detect valvular defects in patients with SLE (e.g., 44 % with TTE versus 60 % with TEE in SLE patients with aPL; 25 % with TTE versus 63 % with TEE in SLE patients without aPL) [15]. Other important points that may explain the variability of the prevalence of valvular disease are the different methodologies used to test aPL and what is considered a positive aPL test in different studies. Due to these limitations, it is difficult to compare studies and establish solid conclusions about the role of aPL in the development of valvular abnormalities

By means of Doppler echocardiography, SLE patients with aPL show a significantly higher prevalence of valvular defects compared to those without aPL [13]. Moreover, almost 90 % of patients with SLE and valvular disease have been found to have aPL compared to 44 % of patients without valvular involvement. However, studies analyzing the association between aPL and valvular disease in SLE patients are contradictory. The majority of studies demonstrated a higher prevalence of valvular abnormalities in patients with SLE and aPL, ranging from 14 to 86 %. In a meta-analysis of 13 studies [16], nearly half of aPL-positive patients with SLE had valve lesions compared with 21 % of aPL-negative SLE patients. Conversely, Roldan et al. [17] and Gabrielli et al. [18] found a similar prevalence of valvular involvement in both aPL-positive and aPL-negative patients with SLE.

Regarding patients with primary APS, echocardiographic studies found heart valve abnormalities in one third of them [13]. As in SLE patients, patients with primary APS had a higher prevalence of valvular defects with TTE compared with healthy individuals (40 % versus 2 %; $p<0.0001$) [13]. However, TEE has a higher sensitivity to detect valvular defects in primary APS patients (73 % with TEE versus 39 % with TTE, $p<0.0005$) (15/11). Unfortunately, the studies with TEE did not include healthy individuals.

A few prospective studies have analyzed the pattern of heart valve lesions over time [13]. Based on these studies, the initial valvular lesions may worsen, improve, disappear, or remain stable over time. Furthermore, new valvular lesions may develop. Espinola-Zavaleta et al. [19] found valve lesions in 71 % of primary APS patients in the initial TEE. After a follow-up of 84 months, valve lesions were unchanged in three cases and new valve lesions were detected in three patients, whereas in six patients the valve lesions had progressed. Turiel et al. [20] evaluated 56 patients with primary APS at baseline, and 47 of them had repeated TEE examinations. Initial valvular involvement was found in 32 (57 %) patients. Over the 5-year follow-up, progression or new cardiac involvement was observed in 17 (36 %) patients. Specifically, 13 (28 %) patients developed valvular lesions [8 (61 %) subjects developed new valvular lesions and 5 (38 %) had worsening lesions]. Interestingly, using multivariate logistic regression analysis, the authors found that high IgG aCL titers (>40 GPL) represented the only independent risk factor for new and progressive cardiac abnormalities in patients with primary APS.

Perez-Villa et al. [21] performed a prospective study in 61 SLE patients with and without APS using TTE. Overall, valvular disease was found in 39 % of patients. After a mean time of 8 years, there was a significant increase in valvular abnormalities at the final echocardiography. The results of a prospective study including 53 patients with APS and previous thrombosis analyzed with TTE with a longer follow-up (more than 10 years) were recently published [22]. The main conclusion was that patients without valvulopathy would have a 93 % likelihood of continued valvulopathy and only a 7 % chance of disappearance of valvular disease during the disease follow-up. Moreover, patients without valvulopathy at initial echocardiography would have a 92 % likelihood of remaining free of valvulopathy. In light of these results, the authors recommended an initial echocardiography in all APS patients at the time of diagnosis, mainly in the presence of arterial thrombosis. With normal valves, serial echocardiographic studies might not be necessary. Conversely, if valvular abnormalities are present, serial echocardiographic studies are warranted in order to detect functional changes that may require surgery.

Unfortunately, no therapeutic trials or prospective clinical studies have specifically addressed the question of whether treatment has any role in the pattern of heart valve lesions over time, and the number of patients who received the different treatments included in the echocardiographic studies is relatively low to allow strong recommendations. Although almost all patients included in the prospective studies were under anticoagulant or antiplatelet treatment, these treatments were unable to reverse established valve lesions or prevent their appearance. In the same sense, immunosuppression had no effect on the evolution of valvular lesions. However, from the few case reports, there is scarce evidence about the possible beneficial effects of corticosteroids and immunosuppression on the treatment of valvular heart disease [13].

A consensus committee developed in 2002 on the occasion of the tenth International Congress on aPL held in Taormina, Sicily, Italy, made the following statements [23]: (1) anticoagulation is recommended for symptomatic patients with valvulopathy; (2) prophylactic antiplatelet therapy may be appropriate for asymptomatic patients (recommended by 13/17 experts in an independent review); and (3) committee members disagreed about whether corticosteroid therapy is helpful, but agreed that distinguishing among presumptive valvulitis (valve thickening on echocardiogram), valve deformity, and vegetations is important as the treatment implications may differ.

More recently, the "Task Force on Catastrophic APS and Non-criteria APS Manifestations," developed in 2010 on the occasion of the 13th International Congress on aPL held in Galveston, Texas, USA, made the following recommendations [15]: (1) In patients with APS and previous thrombosis, mainly with arterial involvement, a TTE is recommended; (2) with normal valves and in the absence of atherosclerotic factors, follow-up controls might not be necessary; (3) if heart valve lesions exist, serial echocardiographic follow-up controls are warranted; and (4) larger studies examining the accuracy of heart valve lesions detected by TEE for the diagnosis of APS are warranted.

Cardiac Surgery in Antiphospholipid Syndrome

Despite all of the above, the actual occurrence of patients requiring an operation to correct a valve defect is uncommon. A literature review confirms that current experience in valve surgery in patients with APS is still scanty and that the majority of the accumulated experience comes in the form of case reports or limited case series. We outlined this in a previous publication [24]. However, the published reports and series do give an overview of organ involvement in patients who were referred for surgical treatment of advanced heart valve disease. Table 38.1 summarizes the organ involvement found by authors in different reports. This confirms that protean manifestations are to be expected in patients with APS requiring valve surgery. Mortality is not to be neglected.

The surgical series and reports published so far are defining a surgical population that is to be considered as on the high-risk side. Single, double, and triple valve surgery has been reported in the past 2 decades in about 20 reports [24–44]. Valve replacement has been commonly performed as many of these patients have advanced disease with severe leaflet and annular involvement precluding at best repair as the first option. Although the replacement option has usually been reported, heart valve operations are not the only one attempted. Although the vast majority of patients with APS suffer from valve disease, coronary bypass graft surgery has also been reported, and additional miscellaneous procedures, too. When valve replacement was not indicated, exploratory operations have also been performed for non-infectious conditions [45].

Aortic and mitral valve replacements are the most frequently performed procedures. They are standardized

Table 38.1 Organ involvements performed

Author	Year	Ref.	Brain	Vasc	Eye	Spleen	Heart	Intestinal	Kidney	P. valve	No TE	Death	FU
Alvarez-Blanco A	1994	[25]								1			
Schumacher M	1995	[26]											
Sakaguchi G	1998	[27]											
Myers GJ	1999	[28]											
Matsuyama K	1999	[29]									1		
Amital H	1999	[46]	1			1			1		1		17 months
Hogan WJ	2000	[47]											
Hasegawa R	2001	[30]											
Kurushima A	2002	[31]		1			1						
Berkun Y	2004	[32]								2		1	8 years
Herrmann M	2004	[33]	1	1	1				1				13 months
Massoudy P	2005	[34]						1				3	1 years
Sasahashi N	2007	[35]									1		26 days
Einav G	2007	[36]											
Hegde VA	2007	[37]	1	1			1						
Wieteska M	2007	[38]											
Colli A	2009	[24]	1	1								2	1 years
Cianciulli TF	2009	[39]									1		10 months
De Agustin JA	2009	[40]									1		
Alaminos P	2010	[41]								1			
Kondo H	2010	[42]	1										
Kim HK	2010	[43]						1					
Ratwat RS	2011	[44]									1		

Ref reference, *P. valve* prosthetic valve, *no TE* no history of thromboembolism, *FU* follow-up

operations, as we currently know, and surgical results according to valve position are quite similar in terms of 30-day mortality regardless of the region, as it can be derived from the available registries. In APS patients, there are worse results as postoperative complications frequently appear in terms of thromboembolic events [24]. One of the reasons may be related to the actual pathophysiological mechanisms because of the deposition of APS antibodies on valve tissue [46]. Whether this can be accepted as an explanation in the presence of valve replacement devices of different designs is still to be clearly defined.

The Main Issues in Cardiac Surgery

There are a few critical issues when considering valve surgery. First, APS is by definition a hypercoagulable state. It has to be remembered that factor XII activation will occur as thrombogenic surfaces are going to be used as part of the routine setup and equipment in cardiac surgery. The most important example to consider is extracorporeal tubing. Also, intraoperative management of anticoagulation is likely to be the most important issue in patients with APS. Attention was drawn to this previously by Hogan et al. concerning a young female patient [47]. Of critical importance is thrombocytopenia as well as the prolonged clotting times. Intraoperative monitoring is a substantial part of the surgical strategy.

The conducting of the operation at our department as part of the strategy across the entire process has included standard cardiopulmonary bypass with full heparinization [activated clotting time (ACT) >450 s] and cardioplegic arrest with intermittent cold blood cardioplegia administered through the aortic root and coronary ostia and/or the retrograde route. Postoperative oral anticoagulation with vitamin K antagonist (VKA) and anticoagulants were started after 48 h postoperatively, and low-molecular-weight heparin was continued until the international normalized ratio (INR)

Table 38.2 Type of operation

Author	Year	Ref.	AVR	MVR	TVR	DVR	TVr	CABG	CABG + O	O	Mortality
Alvarez-Blanco A	1994	[25]		1							–
Schumacher M	1995	[26]		1							No
Sakaguchi G	1998	[27]	1								No
Myers GJ	1999	[28]				1					No
Matsuyama K	1999	[29]	1								No
Amital H	1999	[46]		1							No
Hogan WJ	2000	[47]	1								No
Hasegawa R	2001	[30]		1							–
Kurushima A	2002	[31]						1			No
Berkun Y	2004	[32]	2	7	2	2					Yes (2)
Herrmann M	2004	[33]		1							No
Massoudy P	2005	[34]		1					2	2	Yes (3)
Sasahashi N	2007	[35]	1								No
Einav G	2007	[36]					1				No
Hegde VA	2007	[37]		5				4			No
Wieteska M	2007	[38]								1	No
Colli A	2009	[24]	3	4		1				1	Yes (2)
Cianciulli TF	2009	[39]								1	No
De Agustin JA	2009	[40]								1	No
Alaminos P	2010	[41]		1							No
Kondo H	2010	[42]		1							No
Kim HK	2010	[43]							1		No
Ratwat RS	2011	[44]				1					No

Ref reference, *AVR* aortic valve replacement, *MVR* mitral valve replacement, *TVR* tricuspid valve replacement, *DVR* double valve replacement, *TVr* tricuspid valve repair, *CABG* coronary artery bypass graft, *O* other

reached a range between 2.5 and 3.5. A key component in surgery is a more aggressive management of anticoagulation with ACT lasting twice as long as in regular operations. However, this is a relatively empirical process as the clinical experience is scanty.

Clinical Experience

Our experience has been reported earlier [24]. It now extends to ten clinical cases, with all patients being operated on for valve disease. Two of these patients died, for an in-hospital mortality of 20 %. One of them presented with stroke on the 5th postoperative day, and the second had intracranial bleeding in the form of subdural hematoma that was later followed by carotid artery thrombosis. These two cases are good illustrations of the difficulties in the overall management of patients with APS undergoing cardiac surgery. As stated, protean manifestations and an extreme tendency to thrombotic events in patients are always associated with long-standing steroid therapy. The excellent review of Gorki et al. identified 57 patients who had undergone valve surgery, other than the patients in our own cases, and yielded interesting observations after a meta-analysis of the accumulated experience up to 2007. The first is that the average age of cardiac surgical APS patients is younger than that of the average patient in westernized cardiac surgical units. The second is that there is a trend toward increasing aggressiveness in the intraoperative management of the anticoagulation with more liberal use of heparin and less aggressive reversal by using less protamine sulfate. Finally, the possibility of the eventual appearance of catastrophic APS with multiple vascular occlusions must always be kept in mind [8, 9, 48].

Controversy still exists about how to choose a valve replacement device. Table 38.2 shows the procedures performed by different authors. Our policy has usually been to choose a mechanical valve, and actually six out of ten patients had a mechanical valve implanted. Two had a tissue valve and, and they had uneventful postoperative stays. This is similar to the experience reported in different series. Mechanical valves are usually the first choice considering that these patients will be in oral anticoagulation regimens with or without antiplatelet therapy, an issue that is also currently under discussion. Isolated cases, including one case from our experience [46] (Figs. 38.1, 38.2, and 38.3), may be treated with preservation of the valve, but this is uncommon. A very recent experience by Erdozain et al. [49] that reviewed a multicenter experience with 33 patients treated over a period of 27 years also stressed on similar issues, namely high perioperative morbidity and mortality and the need of the prevention of hemorrhagic and thrombotic complications.

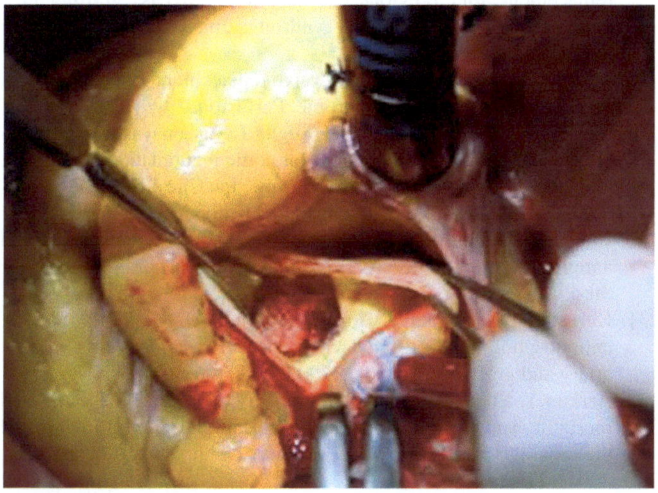

Fig. 38.1 Intraoperative view of an aortic valve mass suggestive of thrombus on a patient with APS (Reproduced with permission from "Cirugía Cardiovascular", Ref. [46])

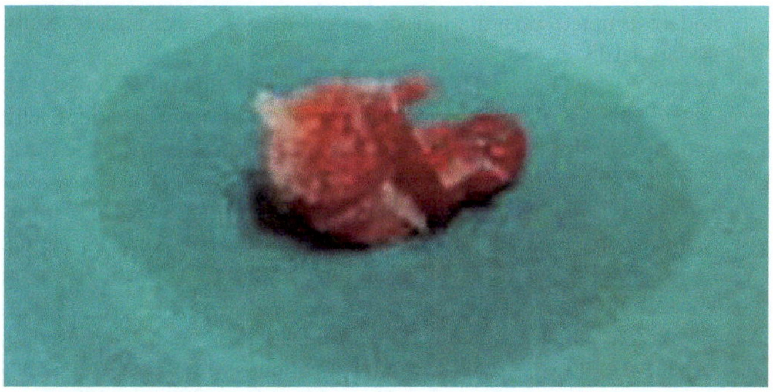

Fig. 38.2 The excised mass, suggestive of thrombus (Reproduced with permission from "Cirugía Cardiovascular", Ref. [46])

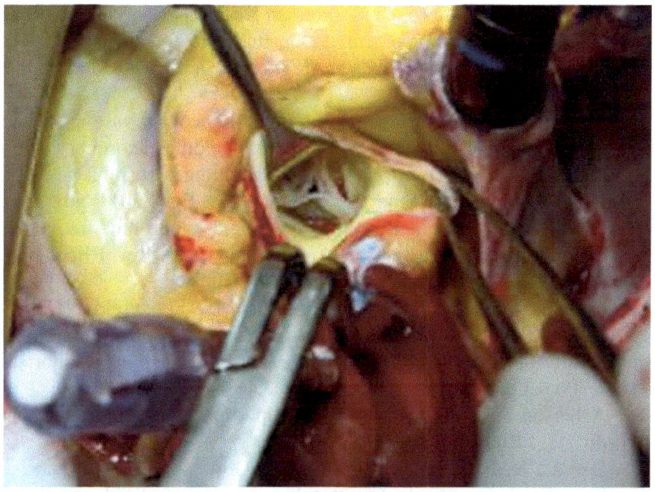

Fig. 38.3 Normal aspect of the aortic valve after excision of the thrombotic mass (Reproduced with permission from "Cirugía Cardiovascular", Ref. [46])

Comments

A brief review of this complex topic from different perspectives, medical and surgical, brings the public's attention to the following considerations that, based on the current body of knowledge, need to be kept in mind concerning this condition:

APS is an uncommon disease that occurs in an small cardiac surgical population.

Specific clinical orientation is needed. This is why specific multidisciplinary teams are to be considered. Individual or collaborative efforts have resulted in the accumulation of useful information [6, 8].

Aggressive intraoperative management is mandatory. Although the evidence is based more on empirical than evidence-based data, there is a trend toward a longer ACT in this patients, who, of course, will eventually need less reversal of anticoagulation.

The patient with APS requiring cardiac surgery requires a difficult decision-making process. This includes problems about the prosthetic valve choice. A thorough discussion is mandatory.

References

1. Lillehei CW, Cohen M, Warden HE, Varco RL. The direct-vision intracardiac correction of congenital anomalies by controlled cross circulation; results in thirty-two patients with ventricular septal defects, tetralogy of Fallot, and atrioventricularis communis defects. Surgery. 1955;38:11–29.
2. Kirklin JW, Du Shane JW, Patrick RT, Donald DE, Hetzel PS, Harshbarger HG, et al. Intracardiac surgery with the aid of a mechanical pump-oxygenator system (Gibbon type): report of eight cases. Proc Staff Meet Mayo Clin. 1955;30:201–6.

3. Byrne JG, Leacche M. The American Heart Association/American College of Cardiology Foundation guideline for coronary artery bypass grafting: 2011 updates. J Thorac Cardiovasc Surg. 2012; 143:35–6.
4. Kurlansky PA, Argenziano M, Dunton R, Lancey R, Nast E, Stewart A, et al. Quality, not volume, determines outcome of coronary artery bypass surgery in a university-based community hospital network. J Thorac Cardiovasc Surg. 2012;143:287–93. Epub 2011 Nov 20.
5. Espinosa G, Cervera R. Antiphospholipid syndrome: frequency, main causes and risk factors of mortality. Nat Rev Rheumatol. 2010;6:296–300.
6. Cervera R, Piette JC, Font J, Khamashta MA, Shoenfeld Y, Camps MT, et al. Antiphospholipid syndrome: clinical and immunologic manifestations and patterns of disease expression in a cohort of 1,000 patients. Arthritis Rheum. 2002;46:1019–27.
7. Asherson RA. The catastrophic antiphospholipid syndrome syndrome. J Rheumatol. 1992;19:508–12.
8. Cervera R, Bucciarelli S, Plasín MA, Gómez-Puerta JA, Plaza J, Pons-Estel G, et al. Catastrophic antiphospholipid syndrome (CAPS): descriptive analysis of a series of 280 patients from the "CAPS Registry". J Autoimmun. 2009;32:240–5.
9. Asherson RA, Cervera R, de Groot P, Erkan D, Boffa MC, Piette JC, et al. Catastrophic antiphospholipid syndrome: international consensus statement on classification criteria and treatment guidelines. Lupus. 2003;12:530–4.
10. Cervera R, Font J, Gómez-Puerta JA, Espinosa G, Cucho M, Bucciarelli S, et al. Validation of the preliminary criteria for the classification of catastrophic antiphospholipid syndrome. Ann Rheum Dis. 2005;64:1205–9.
11. Wilson WA, Gharavi AE, Koike T, Lockshin MD, Branch DW, Piette JC, et al. International consensus statement on preliminary classification criteria for definite antiphospholipid syndrome. Arthritis Rheum. 1999;42:1309–11.
12. Miyakis S, Lockshin MD, Atsumi T, Branch DW, Brey RL, Cervera R, et al. International consensus statement on an update of the classification criteria for definite antiphospholipid syndrome (APS). J Thromb Haemost. 2006;4:295–306.
13. Espinosa G, Fernández de Orueta L, Lluch E, Polvorosa MA, Soro S, Cervera R. Task force report on non-citeria manifestations: cardiac valve disease. In: Erkan D, Pierangeli SS, editors. Antiphospholipid syndrome: insights and highlights from the 13th International Congress on antiphospholipid antibodies. New York: Springer; 2012.
14. Cervera R, Khamashta MA, Shoenfeld Y, et al. Morbidity and mortality in the antiphospholipid syndrome during a 5-year period: a multicentre prospective study of 1000 patients. Ann Rheum Dis. 2009;68:1428–32.
15. Cervera R, Tektonidou MG, Espinosa G, et al. Task force on catastrophic Antiphospholipid Syndrome (APS) and non-criteria APS manifestations (I): catastrophic APS, APS nephropathy and heart valve lesions. Lupus. 2011;20:165–73.
16. Nesher G, Ilany J, Rosenmann D, Abraham AS. Valvular dysfunction in antiphospholipid syndrome: prevalence, clinical features, and treatment. Semin Arthritis Rheum. 1997;27:27–35.
17. Roldan CA, Shively BK, Lau CC, Gurule FT, Smith EA, Crawford MH. Systemic lupus erythematosus valve disease by transesophageal echocardiography and the role of antiphospholipid antibodies. J Am Coll Cardiol. 1992;20:1127–34.
18. Gabrielli F, Alcini E, Di Prima MA, Mazzacurati G, Masala C. Cardiac valve involvement in systemic lupus erythematosus and primary antiphospholipid syndrome: lack of correlation with antiphospholipid antibodies. Int J Cardiol. 1995;51:117–26.
19. Espínola-Zavaleta N, Vargas-Barron J, Comenares-Galvis T, et al. Echocardiographic evaluation of patients with primary antiphospholipid syndrome. Am Heart J. 1999;137:973–9.
20. Turiel M, Sarzi-Puttini P, Peretti R, et al. Five-year follow-up by transesophageal echocardiographic studies in primary antiphospholipid syndrome. Am J Cardiol. 2005;96:574–9.
21. Perez-Villa F, Font J, Azqueta M, et al. Severe valvular regurgitation and antiphospholipid antibodies in systemic lupus erythematosus: a prospective, long-term, follow up study. Arthritis Care Res. 2005;53:460–7.
22. Pardos-Gea J, Ordi-Ros J, Avegliano G, et al. Echocardiography at diagnosis of antiphospholipid syndrome provides prognostic information on valvular disease evolution and identifies two subtypes of patients. Lupus. 2010;19:575–82.
23. Lockshin M, Tenedios F, Petri M, et al. Cardiac disease in the antiphospholipid syndrome: recommendations for treatment. Committee consensus report. Lupus. 2003;12:518–23.
24. Colli A, Mestres CA, Espinosa G, Plasín MA, Pomar JL, Font J, et al. Heart valve surgery in patients with the antiphospholipid syndrome: analysis of a series of nine cases. Eur J Cardiothorac Surg. 2010;37:154–8.
25. Alvarez-Blanco A, Egurbide-Arberas MV, Aguirre-Errasti C. Severe valvular heart disease in a patient with primary antiphospholipid syndrome. Lupus. 1994;3:433–4.
26. Schumacher M, Eber B, Dusleag J, Fruhwald FM, Zweiker R, Pokan R, et al. Thrombosis of a prosthetic mitral valve in the anticardiolipin syndrome. Dtsch Med Wochenschr. 1995;120:795–8.
27. Sakaguchi G, Minami K, Nakayama S, Tsuneyoshi H. Aortic valve replacement after previous coronary artery bypass grafting in a patient with antiphospholipid syndrome. Jpn J Thorac Cardiovasc Surg. 1998;46:257–9.
28. Myers GJ, Hirsch GM. Double valve replacement in a patient with anticardiolipin antibody syndrome. Perfusion. 1999;14:397–401.
29. Matsuyama K, Ueda Y, Ogino H, Sugita T, Matsubayashi K, Nomoto T, et al. Aortic valve replacement for aortic regurgitation in a patient with primary antiphospholipid syndrome. Jpn Circ J. 1999;63:725–6.
30. Hasegawa R, Kitahara H, Watanabe K, Kuroda H, Amano J. Mitral stenosis and regurgitation with systemic lupus erythematosus and antiphospholipid antibody syndrome. Jpn J Thorac Cardiovasc Surg. 2001;49:711–3.
31. Kurushima A, Fukata Y, Horike K, Kanoh M. A difficult case of antiphospholipid syndrome with repeated restenosis of coronary artery and graft. Kyobu Geka. 2002;55:883–6.
32. Berkun Y, Elami A, Meir K, Mevorach D, Naparstek Y. Increased morbidity and mortality in patients with antiphospholipid syndrome undergoing valve replacement surgery. J Thorac Cardiovasc Surg. 2004;127:414–20.
33. Herrmann M, Keysser G, Seige M, Holzhausen HJ, Silber RE, Diez C. Severe, non-infectious mitral valve endocarditis after mitral valve reconstruction in a 32-year old female with primary antiphospholipid syndrome. Z Kardiol. 2004;93:546–54.
34. Massoudy P, Cetin SM, Thielmann M, Kienbaum P, Piotrowski JA, Marggraf G, et al. Antiphospholipid syndrome in cardiac surgery-an underestimated coagulation disorder? Eur J Cardiothorac Surg. 2005;28:133–7.
35. Sasahashi N, Harada H, Saji Y, Marui A, Nishina T, Komeda M. Aortic valve replacement for aortic regurgitation in a patient with antiphospholipid antibody syndrome. Gen Thorac Cardiovasc Surg. 2007;55:293–6.
36. Einav E, Gitig A, Marinescu LM, Tanaka KE, Spevack DM. Valvulitis requiring triple valve surgery as an initial presentation of systemic lupus erythematosus. J Am Soc Echocardiogr. 2007;20(11):1315.e1–3. Epub 2007 Jun 27.
37. Hegde VA, Vivas Y, Shah H, Haybron D, Srinivasan V, Dua A, et al. Cardiovascular surgical outcomes in patients with the antiphospholipid syndrome–a case-series. Heart Lung Circ. 2007;16:423–7.
38. Wieteska M, Szturmowicz M, Kurzyna M, Hajduk B, Biederman A, Torbicki A. Vascular complications in a 51-year-old female with

a primary antiphospholipd syndrome–a case report. Kardiol Pol. 2007;65:50–3.
39. Cianciulli TF, Saccheri MC, Lax JA, Neme RO, Sevillano JF, Maiori ME, et al. Left ventricular thrombus mimicking primary cardiac tumor in a patient with primary antiphospholipid syndrome and recurrent systemic embolism. Cardiol J. 2009;16:560–3.
40. de Agustín JA, Nuñez-Gil IJ, Ruiz-Mateos B, Manzano Mdel C, Vivas D, de Isla LP, et al. Calcified right ventricular thrombus and antiphospholipid syndrome. Eur J Echocardiogr. 2009;10: 471–2.
41. Alaminos García P, Menduiña GMJ, De La Chica Ruiz-Ruano R. Prosthetic valve thrombosis in a patient with antiphospholipid syndrome. Report of one case. Rev Med Chil. 2010;138:330–3.
42. Kondo H, Nakayama M, Ishikawa H. Mitral valve replacement for mitral valve stenosis and insufficiency in a patient with antiphospholipid syndrome and systemic lupus erythematosus; report of a case. Kyobu Geka. 2010;63:1173–5.
43. Kim HW, Hong TH, Moon MH, Jo KH. Postoperative acute superior mesenteric venous thrombosis after cardiac surgery in a patient with anti-phospholipid syndrome. Eur J Cardiothorac Surg. 2010;37:1230.
44. Rawat RS, Mehta Y, Saxena P, Juneja R, Bhan A. Double valve replacement in a patient with antiphospholipid antibody syndrome. Ann Card Anaesth. 2011;14:235–6.
45. García-Valentin A, Colli A, Cartañá R, Pomar JL, Mestres CA. Endocarditis trombótica no bacteriana (Libman-Sachs). Cir Cardiovasc. 2006;13:208.
46. Amital H, Langevitz P, Levy Y, Afek A, Goldberg I, Pras M, et al. Valvular deposition of antiphospholipid antibodies in the antiphospholipid syndrome: a clue to the origin of the disease. Clin Exp Rheumatol. 1999;17:99–102.
47. Hogan WJ, McBane RD, Santrach PJ, Plumhoff EA, Oliver Jr WC, Schaff HV, et al. Antiphospholipid syndrome and perioperative hemostatic management of cardiac valvular surgery. Mayo Clin Proc. 2000;75:971–6.
48. Gorki H, Malinovski V, Stanbridge RDL. The antiphospholipid syndrome and heart valve surgery. Eur J Cardiothorac Surg. 2008;33:168–81.
49. Erdozain JG, Ruiz-Irastorza G, Segura MI, Amigo MC, Espinosa G, Pomar JL, et al. Cardiac valve replacement in patients with antiphospholipid syndrome. Arthritis Care Res (Hoboken). 2012;64(8):1256–60. doi:10.1002/acr.21670.

Part XII

Congenital Heart Diseases

Neurohormonal Factors in Pediatric Heart Surgery

39

Jacek Kolcz

Introduction

Neurohormones are substances produced by neurons that transduce information from both the environment and organism into the cells, tissues, and organs to develop an integrated response to a particular stimulus [1]. The precursors of the signaling particles present in the neuroendocrine system are detected at the most primitive levels of evolution, and some of the amino acid signals, e.g., glutamic acid, are considered to have extraterrestrial origins [2]. The evolution of complex forms of live was originated by the ability of the cells to communicate through secretory substances. After billions of years of evolution, neurohormonal factors take part in maintaining homeostasis in the human organism. All these substances are closely related to each other and can be released by many stimuli, such us external receptor stimuli (ophthalmic, olfactory, auditory), baroreceptors, chemoreceptors, pain, changes in organ perfusion, disturbances of the osmolarity, stretch receptors, inflammatory or immune response, etc. In the field of pediatric cardiac surgery, neurohormonal factors are considered as a part of the neurogenic-inflammatory-endocrine stress response influencing both the preoperative and postoperative periods, playing an important role in early and late pathophysiology, diagnostics, treatment, and monitoring.

There are many definitions of circulatory failure in the core literature. However, the International Society for Heart and Lung Transplantation in its Practice Guidelines for Management of Heart Failure in Children recommends definition reflecting cellular and molecular processes accompanying this condition [3]. A similar definition was proposed by the International Working Group on Acute Heart Failure considering heart failure as a syndrome involving ventricular dysfunction, elevating filing pressures, neurohormonal activation, and worsening symptoms [4]. This model incorporates the complex interactions of the neuroendocrine, paracrine, and immune system pathways. These include the sympathetic nervous system (SNS), renin-angiotensin-aldosterone system (RAAS), hypothalamic-pituitary-adrenal axis, vasopressin, thyroid-stimulating hormone (TSH), natriuretic peptides, cytokines, and other proinflammatory substances, and mediators of endothelial function.

While cardiac dysfunction is not yet associated with overt congestive heart failure (CHF), neurohormonal activation plays a role in the compensatory mechanism for reduced cardiac output, increased atrial pressure, and arterial underfilling. The SNS, hypothalamic-pituitary axis, endothelin system, and RAAS act synergistically to maintain peripheral blood pressure and redistribute blood volume to vital organs. The effects of these mechanisms are antagonized by counter regulatory processes mainly by cholinergic pathway activation and counter-regulatory substances or reflexes that exert many corrective effects. All these mechanisms, if not down-regulated after some time, become detrimental not simply as the result of the heart failure, but also as an important contribution to the progression of circulatory failure. Thus, neurohumoral activation leads to increased myocardial volume and mass in the remodeling process, which is responsible for increased myocardial oxygen demand, myocardial ischemia, impaired contractility, and arrhythmogenesis.

Treating heart failure in a population of patients with congenital heart disease can be quite challenging. In general, evidence for the treatment of decompensated heart failure is skimpy, and the level of evidence decreases with the age of the population. Although there are both medicines blocking neurohormonal activation and strategies using exogenous analogs of neurohormones available, further studies in the field of pediatric heart failure, including neonates, are necessary.

J. Kolcz, MD, PhD, FECTS
Department of Pediatric Cardiac Surgery,
Polish – American Children's Hospital,
Jagiellonian University,
265 Wielicka St, Krakow 30-663, Poland
e-mail: mikolcz@gmail.com

E.A. Gabriel, S.A. Gabriel (eds.), *Inflammatory Response in Cardiovascular Surgery*,
DOI 10.1007/978-1-4471-4429-8_39, © Springer-Verlag London 2013

Sympathetic Nervous System

Sympathetic stimulation exerts many effects on the cardiovascular system by norepinephrine and epinephrine, although the level of epinephrine is not usually elevated in heart failure. Afferent baroreceptor signaling to the brain signals low cardiac output, and efferent sympathetic pathways are activated. The main results of it are vasoconstriction (increased afterload, decreased renal perfusion), increased heart rate and contractility (increased cardiac output and wall stress), and activation of the RAAS. These effects are aimed at the restoration of cardiac output, however, at the expense of increased myocardial oxygen demand, increased intracellular calcium toxicity, and myocardial hypertrophy [5]. Sympathetic overstimulation can cause many undesirable effects such as the expression of fetal genes, apoptosis, necrosis, and remodeling, and high levels of plasma norepinephrine are an independent predictor of mortality [6] (Table 39.1).

The baseline plasma concentrations of catecholamines are higher in neonates compared to older children and adults [7], and age-dependent differences in the clearance rates of sympathomimetic inotropes have also been demonstrated [8]. These features, together with a higher percentage of body water, hypoperfusion of vital organs, systemic inflammatory response, and differences in enzyme activity, determine age-related variation in the hemodynamic response to exogenous catecholamines. Although in the neonatal population there are no appropriate studies, low doses of dopamine (3–5 ug/kg/min) or of epinephrine (0.02–0.05 ug/kg/min) are recommended in acute heart failure. The use of dobutamine and norepinephrine are not advised in neonates [9].

Table 39.1 Sympathetic nervous system activation

Effects of sympathetic stimulation	Cellular effects
Heart	Increased cardiomyocyte calcium entry
Increased contractility (inotropy)	Myocardial hypertrophy
Increased heart rate	Gene expression:
Increased wall stress	Increased expression of fetal genes
Decreased myocardial relaxation (lusitropy)	Decreased expression of calcium metabolism genes
Increased oxygen demand	Apoptosis
Peripheral vessels	Necrosis
Constriction	Fibrosis
Increased afterload	Myocardial hypertrophy/remodeling
Kidney	β1-receptor downregulation
Vasoconstriction	
Sodium retention	
Water retention	
RAAS activation	
Sodium retention	
Water retention	

When catecholamine-resistant hypotension is encountered, a vasopressin infusion may improve systemic vascular resistance (usually 0.01–0.05 units/kg/h).

To decrease of influence of SNS stimulation, β-blocker use has been reported, but in children with HF, the evidence is very limited, and no large placebo-controlled trials are available. The implementation of these drugs in children with large left-to-right shunts improved neurohormonal profiles, decreased respiratory symptoms, and improved growth [10, 11]. Sparse experience on the use of carvedilol in the pediatric population (at an average dose of 0.08 mg/kg/day) has been reported, but the results were equivocal. Interestingly, a significant correlation between the clinical effects of carvedilol and systemic ventricle morphology, with a trend toward having less beneficial effects in patients with a morphologically right ventricle serving as the systemic ventricle, was noted [12, 13].

Endothelin

Endothelins (ET-1,-2,-3) are molecules produced by the endothelium acting as vasoconstrictors and mitogenic factors. In patients with heart failure, their plasma concentrations are increased, and their concentration is proportional to the severity of the disease [14]. Endothelins promote vasoconstriction, inflammation, fibrosis, and hypertrophy in the pulmonary and systemic vasculature.

Plasma ET-1 levels are elevated in patients who have cardiomyopathy or chronic heart failure, and they correlate with severity and prognosis. In particular, the degree of plasma elevation of endothelin correlates with the magnitude of alterations in cardiac hemodynamics and functional class.

Endothelin receptor antagonists cause vasodilation via increased nitric oxide and prostacyclin production, which have antiproliferative properties. Nitric oxide and prostacyclin reduce ET-1 activity by inhibition of pre-pro-ET production. Increased levels of ET-1 have been demonstrated in patients with pulmonary hypertension (PAH) and Eisenmenger syndrome and after cardiopulmonary bypass in children with PAH.

Renin-Angiotensin-Aldosterone Axis

The renin-angiotensin-aldosterone axis exerts many effects on the cardiovascular system (Table 39.2). Neural connexion of the brain and kidneys is stimulated by low sodium, decreased perfusion, and increased alpha-adrenergic activity. It can affect the juxtaglomerular apparatus, increasing renin-protease transforming angiotensinogen to angiotensin I, which is converted within the endothelial cells (particularly concentrated in the lungs) to angiotensin II by angiotensin-

Table 39.2 RAAS activation

Mechanisms	Cellular effects
Constriction of vessels	1. Myocyte hypertrophy
↑ ↑ Afterload	4. Myocyte necrosis
Norepinephrine release	Disorganization of the extracellular matrix
Afterload increase	Apoptosis
Aldosterone	Fetal genes expression
Retention of sodium and water	Myocardial hypertrophy
Vasoconstriction of the efferent arteriole	Left ventricular remodeling
↑ GFR	
Vasoconstriction of the afferent arteriole	
↓ GFR	
Retention of sodium and water	
Vasopressin release	
Retention of sodium and water	

converting enzyme (ACE). Angiotensin II is the most potent vasoconstrictor increasing vascular resistance in stress situations (especially in hypovolemia) and affecting the adrenal cortex, increasing aldosterone production, which increases reclaiming of sodium and water. Its major role is to maintain the circulating volume status [15].

To influence the RAAS axis, ACE inhibitors are used in children with congenital heart defects. Several studies in ventricular level shunts have suggested a possible benefit from ACE inhibitors, presumably due to their relatively selective effect of afterload reduction, increasing systemic blood flow and reducing pulmonary blood flow [16]. A few small studies reported mixed results with respect to the use of ACE inhibitors in patients with single ventricle physiology. Perioperative ACE inhibitor treatment was shown to decrease the severity and duration of pleural effusions after bidirectional cavopulmonary anastomosis surgery [17], although no benefit on exercise performance or cardiac autonomic activity after the Fontan operation was observed [18].

Hypothalamic-Pituitary-Adrenal Axis

Insufficiency of the hypothalamic-pituitary-adrenal axis after pediatric cardiac surgery has been observed, best described as a critical illness related to corticosteroid insufficiency (CIRCI). Together with derangement of other axes, it is considered one of the causes of low cardiac output syndrome in the postoperative period. Many causes of this phenomenon were proposed: brain hypoperfusion, central hypothalamus and pituitary gland insufficiency, tissue resistance to adrenocorticotropic hormone (ACTH), adrenal dysfunction, cyanosis, and tissues immaturities. The CIRCI is diagnosed by a delta cortisol level of 9 g/dl (after 250 g cosyntropin) or a random total cortisol of 10 g/dl. To treat adrenal dysfunction, adrenal function prior to hydrocortisone administration should be tested. Hydrocortisone should be considered in patients with septic shock who have responded poorly to fluid resuscitation and vasopressor agents [19]. Treatment of adrenal dysfunction reduces inotrope requirements, which may reduce low output syndrome in intensive care units and morbidity and improve the neurodevelopmental outcome. The detrimental effects of glucocorticoid therapy should always be considered.

Vasopressin System

Vasopressin is released by the hypothalamus as a result of baroreceptor, osmotic, and neurohormonal stimuli. It normally maintains body fluid balance, vascular tone, and regulates contractility. Heart failure causes a paradoxical increase in AVP. The increased blood volume and atrial pressure in heart failure suggest inhibition of vasopressin secretion, but it does not occur. This phenomenon is related to SNS and RAAS activation overriding the volume and low-pressure cardiovascular receptors and osmotic vasopressin regulation causing an increase in AVP secretion. It contributes to the increased systemic vascular resistance (V1 receptors) and to renal retention of fluid (V2 receptors) [20]. Stimulation of V1 receptors can also cause vasoconstriction of the peripheral vessels, platelet aggregation, and adrenocorticotrophic hormone stimulation. Low-dose arginine infusion initiated in the operating room after complex neonatal cardiac surgery was associated with decreased fluid resuscitation and catecholamine [21].

Growth Hormone

Growth hormone is secreted by the anterior pituitary and mediates its effects via insulin growth factor-1 (IGF-1). Levels of growth hormone are elevated in patients with heart failure as well as in patients with cardiac cachexia. In particular, a recent study showed that treating heart failure patients with growth hormone may result in normalization of the abnormal immunological responses and in suppression of the excessive activation of biochemical apoptotic pathways in the human cardiovascular system.

Thyroid Hormones

Thyroid hormones are stimulated by TSH anterior pituitary secretion. The many actions of thyroid hormones on cardiovascular system are exerted mainly by triiodothyronine (T3). These effects can be divided into genomic and extragenomic actions. T3 binds to the nuclear receptors and activates many genes corresponding to key myocardial functions: myosin heavy chain (MHC), sarcoplasmic reticulum Ca††-ATPase (SERCA2) and its inhibitor phospholamban (affecting cardiac contractile function and diastolic relaxation), voltage-gated Kt channels, b1-adrenergic receptor, guanine nucleotide regulatory proteins, adenylate cyclase, NAt/Kt-ATPase, and Na/Ca exchanger [22]. The main cardiovascular effects of T3 are increased cardiac contractility, reduction of afterload, reduction of vascular resistance, chronotropic effects (increased heart rate), and increased sodium reabsorption, and water improves the atrial filling pressure. All of this increases cardiac output. Low TH levels are common in critical illness of multiple causes, e.g., sepsis, myocardial infarction, and after surgery. Euthyroid sick syndrome is common in pediatric cardiac surgery intensive care units, and the typical physiologic disruptions are reduced, non-pulsatile TSH secretion and T3 reduced by increased conversion of T4 rT3 vs. T3. The total T3 < 0.6 nmol/l can predic: longer mechanical ventilation, longer O_2 supplementation, longer ICU stay, greater use of epinephrine, and greater use of furosemide [23]. Main causes of hypothyroidism in congenital heart surgery population are hemodilution, iodine skin preparations, dopamine administration, and secondary hypothyroidism related to abnormal cerebral perfusion. Transient secondary hypothyroidism occurs in a large number of children after cardiopulmonary bypass operations [24]. The postoperative increase in cardiac output and systolic ventricular function variables was significantly greater after tri-iodothyronine treatment. Patients given tri-iodothyronine after longer cardiopulmonary bypass operations showed improvement in cardiac function. It was also observed after a modified Fontan procedure [25]. T3 has genomic effects that maintain endothelial integrity, such as angiotensin receptors in vascular smooth muscle cells (VSMC). This supports the hypothesis that the vasculature is a principal target for T3 action. T3 decreases resistance in peripheral arterioles. Extragenomic actions include modulating cellular metabolic activities, such as glucose and amino acid transport, ion fluxes at the level of the plasma membrane, and mitochondrial gene expression and function.

Low T3 is also frequently associated with a catabolic pattern characterized by lower insulin levels, higher cortisol levels, lower plasma lipid levels, lower body weight, and lower albumin levels. Furthermore, in asymptomatic and mildly symptomatic patients with non-ischemic left ventricular dysfunction, T3 values and the T3/T4 ratio are linked to both the severity of the left ventricular dysfunction and clinical status, being progressively lower in patients with more depressed ventricular dysfunction (and higher brain natriuretic peptide values).

There is strong evidence that tri-iodothyronine treatment in children after cardiac surgery improves myocardial function without delaying postoperative recovery of thyroid function. What is more, it reduces the postoperative intensive care time [26].

Table 39.3 Mechanisms of action of natriuretic peptides

Systemic effects	Cellular effects
Diuretic and natriuretic action	Antimitogenic action on myocytes
↑ GFR	Reduction in the number of fibroblasts
↓ Retention of sodium and water	Inhibition of left ventricular remodeling
Inhibition of renin secretion	Inhibition of myocardial fibrosis
Inhibition of aldosterone secretion	Inhibition of myocardial hypertrophy
Vasodilation	
Decrease in preload	
Decrease in afterload	
Inhibition of norepinephrine secretion	
Shift of fluid the interstitium	
Decrease in preload	

Counter Regulatory Hormones

There are many counter-regulatory hormones, which are stimulated by stress response (characterized among others by gluconeogenesis, glucogenolysis, relative insulin resistance, reduced insulin-dependent skeletal muscle uptake of glucose, and hyperglycemia). The most important are cortisol, glucagon, epinephrine, and growth hormone.

Cholinergic Pathway

Together with the stimulation of the adrenergic system, the feedback is also started as the antiinflammatory cholinergic pathway [27]. It is comprised of vagus nerve signals leading to acetylcholine interaction with receptors on monocytes and macrophages, resulting in reduced cytokine production [28]. It can prevent tissue injury and improve survival by external stimulation [29, 30]. The cholinergic antiinflammatory pathway exerts a tonic, inhibitory influence on immune responses to infection and tissue injury. Interrupting this pathway produces exaggerated responses to bacterial products and injury [31].

Natriuretic Peptides

The natriuretic peptide system counteracts of some of the effects of neurohormonal activation causing vasodilatation, reduction of aldosterone production (by direct influence on the adrenal gland), increased diuresis and natriuresis, reduction of renin production, decreased vasopressin release, and decreased activation of the sympathetic nervous system. Direct influence of the natriuretic peptides on the myocardium includes prevention of hypertrophy and reduction of fibroblast proliferation [32]. BNP is a natriuretic peptide released in response to ventricular volume expansion and pressure overload (Table 39.3). In normal individuals, BNP levels are elevated immediately after birth, but fall to adult levels by 3 months of age. In the setting of heart failure, BNP levels correlate closely with the NYHA Classification of Heart Failure and with ventricular filling pressures. BNP levels of more than 80 pg/ml have a good specificity and sensitivity in diagnosing heart failure.

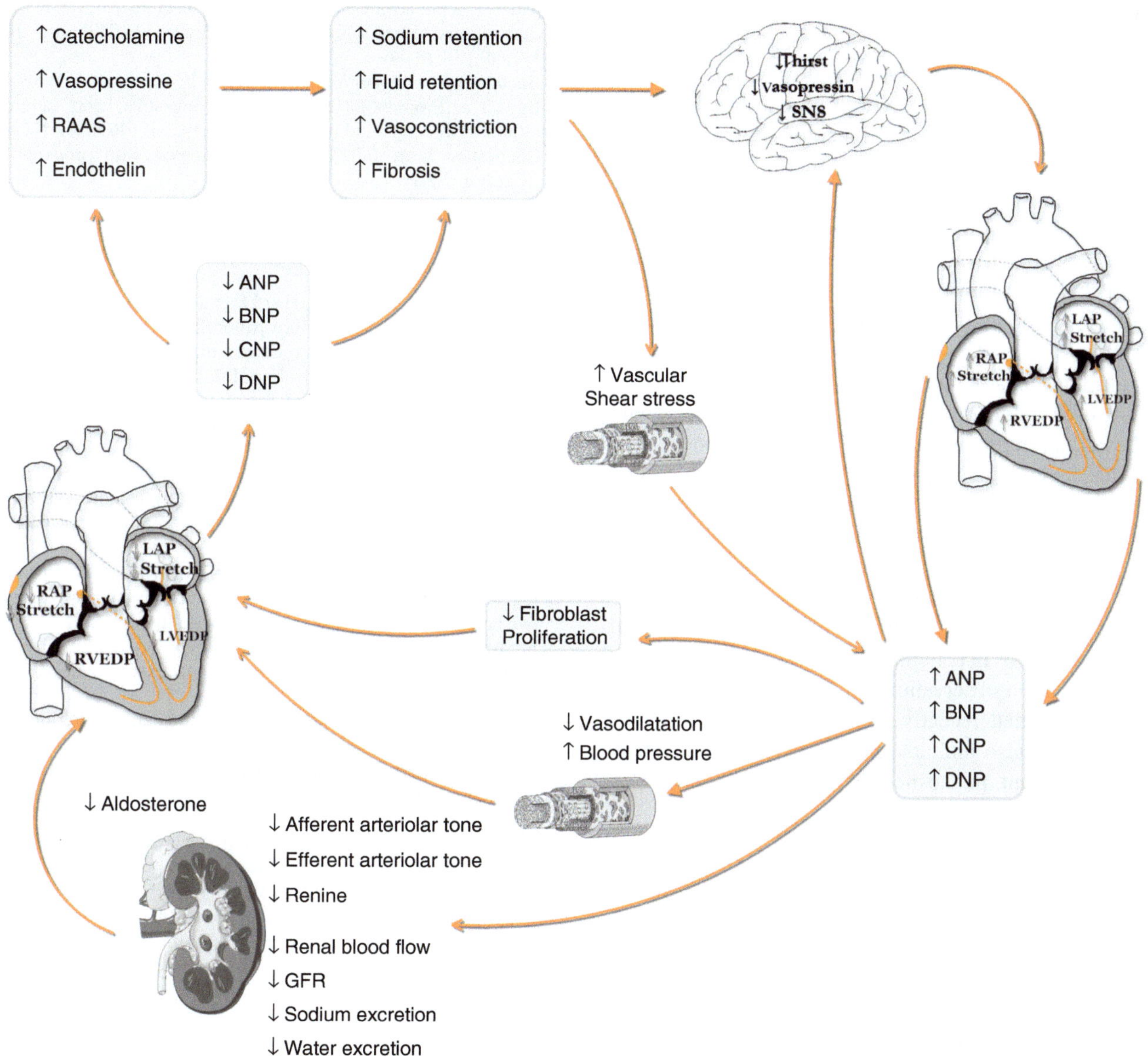

Ryc. Natriuretic factor interactions

Cardiopulmonary bypass in children induces renal and neurohormonal changes similar to those observed in congestive heart failure: upregulation of the RAA axis, increase of renin concentration, and release of vasopressin. These changes are more pronounced in children who undergo palliative procedures for single ventricle lesions (hemi-Fontan, bidirectional Glenn, and Fontan procedures) than in children who undergo biventricular repairs, and the extent of neurohormonal activation after CPB is associated with the severity of fluid retention and development of pleural effusions as well as elevated pulmonary vascular resistance [33, 34].

The endogenous biological activity of the natriuretic hormone system is decreased after the bypass. This is caused by the deficiency of biologically active neurohormones, presence of inactive neurohormones, resistance to natriuretic hormone activity, receptor downregulation, abnormal signal transduction, and increased phosphodiesterase activity [35, 36].

It has been also shown that neurohormones can decrease ischemia-reperfusion injury in multiple tissues, including the heart, by inhibition of angiotensin II and aldosterone, limitation of intracellular Ca^{++} overload, maintenance of ATP stores, and preservation of the myofibril, mitochondrial, and nuclear structure of cardiomyocytes. In clinical trials, the use of natriuretic peptides in the pediatric population showed an improvement of urinary output, increase of the cardiac index, and significant reduction of pulmonary resistance and central venous pressure [37]. There are insufficient data to support the routine use of natriuretic peptides in children. It can be considered in postoperative patients who, despite conventional therapies, have high filling pressures and fluid overload. The diagnostic usefulness of plasma BNP in patients who have symptomatic heart failure is based on observations by many investigators and has been confirmed recently by several large multicenter clinical trials. It also inhibits renin and aldosterone release and is an important diagnostic tool [38].

References

1. Lovejoy D. Neuroendocrinology an integrated approach. Chichester: Wiley; 2005.
2. Brinton KL, Engrand C, Glavin DP, Bada JL, Maurette M. A search for extraterrestrial amino acids in carbonaceous Antarctic micrometeorites. Orig Life Evol Biosph. 1998;28:413–24.
3. Rosenthal D, Chrisant MR, Edens E, Mahony L, Canter C, Colan S, et al. International Society for Heart and Lung Transplantation: practice guidelines for management of heart failure in children. J Heart Lung Transplant. 2004;23:1313–33.
4. Gheorghiade M, Zannad F, Sopko G, Klein L, et al.; for the International Working Group on Acute Heart Failure Syndromes. Acute Heart Failure Syndromes: current state and framework for future research. Circulation. 2005;112:3958–68.
5. Ferrara R, Mastrolilli F, Pasanisi G, Censi S, Aiello ND, Fucili A, et al. Neurohormonal modulation in chronic heart failure. Eur Heart J. 2002;4:D3–11.
6. Stanek B, Frey B, Hulsmann M, et al. Prognostic evaluation of neurohumoral plasma levels before and during beta-blocker therapy in advanced left ventricular dysfunction. J Am Coll Cardiol. 2001; 38(2):436–42.
7. Eliot RJ, Lam R, Leake RD, et al. Plasma catecholamine concentrations in infants at birth and during the first 48 hours of life. J Pediatr. 1980;96:311–5.
8. Allen E, Pettigrew A, Frank D, et al. Alterations in dopamine clearance and catechol- O-methyltransferase activity by dopamine infusions in children. Crit Care Med. 1997;25:181–9.
9. O'Connor CM, Gattis WA, Uretsky BF, et al. Continuous intravenous dobutamine is associated with an increased risk of death in patients with advanced heart failure: insights from the Flolan International Randomized Survival Trial (FIRST). Am Heart J. 1999;138:78–86.
10. Buchhorn R, Hulpke-Wette M, Hilgers R, Bartmus D, Wessel A, Bursch J. Propranolol treatment of congestive heart failure in infants with congenital heart disease: the CHF-PROINFANT trial. Congestive heart failure in infants treated with propanol. Int J Cardiol. 2001;79:167–73.
11. Buchhorn R, Hulpke-Wette M, Ruschewski W, et al. Effects of therapeutic beta blockade on myocardial function and cardiac remodelling in congenital cardiac disease. Cardiol Young. 2003; 13:36–43.
12. Auerbach S, Richmond M, Hsu D, et al. BNP levels predict outcome in pediatric heart failure patients: post hoc analysis of the pediatric carvedilol trial. Circ Heart Fail. 2010;3(5):606–11.
13. Shaddy RE, Boucek MM, Hsu DT, Boucek RJ, Canter CE, Mahony L, et al. Carvedilol for children and adolescents with heart failure: a randomized controlled trial. JAMA. 2007;298: 1171–9.
14. Bauer M, Wilkens H, Langer F, Schneider SO, Lausberg H, Schafers HJ. Selective upregulation of endothelin B receptor gene expression in severe pulmonary hypertension. Circulation. 2002;105: 1034–6.
15. Swedberg K, Eneroth P, Kjekshus J, Wilhelmsen L. Hormones regulating cardiovascular function in patients with severe congestive heart failure and their relation to mortality. CONSENSUS Trial Study Group. Circulation. 1990;82:1730–6.
16. Momma K. ACE inhibitors in pediatric patients with heart failure. Paediatr Drugs. 2006;8:55–69.
17. Thompson LD, McElhinney DB, Culbertson CB, et al. Perioperative administration of angiotensin converting enzyme inhibitors decreases the severity and duration of pleural effusions following bidirectional cavopulmonary anastomosis. Cardiol Young. 2001; 11:195–200.
18. Kouatli AA, Garcia JA, Zellers TM, Weinstein EM, Mahony L. Enalapril does not enhance exercise capacity in patients after Fontan procedure. Circulation. 1997;96:1507–12.
19. Marik PE, et al. Recommendations for the diagnosis and management of corticosteroid insufficiency in critically ill adult patients: consensus statements from an international task force by the American College of Critical Care Medicine. Crit Care Med. 2008;36(6):1937–49.
20. Schrier RW, Abraham WT. Hormones and hemodynamics in heart failure. N Engl J Med. 1999;341(8):577–85.
21. Alten JA, Borasino S, Toms R, Law MA, Moellinger A, Dabal RJ. Early initiation of arginine vasopressin infusion in neonates early initiation of arginine vasopressin infusion in neonates after complex cardiac surgery.After complex cardiac surgery. Pediatr Crit Care Med. 2012;13(3):300–4.
22. Hiroi Y, Kim H-H, Ying H, et al. Rapid nongenomic actions of thyroid hormone. Proc Natl Acad Sci USA. 2006;103:14104e9.

23. Bettendorf M. Transient secondary hypothyroidism in children after cardiac surgery. Pediatr Res. 1997;41:375.
24. Bettendorf M, Schmidt KG, Tiefenbacher U, Grulich-Henn J, Heinrich UE, Schönberg DK. Transient secondary hypothyroidism in children after cardiac surgery. Pediatr Res. 1997;41:375–9.
25. Mainwaring RD, Lamberti JJ, Nelson JC, Billman GF, Carter TL, Shell KH. Effects of tri-iodothyronine supplementation following modified Fontan procedure. Cardiol Young. 1997;7:194–200.
26. Beltendorf M et al. Tri-iodothyronine treatment in children after cardiac surgery: a double-blind, randomised, placebo-controlled study. Lancet. 2000;356:529–34.
27. Tracey KJ. Physiology and immunology of the cholinergic antiinflammatory pathway. J Clin Invest. 2007;117:289–96.
28. Parrish WR, Rosas-Ballina M, Gallowitsch-Puerta M, et al. Modulation of TNF release by choline requires Alpha7 subunit nicotinic acetylcholine receptor-mediated signaling. Mol Med. 2008;14:567–74.
29. Borovikova LV, Ivanova S, Nardi D. Role of vagus nerve signaling in CNI-1493-mediated suppression of acute inflammation. Auton Neurosci. 2000;85:141–7.
30. Mioni C, Bazzani C, Giuliani D, et al. Activation of an efferent cholinergic pathway produces strong protection against myocardial ischemia/reperfusion injury. Crit Care Med. 2005;33:2621–8.
31. Wang H, Yu M, Ochani M, et al. Nicotinic acetylcholine receptor alpha7 subunit is an essential regulator of inflammation. Nature. 2003;421:384–8.
32. Costello JM, Goodman DM, Green TP. A review of the natriuretic hormone system's diagnostic and therapeutic potential in critically ill children. Pediatr Crit Care Med. 2006;7:308–18.
33. Burch M, Lum L, Elliot M, Carter N, Slater D, Smith A, et al. Influence of cardiopulmonary bypass on water balance hormons in children. Br Heart J. 1992;68:309–12.
34. Mainwaring RD, Lamberti JJ, Moore JW, et al. Comparison of the hormonal response after bidirectional Glenn and Fontan procedures. Ann Thorac Surg. 1994;57:59–63.
35. D'Souza SP, Yellon DM, Martin C, Schulz R, Heusch G, Onody A, et al. B-type natriuretic peptide limits infarct size in rat isolated hearts via KATP channel opening. Am J Physiol Heart Circ Physiol. 2003;284:H1592–600.
36. Costello JM et al. Effect of cardiopulmonary bypass and surgical intervention on the natriuretic hormone system in children. J Thorac Cardiovasc Surg. 2005;130:822–9.
37. Hiramatsu T et al. Hemodynamic effects of human atrial natriuretic peptide after modified Fontan procedure. Ann Thorac Surg. 1998;65:761.
38. Abraham WT et al. In-hospital mortality in patients with acute decompensated heart failure requiring intravenous vasoactive medications. J Am Coll Cardiol. 2005;46:57–64.

Antifibrinolytic Therapy in Pediatric Congenital Heart Surgery

40

Ehrenfried Schindler

Preface

For decades, aprotinin was the standard antifibrinolytic drug used in adult and pediatric major surgery [1]. Numerous studies showed that the perioperative loss of blood, and thus the use of homologous blood, could be limited by administering aprotinin. Other antifibrinolytic-acting substances, such as e-aminocapronic acid (EACA) or tranexamic acid (TXA), tended to be misfits in routine clinical practice.

In 2006, the publication of a retrospective study carried out by Managno et al., in which considerable safety concerns were expressed with regard to aprotinin, led to a significant rethinking of its clinical use [2]. Two years later, the results of the BART (Blood Conservation using Antifibrinolytics in a Randomized Trial) study confirmed that there was an increased postoperative mortality associated with the use of aprotinin compared to TXA and EACA [3].

In a few adult studies so far, tranexamic acid has been found to be comparably as effective as aprotinin. Although TXA is a long-known drug available on the market for more than 50 years, the studies connecting the factors of the indication, dosage regimen, and safety are limited, especially in children and infants.

Developmental Hemostasis

In the 1980s, the pioneering work of Andrew and co-workers showed that the coagulation system of children is different from that of adults. They introduced the term "developmental hemostasis" to describe this phenomenon. The study of Andrew and co-worker showed that the concentration of coagulation factors is age-dependent, and therefore reference limits from adult practice cannot be transferred to that for children of 1 to 2 years. Infants up to 6 months can be assumed to have significantly lower plasma levels of certain procoagulants, such as factor II, V, VII, IX, X, XI, and XII. Andrews could show that the inhibitors a_eM and C_1-Inh were increased twofold compared to adults in early childhood. In contrast, the mean plasma concentrations of protein C and HCII were significantly lower than for adults until the early teenage years [4]. The bleeding time in children up to approximately 10 years of age is significantly longer compared to adults. Thromboembolic complications in children following major surgery or prolonged immobilization are rare and usually more likely associated to secondary underlying disorders. The reason for this could be found in the significant reduction of the endogenous thrombin potential (ETP) compared to adults. Children can considered to be protected from thrombosis, but the underlying molecular basis is not yet fully understood [5–8].

Another important fact is that absolute reference range values for coagulation assays in neonates, infants, and children vary with different analyzers and reagent systems. This means that each laboratory should define specific ranges for the children tested there.

Fibrinolytic System in Pediatric Patients

The coagulation system involves a fine balance between coagulation and fibrinolysis to prevent uncontrolled coagulation in vivo. The principle of developmental hemostasis is conferrable to the fibrinolytic part of the coagulation swing. The fibrinolytic system is age-dependent, being different compared to that of adults.

Fibrinolysis is defined as the degradation of intravascular fibrin clots by the action of plasmin, which results from plasminogen hydrolysis. This action is mediated throughout a series of serine proteases that interact to cleave insoluble fibrin into soluble fibrin degradation products [9]. During clot

E. Schindler
Department for Pediatric Anesthesiology,
German Pediatric Heart Center, Asklepios Klinik
Sankt Augustin, Arnold-Janssenstr. 29,
Sankt Augustin 53737, Germany
e-mail: e.schindler@asklepios.com

E.A. Gabriel, S.A. Gabriel (eds.), *Inflammatory Response in Cardiovascular Surgery*,
DOI 10.1007/978-1-4471-4429-8_40, © Springer-Verlag London 2013

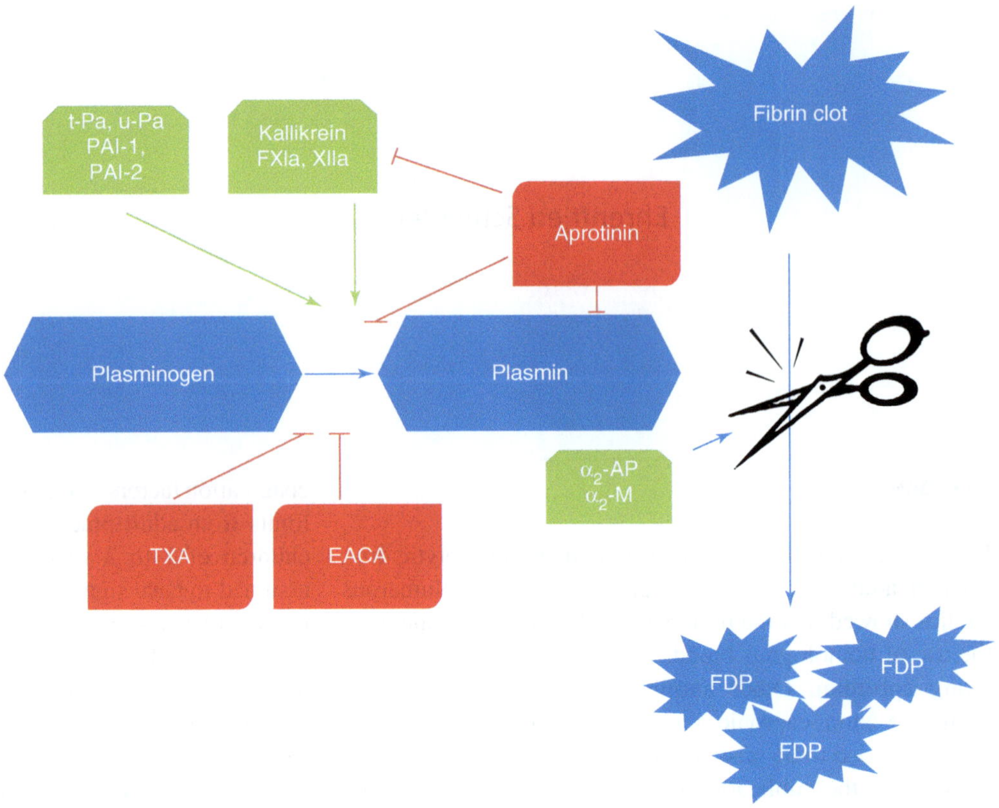

Fig. 40.1 Mechanism of action for tranexamic acid (TXA), e-aminocaproic acid (EACA), and aprotinin during fibrinolysis (*t-PA* tissue-type-plasminogen activator, *u-PA* urokinase type-plasminogen activator, *PAI* plasminogen activator inhibitor, *FDP* fibrin degradation products)

formation, plasminogen is incorporated into the thrombus by binding on fibrin and cell surfaces. The tissue-type plasminogen activator (t-PA) binding is also attracted by fibrin and is also incorporated into the clot formation. There it activates the degradation of plasminogen to plasmin. To prevent excessive fibrinolysis, several modulating substances are present. Plasminogen activator inhibitor-1 and -2 (PAI-1 and PAI-2) regulate fibrin-bound t-PA. Several other molecules fine-tune the fibrinolytic system, such as a_2-antiplasmin(a2-AP), a_2-macroglobulin (a2-M), and thrombin-activated fibrinolysis inhibitor (TAFI), to name the most important (Fig. 40.1).

Studies showed that major components of the coagulation system could be detected in the fetus approximately from 10 weeks of gestation. Immediately after birth, the coagulation system is developed with its all parts, but the blood concentrations are different. Reference values are given by Andrews and were documented in a more recent study by Monagle [4, 6]. One major difference is the concentration of plasminogen, which is reduced by more than half the amount compared to adults. After 6 months of age, the adult concentration is nearly equal, and it remains constant during childhood. t-PA in contrast is significantly increased immediately after birth. Very short after birth the plasma concentration of t-PA is decreasing progressively. There is a rapid increase in t-PA levels after the first period of life, and t-PA levels will reach about 50 % of the adult value during childhood compared to adulthood. Like t-PA, the plasminogen activator inhibitor levels are increased after birth compared to adult values. This may explain why, despite the remarkable

Table 40.1 Changes of reference values over the first month after birth for the coagulation system in healthy children compared to adults. All data are presented in more detail in [4, 6, 9]

Parameter	Day 1	3 month of age	6 month of age
Antithrombin (AT)	⇩	⇘	-
Protein C	⇩	⇘	-
Protein S	⇩	⇘	-
Plasminogen	⇩	⇩	⇩
t-PA	⇧	-	-
PAI-1	⇧	-	-
PAI-2	⇧	-	-
α_2-AP	-	-	
α_2-M	-	-	-

decrease in plasminogen levels, the activity of the fibrinolytic system in infants and very young children is increased compared to adults. The most important differences in the plasma concentration of coagulation molecules compared to that of adults are presented in Table 40.1.

Antifibrinolytic Agents for Children

Aprotinin

Aprotinin is a so-called "serine protease" molecule inhibitor when administered in large doses. Serine molecules can be found in the coagulation pathway and are needed for initiating fibrinolysis [10]. Aprotinin augments and prolongs coagulation initiated by activation of both intrinsic and extrinsic pathways. The main influence on the fibrinolytic system is mediated by blocking kallikrein and the plasmin-activating molecules i-PA, u-PA, and t-PA. Additionally, aprotinin, like other antifibrinolytic drugs, will interfere with the lysine-binding site of plasminogen or plasmin. The effect of t-PA is enhanced more than 400 fold in the presence of fibrin. Several studies showed that aprotinin decreases thrombin formation during surgery with cardiopulmonary bypass. Therefore, it is recommended to start with the aprotinin therapy before fibrin formation has been initiated, which means before the skin incision in major surgery [11].

There are numerous studies on the aprotinin dosage regimes, especially for cardiac or pediatric cardiac surgery. In recent years, "high-dose" schemes were mostly recommended [12].

e-Aminocaproic Acid (EACA)

EACA is not available in all European countries. Comparable to tranexamic acid, EACA reversibly inhibits the transformation of plasminogen to the active protease plasmin. Saturation of the lysine-binding site of plasminogen with EACA displaces plasminogen from the surface of fibrin. Even if plasminogen is transformed into the active component plasmin, it cannot bind to fibrin, and its fibrinolytic action is inhibited [13]. Over 20 years ago, there were reports that high-dose EACA therapy will inhibit the platelet aggregation induced by collagen and ADP [14]. Shortly after the introduction of EACA, serious concerns arose about thromboembolic and renal complications. After a warning message published in the New England Journal of Medicine in 1969, the routine use of EACA dropped, especially for children [15, 16]. A recent large multicenter study including a total of 22,258 patients (25 centers) looking at adverse events associated with aprotinin, TXA, and EACA found no difference in renal failure requiring dialysis in any of the groups. Interestingly, the study favored the TXA group, and comparative analyses suggested similar efficacy of EACA and improved outcomes associated with TXA.

Tranexamic Acid (TXA)

Tranexamic acid has been available for a long time. In Europe, it was introduced for clinical use starting in 1970.

Tranexamic acid is a synthetic derivate of the amino acid lysine that exerts its antifibrinolytic effect through the reversible blockade of lysine-binding sites on plasminogen, thus preventing fibrin degradation. Its main action in the coagulation system is promoting clot stability. Tranexamic acid also preserves platelet function by reducing the effect of plasmin on glycoprotein 1b receptors.

The optimal dosage for TXA to prevent fibrinolysis has not yet been defined for pediatric patients. According to in vitro studies, a concentration of 10 μg/ml can decrease 80 % of t-PA activity, and a concentration of 16 μg/ml can inhibit platelet activation induced by plasmin [17–19]. The concentration of TXA necessary to prevent fibrinolysis in vivo is unknown. A recent study aiming to optimize the dosing schedule in adult patients in cardiac surgery had the objective of achieving a stable plasma concentration >20 μg/ml.

Indication for Antifibrinolytic Agents in Cardiac Surgery

There are many publications on adult cardiac surgery that support the use of antifibrinolytic substances for high-risk patients because of the reduction in the amount of blood products transfused. Less information is available for pediatric open-heart surgery. Moreover, estimation of the effectiveness of the prophylactic use of antifibrinolytics varies a great deal. For example, the study by Davies et al. [20] showed a reduction in neither blood loss nor in the blood products used under aprotinin therapy. Williams et al. [21] also found no effects of aprotinin on newborns with congenital heart defects. However, for Carrel et al. [22] and more recently Murugesan et al. [23], aprotinin had a blood-saving effect in surgery for transposition of the great arteries. Other authors demonstrated a blood-saving effect for all antifibrinolytic agents during repair of cyanotic defects [24]. In conclusion, complex neonatal cardiac surgery, cyanotic defects, and rethoracotomies constitute the three reported indications for using antifibrinolytic drugs for pediatric open-heart surgery. An up-to-date, large multicenter study including a total of 22,258 patients (25 centers) looking at blood saving aspects and adverse events associated with aprotinin, TXA, and EACA found no difference in the rates of renal failure requiring dialysis in any of the groups. The blood-saving aspects of all of the used substances were comparable. Interestingly, the study favored the TXA group, and comparative analyses suggested similar efficacy of EACA and improved outcomes associated with TXA [25].

Dosage and Infusion Schemes of Tranexamic Acid

Up to now, no consensus has been reached about the ideal dosage of TXA for pediatric patients undergoing congenital heart surgery with cardiopulmonary bypass (CPB). When analyzing the existing studies regarding the dosage and efficacy of TXA, it should be noticed that in most of the studies the age range was large, including neonates, infants, children, and adolescents, which makes the results analysis difficult, especially as the results are usually not stratified by age. Additionally, it is important whether the patients are suffering from a cyanotic or non-cyanotic disease because cyanotic heart defects are known to involve platelet dysfunction, and these patients tend to bleed more than non-cyanotic patients. Second, if analyzing efficacy studies, the main clinical endpoints could be blood loss volume, transfusions requirement, coagulation parameters, or a combination of these. Some other endpoints are also found in studies, such as time needed for chest closure, rethoracotomies, platelet activation analysis, and biochemical parameters. Of note, the endpoint blood product transfusion volume may be biased in low weight children since blood products may also be used for hemodynamic reasons and do not always consequently indicate perioperative blood loss. Additionally, in low body weight children, blood must be administered if platelets or fresh frozen plasma have to be given to prevent dilution and therefore low hematocrit values.

Chauhan and coworker could show the efficacy of TXA on blood loss and blood product requirements in three out of four groups with different dosage schemes except one single bolus application of 50 mg/kg [26]. In the four study groups, they have used: group 1, 50 mg/kg TXA at induction of anesthesia; group 2, 10 mg/kg at induction followed by an infusion of 1 mg/kg/h; group 3, 10 mg/kg at induction, 10 mg/kg on bypass, and 10 mg/kg after protamine (end of surgery); group 4, 20 mg/kg at induction and 20 mg/kg after protamine (end of surgery). These results could explain the absence of any significant reduction in the use of blood products in two Canadian studies of Levin and Zonis because they also used a single bolus injection of 50 mg/kg BW [16, 27]. Van der Staak and coworker used TXA continuously in major pediatric surgery. They found a significant reduction in postoperative blood loss and transfusion requirements with a dosage scheme of 4 mg/kg 10 min prior to skin incision followed by an infusion of 1 mg/kg/h for 24 h after surgery [28]. Bulutcu could show a significant decrease in blood loss and blood product requirements with TXA compared to placebo, especially in cyanotic patients [29]. The reported using a high dose scheme of one single bolus of 100 mg/kg followed by 100 mg/kg in the pump prime and 100 mg/kg after CPB. If comparing this high-dose scheme with that of Chauhan, no significant difference could be seen regarding the primary endpoints, allowing the conclusion that the efficacy does not increase dose dependently. Because even in the presence of heparin during cardiopulmonary bypass fibrin formation and therefore activation of coagulation could be assumed, a continuous dosage regimen seems favorable over a single-bolus injection. The most recent regimen used at our institution is based on our own experience [30] and was later modified after pharmacokinetic calculation according to the in-vivo studies of Andersson and Soslau [17, 19]. We now use a single bolus of 10 mg/kg BW followed by a continuous infusion of 3 mg/kg/h, adding 0.1 mg/kg TXA per ml of pump prime volume to the cardiopulmonary bypass circuit.

Timing of Antifibrinolytic Therapy in Pediatric Heart Surgery

Most of the study protocols using antifibrinolytic therapy are focused on different dosage schemes. Considering the mechanism of fibrinolysis and especially antifibrinolytic therapy, the drugs act by binding to the lysine-binding site of plasminogen by interfering with the tissue plasminogen activator. Remember that the potential of t-PA is enhanced more than 400 fold in the presence of fibrin. This means that the activation of the fibrinolytic system must be suppressed before a significant amount of fibrin or fibrin clots have been generated. In the setting of congenital heart surgery, it is therefore considered to be effective to start any antifibrinolytic therapy before skin incision. Data from the available literature do not support the mandatory initiation of antifibrinolytic therapy after skin incision or sternotomy, but strongly suggest starting before the beginning of CPB. Additionally, the initiation of a cardiopulmonary bypass as well as the reversal of heparin to start coagulation with administration of protamine is associated with a significant activation of the coagulation cascade. If not, a_2-antiplasmin will immediately begin degrading plasmin, and a reduction of a_2-antiplasmin is associated with the risk of excessive bleeding [31–34].

Risks and Side Effects

The aforementioned observational study by Mangano et al. published in 2006, observed an increase in the number of cases of renal failure, myocardial infarction, and stroke under aprotinin therapy [2]. In 2007, Mangano, using the same set of data, found an increase in the 5-year mortality rate, which was not the case in the tranexamic acid or in the ε-aminocaproic acid groups [35]. The criticism was that the aprotinin group was at a disadvantage in these observational studies because the high-risk constellation of the patients was countered in 2008 by the data of the prospective, randomized study by Fergusson et al. [3]. This study had to be prematurely abandoned as a distinct trend toward mortality was established. In his publication, Fergusson stated that for aprotinin, the "number needed to harm" is 50. However, in two other more recent studies with a large number of pediatric cardiac surgical patients, Szekely et al., with nearly 700 children, were not able to show that aprotinin was responsible for renal dysfunction [36], and Backer et al., with over 2,500 children, were not able to establish a connection between aprotinin and renal insufficiency, neurological complications, or an increase in mortality [37]. The question is to what extent the data compiled by Mangano and Fergusson in adult surgery can be transferred to the field of pediatric surgery. It is to be noted that in some recent studies, while aprotinin reduced the tendency to bleeding, it was not shown to influence the rate of mortality or to impair organ function. However, the meta-analysis of Brown et al. [38] states that the risks of using aprotinin outweigh the risks of using tranexamic acid, and the authors of a new issue of the Cochrane collaboration overview came to a similar conclusion.

Breuer et al. found an increase (albeit not statistically significant) in the number of seizures in patients treated with tranexamic acid [39]. Data are available from adult cardiac surgery patients, as well as from the field of neurosurgery, indeed showing a connection between the use of tranexamic acid and epileptic seizures. This can be explained by the antagonistic effect of tranexamic acid on GABA receptors [40, 41]. To what extent this aspect affects endpoints such as cerebral ischemia or mortality has yet to be examined. However, this demonstrates the importance, in the "post-aprotinin era," of arousing interest in the safety aspects of other antifibrinolytic alternatives.

The use of antifibrinolytics always naturally interferes with the balance of pro- and anticoagulatory forces. There are justifiable fears that inhibition of fibrinolysis may lead to a thrombotic event. In children with cyanotic defects, activation of fibrinolysis may already be found in the preoperative period. It is difficult to say how often thrombosis occurs when using antifibrinolytic therapy in pediatric cardiac surgery. For both aprotinin and tranexamic acid, the reports are predominantly episodic. Whether tranexamic acid offers an advantage over aprotinin (which is also said to have anticoagulatory characteristics) in this respect has not yet been sufficiently examined. In a study by Jaquiss et al., no thrombotic events were observed in 865 children who underwent cardiac surgery with aprotinin therapy [42]. When one considers that the incidence of thrombosis in the area of the central venous catheter is said to be 20 % in pediatric cardiac surgery patients, one would assume that thrombotic events are probably underdiagnosed. In our study, two patients from the aprotinin group had to undergo rethoracotomy because of thrombosis. However, in comparison with the tranexamic acid group, no significant difference could be determined from this. But there was no control group for comparison [30].

At this point, it is of course interesting to discuss what dose of tranexamic acid should be given to achieve the desired effect and still avoid undesirable side effects.

Convulsive effects following TXA were first shown in animal studies. The mechanism by which TXA can evoke epileptic seizures includes binding to the GABA (γ-aminobutyric acid) binding sites of GABA, and dose-dependent inhibition of the binding of the GABA receptor agonist, muscimol, and consequently antagonistic effects on GABA receptors [41, 43]. These convulsive effects are dose dependent. The convulsive effect of TXA, after application directly in situ in the cortex area or the lumbar spinal cord, is induced by blocking GABA-mediated inhibition in the central nervous system (CSN). Two factors may increase the epileptic effect of TXA: the dose administered and the size of the exposed area. Consequently, the administration of TXA in the CSN or close to the CSN can immediately evoke epileptic seizures.

In the "aprotinin era," the group of cardiac surgical patients was the largest investigated group receiving antifibrinolytic drugs in the adult as well as in the pediatric population. Whereas aprotinin was associated with renal failure, TXA can cause seizures or convulsions in children as well as in adults. In a case series after pediatric neurosurgery, we observed convulsions in four patients postoperativly associated with TXA therapy. The first appearance of convulsions in our case series was in the early postoperative period after neurosurgery between the first 40 min after extubation and the last 5 h post extubation. In most of the pediatric cardiac centers, children below 6 months of age are kept intubated, sedated, and ventilated for at least 6 h after cardiac surgery. It is possible that pathological electroencephalograms (EEG) or silent seizures were not recognized because of ventilation and sedation so that the real number of pathological neurologic events after TXA administration in pediatric cardiac surgery is higher than suspected.

One important message from earlier animal studies was that the convulsive effects of the tranexamic acid are dose-dependent. In our neurosurgical patients, we used a significantly higher dose than described in some other publications (100 mg/kg as a bolus followed by 10 mg/kg/h). Neurotoxic signs occurred in rats at doses starting from 0.5 mg/ml. At 5 mg/ml, two out of six rats showed signs of major toxicity and died. Lastly, at a TXA concentration of 47.5 mg/ml, all the tested rats died. Considering the calculated ratio between concentrations leading to neurotoxic effects estimated in rats and concentrations in the cerebrospinal fluid (CSF) after IV administration of 66 mg/kg TXA in adults or 20 mg/kg in children older than 1 year, it can be concluded that convulsive effects are not expected to be common after this maximum dose [41].

Regarding its use in cardiac surgery, the present data are insufficient to reach a conclusion about a potential risk of TXA inducing a convulsive effect when administered intravenously. Unless there are clinical safety data available, TXA should be indicated carefully in neonates and infants aged less than 12 months of age.

To evaluate the effects of tranexamic acid on death, vascular occlusive events, and blood transfusion in trauma patients, the CRASH-2 study was initiated as a randomized, placebo-controlled multicenter investigation [44]. The results of this study are based on the data of 274 hospitals including 20,211 trauma patients. Although outcome measures on subgroup analysis were considered, no special "children's" group could be created, so data are from adult patients. In the group of patient <25 years, there were only five patients younger than 16 years of age. As an overall result, the conclusion was that the all-cause mortality was significantly reduced with tranexamic acid compared to placebo. No increased risk of non-fatal vascular occlusive events with TXA could be noted. The final conclusions were to recommend TXA for inclusion on the WHO list of Essential Medicines and to consider TXA safe for use in bleeding trauma patients.

References

1. Levy JH, Ramsay JG, Guyton RA. Aprotinin in cardiac surgery. N Engl J Med. 2006;354:1953–7.
2. Mangano DT, Tudor IC, Dietzel C. The risk associated with aprotinin in cardiac surgery. N Engl J Med. 2006;354:353–65.
3. Fergusson DA, Hebert PC, Mazer CD, Fremes S, MacAdams C, Murkin JM, et al. A comparison of aprotinin and lysine analogues in high-risk cardiac surgery. N Engl J Med. 2008;358:2319–31.
4. Andrew M, Vegh P, Johnston M, Bowker J, Ofosu F, Mitchell L. Maturation of the hemostatic system during childhood. Blood. 1992;80:1998–2005.
5. Monagle P. Thrombosis in pediatric cardiac patients. Semin Thromb Hemost. 2003;29:547–55.
6. Monagle P, Barnes C, Ignjatovic V, Furmedge J, Newall F, Chan A, et al. Developmental haemostasis. Impact for clinical haemostasis laboratories. Thromb Haemost. 2006;95:362–72.
7. Monagle P, Ignjatovic V, Savoia H. Hemostasis in neonates and children: pitfalls and dilemmas. Blood Rev. 2010;24:63–8.
8. Monagle P, Massicotte P. Developmental haemostasis: secondary haemostasis. Semin Fetal Neonatal Med. 2011;16:294–300.
9. Albisetti M. The fibrinolytic system in children. Semin Thromb Hemost. 2003;29:339–48.
10. van Oeveren W, Jansen NJ, Bidstrup BP, Royston D, Westaby S, Neuhof H, et al. Effects of aprotinin on hemostatic mechanisms during cardiopulmonary bypass. Ann Thorac Surg. 1987;44:640–5.
11. Royston D. Aprotinin therapy. Br J Anaesth. 1994;73:734–7.
12. Royston D. High-dose aprotinin therapy: a review of the first five years' experience. J Cardiothorac Vasc Anesth. 1992;6:76–100.
13. Verstraete M. Clinical application of inhibitors of fibrinolysis. Drugs. 1985;29:236–61.
14. Green D, Ts'ao CH, Cerullo L, Cohen I, Ruo TI, Atkinson Jr AJ. Clinical and laboratory investigation of the effects of epsilon-aminocaproic acid on hemostasis. J Lab Clin Med. 1985;105:321–7.
15. Ratnoff OD. Epsilon aminocaproic acid–a dangerous weapon. N Engl J Med. 1969;280:1124–5.
16. Zonis Z, Seear M, Reichert C, Sett S, Allen C. The effect of preoperative tranexamic acid on blood loss after cardiac operations in children. J Thorac Cardiovasc Surg. 1996;111:982–7.
17. Andersson L, Nilsson IM, Liedberg G, Nilsson L, Rybo G, Eriksson O, et al. Antifibrinolytic drugs. Comparative studies on trans-4-(aminomethyl)-cyclohexane carbonic acid, aminocapronic acid and p-aminomethylbenzoic acid. Arzneimittelforschung. 1971;21:424–9.
18. Andersson L, Nilsson IM, Olow B. Fibrinolytic activity in man during surgery. Thromb Diath Haemorrh. 1962;7:391–403.
19. Soslau G, Horrow J, Brodsky I. Effect of tranexamic acid on platelet ADP during extracorporeal circulation. Am J Hematol. 1991; 38:113–9.
20. Davies MJ, Allen A, Kort H, Weerasena NA, Rocco D, Paul CL, et al. Prospective, randomized, double-blind study of high-dose aprotinin in pediatric cardiac operations. Ann Thorac Surg. 1997; 63:497–503.
21. Williams GD, Ramamoorthy C, Pentcheva K, Boltz MG, Kamra K, Reddy VM. A randomized, controlled trial of aprotinin in neonates undergoing open-heart surgery. Paediatr Anaesth. 2008;18: 812–9.
22. Carrel TP, Schwanda M, Vogt PR, Turina MI. Aprotinin in pediatric cardiac operations: a benefit in complex malformations and with high-dose regimen only. Ann Thorac Surg. 1998;66:153–8.
23. Murugesan C, Banakal SK, Garg R, Keshavamurthy S, Muralidhar K. The efficacy of aprotinin in arterial switch operations in infants. Anesth Analg. 2008;107:783–7.
24. Schouten ES, van de Pol AC, Schouten AN, Turner NM, Jansen NJ, Bollen CW. The effect of aprotinin, tranexamic acid, and aminocaproic acid on blood loss and use of blood products in major pediatric surgery: a meta-analysis. Pediatr Crit Care Med. 2009;10:182–90.
25. Pasquali SK, Li JS, He X, Jacobs ML, O'Brien SM, Hall M, et al. Comparative analysis of antifibrinolytic medications in pediatric heart surgery. J Thorac Cardiovasc Surg. 2012;143:550–7.
26. Chauhan S, Bisoi A, Kumar N, Mittal D, Kale S, Kiran U, et al. Dose comparison of tranexamic acid in pediatric cardiac surgery. Asian Cardiovasc Thorac Ann. 2004;12:121–4.
27. Levin E, Wu J, Devine DV, Alexander J, Reichart C, Sett S, et al. Hemostatic parameters and platelet activation marker expression in cyanotic and acyanotic pediatric patients undergoing cardiac surgery in the presence of tranexamic acid. Thromb Haemost. 2000;83: 54–9.
28. van der Staak FH, de Haan AF, Geven WB, Festen C. Surgical repair of congenital diaphragmatic hernia during extracorporeal membrane oxygenation: hemorrhagic complications and the effect of tranexamic acid. J Pediatr Surg. 1997;32:594–9.
29. Bulutcu FS, Ozbek U, Polat B, Yalcin Y, Karaci AR, Bayindir O. Which may be effective to reduce blood loss after cardiac operations in cyanotic children: tranexamic acid, aprotinin or a combination? Paediatr Anaesth. 2005;15:41–6.
30. Schindler E, Photiadis J, Sinzobahamvya N, Dores A, Asfour B, Hraska V. Tranexamic acid: an alternative to aprotinin as antifibrinolytic therapy in pediatric congenital heart surgery. Eur J Cardiothorac Surg. 2011;39:495–9.
31. Edmunds Jr LH. Blood-surface interactions during cardiopulmonary bypass. J Card Surg. 1993;8:404–10.
32. Despotis GJ, Joist JH. Anticoagulation and anticoagulation reversal with cardiac surgery involving cardiopulmonary bypass: an update. J Cardiothorac Vasc Anesth. 1999;13:18–29.
33. Edmunds Jr LH, Colman RW. Thrombin during cardiopulmonary bypass. Ann Thorac Surg. 2006;82:2315–22.
34. Chan AK, Leaker M, Burrows FA, Williams WG, Gruenwald CE, Whyte L, et al. Coagulation and fibrinolytic profile of paediatric patients undergoing cardiopulmonary bypass. Thromb Haemost. 1997;77:270–7.
35. Mangano DT, Miao Y, Vuylsteke A, Tudor IC, Juneja R, Filipescu D, et al. Mortality associated with aprotinin during 5 years following coronary artery bypass graft surgery. JAMA. 2007;297: 471–9.
36. Szekely A, Sapi E, Breuer T, Kertai MD, Bodor G, Vargha P, et al. Aprotinin and renal dysfunction after pediatric cardiac surgery. Paediatr Anaesth. 2008;18:151–9.
37. Backer CL, Kelle AM, Stewart RD, Suresh SC, Ali FN, Cohn RA, et al. Aprotinin is safe in pediatric patients undergoing cardiac surgery. J Thorac Cardiovasc Surg. 2007;134:1421–6.
38. Brown JR, Birkmeyer NJ, O'Connor GT. Meta-analysis comparing the effectiveness and adverse outcomes of antifibrinolytic agents in cardiac surgery. Circulation. 2007;115:2801–13.
39. Breuer T, Martin K, Wilhelm M, Wiesner G, Schreiber C, Hess J, et al. The blood sparing effect and the safety of aprotinin compared to tranexamic acid in paediatric cardiac surgery. Eur J Cardiothorac Surg. 2009;35:167–71.

40. Fodstad H. Convulsive seizures following subdural application of fibrin sealant containing tranexamic acid in a rat model. Neurosurgery. 2001;49:479–80.
41. Schlag MG, Hopf R, Zifko U, Redl H. Epileptic seizures following cortical application of fibrin sealants containing tranexamic acid in rats. Acta Neurochir (Wien). 2002;144:63–9.
42. Jaquiss RD, Ghanayem NS, Zacharisen MC, Mussatto KA, Tweddell JS, Litwin SB. Safety of aprotinin use and re-use in pediatric cardiothoracic surgery. Circulation. 2002;106:I90–4.
43. Furtmuller R, Schlag MG, Berger M, Hopf R, Huck S, Sieghart W, et al. Tranexamic acid, a widely used antifibrinolytic agent, causes convulsions by a gamma-aminobutyric acid(A) receptor antagonistic effect. J Pharmacol Exp Ther. 2002;301:168–73.
44. Williams-Johnson JA, McDonald AH, Strachan GG, Williams EW. Effects of tranexamic acid on death, vascular occlusive events, and blood transfusion in trauma patients with significant haemorrhage (CRASH-2) a randomised, placebo-controlled trial. West Indian Med J. 2010;59:612–24.

Thromboembolism in Cyanotic Heart Disease: Mechanisms and Therapies

41

Toshio Nakanishi

Mechanisms of Thrombus Formation

Thrombosis is formed in the presence of an abnormal vascular wall including endothelial damage and dysfunction, altered function of platelets and coagulation factors, and/or abnormal bloodstream. Once the endothelium has been injured and the blood exposed to the thrombogenic matrix, such as collagen, on the vascular wall, platelets adhere to the endothelium via platelet-glycoprotein (GP) interaction with von Willebrand factor on the vascular wall. After platelet adhesion, platelets are activated and bind to fibrinogen via GP 2b/3a receptors, and they release their granules into the bloodstream. Platelet activation and granule secretion result in further platelet aggregation and thrombin generation. Thrombin activates the coagulation cascade and platelets [1–4]. In addition to normal hemostasis, platelet activation may result in the pathologic process of thrombosis and inflammation.

P-selectin is an adhesion molecule found in the secretory granules of platelets [5] and is mobilized to the plasma membrane on activation [2]. P-selectin expressed on platelets may be a direct inducer of procoagulant activity associated with vascular and thrombotic diseases [6].

Endothelial Function

Thrombomodulin is expressed mainly on the surface of vascular endothelial cells. Endothelial thrombomodulin is a key component of the protein C anticoagulant pathway, which facilitates the activation of protein C by thrombin [7–9]. Activated protein C is known to inhibit clotting factors V and VIII. Therefore, thrombomodulin acts as an intrinsic anticoagulant barrier between the blood and endothelium, preventing blood from clotting on the internal surface of vessels. The plasma thrombomodulin level initially increases with acute vascular injury, but it decreases with subsequent downregulation of its production during chronic vessel injury [10]. It was reported that downregulated gene expression of thrombomodulin by rapid atrial pacing induced local coagulation imbalance on the internal surface of the atrial cavity, leading to atrial intramural thrombus formation. Downregulation of this molecule may, therefore, disturb the optimal coagulation balance and promote thrombogenesis.

Cyanotic Congenital Heart Disease

Cyanotic congenital heart disease (CCHD) is associated with an increased risk of stroke and thromboembolism [11, 12]. Ammash and Warnes [12] reported that the incidence of cerebrovascular events were observed in about 14 % of adult patients with CCHD (1/100 patient-years). Conditions that further predispose to thrombosis are (1) after aortopulmonary shunt, especially using a conduit, (2) after the Glenn procedure, (3) after the Fontan procedure, and (4) Eisenmenger syndrome. A recent study using contrast-enhanced computed tomography revealed a high prevalence of pulmonary thrombosis in patients with Eisenmenger syndrome [13]. The precise mechanisms behind the increased incidence of thromboembolism in patients with CCHD have not yet been determined, but endothelial dysfunction, coagulation abnormalities, platelet activation, and an abnormal bloodstream may be underlying factors causing thromboembolism [14, 15].

Platelet Activation

Horigome et al. [16] measured plasma levels of P-selectin and showed that the plasma level of P-selectin was elevated in CCHD. We previously demonstrated that P-selectin

T. Nakanishi, MD
Department of Pediatric Cardiology,
Heart Institute, Tokyo Women's Medical University,
8-1 Kawada-cho, Shinjuku-ku, Tokyo 162-8666, Japan
e-mail: pnakanis@hij.twmu.ac.jp

E.A. Gabriel, S.A. Gabriel (eds.), *Inflammatory Response in Cardiovascular Surgery*,
DOI 10.1007/978-1-4471-4429-8_41, © Springer-Verlag London 2013

expression on the platelets is elevated in patients with CCHD, indicating that platelet activation does exist in CCHD [17]. Some studies failed to demonstrate elevated platelet P-selectin in patients with CCHD [14, 18]. The reason for that is not clear, but different methods of platelet P-selectin measurement may be partly responsible, since P-selectin is rapidly mobilized to the platelet surface and lost in the plasma [19]. Although patients in our study were receiving an antiplatelet drug (aspirin or ticlopidine) or a combination of an antiplatelet and an anticoagulant drug (heparin or warfarin), the platelet P-selectin level was elevated in many patients [17].

Endothelial Dysfunction

Previous studies showed decreased plasma thrombomodulin levels of protein C activity in patients with CCHD [16, 17]. This suggests the presence of impaired endothelial function in patients with CCHD. These data are in agreement with the study of Ferreiro et al. [20] showing that nitric oxide synthesis activity was blunted in patients with CCHD, suggesting that the endothelial function is impaired.

The endothelium may be damaged by the increased shear stress on the vessel wall caused by increased blood viscosity and/or by chronic hypoxemia in CCHD [7]. It has been speculated that in patients with primary pulmonary hypertension, damage to the endothelium leads to a decreased thrombomodulin level [10]. It is likely that in patients with CCHD, the plasma thrombomodulin level may be downregulated by its decreased production due to chronic endothelial injury and persistent hypoxemia.

Endothelial Dysfunction and Platelet Activation

It is possible that the decreased expression of protein C and the increased expression of P-selectin on platelets due to a reduced thrombomodulin level may contribute to the formation of thrombi in patients with CCHD. Recently, Kario et al. [21] demonstrated that endothelial cell damage is a potential risk factor for cerebral infarction. It was also reported that the increased expression of platelet P-selectin associated with a reduced NO level, a marker of endothelial dysfunction, was a risk factor for cerebral infarction in patients with atrial fibrillation [22]. An elevated plasma P-selectin level has been reported in patients with congestive heart failure, primary pulmonary hypertension, and CCHD [18]. The platelet activation under these conditions could be due to the increased shear stress and/or endothelial dysfunction [23]. Horigome et al. [16] reported that the hematocrit value showed a positive correlation with soluble P-selectin, and they speculated that increased shear stress due to hyperviscosity could be a major factor causing platelet activation. The role of hyperviscosity in platelet activation in CCHD should be studied further.

Thromboembolic Events

Increased incidence of thromboembolism and organ infarction has been reported in patients with CCHD [11, 12]. In patients with CCHD <4 years old, the risk of cerebrovascular thrombosis in intracranial veins is increased, and the reported incidence varies from 1.6 to 20 % [11, 12]. Candice et al. [13] reported that a pulmonary artery thrombus was noted in 21 % of patients with Eisenmenger syndrome. We showed previously that the platelet P-selectin level was higher in patients with than in those patients without thromboembolic events in CCHD, suggesting that elevated P-selectin could be a risk factor for cerebral thromboembolism in CCHD [17].

In addition to elevated P-selectin on platelets, we showed plasma levels of thrombin antithrombin complex III (TAT) in patients with thromboembolic events were higher than in those without [17]. Thus, elevated P-selectin and TAT may indicate a high risk of thromboembolism. It should be noted that aspirin alone cannot always inhibit platelet activation.

Fontan Circulation and Thromboembolism

A Fontan circulation is associated with an increased risk of thromboembolism [24–26]. The precise mechanisms by which thrombus is formed in patients after the Fontan procedure remain undetermined, but the process is most likely multifactorial. Possible factors that predispose to thrombus formation after Fontan procedures include an enlarged right atrium, slow blood flow, prosthetic material, atrial arrhythmias, blind cul-de-sacs of the pulmonary artery stump, right-to-left-shunts, and hypercoagulablility. The prevalence of thromboembolic events has been reported to range from 3 to 30 % among Fontan patients [27–29]. The probability of freedom from thromboembolism decreases with the interval after the Fontan procedure [26, 27]. Right atrial volume increases with the interval after atriopulmonary anastomosis. Slow blood flow in the enlarged atrium may further predispose to thrombus formation. However, whether there is a difference in the prevalence of thromboembolism among three types of Fontan procedures (atriopulmonary anastomosis, lateral tunnel, and total cavopulmonary connection) remains to be clarified.

Coagulation

Various abnormalities in the coagulation system have been postulated as mechanisms of the increased incidence of thromboembolism in Fontan patients, including decreased protein C, protein S, and antithrombin III levels [24, 30, 31].

Platelets

Platelets play an important role in thrombus formation, and collagen-induced and adenosine-induced platelet aggregations are elevated in patients after the Fontan procedure [32]. We previously demonstrated that P-selectin expression on platelets is elevated in patients after the Fontan procedure, indicating that platelet activation occurs in Fontan patients [33].

Endothelium

We also showed previously that plasma thrombomodulin levels and protein C activity were decreased in Fontan patients [33], suggesting the presence of impaired endothelial function. Previous studies using near-infrared spectroscopy and flow-mediated vasodilation have suggested that endothelial function in Fontan patients is impaired [34]. The endothelium in Fontan patients may be damaged by increased shear stress on the vessel wall caused by increased blood viscosity and/or by chronic hypoxemia before the Fontan procedure [17]. The negative correlation between thrombomodulin levels and the interval after the Fontan procedure suggests the deterioration of endothelial function over time following the Fontan procedure [33] This may partly explain the high prevalence of thromboembolic events long after the Fontan procedure.

Management of Thrombosis in CCHD

Prophylasis

Prophylactic administration of antiplatelets and anticoagulants in general is not recommended in patients with CCHD. A bleeding tendency exists in patients with CCHD, and the bleeding includes epistaxis, menorrhagia, hemoptysis, and internal pulmonary bleeding, which are sometimes fatal. There is a dilemma between a bleeding tendency and thrombotic disposition in the management of patients with CCHD [11].

Erythroytosis

In patients with CCHD, secondary erythrocytosis due to low systemic oxygen saturation and an increased erythropoietin level is observed. In iron-deficient microcytic erythrocytosis, the erythrocyte is less deformable and the hyperviscosity status is enhanced. Iron-deficient erythrocytosis in patients with CCHD <4 years old predisposes to cerebrovascular thrombosis in the intracranial venous sinuses and veins rather than in the artery [11]. Dehydration enhances the chance of thromboembolic events in children, and treatment for dehydration is important in children with CCHD. Erythrocytosis and hyperviscosity itself do not increase the chance of cerebral thromboembolic events in adults [35], and therefore phlebotomy is not recommended. Phlebotomy causes iron deficiency and ultimately enhances hyperviscosity. The risk factors associated with ceroborovascular events in adults were systemic hypertension, atrial fibrillation, phlebotomy, and iron-deficiency anemia [12], and attempts should be made to eliminate these risk factors. Iron deficiency should be corrected, especially when the mean corpuscular volume is <82, by oral intake of low-dose ferrous sulfate.

Eisenmenger Syndrome

As in Eisenmenger syndrome patients with CCHD, there is a dilemma between bleeding and thromboembolism. Anticoagulation is recommended in patients with idiopathic pulmonary arterial hypertension. However, there are no data supporting routine anticoagulation therapy in patients with Eisenmenger syndrome. Because of the risk of bleeding, prophylactic administration of antiplatelets and anticoagulants is not recommended. Indications for these drugs in patients with Eisenmenger syndrome are (1) frequent episodes of atrial flutter or fibrillation and (2) recurrent thrombotic events.

Shunt

Systemic-to-pulmonary shunt using a conduit (modified Balock-Taussig shunt) is performed as palliation for tetralogy of Fallot and complex congenital heart diseases with severe pulmonary stenosis or pulmonary atresia or hypoplastic left heart syndrome. Beneficial effects of antiplatelets are shown in some studies [36, 37], but not in others [38, 39]. The use of aspirin after shunt placement is recommended in the guideline of the American College of Chest Physicians [40].

Fontan Procedures

There is no consensus regarding the efficacy of antiplatelet and anticoagulant therapy in patients after Fontan procedures. Basically, there are three policies concerning thromboembolism in the management of patients after Glenn and Fontan procedures: (1) no medication, (2) the use of antiplatelets, and (3) the use of anticoagulants. The policy depends on the institution and/or primary physician taking care of patients. Marrone et al. [41] in their meta-analysis reported that the thromboembolic incidence long after extracardiac total cavopulmonary connection (TCPC) with antiplatelet therapy (4.5 %) was similar to that with anticoagulation therapy (5 %). Kaulitz et al. [42] reported that thrombotic events were observed in 7 % of patients long after TCPC, and the incidence was similar among patients without medication, with aspirin, and with warfarin. Cheung et al. [43] also reported similar data. Irrespective of the antithrombotic medication policy, Jacobs and Pourmoghadam [44] emphasized the importance of careful evaluation of thrombosis in the follow-up of post-Fontan patients, including transesophageal echocardiography.

Whether the risk of thromboembolism is high in patients after the Glenn procedure has not been determined. In the presence of right-to-left shunt before Fontan completion, it may be prudent to use antiplatelets and/or anticoagulants in patients after the Glenn procedure [45].

Laboratory Tests

In order to prevent thromboembolic events in patients with CCHD, laboratory tests examining platelet activation, such as the platelet aggregation test and P-selectin, and hypercoagulability, such as TAT, should be performed, and if necessary, appropriate antiplatelet and anticoagulation therapy should be added for each patient. Among antiplatelet medications, clopidogrel is an option [46]. The efficacy of this drug in patients with CCHD remains to be clarified.

References

1. Jurk K, Kehrel BE. Platelets: physiology and biochemistry. Semin Thromb Hemost. 2005;31:381–92.
2. Lefer AM, Weyrich AS, Buerke M. Role of selectins, a new family of adhesion molecules, in ischemia-reperfusion injury. Cardiovasc Res. 1994;28:289–94.
3. Shaun RC. Thrombin signaling and protease-activated receptors. Nature. 2000;407:258–64.
4. Palabrica T, Lobb R, Furie BC, Aronovitz M, Benjamin C, Hsu YM, et al. Leukocyte accumulation promoting fibrin deposition is mediated in vivo by P-selectin on adherent platelets. Nature. 1992;359:848–51.
5. Stenberg PE, McEver RP, Shuman MA, Jacoques YV, Bainton DF. A platelet alpha-granule membrane after activation. J Cell Biol. 1985;101:880–6.
6. Hrachovinová I, Cambien B, Hafezi-Moghadam A, Kappelmayer J, Camphausen RT, Widom A, et al. Interaction of P-selectin and PSGL-1 generates microparticles that correct hemostasis in a mouse model of hemophilia A. Nat Med. 2003;9:1020–5.
7. Walker FJ, Fay PJ. Regulation of blood coagulation by the protein C system. FASEB J. 1992;6:2561–7.
8. Esmon CT. The roles of protein C and thrombomodulin in the regulation of blood coagulation. J Biol Chem. 1989;264:4743–6.
9. Suzuki K, Kusumoto H, Deyashiki Y, Nishioka J, Maruyama I, Zushi M, et al. Structure and expression of human thrombomodulin, a thrombin receptor on endothelium acting as a cofactor for protein C activation. EMBO J. 1987;6:1991–7.
10. Cacoub P, Karmochkine M, Dorent R, Nataf P, Piette JC, Godeau P, et al. Plasma levels of thrombomodulin in pulmonary hypertension. Am J Med. 1996;101:160–4.
11. Perloff JK. Neurologic disorders. In: Perloff JK, Child JS, editors. Congenital heart disease in adults. 2nd ed. Philadelphia: W B Saunders; 1998. p. 237–46.
12. Ammash N, Warnes CA. Cerebrovascular events in adult patients with cyanotic congenital heart disease. J Am Coll Cardiol. 1996;28:768–72.
13. Candice KS, John TG, Eli K, Michelle AH. Pulmonary thrombosis in adults with Eisenmenger syndrome. J Am Coll Cardiol. 2003;42:1982–7.
14. Levin E, Wu J, Devine DV, Alexander J, Reichart C, Sett S, et al. Hemostatic parameters and platelet activation marker expression in cyanotic and acyanotic pediatric patients undergoing cardiac surgery in the presence of tranexamic acid. Thromb Haemost. 2000;83:54–9.
15. Adatia I, Barrow SE, Stratton P, Ritter JM, Haworth SG. Abnormalities in the biosynthesis of thromboxane A2 and prostacyclin in children with cyanotic congenital heart disease. Br Heart J. 1993;69:179–82.
16. Horigome H, Murakami T, Isobe T, Nagasawa T, Matsui A. Soluble P-selectin and thrombomodulin-protein C-Protein S pathway in cyanotic congenital heart disease with secondary erythrocytosis. Thromb Res. 2003;112:223–7.
17. Kajimoto H, Nakazawa M, Murasaki K, Mori Y, Tanoue K, Kasanuki H, et al. Increased thrombogenicity in patients with cyanotic congenital heart disease. Circ J. 2007;71:948–53.
18. Horigome H, Hiramatsu Y, Shigeta O, Nagasawa T, Matsui A. Overproduction of platlet microparticles in cyanotic congenital heart disease with polycythemia. J Am Coll Cardiol. 2002;39:1072–7.
19. Michelson AD, Barnard MR, Hechtman HB, MacGregor H, Connoly RJ, Loscalzo J, et al. In vivo tracking of platelets: circulating degranulated platelets rapidly lose surface P-selectin but continue to circulate and function. Proc Natl Acad Sci. 1996;93:11877–82.
20. Ferreiro CR, Chagas AC, Carvalho MH, Dantas AP, Jatene MB, Bento De Souza LC, et al. Influence of hypoxia on nitric oxide synthase activity and gene expression in children with congenital heart disease: a novel pathophysiological adaptive mechanism. Circulation. 2001;103:2272–6.
21. Kario K, Matsuo T, Kobayashi H, Asada R, Matsuo M. 'Silent' cerebral infarction is associated with hypercoagulability, endothelial cell damage, and high Lp(a) levels in elderly Japanese. Arterioscler Thromb Vasc Biol. 1996;16:734–41.
22. Minamino T, Kitakaze M, Sanada S, Asanuama H, Kurotobi T, Koretsune Y, et al. Increased expression of P-selectin on platelets is a risk factor for silent cerebral infarction in patients with atrial fibrillation: role of nitric oxide. Circulation. 1998;98:1721–7.
23. Merten M, Chow T, Hellums JD, Thiagarajan P. A new role for P-selectin in shear-induced platelet aggregation. Circulation. 2000;102:2045–50.
24. Cromme-Dijkhuis AH, Henkens CM, Bijleveld CM, Hillege HL, Bom VJ, van der Meer J. Coagulation factor abnormalities as possible thrombotic risk factors after Fontan operations. Lancet. 1990;336:1087–90.
25. Stamm C, Friehs I, Mayer Jr JE, Zurakowski D, Triedman JK, Moran AM, et al. Long-term results of the lateral tunnel Fontan operation. J Thorac Cardiovasc Surg. 2001;121:28–41.
26. Freedom RM, Hamilton R, Yoo SJ, Mikailian H, Benson L, McCrindle B, et al. The Fontan procedure: analysis of cohorts and late complications. Cardiol Young. 2000;10:307–31.
27. Seipelt RG, Franke A, Vazquez-Jimenez JF, Hanrath P, von Bernuth G, Messmer BJ, et al. Thromboembolic complications after Fontan procedures: comparison of different therapeutic approaches. Ann Thorac Surg. 2002;74:556–62.

28. Rosenthal DN, Friedman AH, Kleinman CS, Kopf GS, Rosenfeld LE, Hellenbrand WE. Thromboembolic complications after Fontan operations. Circulation. 1995;92(9 Suppl):II287–93.
29. Jahangiri M, Ross DB, Redington AN, Lincoln C, Shinebourne EA. Thromboembolism after the Fontan procedure and its modifications. Ann Thorac Surg. 1994;58:1409–14.
30. Jahangiri M, Shore D, Kakkar V, Lincoln C, Shinebourne E. Coagulation factor abnormalities after the Fontan procedure and its modifications. J Thorac Cardiovasc Surg. 1997;113:989–93.
31. van Nieuwenhuizen RC, Peters M, Lubbers LJ, Trip MD, Tijssen JG, Mulder BJ. Abnormalities in liver function and coagulation profile following the Fontan procedure. Heart. 1999;82:40–6.
32. Ravn HB, Hjortdal VE, Stenbog EV, Emmertsen K, Kromann O, Pedersen J, et al. Increased platelet reactivity and significant changes in coagulation markers after cavopulmonary connection. Heart. 2001;85:61–5.
33. Kajimoto H, Nakazawa M, Murasaki K, Hagiwara N, Nakanishi T. Increased P-selectin expression on platelets and decreased plasma thrombomodulin in Fontan patients. Circ J. 2009;73(9):1705–10. Epub 2009 Jul 28.
34. Jin SM, Noh CI, Bae EJ, Choi JY, Yun YS. Impaired vascular function in patients with Fontan circulation. Int J Cardiol. 2007;120:221–6.
35. Perloff JK, Marelli AJ, Miner PD. Risk of stroke in adults with cyanotic congenital heart disease. Circulation. 1993;87:1954–9.
36. Li JS, Yow E, Berezny KY, Rhodes JF, Bokesch PM, Charpie JR, et al. Clinical outcomes of palliative surgery including a systemic-to-pulmonary artery shunt in infants with cyanotic congenital heart disease: does aspirin make a difference? Circulation. 2007;116:293–7.
37. Motz R, Wessel A, Ruschewski W, Bürsch J. Reduced frequency of occlusion of aorto-pulmonary shunts in infants receiving aspirin. Cardiol Young. 1999;9:474–7.
38. Al Jubair KA, Al Fagih MR, Al Jarallah AS, Al Yousef S, Ali Khan MA, Ashmeg A, et al. Results of 546 Blalock-Taussig shunts performed in 478 patients. Cardiol Young. 1998;8:486–90.
39. Centazzo S, Montigny M, Davignon A, Chartrand C, Fournier A, Marchand T. Use of acetylsalicylic acid to improve patency of subclavian to pulmonary artery Gore-Tex shunts. Can J Cardiol. 1993;9:243–6.
40. Monagle P, Chaimers E, Chan A, Deveber G, Kirkham F, Massicotte P, et al. Antithrombotic therapy in neonates and children. Chest. 2008;133(suppl):887S–968.
41. Marrone C, Galasso G, Piccolo R, de Leva F, Paladini R, Piscione F, et al. Antiplatelet versus anticoagulation therapy after extracardiac conduit Fontan: a systematic review and meta-analysis. Pediatr Cardiol. 2011;32(1):32–9.
42. Kaulitz R, Ziemer G, Rauch R, Girisch M, Bertram H, Wessel A, et al. Prophylaxis of thromboembolic complications after the Fontan operation (total cavopulmonary anastomosis). J Thorac Cardiovasc Surg. 2005;129(3):569–75.
43. Cheung YF, Chay GW, Chiu CS, Cheng LC. Long-term anticoagulation therapy and thromboembolic complications after the Fontan procedure. Int J Cardiol. 2005;102:509–13.
44. Jacobs ML, Pourmoghadam KK. Thromboembolism and the role of anticoagulation in the Fontan patient. Pediatr Cardiol. 2007;28(6):457–64.
45. Binotto MA, Maeda NY, Lopes AA. Evidence of endothelial dysfunction in patients with functionally univentricular physiology before completion of the Fontan operation. Cardiol Young. 2005;15:26–30.
46. Li JS, Yow E, Berezny KY, Bokesch PM, Takahashi M, Graham Jr TP, et al. Dosing of clopidogrel for platelet inhibition in infants and young children: primary results of the Platelet Inhibition in Children On cLOpidogrel (PICOLO) trial. Circulation. 2008;117:553–9.

Endovascular Management of Coarctation of the Aorta

42

Edward B. Diethrich

Introduction

Aortic coarctation has been recognized since the late 1700s [1], but the first and largest post-mortem series appeared in 1928 [2]. Nevertheless, the condition was not commonly diagnosed clinically until the early 1930s. Although de novo lesions in adults are rare, primary aortic coarctation has been documented in patients over a wide range of ages and with varying degrees of severity—in general, the condition presents most commonly in infancy. Aortic coarctation is considered significant if an invasively determined pressure gradient is >20 mmHg at rest or >30 mmHg after exercise in adolescents and adults. Untreated coarctation can cause left ventricular pressure overload and left ventricular hypertrophy, premature coronary artery disease, and, eventually, heart failure.

Successful surgical correction of coarctation of the aorta by resection with end-to-end anastomosis was first described by Crafoord and Nylin in 1945 [3]. Until fairly recently, open surgical repair using either a left thoracotomy with end-to-end anastomosis or end-to-side anastomosis was considered "gold-standard" treatment of coarctation [4–7]. Despite good long-term success, recurrence of coarctation is considerable—as high as 15 % [4–8]. Percutaneous balloon angioplasty was introduced as a treatment in 1981 [9], and we performed one of the early stenting procedures at The Arizona Heart Institute in 1995 [10]. In recent years, stenting (sometimes combined with hybrid repair) has become an accepted treatment for aortic coarctation, reserving surgery for those patients not suited for the endovascular approach or in whom it has failed [11–15].

E.B. Diethrich, MD
Founder and Medical Director of The Arizona Heart Foundation,
Department of Cardiovascular and Endovascular Surgery,
Phoenix, AZ, USA

Patient Selection

Because de novo lesions are rare in adults, most patients who are candidates for endovascular repair have had a previous intervention. Factors to be considered when deciding the most appropriate form of management include age, aortic morphology, any previous surgical or endovascular treatment, and the interventionist's experience. Arch hypoplasia may cause a residual gradient following coarctation repair, particularly if it is severe and this condition represents a significant challenge for successful repair.

Approximately 10 % of patients who underwent surgical repair of neonatal aortic coarctation will develop recurrence as an adult and present with associated aortic diseases. Open repair can be challenging because of complex aortic pathology with the recoarctation, intercostal collateral circulation, and pleural scar tissue from the original operative approach.

Early repair of native coarctation is associated with a lower risk of late hypertension and improved survival, but the risk of recoarctation is higher. Recoarctation with aneurysm or pseudoaneurysm formation is fairly common. Aneurysms may develop at the site of surgical repair or within the proximal aorta and often these are best treated with endovascular therapy; aneurysmal disease distal to a recoarctation is fairly common. Untreated aneurysms carry a considerable risk of aortic rupture. With late repair, there is a greater risk of recurrent hypertension and a lower overall risk of recoarctation; nevertheless, survival and hypertension may still be improved by treating patients who are first diagnosed as adults.

Indications

The presentation of coarctation is dependent on the severity of obstruction and associated cardiac lesions; in general, those diagnosed as infants exhibit congestive heart failure, severe acidosis, and ischemia of the lower extremities. Adolescent and adult patients often present with

E.A. Gabriel, S.A. Gabriel (eds.), *Inflammatory Response in Cardiovascular Surgery*,
DOI 10.1007/978-1-4471-4429-8_42, © Springer-Verlag London 2013

hypertension that is difficult to control, headaches, nosebleeds, leg cramps, muscle weakness, claudication, ischemia of the bowel and lower extremities, and neurologic changes.

Technique

The goal of an endovascular approach to treat coarctation of the aorta is to restore anatomical relief of the obstruction resulting in reduction of the aortic gradient pressures. This concept is exemplified well in Fig. 42.1, which was contributed by one of my former fellows. Endovascular approaches are preferable to open surgery in the vast majority of patients with recoarctation, and balloon angioplasty and stent implantations are widely used [11, 16]; endoluminal grafting (including covered stents) may also be appropriate in selected cases [14]. Both covered and uncovered stents can be used to achieve satisfactory results. At our institution, we use endovascular techniques to provide relief from obstruction at the coarctation site and improve pressures proximally and distally as well as to exclude pericoarctation aneurysms or dissection to minimize the risk of rupture. The average duration of hospitalization following stenting of aortic coarctation is about 2 days, whereas open surgery may require a stay as long as 2 weeks. We strive to avoid disruption of blood flow to the left upper extremity and vertebral circulation, but when subclavian artery coverage is required, a carotid-subclavian bypass prevents vascular compromise to the left upper extremity. All patients with documented coarctation-associated pseudoaneurysms routinely undergo preoperative computed tomography (CT) angiography and Doppler studies to delineate the anatomical and physiological status of their carotid and vertebral arteries and its branches. If the operative procedure entails coverage of the left subclavian artery, we perform elective left carotid-subclavian bypass grafting whenever the right vertebral artery is abnormally small or diseased, or when there is evidence of an incomplete circle of Willis [12]. In the rare case in which the patient has had a left internal mammary artery bypass to the coronary circulation, the carotid-subclavian bypass is also necessary.

Angioplasty

Balloon angioplasty is a widely accepted treatment for patients with native and recurrent coarctation of the aorta in patients older than 6 months of age. The angioplasty procedure stretches and tears the intima and, in some cases, the media of the vessel wall. While ample luminal gain can be achieved, the correct balloon size is key in preventing elastic recoil and inordinate trauma to the vessel. In older patients with degenerative disease and calcification, great care must be taken when dilating the vessel. Indeed, safe use of angioplasty requires a delicate balance, as underdistension of the vessel may cause residual stenosis, and overdistension can result in aortic dissection, rupture, or aneurysm formation. In addition, neointimal proliferation and restenosis may result from vessel wall trauma following intervention. Because of these potential adverse events, stenting (rather than angioplasty alone) has become almost routine at our institution as well as others.

Stenting

Bare stents are generally used to ensure adequate aortic lumen reduction of the pressure gradient and a lower recurrence rate than that seen with angioplasty. Stenting addresses resulting vessel wall trauma from ballooning, prevents elastic recoil, and seals small dissections. Neointimal response and proliferation may be observed following stenting, but stent treatment of coarctation in older children, adolescents, and adults results in immediate hemodynamic benefit [10–13, 15]; in larger vessels, the recurrence rate is very low. Our preference for stenting has been the Palmaz XL 10 series stent (Cordis, Miami Lakes, FL) since for a time it was the only large product available. The IntraStent Max (ev3 Endovascular Inc., Plymouth, MN), approved in 2002, offers another option; however, because of its rounded edges, it results in less pressure in the vessel wall, and migration may be a problem. Other stents, such as the Cheatham-Platinum stent (NuMED, Hopkinton, NY), appear to be highly effective in reducing the coarctation gradient and increasing lesion dilation in both native coarctation and recoarctation but are not yet available in the US [17].

Some technical details regarding the procedure are warranted since mishaps have occurred and caused less-than-favorable results. As the majority of patients will present with recurrent coarctation and a narrow lumen surrounded by scar tissue, our first step after crossing the area with a 0.33-in. Glidewire (Terumo, Somerset, NJ) is an intravascular ultrasound. The exam provides accurate measure of aortic diameters proximal and distal to the coarctation and an exact lumen diameter (Fig. 42.2). A small-diameter balloon (usually no more than 8–10 mm, depending on the degree of stenosis) is used to dilate prior to stent deployment. Serial balloon dilatations are often indicated in heavily calcified, subatretic, or recurrent lesions; however, the major purpose of the balloon is to permit unobstructed passage of the stent deployment system. The large Palmaz stent is loaded by hand crimping onto the delivery balloon. A long sheath is passed across the deployment site, and the mounted stent is centered at the deployment location (usually in the middle of the coarctation). This centering within the sheath is important since sometimes the stent moves on the balloon even after careful crimping. Once positioned, the sheath is

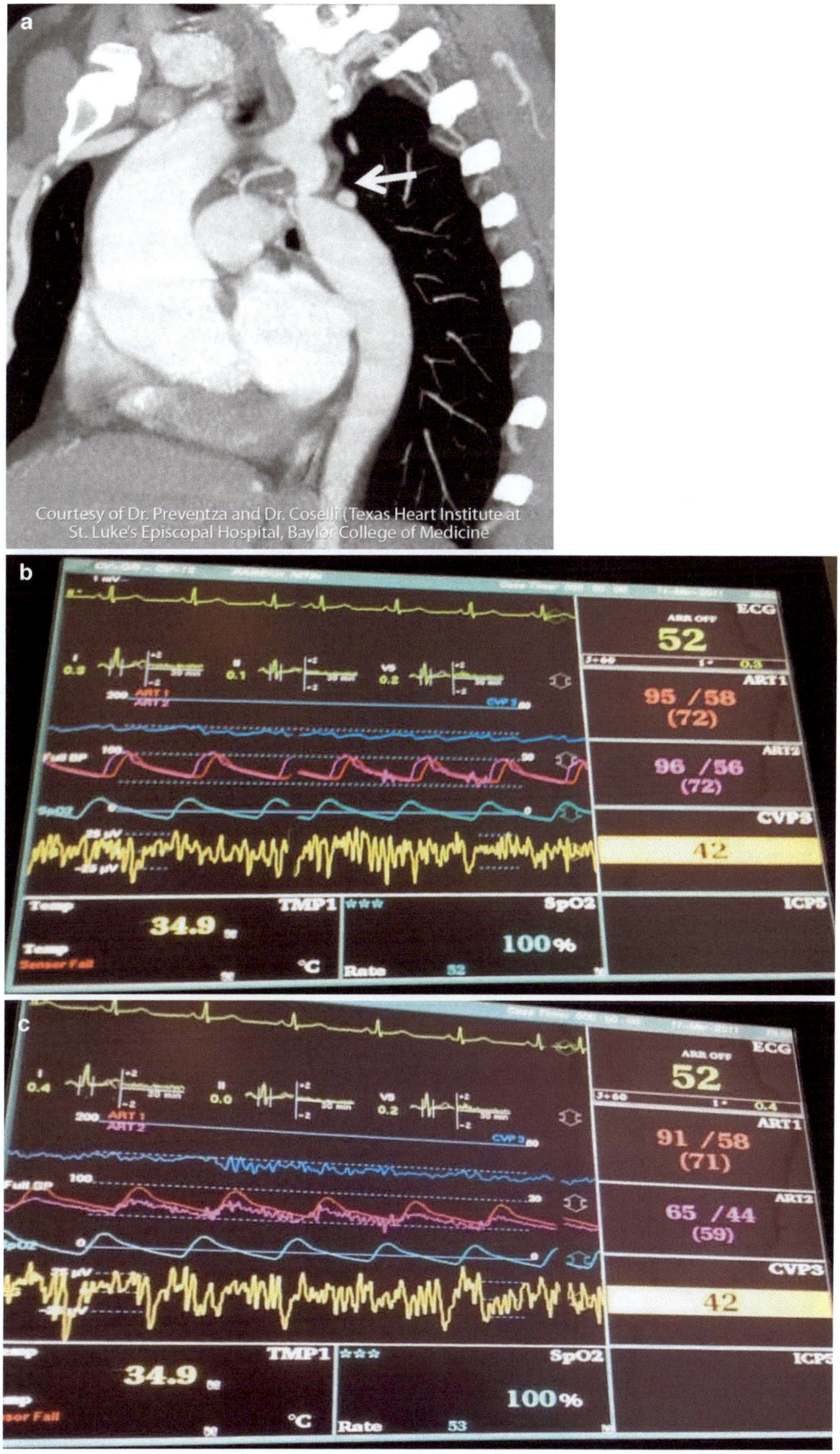

Fig. 42.1 (**a**) Angiogram showing narrow (*arrow*) recurrent coarctation distal to the left subclavian artery (Courtesy of Dr. Preventza and Dr. Coselli [Texas Heart Institute at St. Luke 's Episcopal Hospital, Baylor College of Medicine]). (**b**) Pressure tracings using pigtail catheter proximal to coarctation. (**c**) Tracings distal to coarctation. (**d**) Tracings proximal to coarctation after stent and balloon angioplasty using 12 mm balloon. (**e**) Tracing distal to repair with no pressure gradient. (**f**) Comparison of pre- and postoperative angiograms following successful angioplasty. (**g**) Post-procedure CT examination showing good apposition of stent and satisfactory 14.1 mm residual aortic diameter

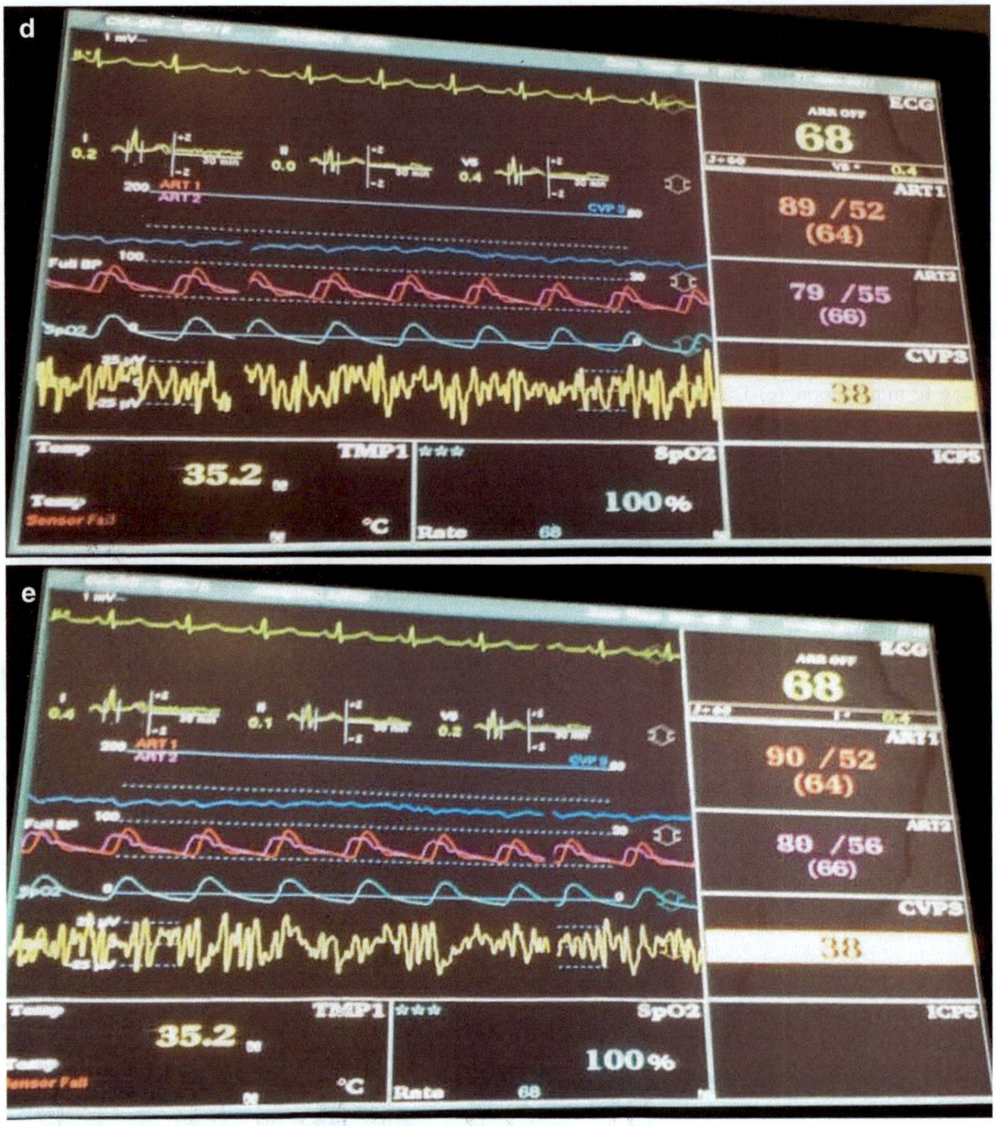

Fig. 42.1 (continued)

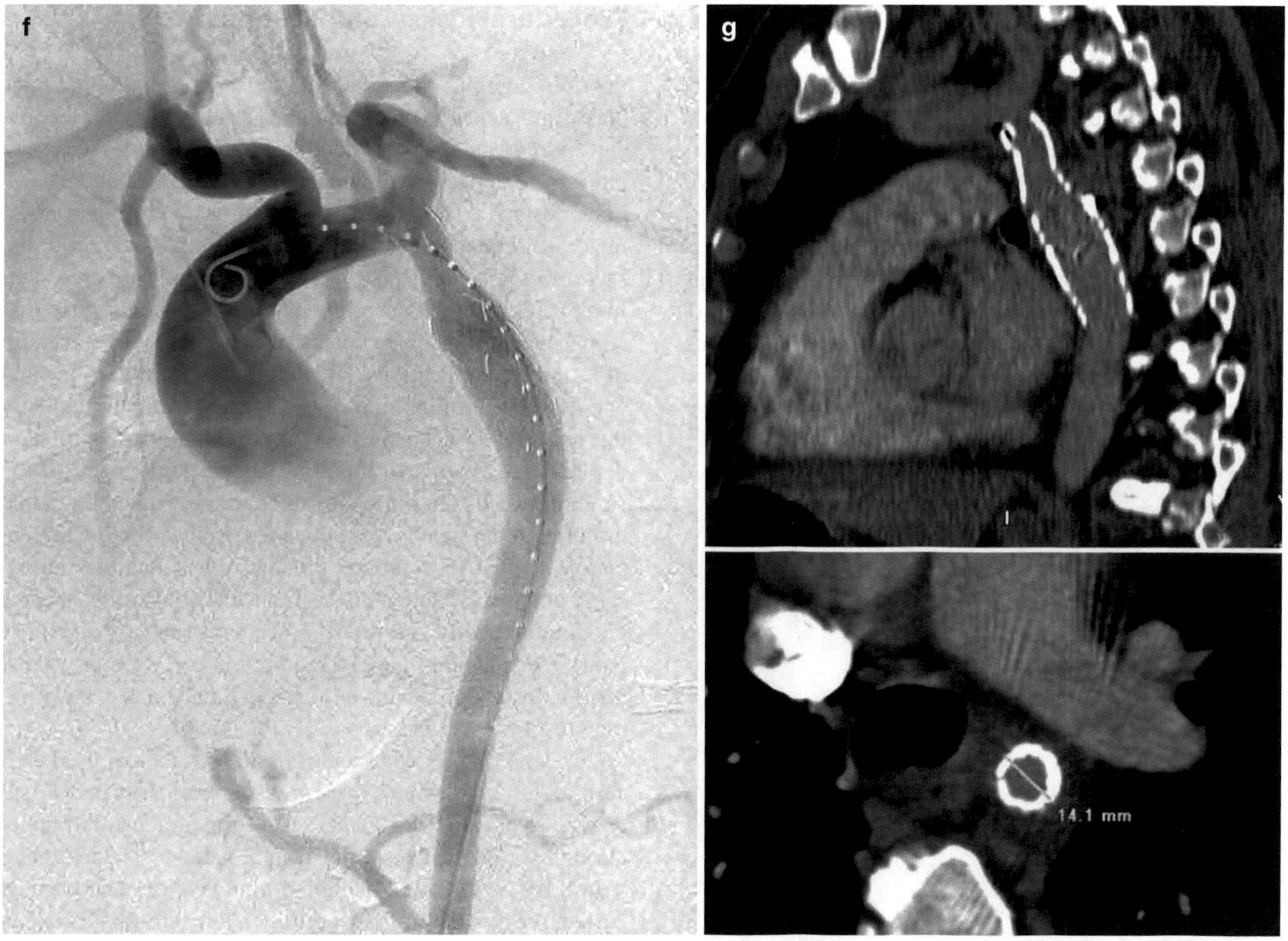

Fig. 42.1 (continued)

retracted to the lower end of the stent, where it prevents the stent from migrating during expansion. When a significant portion of the stent is adequately apposed to the aorta, the sheath is pulled distally, and the balloon is fully expanded. The goal of the procedure is the eradication of the pressure gradient; it is important to understand that a perfect angiographic picture is not necessarily indicative of that achievement. This is nicely illustrated in Figs. 42.3 and 42.4.

Covered Stents

Although both covered and uncovered stents can be used to achieve satisfactory results, covered stents and endoluminal grafts may be used for post-coarctation repair associated with aneurysm formation at or near the site of previous surgery. In patients with a small thoracic aorta, endoluminal grafting may be preferable to stenting because various components and types of endoluminal grafts are available, and the device may be customized as needed [14]. Covered stents are also useful in patients with "tight" native coarctations; in these cases, dilatation of a bare stent may be associated with the risk of dissection or rupture. In addition, older patients in whom the vessel wall appears rigid and less compliant may also benefit from placement of a covered stent. Due to the ever-present potential for aortic dissection and rupture, covered stents should always be available in the endovascular suite as illustrated in Fig. 42.5.

Treatment of Complex Cases

Complex forms of coarctation are frequently managed by anatomic and extra-anatomic bypass techniques commonly referred to as hybrid procedures. These procedures combine classical surgical techniques with endovascular approaches to treat both the recoarctation and its associated pathologies. Figure 42.4a illustrates a frequently observed pattern in which the site of the recoarctation is expanded distally and proximally, even involving the origins of the left subclavian artery. The operative approach (Fig. 42.4b) involved exposure of the left subclavian arteries and carotid arteries with a supraclavicular approach, resection of the proximal subclavian aneurysm with carotid-subclavian, and endoluminal graft exclusion of the entire aneurysm segment (Fig. 42.6).

Another problem encountered in recoarctation is the size discrepancy between the aortic segments adjacent to the narrowed segment. Figure 42.5 shows marked dilation beyond the coarctation with a narrow proximal segment. The repair was accomplished by using separate endografts of different sizes in a customized configuration. Fortunately, endograft design has now evolved enough to include tapered grafts (Fig. 42.7) that are useful in treating complex pathologies.

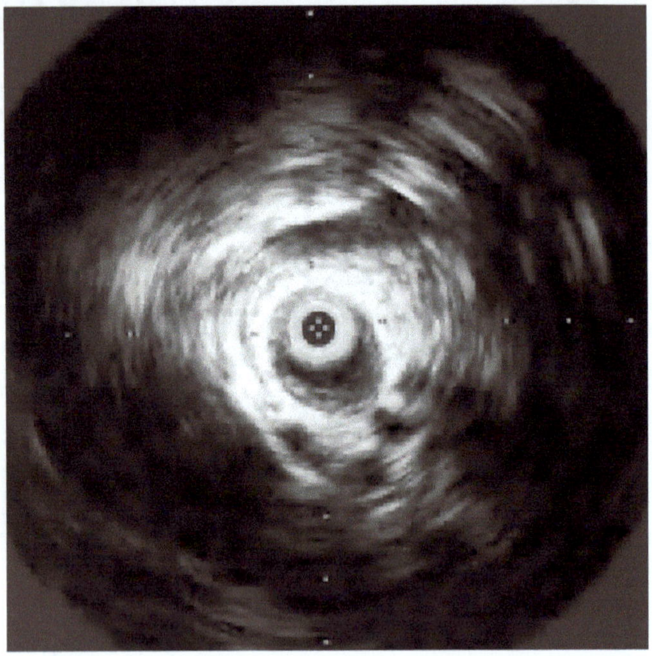

Fig. 42.2 Intravascular ultrasound image showing extremely tight recoarcted aortic area that is almost the same as the diameter of the probe. Such measurements are useful in determining balloon size selection for progressive dilatation of the lesion

Procedural Risks/Complications

Possible complications that may arise from balloon angioplasty and stent placement include aortic rupture, dissection, and pseudoaneurysm formation. Large sheath sizes are required to deliver stents and endoluminal grafts, and the use of hemostatic control devices is advisable to prevent or minimize groin hematomas when appropriate. Acute aortic dissection and aneurysm formation following bare stent implantation can be seen in 10–15 % of patients. Size discrepancies in the device versus the vessel may be the cause of some complications, including stent migration and endoleak. Stent migration is a serious concern and is likely the result of insufficient balloon pre-dilation prior to stent deployment. Excessive force in balloon deployment of the stent may also cause it to slip and migrate. A gentle gradual inflation of the stent is recommended. Reintervention to treat endoleaks that form around the device is sometimes necessary; endoleaks can often be treated by inserting another endoluminal graft. Additional procedures such as coil embolization or plugging may be required in case of a large leak arising from the subclavian artery. Small leaks, however, may resolve spontaneously [12] (Fig. 42.8).

In some cases, when endovascular grafts are used, left carotid–left subclavian bypass procedures must be performed as well to prevent pseudoaneurysm formation and left upper extremity ischemia resulting from coverage of the subclavian artery with an endoluminal graft. Except as indicated earlier, we do not routinely perform a left carotid-subclavian bypass even if the left subclavian artery is covered.

Late hypertension is relatively common, even in the absence of residual or recurrent coarctation. Hypertension that persists after stenting in adult life is likely due to structural and functional abnormalities of the arterial wall, which can result in diminished arterial wall compliance and

Fig. 42.3 Stent deployment can result in distal migration when the coarctation is inadequately dilated and the stenotic region is highly fibrotic. Further stent deployment can result in additional migrations

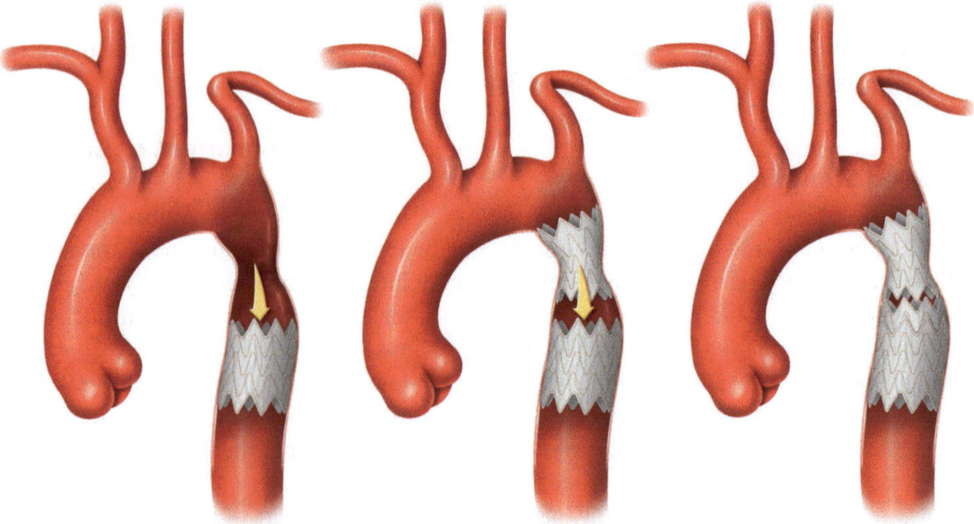

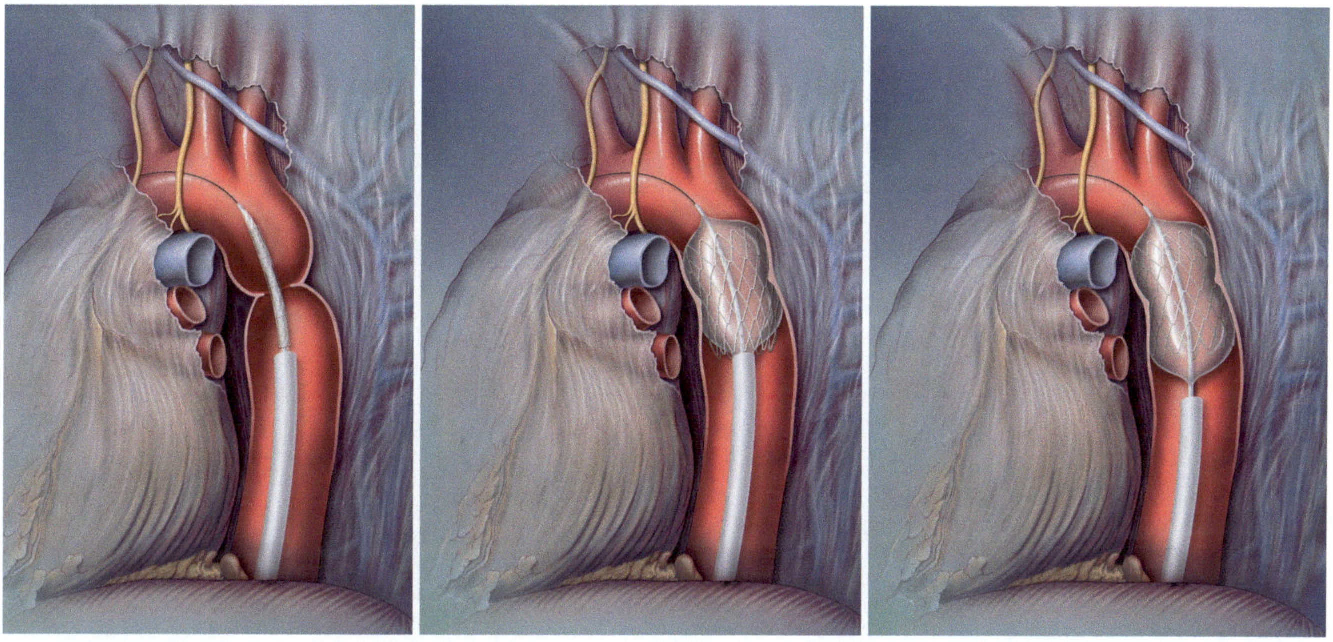

Fig. 42.4 The migration problem can be prevented by placing a sheath across the coarcted area. The sheath is withdrawn, allowing the proximal portion of the stent to deploy and anchor into the stenotic area. The sheath is slowly withdrawn as the balloon is progressively expanded

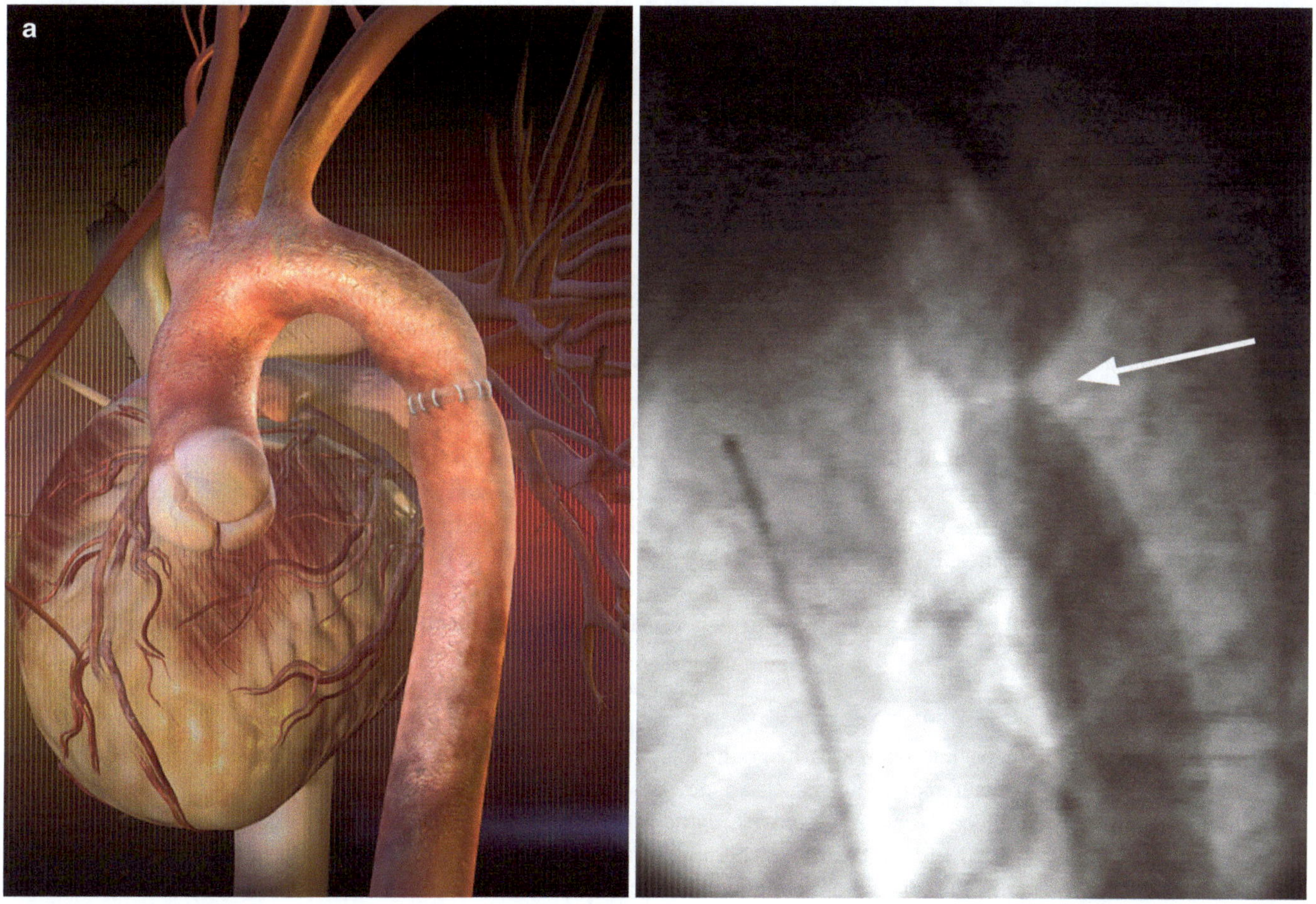

Fig. 42.5 (**a**) Illustration of recoarctation (*arrow*) in an adult previously treated as a child with end-to-end anastomosis. (**b**) Balloon angioplasty and stent deployment resulted in iatrogenic dissection with pseudoaneurysm formation (*arrow*). (**c**) Procedure further complicated by Palmaz stent migration times two. Endoluminal graft deployment closed the pseudoaneurysm and restored normal blood flow distally

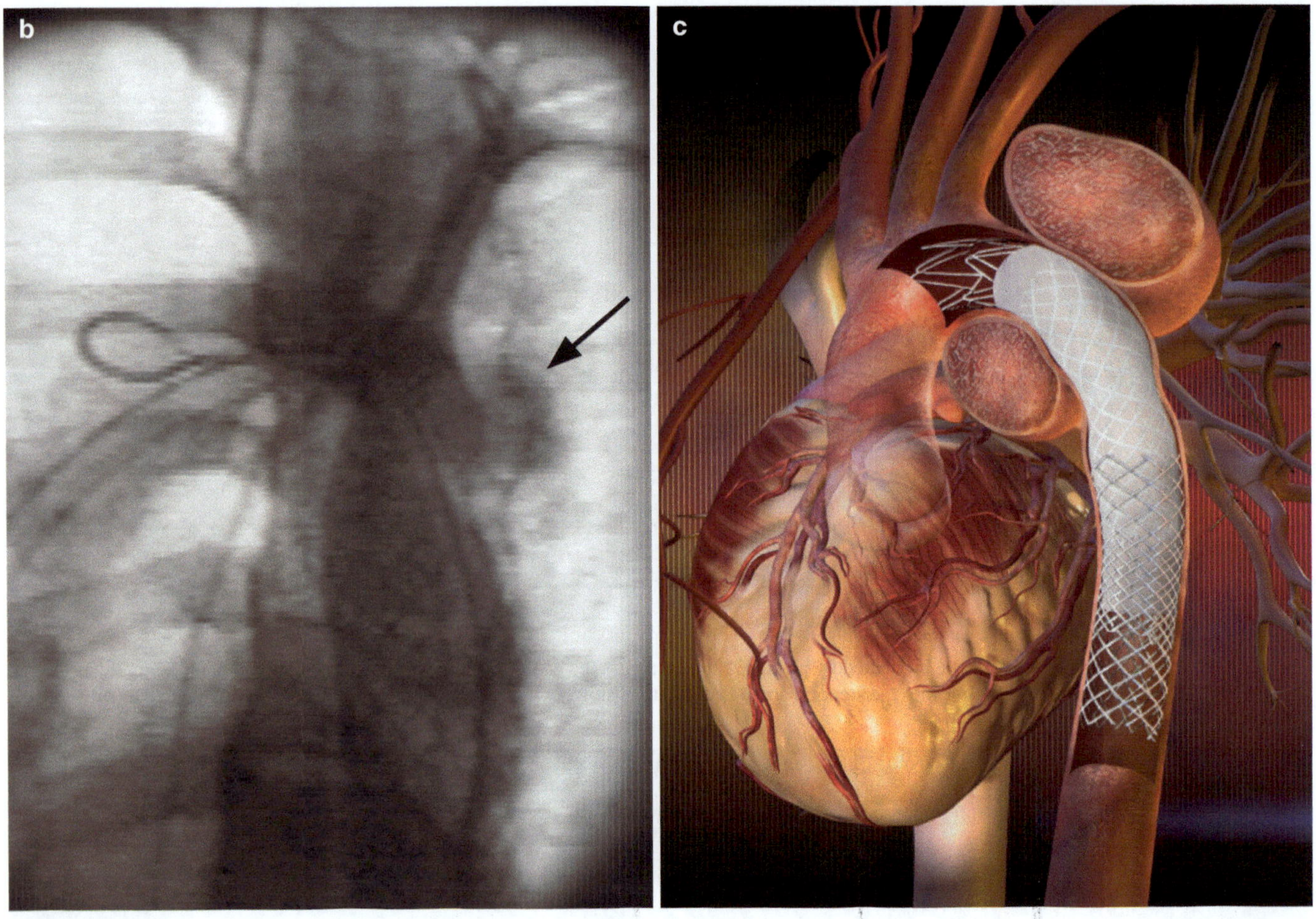

Fig. 42.5 (continued)

increased rigidity. The causes of late hypertension are not known, but decreased aortic compliance, abnormal baroreceptor function, and neuroendocrine activation may be involved. Coarctation may also result in large artery stiffness that reduces the aortic reserve and causes adverse left ventricular remodeling and functional disturbances. If a patient remains hypertensive and has a substantial residual gradient, repeated stent dilatation may be appropriate as the recurrence of hypertension contributes to progression of cerebrovascular disease, aortic rupture, and heart failure.

Procedural Success

Improvement in aortic diameter and decreases in gradients across the coarctation are measures of acute success, as are reductions in symptoms and need for antihypertensive therapy; such results can be achieved with endovascular therapy. In the intermediate term, we have seen anatomical and continued clinical improvements as well; however, recoarctation is a significant concern, and lifelong follow-up in all patients with a history of coarctation is imperative following repair. Our experience indicates both de novo and recurrent aortic coarctations as well as secondary aneurysmal disease can be safely and effectively treated using endovascular therapy; however, additional follow-up in these patients is needed to determine the durability of endovascular therapy. The advent of hybrid procedures has greatly expanded the ability to treat the complex conditions.

Toward the Future

As with any new technology or device, there is always the question of long-term durability. However, in the absence of randomized trial results, there is mounting evidence favoring stent deployment to treat coarctation with approaches that include covered stents. Endoluminal grafts are now an important component in the armamentarium of endovascular specialists. It can be anticipated that minimally invasive endovascular approaches will be considered the gold standard for treating coarctation and recoarctation in the future.

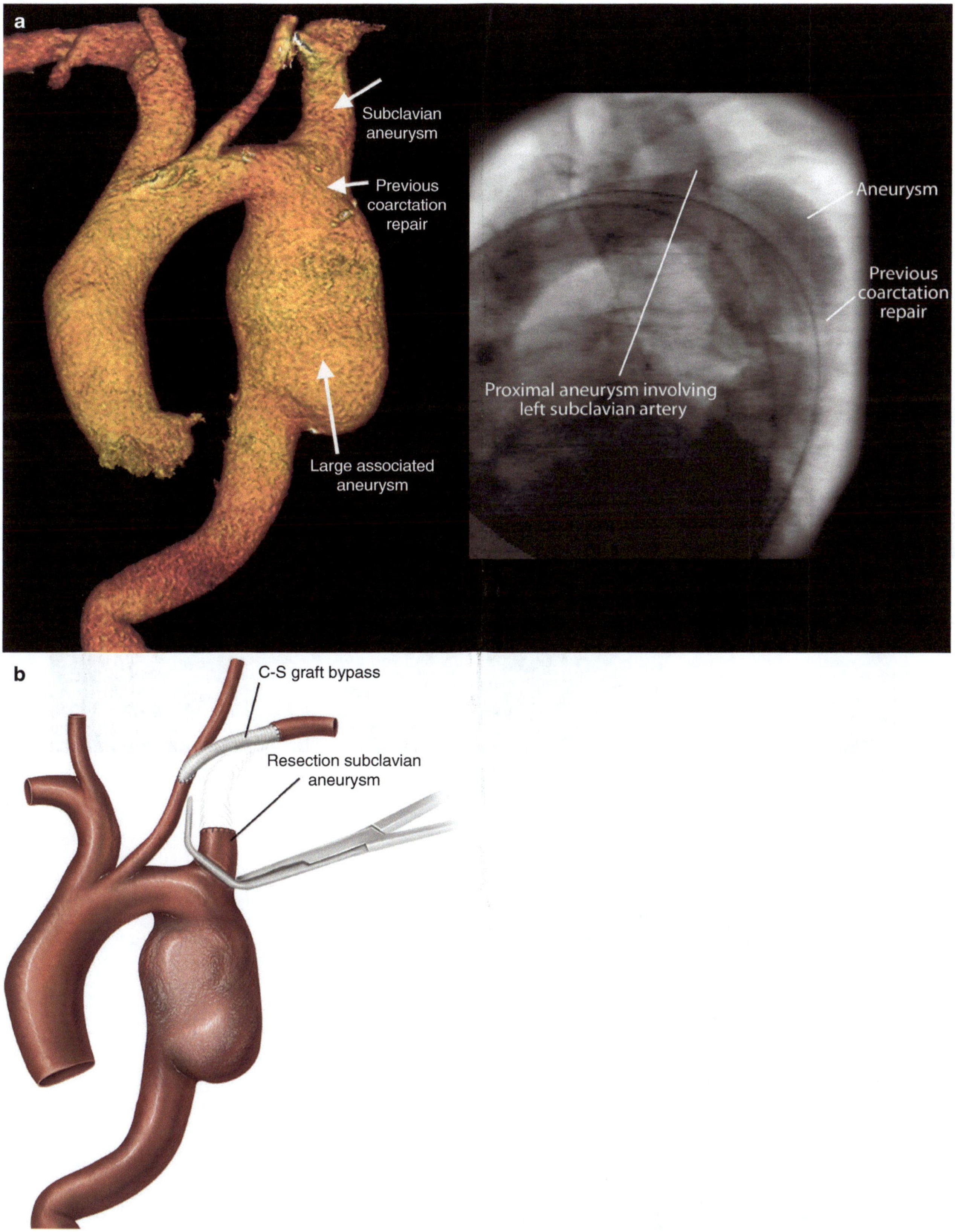

Fig. 42.6 (**a**) Angiogram and CT illustration of recurrent coarctation where a hybrid approach is used for correction. (**b**) Left supraclavicular approach is used to resect proximal subclavian aneurysm with suture closure. Carotid-subclavian bypass restores circulation to left vertebral and subclavian arteries. (**c**) Illustration depicting the hybrid technique to correct complicated recurrent coarctation with diffuse aneurysm formation. (**d**) Endoluminal graft across origin of left subclavian artery and distal to the coarctation isolates the aneurysmal disease. (**e**) A Gianturco Z stent with the barbs removed assure proper apposition of endoluminal graft preventing endoleak. (**f**) Palmaz stent is required to ensure relief of pressure gradient. (**g**) Control angiogram showing complete disease resolution and the effectiveness of the hybrid approach

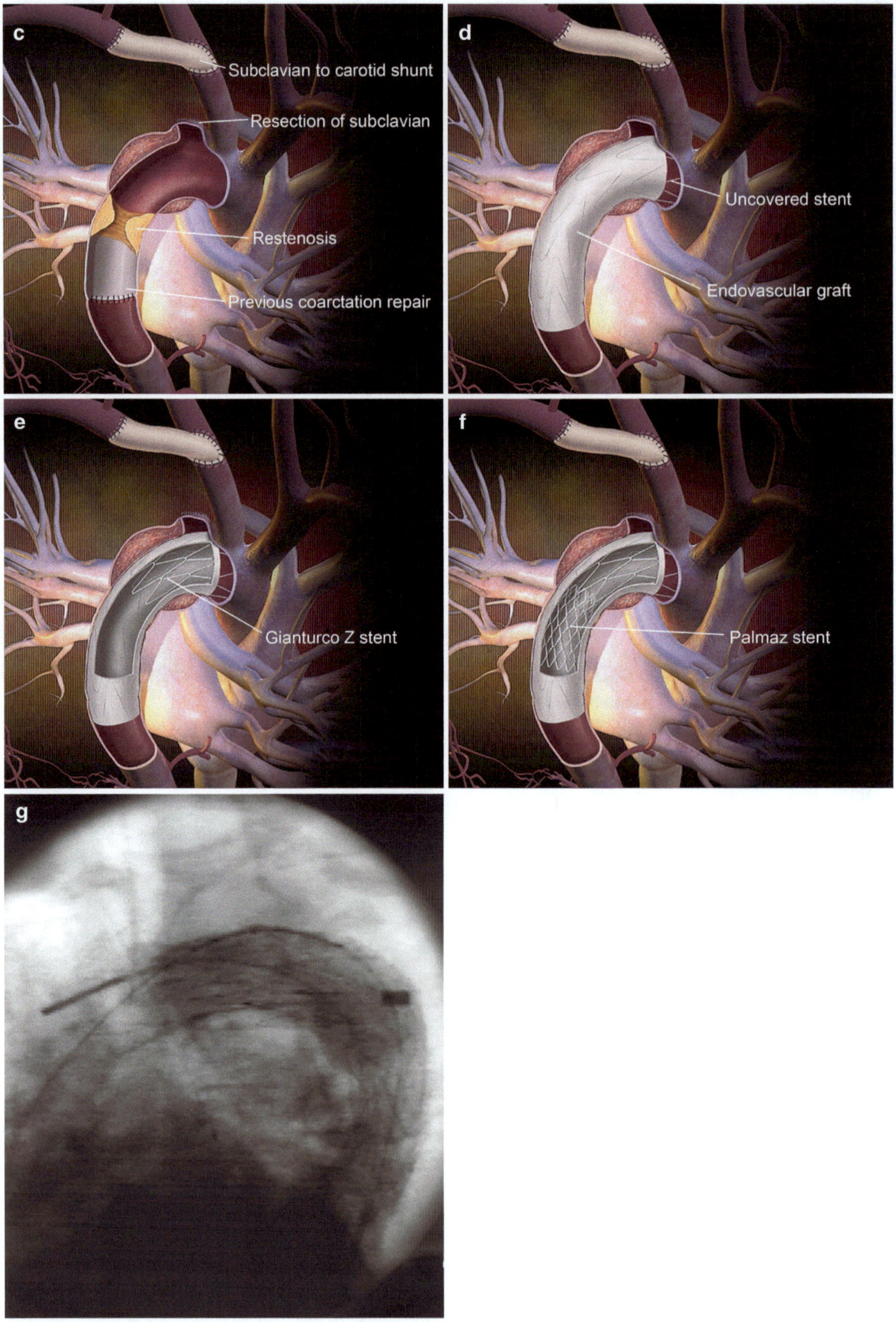

Fig. 42.6 (continued)

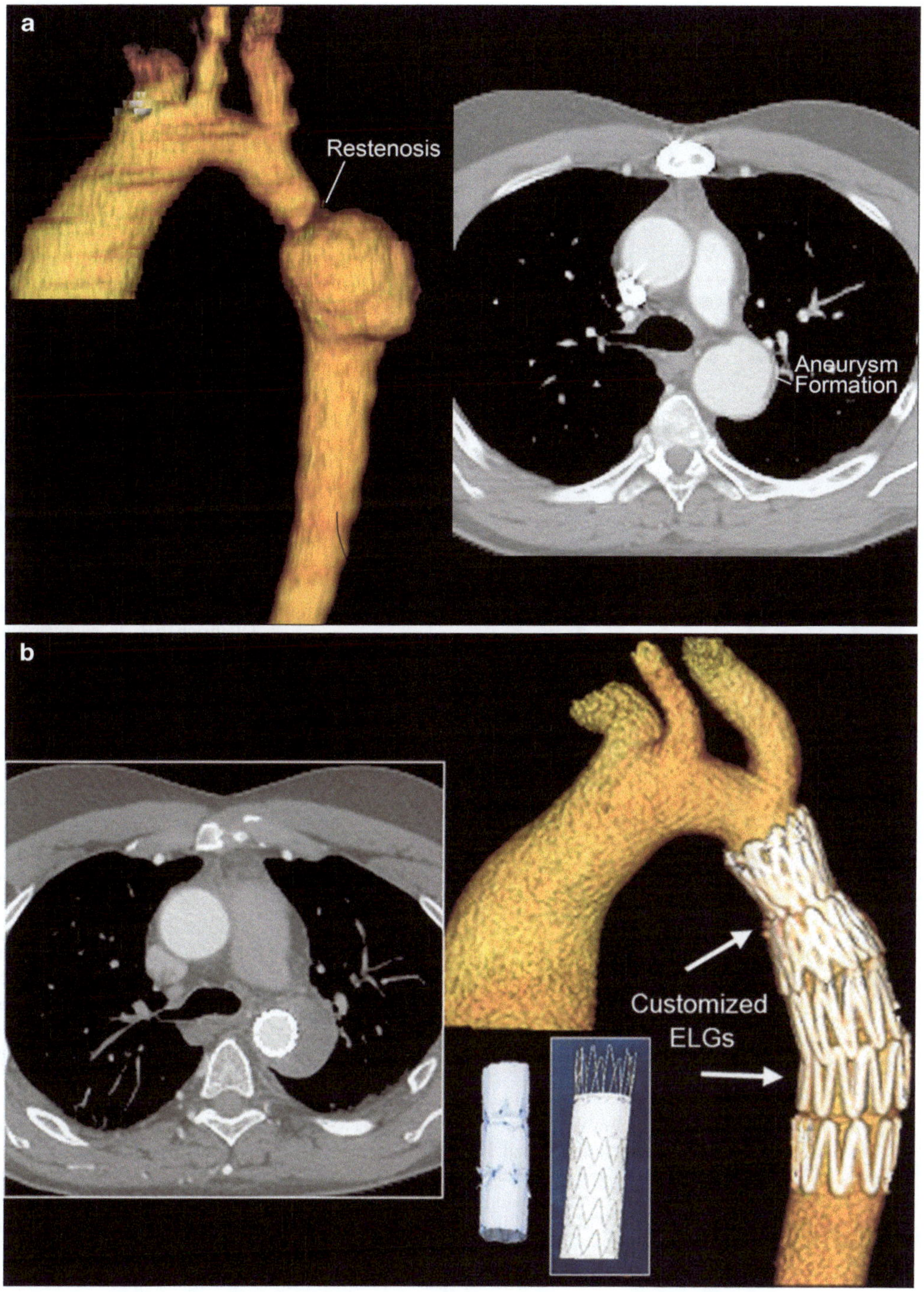

Fig. 42.7 (**a**) This image shows the size discrepancy between the aortic segments adjacent to the coarctation with a small proximal aorta and the marked dilation distally. (**b**) Until recently, the sizing problems required customization using various components of endoluminal grafts and covered stents

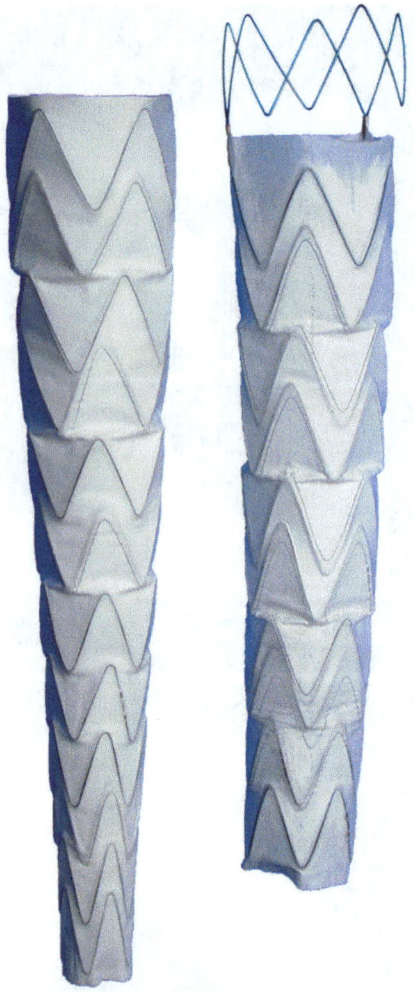

Fig. 42.8 Photograph of new endograft with tapering to accommodate the size discrepancies encountered in complex coarctation repair

References

1. Paris M. Rétrècissement considerable de l'aorte pectorale observé à l'Hotel Dieu de Paris. J Chir Desault. 1791;ii:107.
2. Abbott ME. Statistical study and historical retrospect of 200 recorded cases, with autopsy, of stenosis or obliteration of the descending arch in subjects above the age of two years. Am Heart J. 1928;3:392–421, 574–618.
3. Crafoord C, Nylin G. Congenital coarctation of the aorta and its surgical treatment. J Thorac Surg. 1945;14:347–61.
4. Toro-Salazar OH, Steinberger J, Thomas WI, et al. Long-term follow-up of patients after coarctation of the aorta repair. Am J Cardiol. 2002;89:541–7.
5. Pollack P, Freed MD, Castaneda AR, Norwood WI. Reoperation for isthmic coarctation of the aorta: follow-up of 26 patients. Am J Cardiol. 1983;51:1690–4.
6. Rao PS, Najjar HN, Mardini MK, Solymar L, Thapar MK. Balloon angioplasty for coarctation of the aorta: immediate and long term results. Am Heart J. 1988;15:657–64.
7. Fawzy ME, Dunn B, Galal O, et al. Balloon coarctation angioplasty in adolescents and adults: early and intermediate results. Am Heart J. 1992;24:167–71.
8. Maron BJ, Humphries JO, Rowe RD, Mellits ED. Prognosis of surgically corrected coarctation of the aorta. A 20-year postoperative appraisal. Circulation. 1973;47:119–26.
9. Singer MI, Rowen M, Dorsey TJ. Transluminal aortic balloon angioplasty for coarctation of the aorta in the newborn. Am Heart J. 1982;103(1):131–2.
10. Diethrich EB, Heuser RR, Cardenas JR, Eckert J, Tarlian H. Endovascular techniques in adult aortic coarctation: the use of stents for native and recurrent coarctation repair. J Endovasc Surg. 1995;2(2):183–8.
11. Wheatley 3rd GH, Koullias GJ, Rodriguez-Lopez JA, Ramaiah VG, Diethrich EB. Is endovascular repair the new gold standard for primary adult coarctation? Eur J Cardiothorac Surg. 2010;38(3):305–10.
12. Shennib H, Rodriguez-Lopez J, Ramaiah V, Wheatley G, Kpodonu J, Williams J, et al. Endovascular management of adult coarctation and its complications: intermediate results in a cohort of 22 patients. Eur J Cardiothorac Surg. 2010;37(2):322–7.
13. Kpodonu J, Ramaiah VG, Rodriguez-Lopez JA, Diethrich EB. Endovascular management of recurrent adult coarctation of the aorta. Ann Thorac Surg. 2010;90(5):1716–20.
14. Kpodonu J, Wheatley 3rd GH, Williams JP, Rodriguez-Lopez JA, Ramaiah VG, Diethrich EB. A novel approach for the endovascular repair of the small thoracic aorta: customizing off-the-shelf endoluminal grafts to treat a post-coarctation pseudoaneurysm. Ann Thorac Surg. 2008;85(3):1115–7.
15. Preventza O, Wheatley 3rd GH, Williams J, Hughes K, Ramaiah VG, Rodriguez-Lopez JA, et al. Endovascular approaches for complex forms of recurrent aortic coarctation. J Endovasc Ther. 2006;13(3):400–5.
16. Kische S, Schneider H, Akin I, Ortak J, Rehders TC, Chatterjee T, et al. Technique of interventional repair in adult aortic coarctation. J Vasc Surg. 2010;51(6):1550–9.
17. Erdem A, Akdeniz C, Saritas T, Erol N, Demir F, Karaci A, et al. Cheatham-platinum stent for native and recurrent aortic coarctation in children and adults: immediate and early follow-up results. Anadolu Kardiyol Derg. 2011;11(5):441–9.

Part XIII

Thoracoabdominal Aortic Aneurysm

Inflammatory Response in Open and Endovascular Treatment

43

Edmo Atique Gabriel and Sthefano Atique Gabriel

Patients presenting with aortic aneurysm basically tend to be candidates for two therapeutic approaches using either an open (conventional) or endovascular strategy. Over the last years, another surgical option has been developed, called the hybrid procedure because it encompasses open and endovascular features [1–4].

Regardless of the therapeutic strategy selected for each case, there is a resulting systemic inflammatory response mediated by many factors, such as as cytokines, cellular adhesion molecules, and interleukins. In this setting, it is relevant to remember that the massive presence of intraluminal thrombus is a strong determinant for an intense inflammatory response postoperatively with both therapeutic approaches. In case of endovascular treatment, this inflammatory response is called postimplantation syndrome [5–7].

The most striking difference, in terms of the surgical principle, is that the open approach requires the use of aortic clamping; thus, some complications resulting from ischemia-reperfusion injury are inevitable. Although ischemic injury is a time-dependent process, the resulting inflammatory response takes place even in short procedures. In the endovascular era, devices and technological resources have allowed surgeons to manipulate aortic aneurysm in a risk-free manner [8–10].

Walker et al. designed a very elegant study demonstrating operative complications of open and endovascular procedures that showed better patient outcomes using the endovascular approach (Table 43.1) [11].

The endovascular aortic approach is not free of complications, particularly inflammation. In an attempt to prove this, Gabriel et al. [12] developed clinical research whose main focus was to try to determine the magnitude, intensity, and correlations of the inflammatory response theoretically speculated for the setting of endovascular procedures. The main outcomes of this study are illustrated in Figs. 43.1, 43.2, 43.3, 43.4, 43.5, 43.6, and 43.7. Concerning these figures, we must bear in mind that there is something like an inflammatory response pattern following the deployment of aortic endoprostheses. This pattern is represented by a profile of inflammatory markers as well as "inflammatory time courses" for each marker [12].

To meticulously address the issue of the inflammatory response in the endovascular treatment of aortic aneurysms, Gabriel et al. [13] used data obtained from their previous clinical research to propose the first model of an inflammatory risk score for the endovascular approach. These authors employed classic methodology based on a step-by-step technique, Spearman's test, and logistic regression and ROC curve analysis in order to determine the final variables and their possible cutoff values (Fig. 43.8 and Tables 43.2, 43.3, 43.4, and 43.5). It is important to emphasize that this is a "developing" inflammatory risk score by Gabriel et al. [13], who were trying to meet a need, but the scoring method still needs to be investigated additionaly by new trials.In summary, this risk score model is not definitive and should not be considered as such.

E.A. Gabriel, MD, PhD (✉)
Department of Cardiovascular Surgery, University Nove de Julho, São Paulo, Brazil
e-mail: edag@uol.com.br

S.A. Gabriel, MD
Department of Vascular Surgery, Pontifical Catholic University of Campinas, São Paulo, Brazil

Department of Vascular Surgery, Celso Pierro Hospital and Maternity, Campinas, São Paulo, Brazil
e-mail: sthefanogabriel@yahoo.com.br

E.A. Gabriel, S.A. Gabriel (eds.), *Inflammatory Response in Cardiovascular Surgery*, DOI 10.1007/978-1-4471-4429-8_43, © Springer-Verlag London 2013

Table 43.1 Complications from meta-analysis of 2006 and 2007 national inpatient sample cohorts at only those institutions performing both TEVAR and open repair

	2006					2007				
Variable	Open repair (%)	TEVAR	RR	95 % CI	*p* value	Open repair (%)	TEVAR (%)	RR	95 % CI	*p* value
In-hospital mortality	9.79	1.16 %	8.48	(3.03–23.75)	<0.01	1.35	1.91	0.71	(0.12–4.24)	0.7
Cardiac complications	7.13	1.22 %	5.5	(1.34–25.48)	0.02	10.85	2.02	5.36	(1.82–15.81)	<0.01
Transfusion	32.52	15.77	2.06	(1.22–3.48)	<0.01	29.36	20.68	1.42	(0.77–2.63)	0.26
Hematoma	0	2.91	0	–	–	1.35	3.85	0.35	(0.07–2.63)	0.22
Hemorrhage	7.13	3.45	2.07	(0.41–10.46)	0.38	5.28	1.69	3.12	(0.43–22.71)	0.26
Respiratory complications	23.37	8.29 %	2.82	(1.27–6.25)	0.01	16.01	6.92	2.31	(0.96–5.56)	0.06
Prolonged ventilation	13.41	1.98 %	6.78	(1.51–30.51)	0.01	10.70	2.32	4.61	(0.99–21.46)	0.05
Tracheostomy	0.00	0	–	–	–	7.51	1.91	3.92	(0.79–19.53)	0.09
Acute renal failure	8.35	3.52	2.37	(0.75–7.46)	0.14	6.53	5.16	1.26	(0.29–5.44)	0.75
Postop stroke/TIA	3.66	2.66 %	1.38	(0.31–6.14)	0.67	0.30	2.05	0.14	(0.02–1.36)	0.09
PVC	2.44	4.61 %	0.53	(0.07–4.28)	0.55	0.25	1.78	0.14	(0.01–1.29)	0.08
Sepsis	0.00	0.00 %	–	–	–	0.00	0.34	0	–	–
Graft problem	2.85	4.76 %	0.60	(0.09– 4.01)	0.60	4.05	6.96	0.61	(0.12–3.17)	0.55

CI 95 % confidence interval, *PVC* peripheral vascular complication, *RR* estimated relative risk, *TEVAR* thoracic endovascular aortic repair, *TIA* transient ischemic attack

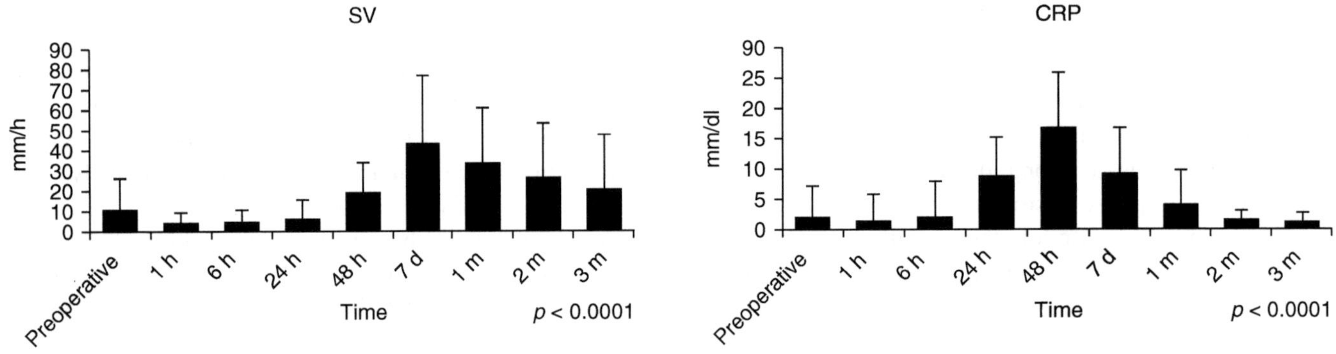

Fig. 43.1 Values of SV and CRP in a period of 3 months

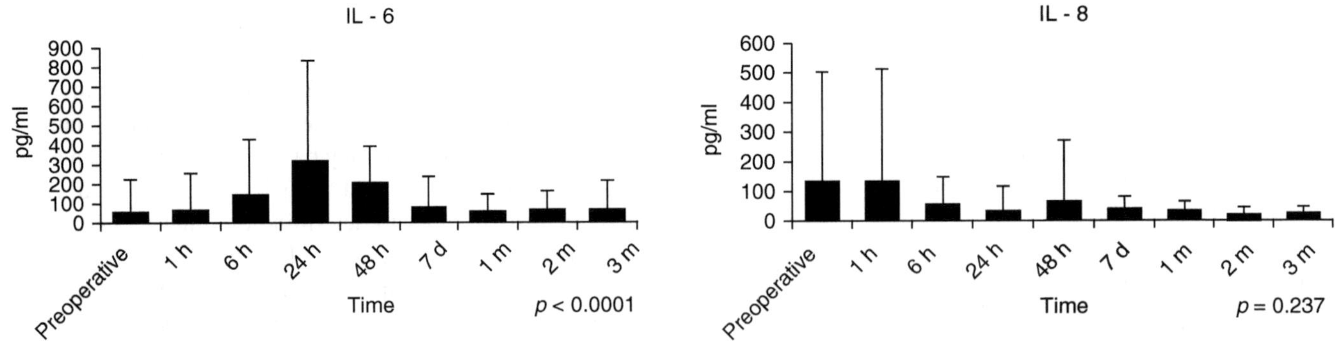

Fig. 43.2 Values of IL-6 and IL-8 in a period of 3 months

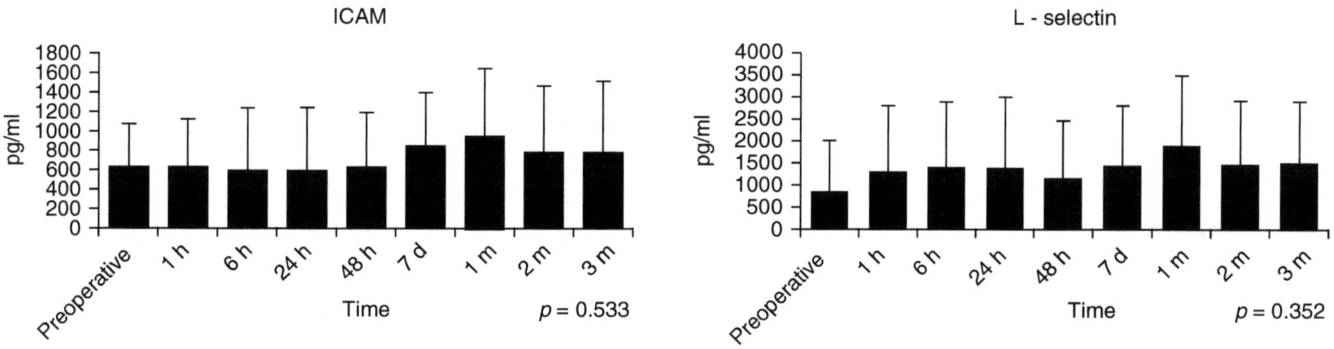

Fig. 43.3 Values of ICAM-1 and L-selectin in a period of 3 months

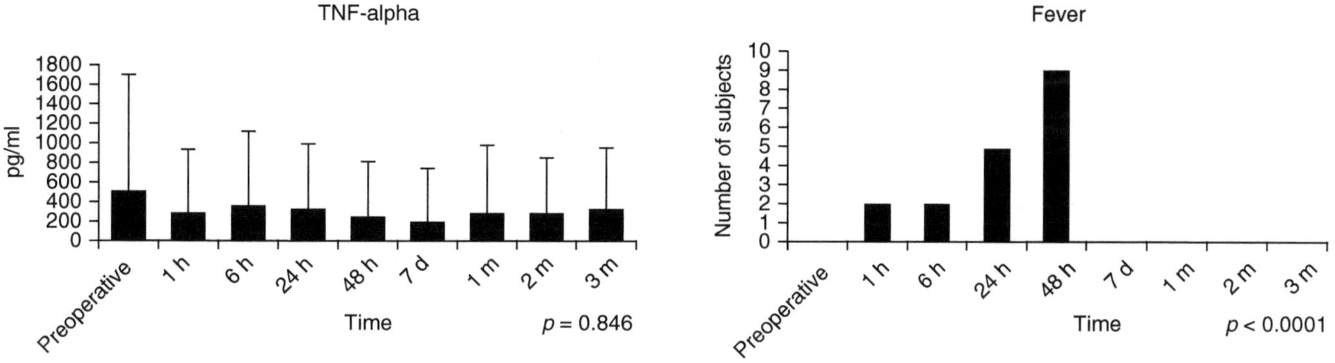

Fig. 43.4 Values of TNF-alpha and frequency of fever episodes in a period of 3 months

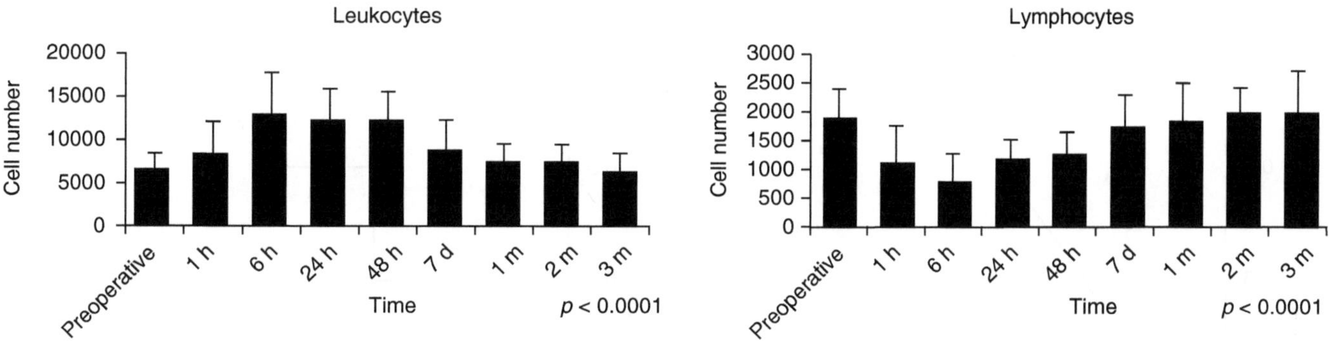

Fig. 43.5 Values of leukocytes and lymphocytes in a period of 3 months

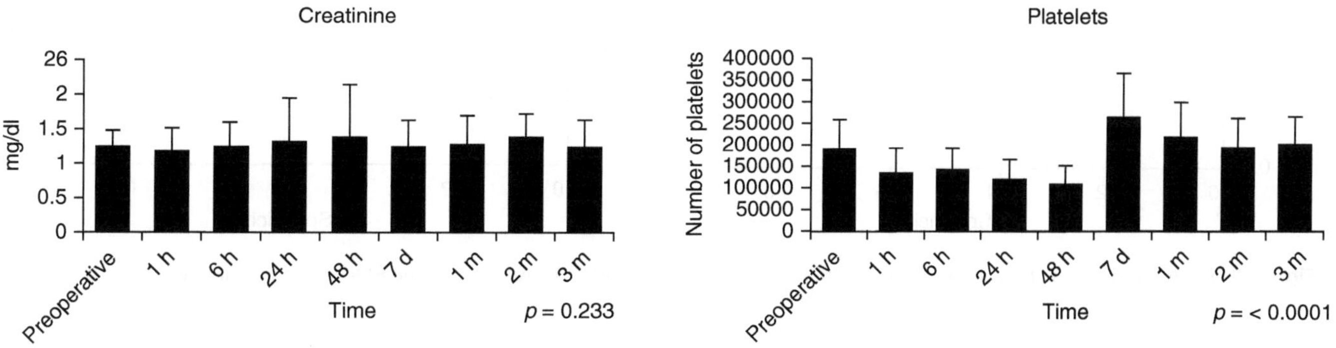

Fig. 43.6 Values of creatinine and platelets in a period of 3 months

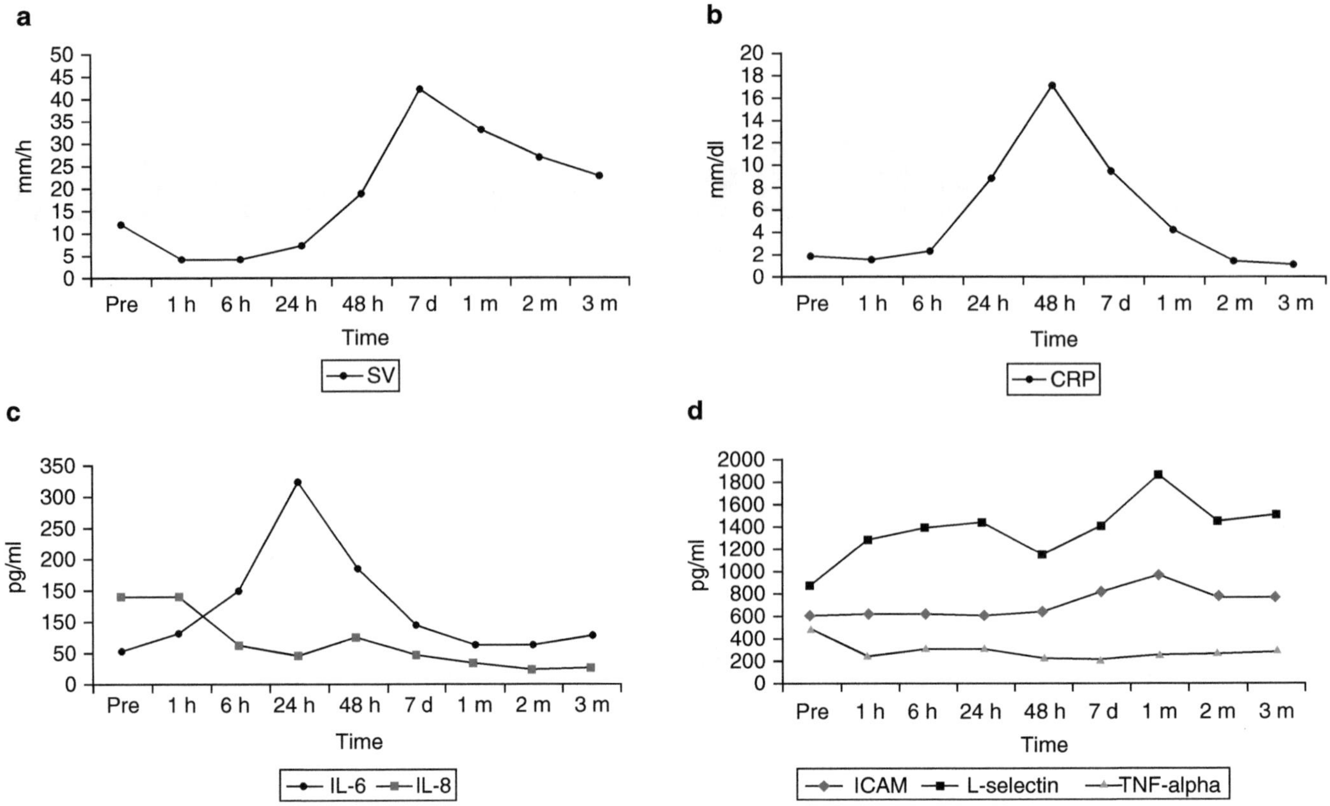

Fig. 43.7 (**a–d**) Inflammatory response curves. (**a**) SV. (**b**) CRP. (**c**) IL-6, IL-8. (**d**) ICAM-1, L-selectin, TNF-alpha

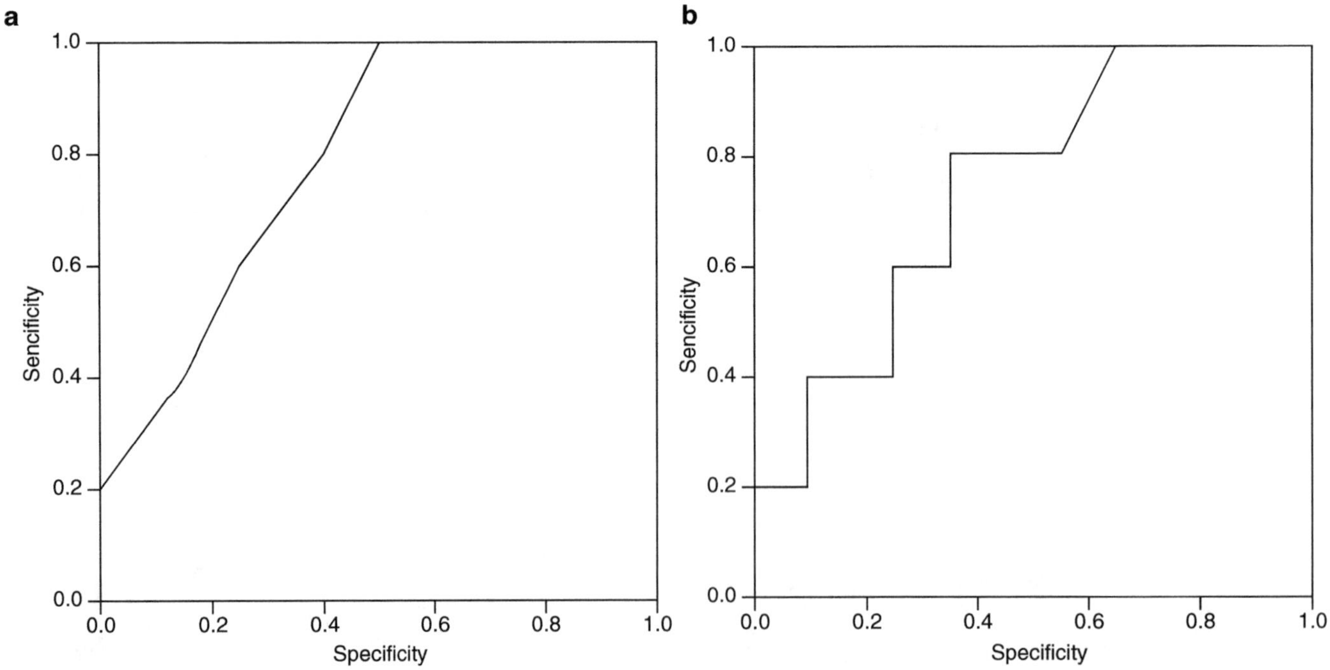

Fig. 43.8 (**a**) Analysis of the ROC curve for the volume of crystalloid solution; (**b**) Analysis of the ROC curve for the pre-operative values of IL-8

Table 43.2 Inflammatory variables and period of greatest prevalence

Variable	Time
Total neutrophil count	24 h
Total lymphocyte count	1 month
Volume of crystalloid solution – ml	[a]
Volume of contrast material – ml	[a]
Transfusion of red blood cells	[a]
Presence of intraluminal thrombi	[b]
Material of endoprosthesis	[b]
Number of endoprostheses	[a]
Velocity of blood sedimentation – mm/h	7 days
C-reactive protein (CRP) – mm/dl	48 h
Interleukin 6 (IL-6) – pg/ml	24 h
Interleukin 8 (IL-8) – pg/ml	Preoperative
Tumoral necrosis factor alpha (TNF-α)-pg/ml	Preoperative
Intercellular adhesion molecule (ICAM-1)-pg/ml	1 month
L-selectin – pg/ml	1 month

[a]Parametric variables related to the intraoperative period
[b]Non-parametric variables

Table 43.3 Candidate variables for the risk score model

Variable	Level of significance (*P*)[a]
Volume of crystalloid solution	0.04
Material of endoprosthesis	0.04
Volume of contrast	0.02
Preoperative IL-8	0.10
ICAM-1 1 month	0.03
L-selectin 1 month	0.06

ICAM intercellular adhesion molecule
[a]Spearman test, $P \leq 20$ %

Table 43.4 Numeric intervals and risk categories

Volume of crystalloid solution (ml)	IL-8 pre (pg/ml)	Risk	Probability (%)
Up to 1,850	Up to 33.53	Mild	Up to 70
1,850–3,250	33.54–53.37	Moderate	71–82
>3,250	>53.37	Severe	>82
3,500	38.7	Severe	86.59[a]

[a]Maximum probability of risk

Table 43.5 Inflammatory risk score

Volume of crystalloid solution (ml)	IL-8 pre (pg/ml)	Risk	Clinical manifestations
Up to 1,850	Up to 33.53	Mild	Fever/leukocytosis
1,850–3,250	33.54–53.37	Moderate	Fever/leukocytosis/ hypotension
>3,250	>53.37	Severe	SIRS/sepsis

SIRS systemic inflammatory response syndrome

References

1. Adams JD, Angle JF, Matsumoto AH, Peeler BB, Arslan B, Cherry KJ, et al. Endovascular repair of the thoracic aorta in the post-FDA approval era. J Thorac Cardiovasc Surg. 2009;137:117–23.
2. Gopaldas RR, Dao TK, LeMaire SA, Huh J, Coselli JS. Endovascular versus open repair of ruptured descending thoracic aortic aneurysms: a nationwide risk-adjusted study of 923 patients. J Thorac Cardiovasc Surg. 2011;142:1010–8.
3. Ferrero E, Ferri M, Viazzo A, Robaldo A, Zingarelli E, Sansone F, et al. Is total debranching a safe procedure for extensive aortic-arch disease? A single experience of 27 cases. Eur J Cardiothorac Surg. 2012;41(1):177–82.
4. Hughes GC, Lee SM, Daneshmand MA, Bhattacharya SD, Williams JB, Tucker Jr SW, et al. Endovascular repair of descending thoracic aneurysms: results with "on-label" application in the post food and drug administration approval era. Ann Thorac Surg. 2010;90: 83–9.
5. Patel HJ, Nguyen C, Diener AC, Passow MC, Salata D, Deeb GM. Open arch reconstruction in the endovascular era: analysis of 721 patients over 17 years. J Thorac Cardiovasc Surg. 2011;141(6): 1417–23.
6. Preventza O, Bavaria J, Ramaiah V, Moser GW, Szeto W, Wheatley III G, et al. Thoracic endografting is a viable option for the octogenarian. Ann Thorac Surg. 2010;90(1):78–82.
7. Cheng D, Martin J, Shennib H, Dunning J, Muneretto C, Schueler C, et al. Endovascular aortic repair versus open surgical repair for descending thoracic aortic disease: a systematic review and meta-analysis of comparative studies. J Am Coll Cardiol. 2010;55(10): 986–1001.
8. Goodney PP, Travis L, Lucas FL, Fillinger MF, Goodman DC, Cronenwett JL, et al. Survival after open versus endovascular thoracic aortic aneurysm repair in an observational study of the Medicare population. Circulation. 2011;124(24):2661–9.
9. Matsagkas MI, Kirou IE, Kouvelos G, Arnaoutoglou EM, Papakostas JC, Katsouras C, et al. Stenting of the descending thoracic aorta: a six-year single center experience. Interact Cardiovasc Thorac Surg. 2011;12(5):789–93.
10. Coselli JS, Gopaldas RR. Ruptured thoracic aneurysms: to stent or not to stent? Circulation. 2010;121(25):2705–7.
11. Walker KL, Shuster JJ, Martin TD, Hess Jr PJ, Klodell CT, Feezor RJ, et al. Practice patterns for thoracic aneurysms in the stent graft era: health care system implications. Ann Thorac Surg. 2010;90:1833–9.
12. Gabriel EA, Locali RF, Romano CC, Duarte AJS, Palma JH, Buffolo E. Analysis of the inflammatory response in endovascular treatment of aortic aneurysms. Eur J Cardiothorac Surg. 2007;31:406–13.
13. Gabriel EA, Locali RF, Matsuoka PK, Romano CC, Duarte AJS, Buffolo E. First inflammatory risk score for aortic endoprostheses. Rev Bras Cir Cardiovasc. 2008;23(4):512–8.

Surgical Treatment of Aortic Aneurysm in Patients with Aortitis

44

Maqsood M. Elahi and Kenton J. Zehr

Introduction

The most common causes of aortitis are the large-vessel vasculitides [giant cell arteritis (GCA) and Takayasu arteritis], although aortitis also is associated with systemic lupus erythematosus, rheumatoid arthritis, the HLA-B27-associated spondyloarthropathies, anti-neutrophil cytoplasmic antibody-associated vasculitides, Behçet's disease, Cogan syndrome, and sarcoidosis. Infectious causes include tuberculosis, syphilis, salmonella, and other bacteria. Acute presentation includes aneurysm rupture, Stanford type A dissection with severe aortic regurgitation, stroke, and myocardial infarction [1, 2]. Isolated aortitis (IA) is a newly recognized condition (i.e., no associated rheumatologic or infectious disease is present), but its differentiation from Takayasu arteritis (TA) is still a challenge.

Most cases of aortitis are non-infectious; however, the possibility of an infectious nature exists, and the treatment regimens widely diverge. In bacterial aortitis, a segment of the aortic wall with preexisting pathology, such as an atherosclerotic plaque or aneurysm sac, is seeded by bacteria via the vasa vasorum [3]. Similarly, tuberculous aortitis, a common problem in the developing world, may occur as a result of direct seeding of the thoracic aorta from adjacent infected tissues such as infected lymph nodes or lung lesions or by miliary spread [4].

M.M. Elahi, MD, PhD
Department of Cardiothoracic Surgery, Glenfield Hospital, Groby Road, Leicester LE3 9QP, UK

K.J. Zehr, MD (✉)
Division of Cardiothoracic Surgery and Center for Aortic Disease, Scott & White Clinic, Texas A & M Health Sciences Center College of Medicine, 2401 S. 31st Street, Temple, TX 76508, USA

Given this, the most common causes of noninfectious aortitis are the large-vessel vasculitides GCA and Takayasu arteritis. Although the epidemiological and clinical features of these two disorders are distinct (see Clinical Presentation), there may be significant overlap in histopathological findings (Fig. 44.1). Both GCA and Takayasu arteritis are associated with an inflammatory cellular infiltrate of the aortic media, adventitia, and vasa vasorum that contains a predominance of lymphocytes, macrophages, and multinucleated giant cells [4, 6]. Over time, scarring of the aortic media and destruction of the elastic lamina occur [6].

A few pathological features can be used to distinguish Takayasu arteritis and GCA. Takayasu arteritis is more commonly associated with extensive intimal and adventitial fibrosis or scarring with resultant luminal narrowing, whereas GCA is more commonly associated with extensive medial inflammation and necrosis and the formation of aortic aneurysms [5, 7]. GCA also is characterized by focal arterial inflammation, and "skip lesions" are common, a finding that can lead to false-negative findings on temporal artery biopsy in patients with associated temporal artery aortitis.

The pathogenesis of both GCA and Takayasu arteritis is unknown. Both are thought to be antigen-driven cell-mediated autoimmune processes, although the specific antigenic stimuli have not been identified [6]. Both GCA and Takayasu arteritis have been associated with specific HLA-linked antigens and a resultant genetic predisposition. In a significant percentage of cases, the diagnosis of aortitis is an incidental histopathological finding because no rheumatologic disorder, infection, or symptoms are attributable directly to the aortitis [7, 8]. Such cases of idiopathic isolated aortitis typically are localized to the ascending thoracic aorta and occur in association with ascending aortic aneurysm. Patchy necrosis of the aortic media is the primary histological finding, along with an inflammatory cellular infiltrate, which may include multinucleated giant cells (Fig. 44.2).

E.A. Gabriel, S.A. Gabriel (eds.), *Inflammatory Response in Cardiovascular Surgery*,
DOI 10.1007/978-1-4471-4429-8_44, © Springer-Verlag London 2013

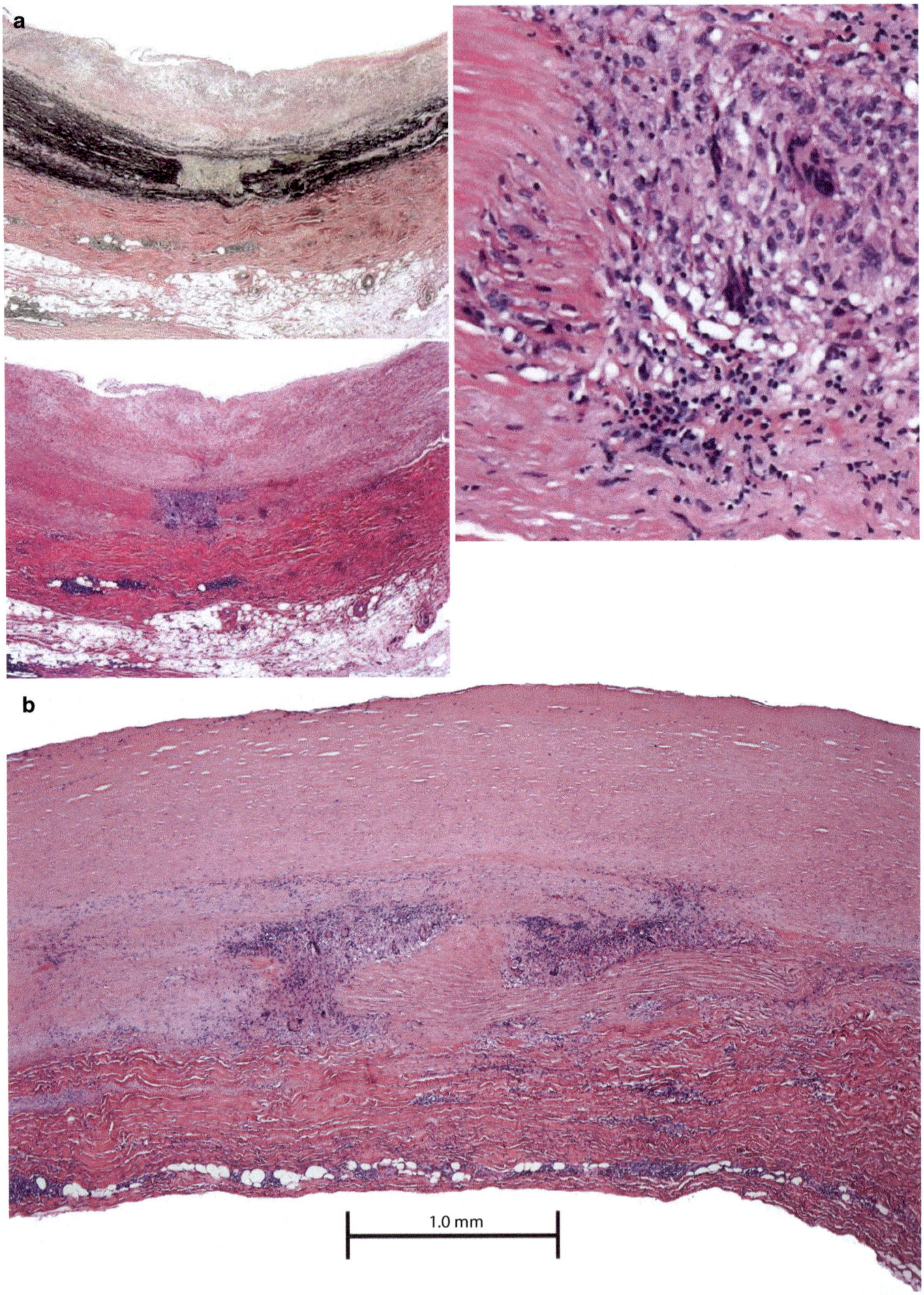

Fig. 44.1 (**a**) Giant cell aortitis shows more active aortitis with similar (but less advanced) medial damage and a punched out area seen in the elastic stain (*top left*). This area corresponds to an area of inflammation (*blue cells*) in the H&E slide (*bottom left*). The *right side* image shows what type of inflammation this is (lymphocytes, macrophages multinucleated giant cells). (**b**) Takayasu arteritis. The pathogenesis of this disease is not well understood. It's generally thought to be autoimmune, but the antigen is unknown. The accepted theory is that the small vasa vasorum that supplies the medial smooth muscle cells (thought to be the caretakers for the elastic scaffolding) are damaged by autoantibodies or self-attacking T cells leading to ischemia in the media and death of the smooth muscle cells. The giant cell inflammation comes in to clean it up, and then collagen scar tissue replaces the elastic tissue in the media causing dilatation and wall thinning. The mechanism is described by Weyand et al. [5]

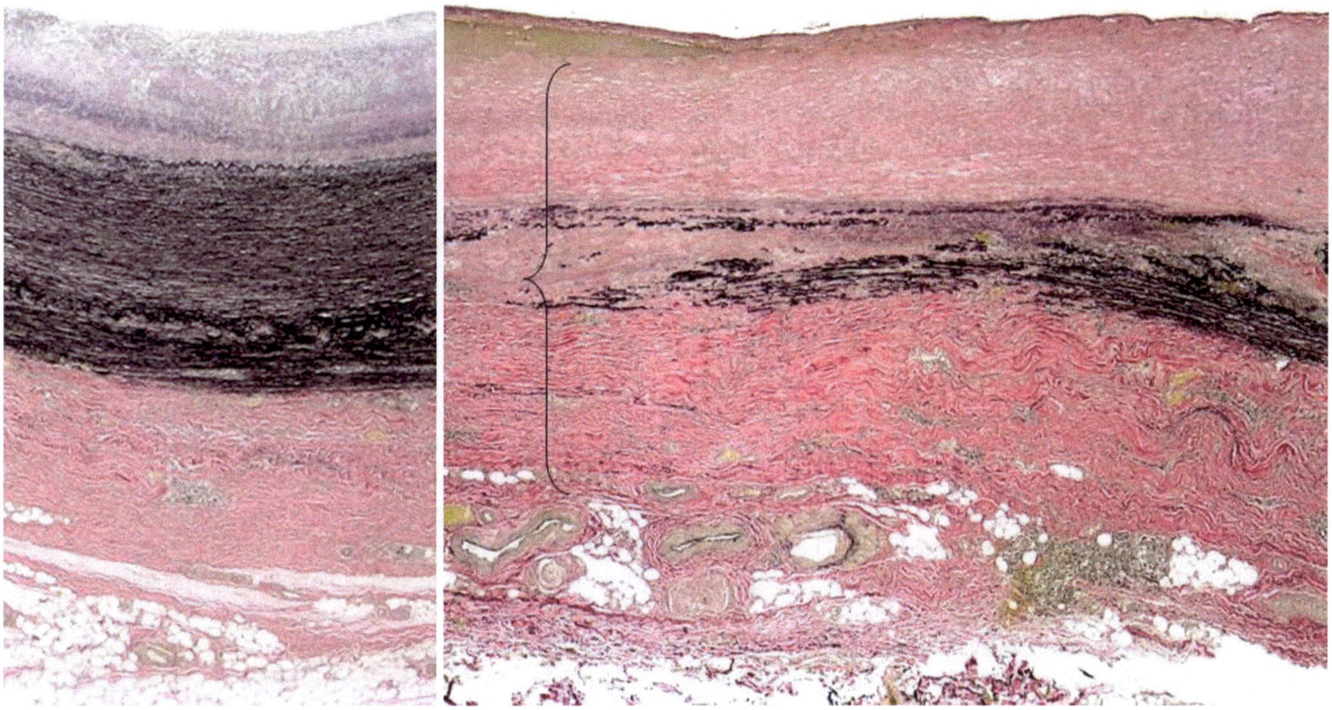

Fig. 44.2 The *left hand side* is taken from the better-preserved or more normal part of the specimen showing the medial layer with a relatively intact elastic scaffolding

Epidemiology

Arteritis was first described clinically in 1890 by Hutchinson [9] and histologically by Horton and associates in 1932 [10] after biopsy of a patient presenting with a swollen, painful temporal artery. The general population prevalence has been reported to be 1 % in a large autopsy series [11], whereas an average annual incidence of 17/100,000 person-years in the local population has been described [12, 13]. Although comparable data on the incidence of aortitis in Western populations or adults are not available, the epidemiology of the large-vessel vasculitides GCA and Takayasu arteritis, the most common causes of aortitis, has been studied in some depth.

Reports have suggested that in the Olmsted County, Minnesota, population, the average age- and sex-adjusted incidence of GCA among individuals ≥50 years during a 50-year period was 18.8 per 100,000 per year [14]. The overall incidence of GCA increased substantially during the 50-year follow-up period of the study, perhaps because of advances in diagnostic modalities. In this cohort, the incidence of GCA was > twofold higher among women than men (24.4 versus 10.3 per 100,000 per year, respectively), and the mean age at the time of diagnosis was 75 years [14]. Few published data are available on the epidemiology of GCA in non-Western countries, although one Japanese study reported a very low prevalence of 1.5 per 100,000 individuals ≥50 years of age [15].

The epidemiology of Takayasu arteritis is not as well characterized as that of GCA. Data from Olmstead County, Minnesota, based on a very small number of cases, estimated an incidence of 2.6 per 1 million residents per year, which is higher than that reported in any other epidemiological series [16]. Although originally described by the Japanese ophthalmologist Dr. Mikoto Takayasu, no data support an increased incidence of this disorder in Japan [17]. In a Cleveland Clinic case series of 1,204 consecutive pathological specimens taken from patients who underwent aortic surgery over 20 years, the prevalence of aortitis on surgical pathology specimens was 4.3 % [8]. Most of the surgeries were performed for aortic aneurysmal disease. In nearly 70 % of patients with evidence of aortitis, no underlying systemic disease was found, and vascular inflammation was a truly incidental finding in most of these cases of isolated idiopathic aortitis [8].

Clinical Presentation

Clinically, presentation of aortitis varies from back or abdominal pain with fever to acute severe aortic insufficiency and to an incidentally identified large thoracic aortic aneurysm. Acute aortic syndromes, including aortic dissection and rupture, can occur in persons with aortitis [18]. Inflammation-associated thrombus formation in the aortic lumen with peripheral embolization also has been reported [19]. The location of aortic inflammation (e.g., ascending thoracic versus abdominal aorta) and the presence of coexisting arteritis in other blood vessels also determine the clinical presentation. Because of the varied presentations of aortitis and the often nonspecific nature of its symptoms and signs, the index of suspicion of the evaluating clinician must be high to establish an accurate diagnosis in a timely fashion. GCA clinically presents as headache, temporal artery abnormalities on physical examination, and elevated markers of inflammation in an older adult. Common manifestations of GCA include polymyalgia rheumatica, scalp tenderness, jaw claudication (resulting from involvement of the branches of the external carotid artery), visual field changes (caused by involvement of the ophthalmic, posterior ciliary, or retinal arteries), and mononeuropathy or polyneuropathy [20]. Coronary GCA, manifest as tapering lesions in the coronary arteries and myocardial infarction, also has been reported [21]. The frequency of aortic involvement in GCA is not known. It is suggested that all patients with temporal GCA who present with symptoms suggestive of extracranial vascular involvement undergo an imaging study to evaluate the aorta and large vessels [20]. An association has been found between a history of GCA and the development of aortic aneurysm, particularly thoracic aortic aneurysm, as a manifestation of extracranial involvement [18]. In the Olmsted County cohort, it is reported that 18 % of patients with GCA and aortic aneurysm were diagnosed with thoracic aortic aneurysm at the time of diagnosis in this population, and most developed aneurysm during follow-up a median of 5.8 years after the initial diagnosis. More than half of the patients with GCA-associated thoracic aneurysm died of acute aortic dissection. In this cohort, GCA also was associated with a >twofold increased (relative risk, 2.4) risk of developing abdominal aortic aneurysm a median of 2.5 years after initial presentation with GCA [13].

Risk factors for the development of aortic and large-vessel complications in GCA have been identified, including the presence of a murmur of aortic insufficiency at diagnosis, concomitant hyperlipidemia, and coronary artery disease [18]. Presentation with classic cranial symptoms and signs of temporal arteritis (i.e., headache, scalp tenderness, abnormal temporal artery pulsations, elevated erythrocyte sedimentation rate) was a negative predictor of an aortic complication [18]. Evidence of GCA also has been identified on histopathological specimens of patients undergoing thoracic aortic aneurysm repair, including those not known to have aortic involvement [7].

In contrast to GCA, Takayasu arteritis is observed to be a much rarer disorder with a predilection for young women. The average age at diagnosis is 25–30 years, and anywhere from 75 to 97 % of patients are female [22, 23]. The most common presentation of Takayasu arteritis includes symptoms resulting from arterial occlusive disease of the aorta, aortic arch, and large vessels. Other common names for Takayasu arteritis, including pulseless disease and aortic arch syndrome, reflect its clinical presentation. Nearly all patients with Takayasu arteritis either present initially or ultimately develop large-vessel manifestations of the disease, including hypertension caused by suprarenal aortic or renal artery occlusive disease, pulse deficits and/or vascular bruits, and upper- and/or lower-extremity claudication [22]. A comprehensive vascular examination, including measurement of blood pressure in both arms and palpitation and auscultation of pulses in all major vascular regions, is a critical component of the clinical evaluation of all patients with suspected Takayasu arteritis. In addition, we recommend measuring blood pressure in all four extremities for such patients. Aortic involvement in Takayasu arteritis is very common, with angiographic abnormalities demonstrated on aortography in nearly all patients [22, 23]. The abdominal aorta is the most common site of involvement, followed by the descending thoracic aorta and aortic arch [22, 23]. At the time of aortography, stenotic lesions in the aorta are most frequently detected, although aortic aneurysm also is common and has been reported in up to 45 % of patients in published case series [22, 23]. Case series also have reported rapid aortic aneurysm expansion, aortic rupture, and the development of aortic aneurysm at the site of anastomoses of prior reconstructive surgery among patients with Takayasu arteritis [24, 25]. Nearly 40 % of patients with Takayasu arteritis develop cardiac abnormalities, including acute myocardial infarction, angina pectoris, and acute aortic insufficiency. In these cases, the cardiac pathology is related directly to the aortic inflammation, including aortic insufficiency as a result of aortic root dilatation and coronary ostial stenoses resulting from aortitis (Fig. 44.3).

Diagnostic Testing

When the diagnosis of aortitis is suspected on the basis of clinical presentation, expedient imaging of the entire aorta with an appropriate modality is critical to establish the diagnosis. Modern imaging tools for the aorta include CTA, MRA, and ultrasonography. CTA and MRA have the advantage of imaging the components of the aortic wall and periaortic structures rather than the lumen only, as is the case of conventional angiography. Invasive aortography generally is reserved for cases in which diagnosis of an acute aortic syndrome is uncertain despite noninvasive imaging or for performance of catheter-based revascularization procedures in select patients. Positron emission tomography (PET) scanning has emerged for targeted imaging of vascular inflammation and may be particularly useful when combined with traditional cross-sectional imaging modalities. CT in the setting of acute aortitis may demonstrate thickening of the aortic wall and periaortic inflammation, although milder degrees of inflammation or wall edema may not be apparent. MRA, generally with gadolinium contrast enhancement, is emerging as a noninvasive imaging

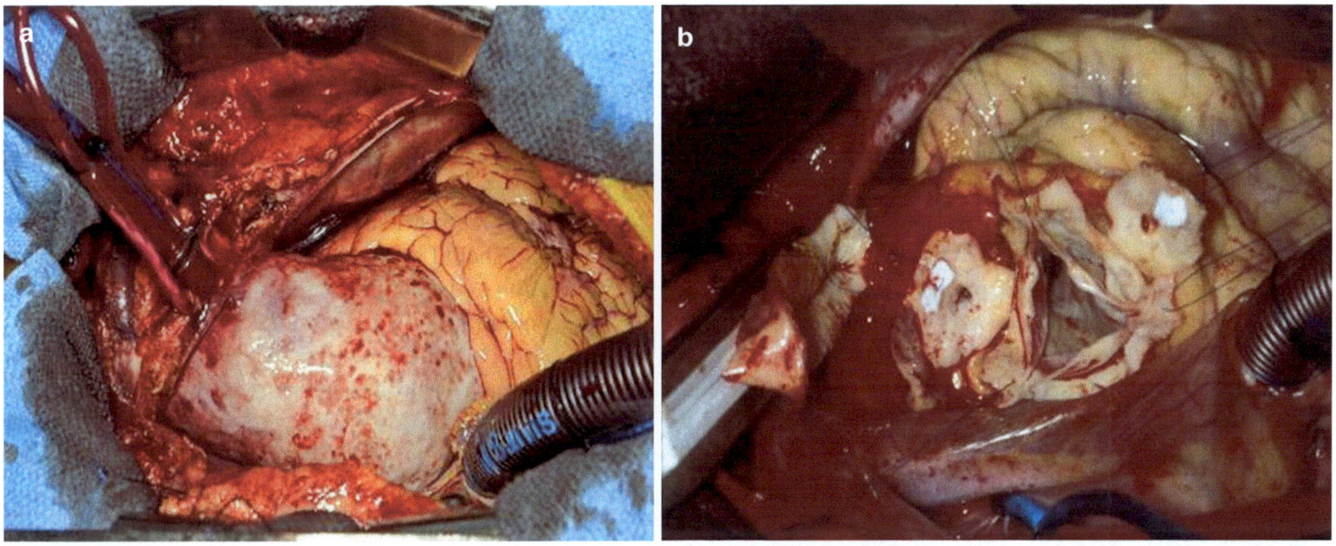

Fig. 44.3 A 7-cm ascending aortic aneurysm involved with giant cell aortitis. Note the glistening cobblestone appearance. Inside view of the coronary buttons and residual involved aorta in a patient with aortic root involvement who was prepared for a valve-preserving aortic root reconstruction. The inflammatory process is grossly evident in the residual aorta, but the morphology of the valve cusps is preserved

modality of choice for aortitis, particularly aortitis associated with GCA and Takayasu arteritis. MR imaging (MRI) may be used to image the entire aorta without radiation exposure or iodinated contrast, and it provides excellent resolution of the aortic wall. Recently, the use of 18-fluorodeoxyglucose (18F-FDG) PET, either alone or in combination with contrast-enhanced CTA or MRA, has emerged as a potential tool for the initial diagnosis and assessment of disease activity of aortitis caused by either GCA or Takayasu arteritis. Recent imaging series have reported a sensitivity of 60–92 % and a specificity of 88–100 % of 18F-FDG PET for diagnosing active inflammation in arteritis, but these studies have been limited by small sample size, heterogeneous patient population, and inconsistent choice of a reference standard [26, 27].

Although generally not used as a primary diagnostic modality for aortitis, abdominal ultrasound or transthoracic or transesophageal echocardiography may demonstrate circumferential thickening of the aortic wall. Abdominal ultrasonography is useful for the diagnosis of abdominal aortic aneurysm occurring as a complication of aortitis or in association with chronic periaortitis or inflammatory aneurysm. In addition, echocardiography plays a key role in the assessment of the aortic root and aortic valve in the setting of aortitis of the ascending thoracic aorta associated with aortic insufficiency and aneurysm formation [28–30].

Laboratory Measurements

Although the diagnosis of aortitis generally is based on clinical presentation and aortic imaging, key laboratory tests are helpful. The initial evaluation of a patient with suspected aortitis should include markers of inflammation, namely erythrocyte sedimentation rate and C-reactive protein, a complete blood count, assessment of kidney and liver function, and blood cultures, to exclude the unlikely but critical diagnosis of infectious aortitis. Additional laboratory testing should be based on the clinical assessment of the patient and the differential diagnosis of the underlying cause. A rheumatologic panel, including anti-nuclear antibodies, antineutrophil cytoplasmic antibodies, and rheumatoid factor, may be helpful in the appropriate clinical setting. Skin testing for tuberculosis and serological testing for syphilis should be completed.

Although the erythrocyte sedimentation rate and C-reactive protein typically are markedly elevated in cases of aortitis caused by GCA and other systemic vasculitides, these inflammatory markers may be unreliable for the prediction of disease activity among patients with Takayasu arteritis [31]. Recent clinical investigation has focused on the identification of novel and more sensitive laboratory markers for disease activity among patients with Takayasu arteritis, with interleukin-6, interleukin-18, and certain matrix metalloproteinases showing promise in small studies [32, 33].

Surgical Management

In our experience, GCA commonly presents as an ascending aortic aneurysm involving the ascending aorta at and above the sinotubular junction and frequently extends into the aortic arch. There is often associated central aortic insufficiency related to effacement of the sinotubular junction. The aortic valve tissue appears to be spared from the vasculitic process.

A surgical strategy of tailoring the operation to address the aortic disease and aortic valve insufficiency can be done with low morbidity and mortality. We advocate that treatment with steroids alone based on assessment of the acute inflammatory process does not seem to protect from aortic involvement. The high incidence of involvement of other parts of the aorta portends close surveillance of the remaining aorta.

Earlier we reported in our published series [34] that a large proportion of patients were asymptomatic at presentation with the aneurysm discovered incidentally on routine physical examination or during workup of an unrelated pathologic process. The question arises whether to serially monitor all patients with temporal arteritis or polymyalgia rheumatica for the development of a thoracic aneurysm or not. In our study [34], evidence of a past history of temporal arteritis or polymyalgia rheumatica was found in 10 of the 37 (27 %) patients. All were treated with steroids for variable periods (6 months to 3 years) depending on the response based on inflammation markers. The mean duration of the diagnosis of temporal arteritis to aortic surgery was 8.9 ± 3.9 years, although most patients had silent vasculitis. In symptomatic patients, the symptoms were related to the aneurysm or the associated aortic regurgitation. This was true even for patients who were previously treated for symptomatic temporal arteritis. This suggests that patients with a history of temporal arteritis should be serially assessed for the development of large vessel disease [13]. Evans and colleagues [13] found 11 of 96 (11.5 %) patients had (2 patients) or developed a thoracic aneurysm (9 patients) during a median time of 5.8 years after the diagnosis of temporal arteritis. On the other hand, Lie [35] made some interesting findings in 72 patients with extracranial giant cell arteritis described to have evidence of temporal arteritis, 67 by biopsy before, concurrent with, or after the diagnosis of aortic and extracranial large vessel giant cell arteritis and 5 by clinical criteria. Lie's study provides evidence that cranial symptoms are often absent in patients with aortitis despite biopsy-proven giant cell involvement of the temporal arteries. Therefore, the presence of symptoms is a suboptimal endpoint to initiate a screening process for aortitis. We recommend that all patients with temporal arteritis be screened for large vessel disease.

Our surgical results have so far been similar to surgery for aneurysms caused by other etiologies when the same algorithm concerning surgery is applied. The usual indication is an ascending aneurysm greater than 5.5 cm or severe aortic regurgitation. The aortic arch or ascending aneurysm is usually cannulated, and femoral cannulation is occasionally performed in patients with tenuous aneurysmal walls. In retrospect, we do not believe there is any contraindication to axillary artery cannulation, and this procedure is preferred in patients in whom arch reconstruction is required to facilitate anterograde cerebral perfusion. The diagnosis is nearly always made by histologic examination. As we gained experience with the clinical entity, a high index of suspicion could be obtained by the gross appearance of the aorta at the time of surgery (Fig. 44.3). If the aneurysm extends into the aortic arch, then replacement is extended to include a partial or complete arch reconstruction. All complete arch reconstructions are and should be done as an elephant trunk procedure in anticipation of the possible need for future descending aortic replacement. In the younger adult patients, valve-sparing aortic root reconstruction should be considered. In our experience, in patients who had their native valves excised, the valve cusps showed no histologic evidence of an inflammatory process [34]. Therefore, the valve can safely be preserved in patients with functionally normal valves.

There is no consensus on the dose and duration of steroid treatment after a histologic diagnosis of giant cell arteritis. Most surgeons recommend treatment with steroids in the active phase of disease. The active phase is determined by either symptomatic vasculitis or elevated markers of inflammation. Our practice is to start prednisolone at a dose of 40–60 mg/day in adults and continue for 6 months to 2 years depending on the response. Cyclophosphamide, azathioprine, or dapsone may be used with steroids if the erythrocyte sedimentation rate does not respond. In our reported series [34], 13 patients received steroid therapy as per the guidelines mentioned. Of these 13 patients, 5 had developed or had progression of an aneurysm in the remaining aorta despite steroid therapy. Of the eight patients who died during follow-up, only one had received steroids after surgery. All three patients who had fatal complication of a thoracic aortic aneurysm during follow-up had not received steroids. Whether aneurysmal dilatation of the remaining aorta and great vessels can be prevented by an aggressive regimen of steroids or antineoplastic agents is unclear. Nevertheless, we recommend a continued aggressive treatment approach in patients with evidence of active disease and computed tomographic scanning on a yearly basis with surgical consideration given at smaller dimensions similar to patients with connective tissue disorders.

Survival

Patients with aneurysms caused by giant cell aortitis carry a high incidence of catastrophic complications. In the Olmstead County population, a study has suggested an incidence of sudden death in 44 % of patients from aortic dissection [13]. Liu and co-workers [2] reported on a series of 23 patients with GCA presenting with dissection; 46 % of patients presented catastrophically. Of these, the 2-week mortality was 80 %. Our earlier series [34] corroborates these data. We reported [34] that in our series 17 patients

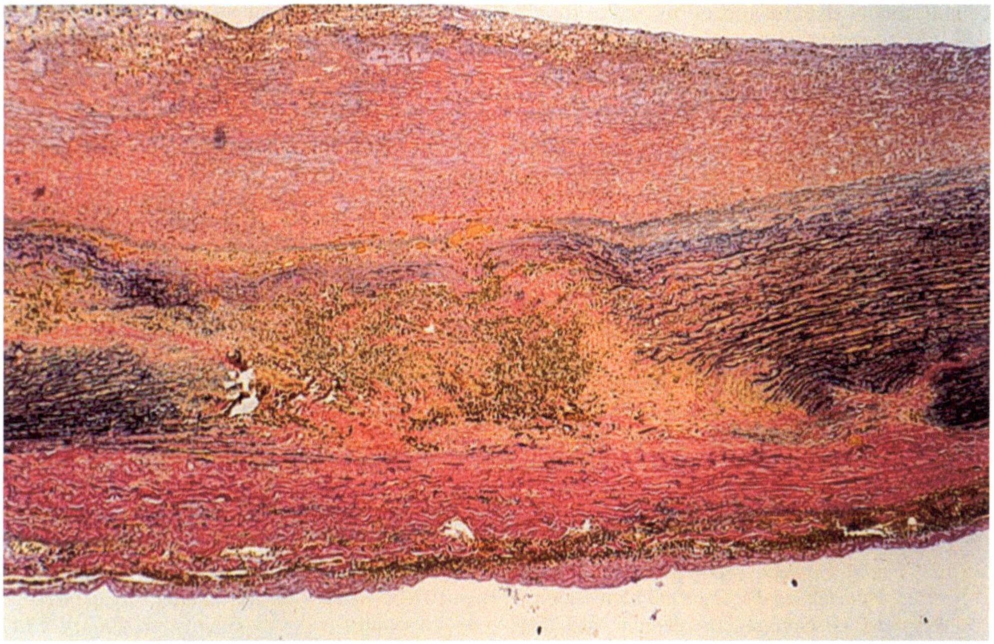

Fig. 44.4 Photomicrograph of a cross-section through the aortic wall showing near-complete disruption of the elastic fibers and media by the inflammatory giant cell process

had aneurysmal involvement of the descending or thoracoabdominal aorta. Out of these, five patients died. Three were caused by complications of a thoracic aortic aneurysm, two had documented rupture, and one had a localized rupture with a thoracic hematoma that contributed to the development of disseminated intravascular coagulation. All three patients had aneurysms of less than 6 cm in diameter. One patient died suddenly, and an autopsy was not performed. The histology of this disease suggests that patients often have a near-complete disruption of the elastic medial layer, as outlined in Fig. 44.4. This may predispose patients to rupture and dissection before the aneurysm achieves the standard sizes for usual intervention.

Eklund and coworkers [36] reported on a patient who presented with an aortic rupture 3 cm above the valve annulus with a normal-sized aorta but marked thinning of the aortic media. The patient had been treated for 5 years with a maintenance dose of 5 mg/day of prednisolone after achieving a normal erythrocyte sedimentation rate. There is no doubt that close surveillance of the remaining aorta in this patient population is necessary. However, the overall survival rate in a cohort of patients undergoing aneurysm operation on the proximal thoracic aorta has been reported to be 90.6 % with a median follow-up time of 15.4 months [37]. This is similar to the 87 % 1-year survival rate from a Swedish population-based study [38]. We have so far demonstrated an overall survival of 97.2 % with a mean follow-up of 2.8 ± 2.3 years [34]. Our actuarial survival in 37 patients at 4 years is 74 % (95 % confidence interval, 57–94 %; Fig. 44.5) at a mean follow-up of 3.8 ± 2.3 years [34]. No patients from the surviving cohort required aortic value replacement.

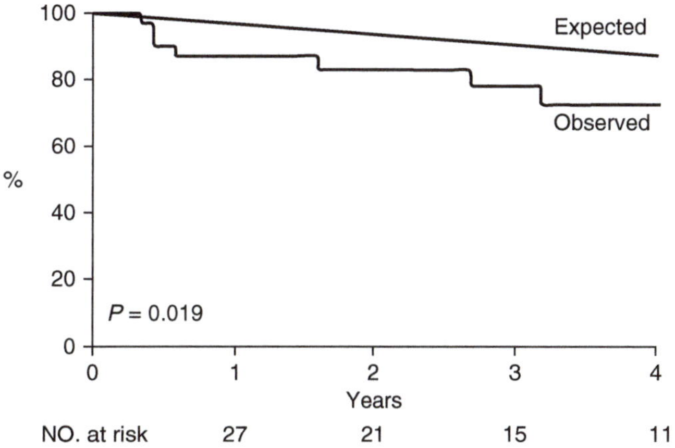

Fig. 44.5 Survival curve of patients undergoing surgical repair compared with the expected survival of our age- and sex-matched regional population (Adapted from Ref. [34] with permission)

Conclusion

Most of the factors predictive of large-artery stenosis are identified in this chapter. Diminished pulse or blood pressure and/or claudication of an arm, TIA or stroke, and diplopia are all predictive of large-artery stenosis, and an aortic insufficiency murmur could be predictive of aortic aneurysm and/or aortic dissection. The presence of any of these symptoms should prompt further evaluation for possible large artery complication. The negative association of cranial symptoms and a higher ESR at the time of diagnosis of GCA with large-artery stenosis, and the borderline association of polymyalgia rheumatic-type symptoms with large-artery stenosis, might somewhat help in risk stratifying patients with GCA for the development of large-artery complications. Surgical tailoring to address the aortic disease and aortic valve insufficiency and steroid therapy based on assessment of the acute inflammatory process can be implemented with low morbidity and mortality. However, a standardized, prospective, large-scale study is needed to better determine factors and outcomes predictive of such anomaly.

References

1. Evans JM, Bowles CA, Bjornsson J, Mullany CJ, Hunder GG. Thoracic aortic aneurysm and rupture in giant cell arteritis: a descriptive study of 41 cases. Arthritis Rheum. 1994;37:1539–47.
2. Liu G, Shupak R, Chiu BKY. Aortic dissection in giant-cell arteritis. Semin Arthritis Rheum. 1995;25:160–71.
3. Foote EA, Postier RG, Greenfield RA, Bronze MS. Infectious aortitis. Curr Treat Options Cardiovasc Med. 2005;7:89–97.
4. Virmani R, Burke A. Nonatherosclerotic diseases of the aorta and miscellaneous disease of the main pulmonary arteries and large veins. In: Silver M, Gotlieb A, Schoen F, editors. Cardiovascular pathology. 3rd ed. Philadelphia, Pa: Churchill Livingstone; 2001. p. 107–37.
5. Weyand CM, Goronzy JJ. Medium- and large-vessel vasculitis. N Engl J Med. 2003;349:160–9.
6. Gravanis MB. Giant cell arteritis and Takayasu aortitis: morphologic, pathogenetic and etiologic factors. Int J Cardiol. 2000;75:21–33.
7. Miller DV, Isotalo PA, Weyand CM, Edwards WD, Aubry MC, Tazelaar HD. Surgical pathology of noninfectious ascending aortitis: a study of 45 cases with emphasis on an isolated variant. Am J Surg Pathol. 2006;30:1150–8.
8. Rojo-Leyva F, Ratliff NB, Cosgrove 3rd DM, Hoffman GS. Study of 52 patients with idiopathic aortitis from a cohort of 1,204 surgical cases. Arthritis Rheum. 2000;43:901–7.
9. Hutchinson J. Diseases of the arteries: on a peculiar form of thrombotic arteritis of the aged which is sometimes productive of gangrene. Arch Surg (Lond). 1890;1:323–9.
10. Horton BT, Magath TB, Brown GE. An undescribed form of arteritis of the temporal vessels. Mayo Clin Proc. 1932;7:700–1.
11. Ostberg G. Temporal arteritis in a large necropsy series. Ann Rheum Dis. 1971;30:224–35.
12. Machado EB, Michet CJ, Ballard DJ, et al. Trends in incidence and clinical presentation of temporal arteritis in Olmstead County, Minnesota, 1950–1985. Arthritis Rheum. 1988;31:745–9.
13. Evans JM, O'Fallon WM, Hunder GG. Increased incidence of aortic aneurysm and dissection in giant cell (temporal) arteritis: a population based study. Ann Intern Med. 1995;122:502–7.
14. Salvarani C, Crowson CS, O'Fallon WM, Hunder GG, Gabriel SE. Reappraisal of the epidemiology of giant cell arteritis in Olmsted County, Minnesota, over a fifty-year period. Arthritis Rheum. 2004;51:264–8.
15. Kobayashi S, Yano T, Matsumoto Y, Numano F, Nakajima N, Yasuda K, et al. Clinical and epidemiologic analysis of giant cell (temporal) arteritis from a nationwide survey in 1998 in Japan: the first government-supported nationwide survey. Arthritis Rheum. 2003;49:594–8.
16. Hall S, Barr W, Lie JT, Stanson AW, Kazmier FJ, Hunder GG. Takayasu arteritis: a study of 32 North American patients. Medicine (Baltimore). 1985;64:89–99.
17. Koide K. Takayasu arteritis in Japan. Heart Vessels Suppl. 1992; 7:48–54.
18. Nuenninghoff DM, Hunder GG, Christianson TJ, McClelland RL, Matteson EL. Incidence and predictors of large-artery complication (aortic aneurysm, aortic dissection, and/or large-artery stenosis) in patients with giant cell arteritis: a population-based study over 50 years. Arthritis Rheum. 2003;48:3522–31.
19. Silver AS, Shao CY, Ginzler EM. Aortitis and aortic thrombus in systemic lupus erythematosus. Lupus. 2006;15:541–3.
20. Salvarani C, Cantini F, Boiardi L, Hunder GG. Polymyalgia rheumatic and giant-cell arteritis. N Engl J Med. 2002;347: 261–71.
21. Jang JJ, Gorevic PD, Olin JW. Images in vascular medicine: giant cell arteritis presenting with acute myocardial infarction. Vasc Med. 2007;12:379.
22. Mwipatayi BP, Jeffery PC, Beningfield SJ, Matley PJ, Naidoo NG, Kalla AA, et al. Takayasu arteritis: clinical features and management: report of 272 cases. ANZ J Surg. 2005;75:110–7.
23. Park MC, Lee SW, Park YB, Chung NS, Lee SK. Clinical characteristics and outcomes of Takayasu's arteritis: analysis of 108 patients using standardized criteria for diagnosis, activity assessment, and angiographic classification. Scand J Rheumatol. 2005;34:284–92.
24. Sueyoshi E, Sakamoto I, Hayashi K. Aortic aneurysms in patients with Takayasu's arteritis: CT evaluation. AJR Am J Roentgenol. 2000;175:1727–33.
25. Miyata T, Sato O, Koyama H, Shigematsu H, Tada Y. Long-term survival after surgical treatment of patients with Takayasu's arteritis. Circulation. 2003;108:1474–80.
26. Webb M, Chambers A, Al-Nahhas A, Mason JC, Maudlin L, Rahman L, et al. The role of 18F-FDG PET in characterising disease activity in Takayasu arteritis. Eur J Nucl Med Mol Imaging. 2004;31:627–34.
27. Walter MA, Melzer RA, Schindler C, Muller-Brand J, Tyndall A, Nitzsche EU. The value of [18F]FDG-PET in the diagnosis of large vessel vasculitis and the assessment of activity and extent of disease. Eur J Nucl Med Mol Imaging. 2005;32:674–81.
28. Soto ME, Espinola-Zavaleta N, Ramirez-Quito O, Reyes PA. Echocardiographic follow-up of patients with Takayasu's arteritis: five-year survival. Echocardiography. 2006;23:353–60.
29. Harris KM, Malenka DJ, Plehn JF. Transesophageal echocardiographic evaluation of aortitis. Clin Cardiol. 1997;20:813–5.
30. Tsui KL, Lee KW, Chan WK, Chan HK, Hon SF, Leung TC, et al. Behcet's aortitis and aortic regurgitation: a report of two cases. J Am Soc Echocardiogr. 2004;17:83–6.
31. Salvarani C, Cantini F, Boiardi L, Hunder GG. Laboratory investigations useful in giant cell arteritis and Takayasu's arteritis. Clin Exp Rheumatol. 2003;21:S23–8.
32. Park MC, Lee SW, Park YB, Lee SK. Serum cytokine profiles and their correlations with disease activity in Takayasu's arteritis. Rheumatology (Oxford). 2006;45:545–8.
33. Matsuyama A, Sakai N, Ishigami M, Hiraoka H, Kashine S, Hirata A, et al. Matrix metalloproteinases as novel disease markers in Takayasu arteritis. Circulation. 2003;108:1469–73.
34. Zehr KJ, Mathur A, Orszulak TA, Mullany CJ, Schaff HV. Surgical treatment of ascending aortic aneurysms in patients with giant cell aortitis. Ann Thorac Surg. 2005;79(5):1512–7.
35. Lie JT. Aortic and extracranial large vessel giant cell arteritis: a review of 72 cases with histopathologic documentation. Semin Arthritis Rheum. 1995;24:422–31.
36. Eklund E, Valdemarsson S. Rupture of a non-aneurysmatic aortic trunk in a patient with giant cell arteritis. Ann Rheum Dis. 1998; 57:442–3.
37. Liang KP, Chowdhary VR, Michet CJ, Miller DV, Sundt TM, Connolly HM, et al. Noninfectious ascending aortitis: a case series of 64 patients. J Rheumatol. 2009;36(10):2290–7.
38. Olsson C, Eriksson N, Stahle E, Thelin S. Surgical and long-term mortality in 2634 consecutive patients operated on the proximal thoracic aorta. Eur J Cardiothorac Surg. 2007;31:963–9.

Part XIV

Heart and Lung Transplantation

Cytokine Profile in Heart Transplantation

45

Ahmet Ruchan Akar, Serkan Durdu, Bahadır Inan, and Mustafa Sırlak

Brief Historical Review

The founder of modern organ transplantation is Alexis Carrel (1873–1944) because of his extensive work on vascular anastomosis and accomplishment of the first successful heart transplantation (HT) in a canine model using carotid artery and jugular vein anastomosis in 1905 [1]. The realization of the first human-to-human HT was closely related to the work of Norman Shumway and Richard Lower at Stanford University, who described the technique for orthotopic canine HT [2, 3]. Shumway and colleagues not only worked extensively on an efficient surgical technique for HT, but also performance characteristics of the allograft and control of allograft rejection [2, 4–10]. However, Christiaan N. Barnard (1922–2001) performed the world's first successful human-to-human HT in Groote Schuur Hospital, Cape Town, in 1967 [11]. The immunosuppressive regimen of Barnard and colleagues in their first three patients included corticosteroids, azathioprine, local irradiation to the transplanted heart, and antilymphocyte globulin [12, 13]. Dr. Barnard [12] pointed out that "one day this problem will be solved, we will be able to induce tolerance in our patients and organ transplantation will be a curative and not a palliative procedure." Between 1968 and1970, a total of 166 (102, 48, and 16 annually) HTs were performed worldwide with unacceptably high mortality rates due to either rejection or infection [14]. These unfavorable outcomes led to the investigation of new immunosuppressive regimens, and most centers have stopped practicing HT. Another milestone in immunosuppression was reached in 1972 when cyclosporine was discovered in Basel, Switzerland, and subsequently approved for clinical use in 1983 [15–19]. During that period, only Shumway and his team continued using HT at Stanford University and performed 227 HT procedures between 1968 and 1981 [20]. Today, HT provides the gold standard treatment modality for patients with end-stage heart failure [21]. Since 1967, over 100,000 HTs have been performed worldwide. In the last decade, between 3,600 and 3,850 HTs have been performed in 388 countries registered with International Society of Heart and Lung transplantation (ISHLT) Registry [21, 22].

According to the ISHLT Registry, the 30-day and 1-year mortality after HT are 8 and 14 %, respectively. The UK transplant registry reported that 20 % of patients who get the chance to have HT die within the first year of transplantation. Following the first year, there is a constant mortality rate of 3–4 % per year. Moreover, it has been generally agreed that the 5-year survival rate for heart transplantation is around 65–70 % [23]. Median survival is 11 years for the entire cohort of adult and pediatric heart recipients in the ISHLT Registry. Major complications following HT are perioperative ischemic injury, allograft rejection, infection, lymphoproliferative disease, and cardiac allograft vasculopathy. Cell-to-cell communication via cytokine networks has an active role in immune responses following heart transplantation. Furthermore, the correlation between the cytokine profile and clinical outcomes after HT is under intense research.

A.R. Akar, MD, FRCS CTh (✉) • S. Durdu, MD, PhD
Department of Cardiovascular Surgery,
Heart Center, Ankara University School of Medicine,
Dikimevi, Ankara 06340, Turkey

Department of Multi-disciplinary Stem Cell and Regenerative Medicine, Stem Cell Institute, Ankara University, Ankara, Turkey
e-mail: akarruchan@gmail.com; akar@ankara.edu.tr

B. Inan, MD
Department of Cardiovascular Surgery,
Heart Center, Ankara University School of Medicine,
Dikimevi, Ankara 06340, Turkey

M. Sırlak, MD
Department of Cardiovascular Surgery, Heart Center,
Ankara University School of Medicine,
Ankara, Turkey

E.A. Gabriel, S.A. Gabriel (eds.), *Inflammatory Response in Cardiovascular Surgery*,
DOI 10.1007/978-1-4471-4429-8_45, © Springer-Verlag London 2013

Cytokine Release During Donor Brain Death

Acute brain death is associated with the release of catecholamines and substantial decreases in free thyroxine and T3, cortisol, insulin, and antidiuretic hormone levels, leading to diabetes insipidus. Furthermore, change from aerobic to anaerobic metabolism and increases in inflammatory cytokines are common [24]. Recently, de Vries and colleagues demonstrated that donor brain death is associated with inflammatory cytokine release upon reperfusion [25]. In this study, the investigators showed prompt release of inflammatory cytokines, including G-CSF, IL-6, IL-9, IL-16, and MCP-1 after reperfusion of kidneys from brain-dead donors in contrast to kidneys from living and cardiac dead donors [25].

Early Postoperative Systemic Inflammatory Response

Heart transplantation is associated with systemic inflammatory response triggered by oxidative stress and enhanced production of glycoprotein messengers, namely cytokines [26]. The cytokine milieu in the early postoperative period is triggered by several factors, including surgical trauma, exposure of blood to extracorporeal artificial surfaces, ischemia/reperfusion injury, sheer stress, and release of endotoxin [27, 28]. Cell-to-cell contact, immune complexes/autoantibodies, local complement activation, microorganisms, reactive oxygen species, and donor DNA also promote cytokine expression after HT. The release of cytokines (IL-1, IL-6, and IL-8) and complement fragments (C3a, C5a, membrane attack complex) during cardiopulmonary bypass (CPB) activates the vascular endothelium via endothelial cell adhesion molecules and causes functional changes in endothelial cells. IL-1, tumor necrosis factor-alpha (TNF-α), and IL-6 have significant roles in driving the acute-phase response. Frering and colleagues showed that normothermic CPB is associated with IL-6 and IL-8 production, which is similar to hypothermic CPB; however, plasma levels of TNF-α and IL-1-β remained undetectable after normothermic CPB [29]. IL-1-β and TNF-α stimulate procoagulant activity of endothelial cells. Both inhibit the thrombomodulin/protein C anticoagulant pathway and stimulate production of type I plasminogen activator inhibitor. The cardiac allograft is a major source of cytokines after HT associated with activated T lymphocytes and macrophages and elevated coronary sinus levels of TNF-alpha, IL-6, and high soluble IL-2 receptor levels [30].

Hyperacute Rejection

The major blood group (ABO) antigens are the targets of a dramatic hyperacute rejection process. Recognition of blood group antigens on the endothelial surface of the graft vessels by recipient "natural" antibodies activates the complement and coagulation cascades, resulting in rapid graft thrombosis and ischemia. B cell maturation, proliferation, activation, and survival require particular cytokines (TNF superfamily cytokines, BLyS and APRIL).

Acute Cellular Rejection

Within the first year, approximately 20–40 % of heart transplant recipients experience at least one episode of acute cellular rejection (ACR) [31, 32]. In a recent cohort between 2001 and 2009, hospitalization for rejection treatment was required in 26 % of patients within 1 year and in 44 % of patients within 5 years after HT [21]. Younger and female recipients were at a higher risk of rejection [21]. Alloreactivity in retransplant candidates, blood product recipients, previous LVAD recipients, and multiparous women is increased because of repeated B- and T-cell exposure to alloantigens.

The major histocompatibility complex (MHC) proteins (human leukocyte antigens in humans) and ABO blood antigens are the primary targets of the allogeneic immune response. The rejection of transplanted heart is mainly a T-lymphocyte (T-cell)-mediated event, although humoral (B-cell) responses may also contribute [33]. T cells, B cells, and antigen-presenting cells (APCs) all participate in the production of cytokines. Indeed, cytokines play a critical role in orchestrating acute cellular rejection. Furthermore, non-immune endothelial cells via lymphokines further modulate the immune response.

CD34+ T helper (Th) cells and their committed Th counterparts, namely Th1, Th2, and Th17 subsets, and regulatory T cells (Tregs) are the active actors of acute cardiac cellular rejection (Fig. 45.1) [34]. Figure 45.1 shows the principal features of the APC/CD34+ Th cell interaction and recognition of alloantigens by CD34 T cells. The Th1 subset preferentially produces IL-2, IFN-γ, and TNF-α. Th1 cytokines activate macrophages, promoting delayed-type hypersensitivity (DTH) reactions. The Th2 subset produces IL-4, IL-5, IL-10, and IL-13. Both subsets contribute to the production of IL-3, TNF-α, and granulocyte-macrophage colony-stimulating factor (GMCSF). In contrast, Tregs have an antiinflammatory role and are responsible for self-tolerance. Although several studies [35] have highlighted the link between IL-17 and allograft rejection, the impact of Th17 cells on transplant outcomes requires further investigation. Through their developmental stages, T cells require cytokine release. These steps include bone marrow stem cell differentiation and proliferation, thymic education leading to central tolerance [36], and maturation after primary or secondary antigen exposure. In brief, direct allorecognition by T cells mediates acute rejection.

Initially, donor's antigen-presenting cells (APC) recognize donor-derived antigens located on the cells of the allograft. APCs migrate from the allograft to the recipient

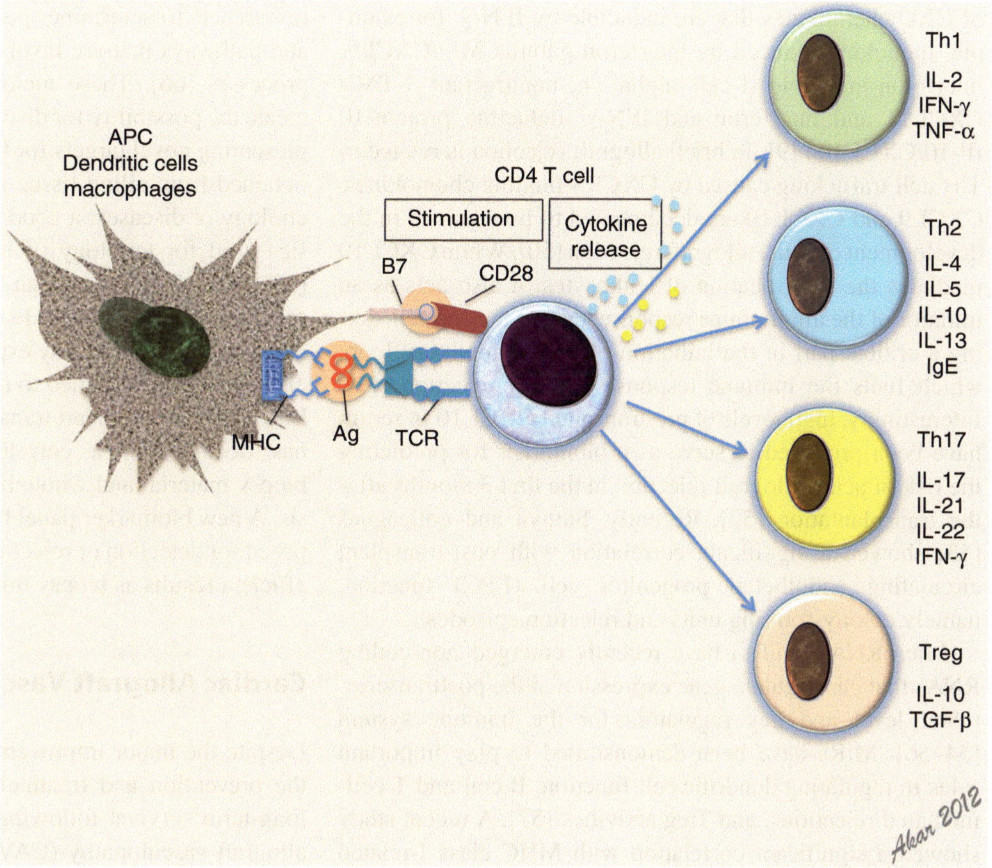

Fig. 45.1 Immature dendritic cells mature into antigen-presenting cells (*APCs*) within recipients' lymph nodes and spleen. APCs present donor alloantigens on their class II MHC molecules. CD4 helper T cells recognize alloantigens with the use of their surface immunoglobulins and MHC class II molecules. Activated subgroups of helper T cells have distinct cytokine profiles to promote rejection or tolerance. *APC* antigen-presenting cell, *MHC* major histocompatibility complex, *TCR* T-cell receptor, *IL* Interleukin, *IFN-γ* interferon-γ, *Treg* regulatory T cell, *TGF-β* transforming growth factor β

lymphoid tissue and present donor major histocompatibility complex class II and B7 complex to the recipient's T-cells for direct allorecognition [32, 33]. Allorecognition is mediated by the recognition of foreign MHC molecules on the surface of donor cells by recipient dendritic cells [37]. T cell-dendritic cell interaction requires local cytokine expression. Intracellular activation of calcineurin leads to production of IL-2. In fact, blockade of IL-2R has been used as an effective therapeutic strategy promoting allograft survival [38].

Active APCs produce IL-12. IL-12 initiates CD4+Th1 activation and stimulates the development of activated CD8+ cells and interferon (IFN)-γ production both in vivo and in vitro [39, 40]. IFN-γ activates macrophages, upregulates the expression of MHC class II antigen, and promotes allograft rejection [41]. In their enlightening study, Saiura and colleagues have revealed a distinct upregulating effect on the genes that are involved in the inflammatory process after HT, while failing to document any conclusive findings on the regulation of chemokine ligand 9 and chemokine ligand 10 in mice. They also reported upregulation of allograft inflammatory factor-1 throughout the investigated time points (days 3, 5, and 7) following HT. Most importantly, samples taken from patients with acute graft rejection displayed the central role of IFN-γ in inducing several chemokines. Macrophage inflammatory protein 1 alpha expression is shown to increase during rejection in both wild-type and IFN-γ-deficient mice, while the rejection process in IFN-γ-deficient mice did not show increased expressions of CXCL9 and CXCL10 [42].

IL-12 and -23 share the p40 subunit and are crucial for the development of T helper (Th) 1 and Th17 cell responses in acute graft rejection [43]. Th17 cells, a recently identified CD4+ effector T cell subset, produce proinflammatory IL-17 in both mice and humans [44]. Furthermore, Xie and colleagues [43] demonstrated effective inhibition of Th1 and Th17 cell responses after treatment with an anti-IL-12/23p40 antibody in vivo mouse model of acute cardiac allograft rejection. Recently, Wang and colleagues [45] demonstrated that the levels of Th1, Th17, and FoxP3+ CD4+ T cells and their specific transcription factors increased in patients with acute rejection after HT and were associated with rejection grades.

T-helper 1 (Th1)-type cytokines (e.g., IL-2, IFN-γ, IL-12, TNF-α) are closely linked in the elimination of intracellular infections and mediating allograft rejection [46]. TNF-α -308 SNP is associated with acute cellular rejection following HT [47]. In contrast, the Th2 cytokine profile (IL-4, -5, and -10) is associated with allograft tolerance. For example, IL-10 promoter at positions −1,082, −819, and −592 correlates with increased IL-10 production [48]. Allograft rejection is characterized by CXCR3 carrying T cells and, more importantly, release of Th1-related cytokines and expression of CXC chemokines that are inducible by IFN-γ, for example, monokine induced by interferon gamma Mig/CXCL9, interferon-inducible T-cell alpha chemoattractant I-TAC/CXCL11 and interferon and IFN-γ -inducible protein-10 IP-10/CXCL10 [49]. In brief, allograft rejection is related to Th1 cell trafficking caused by CXCR3-binding chemokines. CXCL9 and CXCL10 are documented to be involved in the development of acute allograft rejection [50]. While CXCL10 mediates the congregation of leukocytes, it also acts as an initiator of the alloimmune response against the antigen, taking a critical part in the initiation of an inflammatory loop, which fuels the immune response in graft rejection [51]. Interestingly, high levels of pre-transplant CXCL10 in serum have been proposed to serve as a biomarker for predicting the risk of acute allograft rejection in the first 3 months after the transplantation [52]. Recently, Sathya and colleagues [53] showed a significant correlation with post-transplant circulating endothelial progenitor cell (EPC) function, namely colony-forming units and rejection episodes.

MicroRNAs (miRs) have recently emerged non-coding RNAs that can regulate gene expression at the posttranscriptional level and key regulators for the immune system [54–56]. MiRs have been demonstrated to play important roles in regulating dendritic cell function, B cell and T cell-mediated rejections, and Treg activities [57]. A recent study showed a significant correlation with MHC class I-related gene A (MICA) upregulation and histological evidence of severe rejection after HT in 44 patients [58].

Diagnosis of Rejection

Endomyocardial biopsy (EMB) is currently the gold standard method for detection and confirmation of the allograft rejection. Several methods have been proposed for an accurate diagnosis, yet none so far has proven to be adequate or specific enough to replace the status quo [59]. The necessity to replace endomyocardial biopsy is to avoid an invasive method and to provide the clinician with a tool with fast and accurate results. In current practice, major adjunct methods are used for monitoring rejection, such as electrocardiography, electrophysiology, radio-isotopic techniques, cyto-immunologic monitoring, and magnetic resonance imaging [60, 61]. Among the proposed biochemical markers are urinary polyamines [61], neopterins [62], prolactin [63], beta-2-microglobulins [64], and brain natriuretic peptide (BNP) [65], none of which had fulfilled the need for sensitivity.

New high-throughput analyses that utilize protein or gene expression analysis techniques, cell-mediated immune assays, and fluorescence-activated cell sorter analysis of cellular subpopulations have the potential to provide the clinicians with more accurate markers of allograft rejection. Advancements in microarray technologies and bioinformatics allow researchers to determine specific proteins, genes, metabolites and pathways that are involved in normal and dysfunctional processes [66]. These major methodological developments create the possibility for discovery of new markers, while also presenting novel targets for therapy. Human biopsy materials obtained from ailing tissue are being used to investigate the etiology of diseases; a good example would be cardiac biopsies used for tetralogy of Fallot [67] and atrial fibrillation [68]. New biomarkers can be developed by utilizing such methodologies and provide stepping stones for new therapy options. DNA microarray experiments involving animal models have been performed to understand the Brown Norway to Lewis heterotopic heart transplant model [69]. A recent study has documented a correlation between endomyocardial biopsy material and whole blood by using microarray analysis. A new biomarker panel from whole blood samples is proposed for detection of rejection, which was claimed to have as efficient results as biopsy microarray [70].

Cardiac Allograft Vasculopathy

Despite the major improvements that have been achieved in the prevention and treatment of acute transplant rejection, long-term survival following HT has not improved. Cardiac allograft vasculopathy (CAV) is the major long-term limitation of HT survivors [71, 72]. Despite a 2–4 % recent decrease in the cumulative incidence of CAV, the prevalence of CAV still remains high. CAV is detectable by angiography in 8 % of the patients within the first year, 20 % at 3 years, 32 % at 5 years, and 45 % at 8 years following HT [21]. Briefly, CAV is the leading cause of late morbidity and mortality in HT patients, accounting for 30 % mortality in the first 5 years [21]. The pathogenesis of CAV is not fully elucidated. Indeed, CAV is a complex, multifactorial phenomenon. Immunologic (indirect allorecognition, upregulation of cytokines and cytokine-related adhesion molecules, focal inflammation, and vasculitis) and nonimmunologic factors (repetitive vascular injury) may play critical roles in the process [32, 73–75].

EMB and coronary angiography provide effective but invasive monitoring methods for CAV in cardiac transplantation recipients. Histologically CAV is characterized by a concentric and diffuse intimal thickening composed of T cells, macrophages, and modified smooth muscle cells beneath an activated endothelium in epicardial and intramural coronary arteries along their entire lengths [76–83]. The disease begins as concentric fibrous intimal thickening caused by myofibroblast proliferation and fibrosis mainly in the proximal region of epicardial arteries [80]. Following the first year of HT, intermediate lesions with intimal lipid-filled cell accumulation can be detected. In long-term survivors, fibrous and fibrofatty intimal lesions often diffusely involve large and small epicardial and intramural arteries [80–83]. Late increase in TNF-α and IFN-γ in endomyocardial biopsies precedes the development of CAV [84]. van Loosdregt and colleagues demonstrated abundant CD4+ T cells that express HLA DR in transplanted hearts with CAV [85]. IL-17 has been shown to be critical in TGFbeta-driven allograft fibrosis [86]. Recently, elevated levels of circulating smooth muscle progenitor cells (SPCs), but not EPCs, and elevated plasma CXCL12 concentrations were found in CAV patients in contrast to patients without CAV [87]. Furthermore, the presence of coronary inflammatory plaque as assessed by virtual histology intravascular ultrasound (VH-IVUS) was associated with early recurrent rejection and with subsequent progression of CAV [88]. Metabolic syndrome is associated with endothelial dysfunction and increases the risk of CAV [89]. New-generation immunosuppressive drugs and immunomodulatory medication may have beneficial effects on coronary microvasculature following heart transplantation [90].

Conflicts of Interest There is no undisclosed ethical problem or conflict of interest related to the submitted manuscript.

References

1. Carrel A, Guthrie CC. The transplantation of veins and organs. Am Med. 1905;10:1101–2.
2. Lower RR, Shumway NE. Studies on orthotopic homotransplantation of the canine heart. Surg Forum. 1960;11:18–9.
3. Shumway NE, Lower RR. Topical cardiac hypothermia for extended periods of anoxic arrest. Surg Forum. 1960;10:563–6.
4. Shumway NE, Angell WW, Wuerflein RD. Progress in transplantation of the heart. Transplantation. 1967;5(Suppl):900–3.
5. Shumway NE, Lower RR, Angell WW. Present status of cardiac transplantation. Angiology. 1966;17(5):289–91.
6. Shumway NE, Lower RR, Stofer RC. Transplantation of the heart. Adv Surg. 1966;2:265–84.
7. Shumway NE. Transplantation of the heart. Surg Gynecol Obstet. 1963;117:361–2.
8. Shumway NE. Cardiac transplantation. Heart Bull. 1963;12:57–60.
9. Lower RR, Stofer RC, Hurley EJ, Dong Jr E, Cohn RB, Shumway NE. Successful homotransplantation of the canine heart after anoxic preservation for seven hours. Am J Surg. 1962;104:302–6.
10. Lower RR, Stofer RC, Hurley EJ, Shumway NE. Complete homograft replacement of the heart and both lungs. Surgery. 1961;50:842–5.
11. Barnard CN. The operation. A human cardiac transplant: an interim report of a successful operation performed at Groote Schuur Hospital, Cape Town. S Afr Med J. 1967;41(48):1271–4.
12. Barnard CN. Human heart transplantation. Can Med Assoc J. 1969;100(3):91–104.
13. Barnard MS, van Heerden J, Hope A, O'Donovan TG, Barnard CN. Total body perfusion for cardiac transplantation. S Afr Med J. 1969;43(3):64–7.
14. Brink JG, Hassoulas J. The first human heart transplant and further advances in cardiac transplantation at Groote Schuur Hospital and the University of Cape Town – with reference to: the operation. A human cardiac transplant: an interim report of a successful operation performed at Groote Schuur Hospital, Cape Town. Cardiovasc J Afr. 2009;20(1):31–5.
15. Wallwork J, McGregor CG, Wells FC, Cory-Pearce R, English TA. Cyclosporin and intravenous sulphadimidine and trimethoprim therapy. Lancet. 1983;1(8320):366–7.
16. White DJ, Calne RY. The use of cyclosporin a immunosuppression in organ grafting. Immunol Rev. 1982;65:115–31.
17. Jamieson SW, Burton NA, Bieber CP, Reitz BA, Oyer PE, Stinson EB, et al. Cardiac-allograft survival in primates treated with cyclosporin A. Lancet. 1979;1(8115):545.
18. Calne RY, White DJ, Rolles K, Smith DP, Herbertson BM. Prolonged survival of pig orthotopic heart grafts treated with cyclosporin A. Lancet. 1978;1(8075):1183–5.
19. Cooley DA, Frazier OH, Kahan BD. Cardiac transplantation with the use of cyclosporin a for immunologic suppression. Tex Heart Inst J. 1982;9(3):247–51.
20. Pennock JL, Oyer PE, Reitz BA, Jamieson SW, Bieber CP, Wallwork J, et al. Cardiac transplantation in perspective for the future. Survival, complications, rehabilitation, and cost. J Thorac Cardiovasc Surg. 1982;83(2):168–77.
21. Stehlik J, Edwards LB, Kucheryavaya AY, Benden C, Christie JD, Dobbels F, et al. The Registry of the International Society for Heart and Lung Transplantation: Twenty-eighth Adult Heart Transplant Report – 2011. J Heart Lung Transplant. 2011;30(10):1078–94. doi:10.1016/j.healun.2011.08.003.
22. Stehlik J, Edwards LB, Kucheryavaya AY, Aurora P, Christie JD, Kirk R, et al. The Registry of the International Society for Heart and Lung Transplantation: twenty-seventh official adult heart transplant report–2010. J Heart Lung Transplant. 2010;29(10):1089–103. doi:10.1016/j.healun.2010.08.007.
23. Taylor DO, Edwards LB, Boucek MM, Trulock EP, Waltz DA, Keck BM, et al. Registry of the International Society for Heart and Lung Transplantation: twenty-third official adult heart transplantation report–2006. J Heart Lung Transplant. 2006;25(8):869–79. doi:10.1016/j.healun.2006.05.002. S1053-2498(06)00399-8 [pii].
24. Novitzky D, Cooper DK, Rosendale JD, Kauffman HM. Hormonal therapy of the brain-dead organ donor: experimental and clinical studies. Transplantation. 2006;82(11):1396–401. doi:10.1097/01.tp. 0000237195.12342.f1.
25. de Vries DK, Lindeman JH, Ringers J, Reinders ME, Rabelink TJ, Schaapherder AF. Donor brain death predisposes human kidney grafts to a proinflammatory reaction after transplantation. Am J Transplant. 2011;11(5):1064–70. doi:10.1111/j.1600-6143.2011.03466.x.
26. Kubala L, Ciz M, Vondracek J, Cerny J, Nemec P, Studenik P, et al. Perioperative and postoperative course of cytokines and the metabolic activity of neutrophils in human cardiac operations and heart transplantation. J Thorac Cardiovasc Surg. 2002;124(6):1122–9. doi:10.1067/mtc.2002.125814.
27. Butler J, Rocker GM, Westaby S. Inflammatory response to cardiopulmonary bypass. Ann Thorac Surg. 1993;55(2):552–9.
28. Knudsen F, Andersen LW. Immunological aspects of cardiopulmonary bypass. J Cardiothorac Anesth. 1990;4(2):245–58.
29. Frering B, Philip I, Dehoux M, Rolland C, Langlois JM, Desmonts JM. Circulating cytokines in patients undergoing normothermic cardiopulmonary bypass. J Thorac Cardiovasc Surg. 1994;108(4):636–41.
30. Fyfe A, Daly P, Galligan L, Pirc L, Feindel C, Cardella C. Coronary sinus sampling of cytokines after heart transplantation: evidence for macrophage activation and interleukin-4 production within the graft. J Am Coll Cardiol. 1993;21(1):171–6.
31. Patel JK, Kobashigawa JA. Should we be doing routine biopsy after heart transplantation in a new era of anti-rejection? Curr Opin Cardiol. 2006;21(2):127–31. doi:10.1097/01.hco.0000210309.71984.30.
32. Costanzo MR, Dipchand A, Starling R, Anderson A, Chan M, Desai S, et al. The International Society of Heart and Lung Transplantation Guidelines for the care of heart transplant recipients. J Heart Lung Transplant. 2010;29(8):914–56. doi:10.1016/j.healun.2010.05.034.
33. Lindenfeld J, Miller GG, Shakar SF, Zolty R, Lowes BD, Wolfel EE, et al. Drug therapy in the heart transplant recipient: part I: cardiac rejection and immunosuppressive drugs. Circulation. 2004;110(24):3734–40. doi:10.1161/01.CIR.0000149745.83186.89.

34. Afzali B, Lombardi G, Lechler RI, Lord GM. The role of T helper 17 (Th17) and regulatory T cells (Treg) in human organ transplantation and autoimmune disease. Clin Exp Immunol. 2007;148(1):32–46. doi:10.1111/j.1365-2249.2007.03356.x.
35. Chadha R, Heidt S, Jones ND, Wood KJ. Th17: contributors to allograft rejection and a barrier to the induction of transplantation tolerance? Transplantation. 2011;91(9):939–45. doi:10.1097/TP.0b013e3182126eeb.
36. Starr TK, Jameson SC, Hogquist KA. Positive and negative selection of T cells. Annu Rev Immunol. 2003;21:139–76. doi:10.1146/annurev.immunol.21.120601.141107.
37. Lechler R, Ng WF, Steinman RM. Dendritic cells in transplantation – friend or foe? Immunity. 2001;14(4):357–68.
38. Vincenti F, Kirkman R, Light S, Bumgardner G, Pescovitz M, Halloran P, et al. Interleukin-2-receptor blockade with daclizumab to prevent acute rejection in renal transplantation. Daclizumab Triple Therapy Study Group. N Eng J Med. 1998;338(3):161–5. doi:10.1056/NEJM199801153380304.
39. Manetti R, Parronchi P, Giudizi MG, Piccinni MP, Maggi E, Trinchieri G, et al. Natural killer cell stimulatory factor (interleukin 12 [IL-12]) induces T helper type 1 (Th1)-specific immune responses and inhibits the development of IL-4-producing Th cells. J Exp Med. 1993;177(4):1199–204.
40. Gately MK, Desai BB, Wolitzky AG, Quinn PM, Dwyer CM, Podlaski FJ, et al. Regulation of human lymphocyte proliferation by a heterodimeric cytokine, IL-12 (cytotoxic lymphocyte maturation factor). J Immunol. 1991;147(3):874–82.
41. Atalar K, Afzali B, Lord G, Lombardi G. Relative roles of Th1 and Th17 effector cells in allograft rejection. Curr Opin Organ Transplant. 2009;14(1):23–9. doi:10.1097/MOT.0b013e32831b70c2.
42. Saiura A, Kohro T, Yamamoto T, Izumi A, Wada Y, Aburatani H, et al. Detection of an up-regulation of a group of chemokine genes in murine cardiac allograft in the absence of interferon-gamma by means of DNA microarray. Transplantation. 2002;73(9):1480–6.
43. Xie A, Wang S, Zhang K, Wang G, Ye P, Li J, et al. Treatment with interleukin-12/23p40 antibody attenuates acute cardiac allograft rejection. Transplantation. 2011;91(1):27–34.
44. Yuan X, Paez-Cortez J, Schmitt-Knosalla I, D'Addio F, Mfarrej B, Donnarumma M, et al. A novel role of CD4 Th17 cells in mediating cardiac allograft rejection and vasculopathy. J Exp Med. 2008;205(13):3133–44. doi:10.1084/jem.20081937.
45. Wang S, Li J, Xie A, Wang G, Xia N, Ye P, et al. Dynamic changes in Th1, Th17, and FoxP3+ T cells in patients with acute cellular rejection after cardiac transplantation. Clin Transplant. 2011;25(2):E177–86. doi:10.1111/j.1399-0012.2010.01362.x.
46. McNally CM, Luckhurst E, Penny R. Cell free serum interleukin-2 receptor levels after heart transplantation. J Heart Lung Transplant. 1991;10(5 Pt 1):769–74.
47. Hutchinson IV, Turner D, Sankaran D, Awad M, Pravica V, Sinnott P. Cytokine genotypes in allograft rejection: guidelines for immunosuppression. Transplant Proc. 1998;30(8):3991–2.
48. Densem CG, Hutchinson IV, Yonan N, Brooks NH. Influence of interleukin-10 polymorphism on the development of coronary vasculopathy following cardiac transplantation. Transpl Immunol. 2003;11(2):223–8. doi:10.1016/S0966-3274(03)00015-7.
49. Tellides G. Th1 adaptive immune responses in cardiac graft arteriosclerosis: deleterious or beneficial? Circulation. 2006;114(15):1561–4. doi:10.1161/CIRCULATIONAHA.106.651521.
50. El-Sawy T, Fahmy NM, Fairchild RL. Chemokines: directing leukocyte infiltration into allografts. Curr Opin Immunol. 2002;14(5):562–8.
51. Campbell JD, Gangur V, Simons FE, HayGlass KT. Allergic humans are hyporesponsive to a CXCR3 ligand-mediated Th1 immunity-promoting loop. FASEB J. 2004;18(2):329–31. doi:10.1096/fj.02-0908fje.
52. Crescioli C, Buonamano A, Scolletta S, Sottili M, Francalanci M, Giomarelli P, et al. Predictive role of pretransplant serum CXCL10 for cardiac acute rejection. Transplantation. 2009;87(2):249–55. doi:10.1097/TP.0b013e3181919f5d.
53. Sathya CJ, Sheshgiri R, Prodger J, Tumiati L, Delgado D, Ross HJ, et al. Correlation between circulating endothelial progenitor cell function and allograft rejection in heart transplant patients. Transpl Int. 2010;23(6):641–8. doi:10.1111/j.1432-2277.2009.01043.x.
54. Bartel DP, Chen CZ. Micromanagers of gene expression: the potentially widespread influence of metazoan microRNAs. Nat Rev Genet. 2004;5(5):396–400. doi:10.1038/nrg1328.
55. Lu LF, Liston A. MicroRNA in the immune system, microRNA as an immune system. Immunology. 2009;127(3):291–8. doi:10.1111/j.1365-2567.2009.03092.x.
56. Xiao C, Rajewsky K. MicroRNA control in the immune system: basic principles. Cell. 2009;136(1):26–36. doi:10.1016/j.cell.2008.12.027.
57. Shan J, Feng L, Luo L, Wu W, Li C, Li S, et al. MicroRNAs: potential biomarker in organ transplantation. Transpl Immunol. 2011;24(4):210–5. doi:10.1016/j.trim.2011.03.004.
58. Suarez-Alvarez B, Lopez-Vazquez A, Gonzalez MZ, Fdez-Morera JL, Diaz-Molina B, Blanco-Gelaz MA, et al. The relationship of anti-MICA antibodies and MICA expression with heart allograft rejection. Am J Transplant. 2007;7(7):1842–8. doi:10.1111/j.1600-6143.2007.01838.x.
59. Hosenpud JD. Noninvasive diagnosis of cardiac allograft rejection. Another of many searches for the grail. Circulation. 1992;85(1):368–71.
60. Kemkes BM, Schutz A, Engelhardt M, Brandl U, Breuer M. Noninvasive methods of rejection diagnosis after heart transplantation. J Heart Lung Transplant. 1992;11(4 Pt 2):S221–31.
61. Carrier M, Russell DH, Davis TP, Emery RW, Copeland JG. Urinary polyamines as markers of cardiac allograft rejection. A clinical evaluation. J Thorac Cardiovasc Surg. 1988;96(5):806–10.
62. Smillie AE, Rigby RJ, Petrie JJ. Monitoring the response to antirejection therapy with serum neopterin. Transplant Proc. 1989;21(1 Pt 2):1869–70.
63. Carrier M, Russell DH, Wild JC, Emery RW, Copeland JG. Prolactin as a marker of rejection in human heart transplantation. J Heart Transplant. 1987;6(5):290–2.
64. Goldman MH, Landwehr DM, Lippman R, Hess M, Wolfgang T, Szentpetery S, et al. Beta 2 microglobulins in rejection and cytomegalovirus infection in a cardiac transplant recipient. Transplant Proc. 1982;14(2):437–9.
65. Hammerer-Lercher A, Mair J, Antretter H, Ruttmann E, Poelzl G, Laufer G, et al. B-type natriuretic peptide as a marker of allograft rejection after heart transplantation. J Heart Lung Transplant. 2005;24(9):1444. doi:10.1016/j.healun.2004.08.018.
66. Cubukcuoglu Deniz G, Durdu S, Akar AR, Ozyurda U. Biotechnology and stem cell research: a glance into the future. Anadolu Kardiyol Derg. 2008;8(4):297–302.
67. Sharma HS, Peters TH, Moorhouse MJ, van der Spek PJ, Bogers AJ. DNA microarray analysis for human congenital heart disease. Cell Biochem Biophys. 2006;44(1):1–9. doi:10.1385/CBB:44:1:001.
68. Ohki R, Yamamoto K, Ueno S, Mano H, Misawa Y, Fuse K, et al. Gene expression profiling of human atrial myocardium with atrial fibrillation by DNA microarray analysis. Int J Cardiol. 2005;102(2):233–8. doi:10.1016/j.ijcard.2004.05.026.
69. Stegall M, Park W, Kim D, Kremers W. Gene expression during acute allograft rejection: novel statistical analysis of microarray data. Am J Transplant. 2002;2(10):913–25.
70. Hollander Z, Lin D, Chen V, Ng R, Wilson-McManus J, Ignaszewski A, et al. Whole blood biomarkers of acute cardiac allograft rejection: double-crossing the biopsy. Transplantation. 2010;90(12):1388–93. doi:10.1097/TP.0b013e3182003df6.
71. Mitchell RN. Allograft arteriopathy: pathogenesis update. Cardiovasc Pathol. 2004;13(1):33–40. doi:10.1016/S1054-8807(03)00108-X.
72. Almenar-Bonet L. Spanish Heart Transplantation Registry. 18th official report of the Spanish Society of Cardiology Working Group on Heart Failure, Heart Transplantation and Associated Therapies (1984–2006). Rev Esp Cardiol. 2007;60(11):1177–87.

73. Julius BK, Attenhofer Jost CH, Sutsch G, Brunner HP, Kuenzli A, Vogt PR, et al. Incidence, progression and functional significance of cardiac allograft vasculopathy after heart transplantation. Transplantation. 2000;69(5):847–53.
74. Mehra MR, Jessup M, Gronda E, Costanzo MR. Rationale and process: International Society for Heart and Lung Transplantation guidelines for the care of cardiac transplant candidates–2006. J Heart Lung Transplant. 2006;25(9):1001–2. doi:10.1016/j.healun.2006.06.006.
75. Schmauss D, Weis M. Cardiac allograft vasculopathy: recent developments. Circulation. 2008;117(16):2131–41. doi:10.1161/CIRCULATIONAHA.107.711911.
76. Salomon RN, Hughes CC, Schoen FJ, Payne DD, Pober JS, Libby P. Human coronary transplantation-associated arteriosclerosis. Evidence for a chronic immune reaction to activated graft endothelial cells. Am J Pathol. 1991;138(4):791–8.
77. Hosenpud JD, Shipley GD, Wagner CR. Cardiac allograft vasculopathy: current concepts, recent developments, and future directions. J Heart Lung Transplant. 1992;11(1 Pt 1):9–23.
78. Hosenpud JD. Immune mechanisms of cardiac allograft vasculopathy: an update. Transpl Immunol. 1993;1(4):237–49.
79. Hosenpud JD, Everett JP, Morris TE, Mauck KA, Shipley GD, Wagner CR. Cardiac allograft vasculopathy. Association with cell-mediated but not humoral alloimmunity to donor-specific vascular endothelium. Circulation. 1995;92(2):205–11.
80. Johnson DE, Gao SZ, Schroeder JS, DeCampli WM, Billingham ME. The spectrum of coronary artery pathologic findings in human cardiac allografts. J Heart Transplant. 1989;8(5):349–59.
81. Heroux AL, Silverman P, Costanzo MR, O'Sullivan EJ, Johnson MR, Liao Y, et al. Intracoronary ultrasound assessment of morphological and functional abnormalities associated with cardiac allograft vasculopathy. Circulation. 1994;89(1):272–7.
82. Kofoed KF, Czernin J, Johnson J, Kobashigawa J, Phelps ME, Laks H, et al. Effects of cardiac allograft vasculopathy on myocardial blood flow, vasodilatory capacity, and coronary vasomotion. Circulation. 1997;95(3):600–6.
83. Behrendt D, Ganz P, Fang JC. Cardiac allograft vasculopathy. Curr Opin Cardiol. 2000;15(6):422–9.
84. Ueland T, Sikkeland LI, Yndestad A, Eiken HG, Holm T, Guevara C, et al. Myocardial gene expression of inflammatory cytokines after heart transplantation in relation to the development of transplant coronary artery disease. Am J Cardiol. 2003;92(6):715–7.
85. van Loosdregt J, van Oosterhout MF, Bruggink AH, van Wichen DF, van Kuik J, de Koning E, et al. The chemokine and chemokine receptor profile of infiltrating cells in the wall of arteries with cardiac allograft vasculopathy is indicative of a memory T-helper 1 response. Circulation. 2006;114(15):1599–607. doi:10.1161/CIRCULATIONAHA.105.597526.
86. Faust SM, Lu G, Marini BL, Zou W, Gordon D, Iwakura Y, et al. Role of T cell TGFbeta signaling and IL-17 in allograft acceptance and fibrosis associated with chronic rejection. J Immunol. 2009;183(11):7297–306. doi:10.4049/jimmunol.0902446.
87. Schober A, Hristov M, Kofler S, Forbrig R, Lohr B, Heussen N, et al. CD34+ CD140b+ cells and circulating CXCL12 correlate with the angiographically assessed severity of cardiac allograft vasculopathy. Eur Heart J. 2011;32(4):476–84. doi:10.1093/eurheartj/ehq402.
88. Raichlin E, Bae JH, Kushwaha SS, Lennon RJ, Prasad A, Rihal CS, et al. Inflammatory burden of cardiac allograft coronary atherosclerotic plaque is associated with early recurrent cellular rejection and predicts a higher risk of vasculopathy progression. J Am Coll Cardiol. 2009;53(15):1279–86. doi:10.1016/j.jacc.2008.12.041.
89. Sanchez-Gomez JM, Martinez-Dolz L, Sanchez-Lazaro I, Almenar L, Sanchez-Lacuesta E, Munoz-Giner B, et al. Influence of metabolic syndrome on development of cardiac allograft vasculopathy in the transplanted heart. Transplantation. 2012;93(1):106–11. doi:10.1097/TP.0b013e3182398058.
90. Tona F, Marra MP, Fedrigo M, Famoso G, Bellu R, Thiene G, et al. Recent developments on coronary microvasculopathy after heart transplantation: a new target in the therapy of cardiac allograft vasculopathy. Curr Vasc Pharmacol. 2012;10(2):206–15.

Platelet Activation After Lung Transplantation

46

David Sternberg and Joshua Sonett

Introduction

Initially recognized for their central role in thrombosis, there has been an emerging understanding that platelets also play an important role in both the innate as well as the adaptive immune response. The profound impact and putative role of platelet activation in both acute and chronic allograft failure after lung transplant are just beginning to be truly appreciated. To understand this multifactorial interaction, one must first understand the basics of platelet physiology. Produced through a budding process by megakaryocytes in the bone marrow, platelets have an average lifespan of 5–10 days. Normally, there are approximately $200–400 \times 10^3$ circulating platelets per microliter. The average volume of each platelet is approximately 7 fl, giving each anucleate cell an average surface area of 8 μm^2. This important fact implies that the total surface area of platelets outnumbers that of all other circulating leukocyte types combined [1].

Each platelet is composed of an open canalicular system as well as three biochemically distinct cellular compartments, alpha granules, dense granules, and lysozomes. During platelet activation, an exocytosis process causes the release of over 300 proteins, many of which directly modulate the immune system [2, 3]. Alpha granules, in particular, contain high concentrations of platelet factor 4 (PF4) and β-thromboglobulin [4–7]. These platelet-derived CXC chemokines bind chemokine receptor CXCR1 and CXCR2, and, in the presence of TNF-α, induce neutrophil adhesion to endothelium [8, 9]. Platelets simultaneously release a variety of proinflammatory cytokines, such as interleukin-1, which further upregulates endothelial adhesion receptors, as well as the powerful immune chemoattractants, interleukin 8, MCP-1, and RANTES [10–14]. Release of ADP, serotonin, and thromboxane A2 further upregulates local inflammatory processes and induces endothelial permeability and vasoconstriction [15–17].

D. Sternberg, MD (✉)
Lung Transplant Program, Henry Ford Health System, K-14 2799 West Grand Blvd, Detroit, MI 48202, USA
e-mail: dsternb1@hfhs.org

J. Sonett, MD
Lung Transplant Program, General Thoracic Surgery, Columbia University Medical Center, PH Room 104, 14th Floor, 622 West 168th St, New York, NY 10032, USA
e-mail: js2106@columbia.edu

Platelet Activation

During platelet activation, the conformational status and concentration of a variety of surface receptors are altered by activation of endogenous biochemical circuits and by the exocytic process itself. The most abundant surface receptor, integrin $\alpha_{IIb}\beta_3$, undergoes a conformational change during platelet activation that is referred to as "inside out" when initiated by intracellular ligand binding or "outside in" when mediated by engagement of external signaling domains [18–20]. Activated $\alpha_{IIb}\beta_3$ binds fibrinogen, which crosslinks activated platelets, forming platelet aggregates, and also mediates adhesion to intercellular adhesion molecules (ICAMS), which are expressed on endothelial surfaces [21, 22]. Platelets also express integrin $\alpha_2\beta_1$, which is a collagen receptor that mediates platelet activation upon co-stimulation by GPVI [23, 24]. This is an important nexus between the thrombotic and inflammatory pathways. Similarly, GP1b-IX binds von Willebrand factor, which induces platelet activation, cross-linking, and aggregate formation [25, 26]. P-Selectin is an important transmembrane receptor nominally stored in α-granules whose concentration on the platelet surface rapidly increased after exocytosis. P-selectin binds P-selectin glycoprotein ligand-1 (PSGL-1), which is expressed on leukocytes and represents an important mechanism by which activated platelets initiate and form aggregates with leukocytes [27–29]. Recently, relatively high concentrations of Toll-like receptors (TLRs), types 2, 4, and 9, have also been reported on platelets [30, 31]. These ancient receptors are expressed on immune cells and recognize common conserved

E.A. Gabriel, S.A. Gabriel (eds.), *Inflammatory Response in Cardiovascular Surgery*,
DOI 10.1007/978-1-4471-4429-8_46, © Springer-Verlag London 2013

microbial motifs; they thus represent a form of innate non-self recognition. This discovery supports a role for platelets upstream in the innate immune response [32]. Thus, platelet activation is a key early event that links, recruits, and ultimately upregulates both leukocytes and endothelial cells in both the thrombotic as well as the immune pathways.

Circulating platelets form immunologically active aggregates with leukocytes, particularly monocytes [25]. Other than aggregate formation, however, the presence of these activated platelets strongly affects leukocyte function. After binding, NF-kappa B translocates to the monocyte nucleus, signifying that the master cellular control switch has been set to a proinflammatory setting [33]. Interleukin-8, tumor necrosis factor-α, and MCP-1 production are all strongly upregulated, as is surface expression of PSGL-1 and CD-16, which increases the adhesive capacity of monocytes to the vascular endothelium [34–37]. Platelets also directly bind and interact with endothelial cells in a highly reflexive manner. Activated endothelial surfaces express PSGL-1, P-selectin, ICAM-1,GP-1b, as well as the important co-stimulatory CD-40 receptor, which mediate stable platelet and platelet-leukocyte aggregate adhesion to the endothelium [38, 39]. CD40 ligand is stored in platelet granules and released shortly after $\alpha_{IIb}\beta_3$ ligand engagement [40, 41]. Platelet factor 4 release has also been shown to stimulate NF-kappa B nuclear migration, activating a proinflammatory endothelial phenotype that is hallmarked by the release of P-selectin-laden Weibel-Palade bodies [42]. A multidirectional relationship among the platelets, leukocytes, and endothelium thus exists whereby any participant can recruit and stimulate the other party and thus induce or propagate local inflammatory signals.

Clinical Consequences of Platelet Activation

The clinical consequences of platelet activation have long been recognized for their importance in thrombotic vascular disease. Recently, however, recognition that platelet activation may be important in inflammatory disease is gaining traction as well. Platelets have been implicated in the development of acute lung injury (ALI) and acute respiratory distress syndrome (ARDS). Analysis of lung biopsy specimens in these patients shows platelet aggregate deposition in both ARDS patients and those with ALI after acid aspiration [43, 44]. Idell and Niewiarowski have shown that the degree of platelet activation, inferred from the concentration of platelet α-granule specific proteins in bronchial lavage fluid, correlated well with clinical severity scores [45]. Furthermore, murine models of ALI have shown that inhibiting P-selectin-mediated platelet neutrophil interactions abrogate lung injury after intrapulmonary acid instillation [46]. Support for a pathological role in pulmonary leukocyte trafficking is also derived from asthmatic bronchial biopsy specimens [47]. Indeed, allergen challenging of asthmatic patients increases peripheral circulating activated platelet leukocyte complexes while transfusing thrombocytopenic murine models of asthma restored pulmonary inflammation [48]. Multiple lines of evidence, including increases in platelet-derived soluble CD40L, also suggest that platelets participate in the chronic pulmonary inflammatory processes that are the hallmark of cystic fibrosis (CF) [49, 50]. Platelets have also been implicated in the pathophysiology of primary pulmonary hypertension (PPH), although the exact mechanism remains unclear [51]. Many patients with PPH have chronic levels of thrombocytopenia, and clinical studies suggest 87 % of adult patients with PPH have abnormal platelet aggregration [52]. Indeed, high concentrations of platelet-derived soluble CD40L have been reported in PPH patients [53]. Injured pulmonary arterial endothelium is a central thesis in this disease, but platelets also seem to be recruited and operative within this process [51]. Reports of platelet activation as a contributory event in the pathophysiology of sepsis have been suggestive, but far from conclusive. Reports of increased platelet aggregation in sepsis have been inconsistent, although more recent evidence seems to support the case for diffuse platelet activation and aggregate formation with pulmonary trapping [54–57]. Furthermore, inhibition of platelet neutrophil binding mitigates sepsis, at least in animal models of abdominal sepsis [58]. It seems highly likely then, especially since the discovery of Toll-like receptors on their surface, that platelets participate in the physiology of sepsis, although the exact role has yet to be fully elucidated.

Platelet Activation After Transplant

A putative role for platelet activation during acute post-transplant graft dysfunction after solid organ transplant has also been scrutinized. Ischemia and reperfusion injury (I/RI) is thought to injure the vascular endothelium and induce a global “activated” phenotype. Injured endothelium expresses platelet receptors that mediate platelet as well as leukocyte adhesion and could be an important injury mechanism. After liver transplant in a rat model, platelets have been shown to mediate endothelial apoptosis in hepatic sinusoids [59–61]. Another interesting observation from this model was the discovery that thrombocytopenia inversely correlated strongly with ischemic time. Additionally, after reperfusion injury in a clinical study, increased concentrations of activated platelets can be detected in the circulation for days, unlike control transplants without reperfusion injury [62]. Platelet deposition has been reported in livers, kidney, intestine, and pancreas grafts and in rat cardiac allografts [63–66]. Platelet deposition has also now been linked with overall graft function. For example, increased platelet deposition correlated with elevated post-transplant creatinine after kidney transplantation [65]. Thrombocytopenia has been observed after liver transplant and correlates poorly with survival.

Platelet activation also seems to be a key injury mechanism during allo- or xenograft hyperacute rejection [67–69]. It is known that both complement and humoral mechanisms strongly activate platelets and co-injure vascular endothelium during hyperacute rejection. Vascular permeability, tissue edema, and leukocyte infiltration all ensue. Simultaneous platelet-mediated activation of the coagulation cascade causes a microthrombotic failure of organ perfusion and graft loss. Platelet activation lies at the fulcrum of these events and has thus served as an appealing therapeutic target, given its key role in both pathways. Multiple groups have reported prolonged graft function and therefore partial success with the use of $\alpha_{IIb}\beta_3$ antagonists in cardiac xenograft models [70, 71]. Similarly, blockade of GP1b-mediated platelet aggregation, inhibition of ADP-mediated platelet activation, and platelet-activating factor antagonism have all prolonged cardiac xenograft failure [72–74]. Platelet antagonism with GP1b and $\alpha_{IIb}\beta_3$ inhibitors has also been favorably evaluated in rabbit to dog and guinea pig to rat lung xenotransplant models as well as isolated guinea pig lungs perfused with whole heparinized human blood [75, 76].

Platelet Activation and Pulmonary Reperfusion Injury

Lung grafts, in particular, are a cogent model to study platelet endothelial cell interaction because of the high degree of vascularity, low pressure/high flow perfusion characteristics, and exquisite organ sensitivity to edema. Reperfusion injury can be studied in situ after cross-clamping the pulmonary artery for a variable period of time and then permitting reperfusion for further periods of time, or it can be studied after transplantation. Although studied directly in humans after lung transplant, this has proven to be exceedingly hard to do directly for a variety of reasons. First, all grafts used in clinical lung transplant are exposed to variable periods of a severely deranged hormonal and neuroendocrine environment after brain death that could stimulate endothelial dysfunction and predispose to platelet activation well before the transplant is contemplated. Second, since no two transplants have exactly the same periods of ischemia, consistent data collection is challenging. Third, the use of cardiopulmonary bypass itself causes platelet activation and deposition in the lungs. Fourth, patients that come to lung transplant themselves suffer a variety of ailments, some of which are thought to involve variable degrees of platelet activation, such as primary pulmonary hypertension. Fifth, some patients, such as those with interstitial lung disease, are heavily immunosuppressed prior to transplant, and this may effect platelet leukocyte interaction in the graft during reperfusion injury. Sixth, it is impractical to obtain lung biopsies at meaningful time frames after transplant, as these patients have already been transported to the intensive care unit.

Despite these limitations, much has been learned, both from animal studies and from clinical investigations. Platelet deposition was first reported in a careful pathological study of canine lung grafts as early as 1978 by Hoyer et al. [77]. This observation was later repeated in humans when Zenati performed post-mortem analysis of five lung transplant recipients who succumbed to primary graft failure in 1990 [78]. In 1997, Okada observed increasing platelet deposition in rat lung grafts with incrementally prolonged ischemic times [79]. He also made the important observation that ischemia time correlated with the severity of reperfusion injury, determined functionally and via histological severity scores. When the platelet inhibitor, beraprost sodium, was administered prior to lung transplant in rats, reperfusion injury – measured morphologically by the severity of capillary congestion, tissue edema, and graft flow – were all improved in comparison to untreated control animals [80]. This led to a specific focus on P-selectin-mediated signaling because it is critical for platelet adhesion to endothelial surfaces as well as the recruitment of leukocytes into immunologically active aggregates with platelets. In 1997, Naka et al. used an antibody to abrogate P-selectin signaling and P-selectin-deficient lines of Lewis rats to study reperfusion injury after transplant. He reported improved oxygenation, pulmonary vascular resistance, and overall survival in isogenic animals in lung grafts in animals without intact P-selectin signaling [81]. These results were supported by Roberts who also blocked P-selectin binding and then directly observed a decrease in platelet rolling and adhesion in sub-pleural arterioles after 2 h of warm ischemia in rabbits [82]. In 2004, Colombat directly observed platelet aggregation and increased surface P-selectin expression in human lung grafts after 15–30 min of reperfusion [83]. Furthermore, Colombat noted that increased P-selectin expression correlated with clinical markers of primary graft dysfunction, such as prolonged mechanical ventilation, decreased oxygenation, and pulmonary edema assessed by chest radiograph [83]. In 2008, we reported increased concentrations of two circulating markers of platelet activation, soluble P-selectin and soluble CD40 ligand, as well as increased concentrations of circulating platelet-monocyte aggregates 6 h after clinical lung transplantation [84]. In 2009, Kawut reported a correlation between increased soluble P-selectin levels and primary graft dysfunction at both 6 and 24 h after lung transplant [85]. Thus, a significant body of evidence in both clinical lung transplant and a variety of animal models supports a central critical role for platelet activation in pulmonary reperfusion injury.

Anti-Platelet Therapy and Transplant

Despite the theoretical appeal of an antagonist of platelet activation from a reperfusion-oriented perspective, unfortunately and yet quite legitimately, concerns regarding hemorrhage have limited surgical enthusiasm for many of these antiplatelet agents. However, despite the elegant, intricate, and reflexive nature of the inflammatory and thrombotic pathways, it cannot be wholly and honestly said that the two pathways are necessarily inseparable. Furthermore, because the therapeutic intent would be diminution of platelet activation without complete incapacitation, there may be a clinical safety margin of platelet inhibition before a point where surgical blood loss might become inelegant. Platelet inhibitors in routine use that do not pose significant surgical challenges, such as aspirin or persantine, may be useful in this regard, but this question has not yet been extensively studied after lung transplant [86, 87]. Additional targets such as CD40 ligand, CD 154, PDGL-1, and platelet activating factor, have been suggested because these molecules specifically focus on platelet-endothelial interaction and not platelet co-aggregation, cross-linking, and clot nucleation [67, 88].

Conclusion

Lung transplant remains the most successful option for patients with irreversible symptomatic respiratory failure. However, primary graft dysfunction after transplant causes a high degree of morbidity and further predisposes to chronic rejection, graft loss, and death. A significant body of evidence has now established platelet activation as a key event in a variety of pathological inflammatory states that affect the lungs and solid organ transplants. Evidence that directly implicates platelets in pulmonary reperfusion injury is mounting to such an extent that, despite surgical fear of platelet inhibitors, these little cells can no longer be ignored from an immunological point of view. Much bench work remains to be done before the surgical apprehension of platelet inhibition can be assuaged by dreams of smoother postoperative graft function.

References

1. Bonfanti R, Furie BC, Furie B, Wagner DD. PADGEM (GMP140) is a component of Weibel Palade bodies of human endothelial cells. Blood. 1989;73:1109–12.
2. Coppinger JA CG, Toomey S, Kislinger T, Belton O, McRedmond JP, Cahill DJ, et al. Characterization of the proteins released from activated platelets leads to localization of novel platelet proteins in human atherosclerotic lesions. Blood. 2004;103:2096–104.
3. Italiano Jr JE, Battinelli EM. Selective sorting of alpha-granule proteins. J Thromb Haemost. 2009;7 Suppl 1:173–6.
4. Brandt E, Ludwig A, Petersen F, Flad HD. Platelet-derived CXC chemokines: old players in new games. Immunol Rev. 2000;177: 204–16.
5. Power CA, Furness RB, Brawand C, Wells TN. Cloning of a full-length cDNA encoding the neutrophil-activating peptide ENA-78 from human platelets. Gene. 1994;151:333–4.
6. Ravindran R, Krishnan LK. A biochemical study on the effect of proteolysis of beta-thromboglobulin proteins released from activated platelets on fibroblast proliferation. Pathophysiol Haemost Thromb. 2007;36:285–9.
7. Resmi KR, Krishnan LK. Protease action and generation of beta-thromboglobulin-like protein followed by platelet activation. Thromb Res. 2002;107:23–9.
8. Kasper B, Brandt E, Bulfone-Paus S, Petersen F. Platelet factor 4 (PF-4)-induced neutrophil adhesion is controlled by src-kinases, whereas PF-4-mediated exocytosis requires the additional activation of p38 MAP kinase and phosphatidylinositol 3-kinase. Blood. 2003;103:1602–10.
9. Petersen F, Bock L, Flad HD, Brandt E. Platelet factor 4-induced neutrophil-endothelial cell interaction: involvement of mechanisms and functional consequences different from those elicited by interleukin-8. Blood. 1999;94:4020–8.
10. Hawrylowicz CM, Santoro SA, Platt FM, Unanue ER. Activated platelets express IL-1 activity. J Immunol. 1989;143:4015–8.
11. Hawrylowicz CM HG, Feldmann M. Platelet-derived interleukin 1 induces human endothelial adhesion molecule expression and cytokine production. J Exp Med. 1991;174:785–90.
12. Kameyoshi Y, Dörschner A, Mattel AI, Christopher E, Schroder JM. Cytokine RANTES released by thrombin-stimulated platelets is a potent attractant for human eosinophils. J Exp Med. 1992;176: 587–92.
13. Klinger MH WD, Bubel S, Sticherling M, Schröder JM, Kühnel W. Immunocytochemical localization of the chemokines RANTES and MIP-1 alpha within human platelets and their release during storage. Int Arch Allergy Immunol. 1995;107:541–6.
14. Schober A, Zernecke A, Liehn EA, von Hundelshausen P, Knarren S, Kuziel WA, et al. Crucial role of the CCL2/CCR2 axis in neointimal hyperplasia after arterial injury in hyperlipidemic mice involves early monocyte recruitment and CCL2 presentation on platelets. Circ Res. 2004;95:1125–33.
15. Ashby B, Daniel J, Smith JB. Mechanisms of platelet activation and inhibition. Hematol Oncol Clin North Am. 1990;4:1–26.
16. Li Z, Delaney M, O'Brien KA, Du X. Signaling during platelet adhesion and activation. Arterioscler Thromb Vasc Biol. 2010;30:2341–9.
17. Offermanns S. Activation of platelet function through G protein-coupled receptors. Circ Res. 2006;99:1293–304.
18. Tadokoro S, Shattil SJ, Eto K, Tai V, Liddington RC, de Pereda JM, et al. Talin binding to integrin beta tails: a final common step in integrin activation. Science. 2003;302:103–6.
19. Moser M, Nieswandt B, Ussar S, Pozgajova M, Fässler R. Kindlin-3 is essential for integrin activation and platelet aggregation. Nat Med. 2008;14:325–30.
20. Leisner TM, Wencel-Drake J, Wang W, Lam SC. Bidirectional transmembrane modulation of integrin alphaIIbbeta3 conformations. J Biol Chem. 1999;274:12945–9.
21. Li JM, Podolsky RS, Rohrer MJ, Cutler BS, Massie MT, Barnard MR, et al. Adhesion of activated platelets to venous endothelial cells is mediated via GPIIb/IIIa. J Surg Res. 1996;61:543–8.
22. Bombeli T, Schwartz BR, Harlan JM. Adhesion of activated platelets to endothelial cells: evidence for a GPIIbIIIa-dependent bridging mechanism and novel roles for endothelial intercellular adhesion molecule 1 (ICAM-1), alphavbeta3 integrin, and GPIbalpha. J Exp Med. 1998;187:329–39.
23. Clemetson KJ, Clemetson JM. Platelet collagen receptors. Thromb Haemost. 2001;86:189–97.
24. Ezumi Y, Shindoh K, Tsuji M, Takayama H. Physical and functional association of the Src family kinases Fyn and Lyn with the collagen receptor glycoprotein VI-Fc receptor gamma chain complex on human platelets. J Exp Med. 1998;188:267–76.

25. Arya M, López JA, Romo GM, Cruz MA, Kasirer-Friede A, Shattil SJ, et al. Glycoprotein Ib-IX-mediated activation of integrin alpha(IIb)beta(3): effects of receptor clustering and von Willebrand factor adhesion. J Thromb Haemost. 2003;1:1150–7.
26. Du X. Signaling and regulation of the platelet glycoprotein Ib-IX-V complex. Curr Opin Hematol. 2007;14(3):262–9.
27. Yang J, Furie BC, Furie B. The biology of P-selectin glycoprotein ligand-1: its role as a selectin counterreceptor in leukocyte-endothelial and leukocyte-platelet. Thromb Haemost. 1999;81:1–7.
28. Diacovo TG, Roth SJ, Buccola JM, Bainton DF, Springer TA. Neutrophil rolling, arrest, and transmigration across activated, surface-adherent platelets via sequential action of P-selectin and the beta 2-integrin CD11b/CD18. Blood. 1996;183:1193–203.
29. Palabrica T, Lobb R, Furie BC, Aronivitz M, Benjamin C, Hsu Y-M, et al. Leukocyte accumulation promoting fibrin deposition is mediated in vivo by P-selectin on adherent platelets. Nature. 1992;359:848–51.
30. Cognasse F, Hamzeh H, Chavarin P, Acquart S, Genin C, Garraud O. Evidence of Toll-like receptor molecules on human platelets. Immunol Cell Biol. 2005;83:196–8.
31. Aslam R, Speck ER, Kim M, Crow AR, Bang KW, Nestel FP, et al. Platelet Toll-like receptor expression modulates lipopolysaccharide-induced thrombocytopenia and tumor necrosis factor-alpha production in vivo. Blood. 2006;107:637–41.
32. Cox D, Kerrigan S, Watson SP. Platelets and the innate immune system: mechanisms of bacterial-induced platelet activation. J Thromb Haemost. 2011;9:1097–107.
33. Dixon DA, Tolley ND, Bemis-Standoli K, Martinez ML, Weyrich AS, Morrow JD, et al. Expression of COX-2 in platelet-monocyte interactions occurs via combinatorial regulation involving adhesion and cytokine signaling. J Clin Invest. 2006;116:2727–38.
34. da Costa Martins PA, van Gils JM, Mol A, Hordijk PL, Zwaginga JJ. Platelet binding to monocytes increases the adhesive properties of monocytes by up-regulating the expression and functionality of beta1 and beta2 integrins. J Leukoc Biol. 2006;79:499–507.
35. Weyrich AS MT, McEver RP, Prescott SM, Zimmerman GA. Monocyte tethering by P-selectin regulates monocyte chemotactic protein-1 and tumor necrosis factor-α secretion. J Clin Invest. 1995;95:2297–303.
36. Weyrich AS, Elstad MR, McEver RP, McIntyre TM, Moore KL, Morrissey JH, et al. Activated platelets signal chemokine synthesis by human monocytes. J Clin Invest. 1996;97:1525–34.
37. Passacquale G, Vamadevan P, Pereira L, Hamid C, Corrigall V, Ferro A. Monocyte-platelet interaction induces a pro-inflammatory phenotype in circulating monocytes. PLoS One. 2011;6:e25595.
38. Langer HF, Gawaz M. Platelet-vessel wall interactions in atherosclerotic disease. Thromb Haemost. 2008;99:480–6.
39. Gawaz M, Brand K, Dickfeld T, Pogatsa-Murray G, Page S, Bogner C, et al. Platelets induce alterations of chemotactic and adhesive properties of endothelial cells mediated through an interleukin-1-dependent mechanism. Implications for atherogenesis. Atherosclerosis. 2000;148:75–85.
40. May AE, Kälsch T, Massberg S, Herouy Y, Schmidt R, Gawaz M. Engagement of glycoprotein IIb/IIIa (alpha(IIb)beta3) on platelets upregulates CD40L and triggers CD40L-dependent matrix degradation by endothelial cells. Circulation. 2002;106:2111–7.
41. Henn V, Slupsky JR, Gräfe M, Anagnostopoulos I, Förster R, Müller-Berghaus G, et al. CD40 ligand on activated platelets triggers an inflammatory reaction of endothelial cells. Nature. 1998;391:591–4.
42. Yu G, Rux AH, Ma P, Bdeir K, Sachais BS. Endothelial expression of E-selectin is induced by the platelet-specific chemokine platelet factor 4 through LRP in an NF-kappaB-dependent manner. Blood. 2005;105:3545–51.
43. Bone RC, Francis P, Pierce AK. Intravascular coagulation associated with the adult respiratory distress syndrome. Am J Med. 1976;61:585–9.
44. Zarbock A, Ley K. The role of platelets in acute lung injury (ALI). Front Biosci. 2009;1:150–8.
45. Idell S, Maunder R, Fein AM, Switalska HI, Tuszynski GP, McLarty J, et al. Platelet-specific alpha granule proteins and thrombospondin in bronchoalveolar lavage in the adult respiratory distress syndrome. Chest. 1989;96:1125–32.
46. Zarbock A, Singbartl K, Ley K. Complete reversal of acid-induced acute lung injury by blocking of platelet-neutrophil aggregation. J Clin Invest. 2006;116:3211–9.
47. Jeffery PK, Wardlaw A, Nelson FC, Collins JV, Kay AB. Bronchial biopsies in asthma: an ultrastructural, quantitative study and correlation. With hyperreactivity. Am Rev Respir Dis. 1989;140:1745–53.
48. Pitchford SC, Yano H, Lever R, Riffo-Vasquez Y, Ciferri S, Rose MJ, et al. Platelets are essential for leukocyte recruitment in allergic inflammation. J Allergy Clin Immunol. 2003;112:109–18.
49. O'Sullivan BP, Michelson A. The inflammatory role of platelets in cystic fibrosis. Am J Respir Crit Care Med. 2006;173:483–90.
50. Falco A, Romano M, Lapichino L, Collura M, Davi G. Increased soluble CD40 ligand levels in cystic fibrosis. J Thromb Haemost. 2004;2:557–60.
51. Herve P, Humbert M, Sitbon O, Parent F, Nunes H, Legal C, et al. Pathobiology of pulmonary hypertension. The role of platelets and thrombosis. Clin Chest Med. 2001;22:451–8.
52. Friedman R, Mears J, Barst RJ. Continuous infusion of prostacyclin normalizes plasma markers of endothelial cell injury and platelet aggregation in primary pulmonary hypertension. Circulation. 1997;96:2782–4.
53. Damås JK, Otterdal K, Yndestad A, Aass H, Solum NO, Frøland SS, et al. Soluble CD40 ligand in pulmonary arterial hypertension: possible pathogenic role of the interaction between platelets and endothelial cells. Circulation. 2004;110:999–1005.
54. Yaguchi A, Lobo FL, Vincent JL, Pradier O. Platelet function in sepsis. J Thromb Haemost. 2004;2:2096–102.
55. Gawaz M, Dickfeld T, Bogner C, Fateh-Moghadam S, Neumann FJ. Platelet function in septic multiple organ dysfunction syndrome. Intensive Care Med. 1997;23:379–85.
56. Saba HI, Saba SR, Morelli G, Hartmann RC. Endotoxin mediated inhibition of human platelet aggregation. Thromb Res. 1984;34:19–33.
57. Ogura H, Kawasak T, Tanaka H, Koh T, Tanaka R, Ozeki Y, et al. Activated platelets enhance microparticle formation and platelet-leukocyte interaction in severe trauma and sepsis. J Trauma. 2001;50:801–9.
58. Asaduzzaman M, Lavasani S, Rahman M, Zhang S, Braun OO, Jeppsson B, et al. Platelets support pulmonary recruitment of neutrophils in abdominal sepsis. Crit Care Med. 2009;37:1389–96.
59. Sindram D, Porte RJ, Hoffman MR, Bentley RC, Clavien PA. Platelets induce sinusoidal endothelial cell apoptosis upon reperfusion of the cold ischemic rat liver. Gastroenterology. 2000;118:183–91.
60. Cywes R, Packham MA, Tietze L, Sanabria JR, Harvey PR, Phillips MJ, et al. Role of platelets in hepatic allograft preservation injury in the rat. Hepatology. 1993;18:635–47.
61. Ilona TA, Pereboom I, Lisman T, Porte RJ. Platelets in liver transplantation: friend or foe? Liver Transpl. 2008;14:923–31.
62. Esch JS, Jurk K, Knoefel WT, Roeder G, Voss H, Tustas RY, et al. Platelet activation and increased tissue factor expression on monocytes in reperfusion injury following orthotopic liver transplantation. Platelets. 2010;21:348–59.
63. Jassem W, Koo D, Cerundolo L, Rela M, Heaton ND, Fuggle SV. Cadaveric versus living-donor livers: differences in inflammatory markers after transplantation. Transplantation. 2003;76:1599–603.
64. Massberg S, Enders G, Leiderer R, Eisenmenger S, Vestweber D, Krombach F, et al. Platelet- endothelial cell interactions during ischemia/reperfusion: the role of P-selectin. Blood. 1998;92:507–15.

65. Koo DD, Welsh K, Roake JA, Morris PJ, Fuggle SV. Ischemia/reperfusion injury in human kidney transplantation: an immunohistochemical analysis of changes after reperfusion. Am J Pathol. 1998;153:557–66.
66. Lefer AM CB, Scalia R, Lefer DJ. Synergism between platelets and neutrophils in provoking cardiac dysfunction after ischemia and reperfusion: role of selectins. Circulation. 1998;98:1322–8.
67. Kirk AD, Morrell CN, Baldwin 3rd WM. Platelets influence vascularized organ transplants from start to finish. Am J Transplant. 2009;9:14–22.
68. Bustos M, Saadi S, Platt JL. Platelet-mediated activation of endothelial cells: implications for the pathogenesis of transplant rejection. Transplantation. 2001;72:509–15.
69. Daniels LJ, Platt JL. Hyperacute xenograft rejection as an immunologic barrier to xenotransplantation. Kidney Int Arch Allergy Immunol. 1997;51:S28.
70. Candinas D, Lesnikoski BA, Hancock WW, Otsu I, Koyamada N, Dalmasso AP, et al. Inhibition of platelet integrin GPIIbIIIa prolongs survival of discordant cardiac xenografts. Transplantation. 1996;62:1–5.
71. Lesnikoski BA, Candinas D, Hancock WW, Otsu I, Siegel J, Bach FH, et al. Inhibition of platelet GPIIbIIIa prolongs survival of discordant cardiac xenografts. Transplant Proc. 1996;28:703.
72. Chen G, Wei Q, Wang XM, Wang WY, Xiong YL, Chen S. TMVA, a novel GPIb-binding protein, significantly prevents platelet microthrombi formation and prolongs discordant cardiac xenograft survival. Xenotransplantation. 2004;11:203.
73. Koyamada N, Miyatake T, Candinas D, Hechenleitner P, Siegel J, Hancock WW, et al. Apyrase administration prolongs discordant xenograft survival. Transplantation. 1996;62:1739–43.
74. Makowka L, Chapman FA, Cramer DV, Qian SG, Sun H, Starzl TE. Platelet activating factor and hyperacute rejection. The effect of a platelet-activating factor antagonist, SRI 63–441, on rejection of xenografts and allografts in sensitized hosts. Transplantation. 1990;50:359.
75. Nonaka M, Kadokura M, Kunimura T, Kataoka D, Yamamoto S, Michihata T, et al. Organ perfusion combined with platelet aggregation inhibitor reduce IgM deposition and hyperacute xenorejection in a guinea pig-to-rat lung transplantation model. Transplant Proc. 2002;34:2749–51.
76. Onozuka N, Harada O, Kobayashi M, Suto T, Fukuda A, Sudo Y, et al. Effect of prostacyclin and glycoprotein IIb/IIIa inhibitor on hyperacute rejection in a rabbit-to-dog lung xenotransplant model. Transplant Proc. 2003;35:531–2.
77. Hoyer J, Lebreui G, Sicardi F, Noirclerc M. Effects of experimental lung transplantation on blood coagulation and platelets. Eur Surg Res. 1974;6:110–6.
78. Zenati M, Yousem SA, Dowling RD, Stein KL, Griffith BP, Zenati M, et al. Primary graft failure following pulmonary transplantation. Transplantation. 1990;50:165–7.
79. Okada Y, Marchevsky AM, Zuo XJ, Pass JA, Kass RM, Matloff JM, et al. Accumulation of platelets in rat syngeneic lung transplants: a potential factor responsible for preservation-reperfusion injury. Transplantation. 1997;64:801–6.
80. Okada Y, Marchevsky AM, Kass RM, Matloff JM, Jordan SC. A stable prostacyclin analog, beraprost sodium, attenuates platelet accumulation and preservation-reperfusion injury of isografts in a rat model of lung transplantation. Transplantation. 1998;66:1132–6.
81. Naka Y, Toda K, Kayano K, Oz MC, Pinsky DJ. Failure to express the P-selectin gene or P-selectin blockade confers early pulmonary protection after lung ischemia or transplantation. Proc Natl Acad Sci USA. 1997;94:757–61.
82. Roberts AM, Ovechkin A, Mowbray JG, Robinson TW, Lominadze D. Effects of pulmonary ischemia-reperfusion on platelet adhesion in subpleural arterioles in rabbits. Microvasc Res. 2004;67:29–37.
83. Colombat M, Castier Y, Lesèche G, Rufat P, Mal H, Thabut G, et al. Early expression of adhesion molecules after lung transplantation: evidence for a role of aggregated P-selectin-positive platelets in human primary graft failure. J Heart Lung Transplant. 2004;23:1087–92.
84. Sternberg DI, Shimbo D, Kawut SM, Sarkar J, Hurlitz G, D'Ovidio F, et al. Platelet activation in the postoperative period after lung transplantation. J Thorac Cardiovasc Surg. 2008;135:679–84.
85. Kawut SM, Okun J, Shimbo D, Lederer DJ, De Andrade J, Lama V, et al. Soluble p-selectin and the risk of primary graft dysfunction after lung transplantation. Chest. 2009;136:237–44.
86. Grotz W, Siebig S, Olschewski M, Strey CW, Peter K. Low-dose aspirin therapy is associated with improved allograft function and prolonged allograft survival after kidney transplantation. Transplantation. 2004;77:1848–53.
87. Murphy GJ, Taha R, Windmill DC, Metcalfe M, Nicholson ML. Influence of aspirin on early allograft thrombosis and chronic allograft nephropathy following renal transplantation. Br J Surg. 2001;88:261–6.
88. Wittwer T, Grote M, Oppelt P, Franke U, Schaefers HJ, Wahlers T. Impact of PAF antagonist BN 52021 (Ginkolide B) on post-ischemic graft function in clinical lung transplantation. J Heart Lung Transplant. 2001;20:358–63.

Role of BNP in Pediatric Heart Transplantation

47

Marcelo Biscegli Jatene and Estela Azeka

Introduction

The role of hormonal changes and biomarkers has been studied after heart transplantation; they include B-type natriuretic peptide (BNP), atrial natriuretic peptide (ANP), adrenomedullin (ADM), cardiac troponin T (cTnT), C-reactive protein (CRP), endothelial growth factor, glycoprotein 130, and cytokines, such as tumor necrosis factor α (TNF), interleukin 1 beta (IL-1ß), and interleukin 6 (IL-6) [1].

Studies with electron microscopy of atrial and ventricular muscle cells made by Kisch in 1963 [2] and Jamieson and Palade in 1964 [3] marked the beginning of the research on polypeptide hormones called natriuretic factors and the atrial natriuretic factor (ANF). In 1981, Bold [4] experimentally tested the actions of these polypeptides. They had a characteristically high biological natriuretic response, drop in blood pressure, and increased hematocrit values [4–7].

Natriuretic peptides are a family that consists of three main components: atrial natriuretic peptide (ANP), brain natriuretic peptide (BNP), and C-type natriuretic peptide (CNP), in addition to urodilatin, a peptide found in the urine [4–7].

In 1983, de Bold and Flynn [8], after isolating and sequencing BNP, started their studies on the correlation between serum levels of circulating BNP and the diagnosis and treatment of heart failure.

Brain natriuretic peptide (BNP) is homologous to ANP hormone (neurohormone released by atrial myocytes and to a lesser extent in the ventricles), and the physiologically active portion consists of 32 amino acids [9].

M.B. Jatene, MD (✉)
Pediatric Cardiothoracic Surgery Unit, Heart Institute (InCor), University of Sao Paulo Medical School, Av. Eneas de Carvalho Aguiar, 44, 2nd Floor – Block 2, Room 5, 05403-000 Sao Paulo, Brazil
e-mail: mbjatene@uol.com.br

E. Azeka, MD, PhD
Pediatric Cardiology and Adult Congenital Heart Disease Unit, Heart Institute (InCor), University of Sao Paulo Medical School, Sao Paulo, Brazil

It has been identified in the brain and subsequently in the heart, mainly in the myocytes of the ventricle. Studies have shown low plasma concentrations under physiological settings, with a significant increase in pathological situations, such as ventricular hypertrophy and heart failure [9].

It has been shown that the concentration of BNP is less than 20 % of the levels of ANP in normal individuals, but can equal or exceed these levels in patients with congestive heart failure [10].

NT pro-BNP is an inactive metabolite of the pro-BNP peptide, and it has been described to be useful for the evaluation of heart failure and the prognostic outcome of heart transplant candidates [11] because of its greater serum stability and not being metabolized by neuropeptidase. Furthermore, it seems to have a longer half-life than BNP [7].

A study conducted in healthy subjects showed increased levels of BNP with age and in females. The authors concluded that 90 % of healthy young adults present BNP values smaller than 25 pg/ml and NT pro-BNP smaller than or equal to 70 pg/ml [7].

In 2006, Soldin et al. evaluated 808 persons for –21 years, with a significant number of subjects in each age group, showing high levels of BNP in neonates (1,585 pg/ml) and in children up to 6 months (263 pg/ml), with little variation in the other age groups. In this study, no difference was observed between genders, and the 95th percentile was around 100 pg/ml [12].

The secretion of BNP is regulated by the myocardial wall tension, and its plasma levels are elevated in systolic and/or diastolic heart failure and in cases of volume overload, providing a predictor of the development of heart failure and cardiovascular mortality [13–19].

Elevated serum levels of BNP (greater than 200 pg/ml) showed 100 % sensitivity and specificity of 97.1 %, a positive predictive value of 97.3 %, and a negative predictive value of 100 % for diagnosing decompensated heart failure in adult patients, and 80 % sensitivity and specificity of 86 % as a predictor of mortality. In some studies, BNP is related to increased central venous pressure and pulmonary capillary wedge pressure [20–22].

E.A. Gabriel, S.A. Gabriel (eds.), *Inflammatory Response in Cardiovascular Surgery*, DOI 10.1007/978-1-4471-4429-8_47, © Springer-Verlag London 2013

BNP is present in high levels in children with congenital heart disease with volume overload and/or myocardial dysfunction and in patients with cardiomyopathies [23–26].

BNP and Heart Transplantation

Heart transplantation has been a therapeutic option in patients with heart failure refractory to conventional therapy and in patients with complex congenital heart disease [27, 28].

The first heart transplant in humans was performed by Barnard et al. in 1967, and Kantrovitz et al. performed the first transplantation in a newborn in the same year [29, 30].

The absence of immunosuppressive drugs effective in the prophylaxis, treatment of rejection, and the difficulty in diagnosis resulted in a decrease in the number of procedures before 1980. The introduction of cyclosporine as an immunosuppressive drug in the 1980s [31] as well as increased survival has led many centers to re-initiate their programs.

Despite the significant improvement in survival, rejection [hyperacute, acute humoral (vascular), acute cellular, and chronic (allograft vasculopathy)] has been described up to 70 % of deaths within 5–10 years after transplant [1].

Hyperacute rejection is less frequent and may occur immediately after extracorporeal circulation. It is caused by antibodies to the ABO system and to histocompatibility antigens (HLA). This is a serious event that can lead to graft loss [1].

Acute rejection is observed, especially in the first 6 months post-transplant. It is mediated by T cells. The patient may be asymptomatic or have nonspecific symptoms to low cardiac output due to graft failure. Endomyocardial biopsy is the gold standard for the diagnosis and determines the intensity and distribution of the cellular infiltrate in the myocardium as well as whether myocardial necrosis is present [1].

The humoral or vascular rejection is mediated by antibodies against the T cells and antibodies directed against the HLA antigens and endothelial cells of the donor. It is more common in already sensitized patients who have received blood products prior to transplantation or have a history of pregnancy or use of mechanical ventricular assist support before transplantation. These patients may present with severe hemodynamic compromise related to ventricular dysfunction due to diffuse ischemia [1].

Some biological markers such as BNP have been compared with the findings of endomyocardial biopsy in the diagnosis of cellular rejection; however, the results are still controversial, especially in pediatric patients [32].

The blood level of BNP has been shown to be a factor indicative of rejection and appears to be related to ventricular remodeling after orthotopic cardiac transplantation. In multivariate analysis, independent predictors of elevated BNP were changes in the diastolic function and/or systolic echocardiogram, elevated pulmonary capillary wedge pressure, reduction of the cardiac index score, and presence of symptoms of fatigue and dyspnea [33].

Ationu et al. [34] studied the gene expression of ventricular and atrial natriuretic peptide in patients undergoing heart transplantation and found that these peptides may be involved in ventricular remodeling after transplantation.

Studies evaluating blood levels of BNP and endomyocardial biopsy showed accuracy in the detection of rejection episodes, increasing according to the degree of rejection, with values ranging from 101 to 194 pg/ml in rejection grade 0–3 A and levels of 1,144–1,843 pg/ml in more severe degrees of rejection, negative predictive value of 98 %, and a cutoff value of 130 pg/ml [35].

In the adult population, studies show that blood levels of BNP remain high in the first 2 months after transplantation, preventing the diagnosis of rejection, with its levels reducing progressively over a 6-month period, at which point correlation with the histological rejection can be observed [36].

Martinez et al. evaluated BNP levels measured consecutively 9–12 months after transplantation in relation to the following events: death, late rejection (after first year), and graft dysfunction. The authors found a higher number of events in the group with BNP levels that had increased by more than 20 % [36].

Lan et al. [37] reported a study conducted in 44 children who underwent orthotopic heart transplantation. The peptide levels remained high after the transplants, with decreased levels to lower values of 100 pg/ml at 14 weeks in a follow-up period of 171 months.

Claudius et al. [38] found that serum levels of BNP are elevated in children after heart transplantation with symptomatic ventricular dysfunction because of rejection or coronary artery disease after transplantation.

Rousseau et al. [39] compared blood levels of BNP and histological findings of endomyocardial biopsy, showing a correlation between elevated natriuretic peptide levels above 100 pg/ml and the presence of rejection.

Sylos et al. [32] studied the role of BNP after pediatric transplantation and concluded that children could be asymptomatic at allograft rejection episodes. The BNP level was statistically different in patients in the allograft rejection group, and its evaluation could be an additional method to assess the diagnosis of allograft rejection.

Coronary heart disease after transplantation, called graft vascular disease, is one of the main factors affecting the survival of adults and children undergoing heart transplantation [1]. Studies show that the incidence of graft vascular disease varies from 30 to 50 % depending on the post-transplant period of evolution examined and on the immunosuppressive regimen. Factors associated with a higher incidence of coronary artery disease and graft loss are older age of the recipient, a greater number of rejections, and the presence of late rejection and moderate to severe coronary artery disease detected by angiography and intravascular ultrasound [1].

The evaluation of graft coronary artery disease by angiography is recommended after the first year of transplantation and in the presence of symptoms of heart failure, arrhythmia, chest pain, or syncope [1]. There are reports of a correlation between graft coronary artery disease and increased serum levels of BNP in the adult population [1].

In conclusion, BNP has potential beneficial effects and prognostic value after heart transplantation; however, future investigations are needed to better understand its role and relation to the inflammatory process.

References

1. Rejeição após transplante cardíaco pediátrico. Utilidade do Peptídeo Natriurético tipo B (BNP). Tese de Doutorado – Cardiologia – Faculdade de Medicina USP; 2005.
2. Kisch B. A significant electron microscopic difference between the atria and the ventricles of the mammarian heart. Exp Med Surg. 1963;21:193–221.
3. Jamieson JD, Palade GE. Specific granules in atrial muscle cells. J Cell Biol. 1964;23:151–72.
4. de Bold AJ, Borenstein HB, Veress AT, Sonenberg H. A rapid and potent natriuretic response to intravenous injection of atrial myocardial extracts in rats. Life Sci. 1981;28:89.
5. Wilkins MR, Redondo J, Brown LA. The natriuretic peptide family. Lancet. 1997;349:1307.
6. Endlich K, Forssmann WG, Steinhausen M. Effects of urodilatin in the rat kidney: comparison with ANF and interaction with vasoactive substances. Kidney Int. 1995;47:1558.
7. Daniels L, Maisel AS. Natriuretic peptides. J Am Coll Cardiol. 2007;50(25):2357–68.
8. Flynn TG, de Bold ML, de Bold AJ. The amino acid sequence of an atrial peptide with potent diuretic and natriuretic properties. Biochem Biophys Res Commun. 1983;117(3):859–65.
9. Maack T. The broad homeostatic role of natriuretic peptides. Arq Bras Endocrinol Metabol. 2006;50(2):198–207.
10. Davidson NC, Struthers AD. Brain natriuretic peptide. J Hypertens. 1994;12:329.
11. Rothemburger M, Stypmann J, Hoffmeier A, Berendes E, Etz C, Pioux A, et al. Aminoterminal pro type B natriuretic peptide as a predictive and prognostic marker in patients with chronic heart failure. J Heart Lung Transplant. 2004;23(10):1189–97.
12. Soldin SJ, Soldin OP, Boyajian AJ, Madeleine ST. Pediatric brain natriuretic and N-terminal pro-brain natriuretic peptide reference intervals. Clin Chim Acta. 2006;366:304–8.
13. Troughton RW, Prior DL, Pereira JJ, Martin M, Fogarty A, Morehead A, et al. Plasma brain natriuretic peptide levels in systolic heart failure: importance of left ventricular diastolic function and right ventricular systolic function. J Am Coll Cardiol. 2004;43(3):416–22.
14. Bibbins-Domingo K, Ansari M, Schiller NB, Massie B, Whooley MA. B-natriuretic peptide and ischemia in patients with stable coronary disease. Circulation. 2003;108(24):2987–92.
15. Mayer SA, De Lemos JA, Murphy SA, Brooks S, Robert BJ, Grayburn PA. Comparison of B-natriuretic peptide levels in patients with heart failure versus without mitral regurgitation. Am J Cardiol. 2004;15(8):1002–6.
16. Kruger S, Graf J, Kumz D, Stickel T, Hanrath P, Jansens U. Brain natriuretic peptide levels predict functional capacity in patients with chronic heart failure. J Am Coll Cardiol. 2002;21(4):718–22.
17. Tang WH, Girod JP, Lee MJ, Starling RC, Ypung JB, Van Lente F, et al. Plasma brain natriuretic peptide levels in ambulatory patients with established chronic symtomatic systolic heart failure. Circulation. 2003;208(24):2964–6.
18. Wang TJ, Larson MG, Levy D, Benjamin E, Leip EP, Omland T, et al. Plasma natriuretic peptide levels and the risk of cardiovascular events and death. N Engl J Med. 2004;350(7):655–63.
19. Groenning B, Raymond I, Hildebrandt PR, Nilsson JC, Baumann M, Pedersen F. Diagnostic and prognostic evaluation of left ventricular systolic heart failure by plasma N terminal pro-brain natriuretic peptide concentration in a large sample of general population. Heart. 2004;90(3):297–303.
20. Villacorta H, Duarte NM, Carrano A, Mesquita ET, Dohmann HJ, Ferreira FE. The role of B-type natriuretic peptide in the diagnosis of congestive heart failure in patients presenting to an emergency department with dyspnea. Arq Bras Cardiol. 2002;79(6):564–8.
21. Akioka K, Takeuchi K, Yanagi S, Hirota K, Sakamoto K, Yoshimura T, et al. Prognostic value of Doppler transmitral flow patterns and cardiac natriuretic peptides in patients with chronic congestive heart failure admitted for episodes of acute decompensation. Heart Vessels. 2000;15(2):53–60.
22. Westerling A, Wahlander H, Lindstedt G, Lundberg PA, Holmgren D. Clinical signs of heart failure are associated with increased levels of natriuretic peptide types B and A in children with congenital heart defects or cardiomyopathy. Acta Paediatr. 2004;93(3):340–5.
23. Kunni O, Kamada M, Ohtsuki S, Araki T, Kataoka K, Kageyama M, et al. Plasma brain natriuretic peptide and the evaluation of volume overload in infants and children with congenital heart disease. Acta Med Okayama. 2003;57(4):191–7.
24. Redfield MM, Rodeheffer RJ, Jacobsen SJ, Mahoney DW, Bailey KR, Burnett Jr JC. Plasma brain natriuretic peptide concentration; impact of age and gender. J Am Coll Cardiol. 2002;40(5):976–82.
25. Cowley CG, Bradley JD, Shaddy RE. B-type natriuretic peptide levels in congenital heart disease. Pediatr Cardiol. 2004;25(4):336–40.
26. Koch A, Singer H. Normal values of B-type natriuretic peptide in infants, children and adolescents. Heart. 2003;89(8):874–8.
27. Azeka E, Barbero-Marcial M, Jatene M, Auler JO, Ramires JA. Eight years experience of pediatric heart transplantation: clinical outcome using non-invasive methods for the evaluation of acute rejection. Pediatr Transplant. 2002;6(3):208–13.
28. Jatene MB, Miana LA, Pessoa AJ, Riso A, Azeka E, Tanamati C, et al. Pediatric heart transplantation in refractory cardiogenic shock: a critical analysis of feasibility, applicability and results. Arq Bras Cardiol. 2008;90(5):329–33.
29. Barnard CN. The operation. A human cardiac transplant: an interim report of a successful operation performed at Groote Schuur Hospital, Cape Town. S Afr Med J. 1967;41(48):1271–4.
30. Kantrowitz A, Haller JD, Joos H, Cerruti MM, Carstensen HE. Transplantation of the heart in an infant and an adult. Am J Cardiol. 1968;22:782–90.
31. Modry DL, Oyer PE, Jamieson SW, Stinson EB, Baldwin JC, Reitz BA, et al. Cyclosporine in heart and heart-lung transplantation. Can J Surg. 1985;28(3):274–80, 282.
32. Sylos C, Azeka E, Kajita L, Benvenutti L, Strunz CC, Branco KC, et al. B-type natriuretic peptide assessment in the diagnosis of rejection after pediatric heart transplant. Arq Bras Cardiol. 2009;92(3):215–26.
33. Hervas I, Almenar L, Perez-Pastor JL, Chirivella M, Osa A, Martinez-Doltz P, et al. Radioimmunometric assay of B-type natriuretic peptide (BNP) in heart transplantation: correlation between BNP determination and biopsy grading of rejection. Nucl Med Commun. 2003;24(8):925–31.

34. Ationu A, Sorensen K, Whitehead B, Singer D, Burch M, Carter ND. Ventricular expression of brain natriuretic peptide gene following orthotopic cardiac transplantation in children – a three year follow up. Cardiovasc Res. 1993;27(12):2135–9.
35. Hammerer-Lercher A, Mair J, Antretter H, Ruttmann E, Poeltzl G, Laufer G, et al. B-type natriuretic peptide as a marker of allograft rejection after heart transplantation. J Heart Lung Transplant. 2005;24(9):1444–7.
36. Martinez-Doltz L, Almenara L, Hervas I, Moro J, Aguero J, Sanchez-Lazaro I, et al. Prognostic relationship between two serial determination of B-type natriuretic peptide and medium-long term events in heart transplantation. J Heart Lung Transplant. 2008;27(7):735–40.
37. Lan YT, Chang RK, Alejos JC, Burch C, Wetzel GT. B-type natriuretic peptide in children after cardiac transplantation. J Heart Lung Transplant. 2004;23(5):558–63.
38. Iene Claudius MD, Yueh-Tze Lan MD, Chang RK, Wetzel GT, Alejos J. Usefulness of B-type natriuretic peptide as a noninvasive screening tool for cardiac allograft pathology in pediatric heart transplant recipients. Am J Cardiol. 2003;92(11):1368–70.
39. Rossano JW, Denfield SW, Kim JJ, Price JF, Jefferies JJ, Decker JA, et al. B-type natriuretic peptide is a sensitive screening test for acute rejection in pediatric heart transplant patients. Pediatr Transplant. 2008;27(6):649–54.

48 Nutritional Factors, Oxidative Stress and Lung Transplantation

Janet Madill, Bianca Arendt, Chung-Wai Chow, and Johane Allard

Introduction

Transplantation is the only treatment of choice for end-stage lung disease patients. This procedure is labor-intensive, expensive, and driven by the availability of organ donation. Considering the ongoing significant organ donor shortage, it is important to ensure that each transplant candidate will survive and achieve the maximum long-term outcome. Unfortunately, there are still challenging long-term complications associated with lung transplant recipients, and research is ongoing to maximize medical treatment.

In lung transplantation, the long-term outcome is hampered by the development of bronchiolitis obliterans syndrome (BOS). Although the survival rate at 1 year is 80 %, this rapidly decreases to 50 % at 5 years post-transplant because of BOS [1]. Medical and pharmacological approaches to prevent these long-term complications are improving, but the success is limited. The main reason for this limited success is the complex pathogenesis of BOS, which can be associated with ischemia-reperfusion injury [2], immunological reactions [3], acute and chronic rejection [4–9], inflammation [10], and concomitant infections [11]. Oxidative stress may contribute to BOS pathogenesis and induce further tissue injury and inflammation. Oxidative stress can be influenced by several factors, including nutrition.

We have previously reported that oxidative stress may play a role in the pathogenesis of BOS in lung transplant recipients [12]. Considering that oxidative stress can be associated with nutritional factors, this chapter will focus on antioxidants and antioxidant studies in relation to lung disease and lung transplantation.

J. Madill, PhD, RD (✉)
Assistant Professor, Brescia University College, Western University, London, Ontario
e-mail: jmadill7@uwo.ca

C. Chow, MD
Lung Transplant Program, University of Toronto, Toronto, ON, Canada

B. Arendt, PhD • J. Allard, MD
Department of Medicine, University Health Network (UHN), Toronto, ON, Canada

Oxidative Stress

The role of oxygen is double-edged. It is utilized in the metabolic processes that provide energy for cell functions and in this process generates toxic free radicals [13]. Under normal conditions, these free radicals, which include reactive oxygen species (ROS) and reactive nitrogen species (RNS), are efficiently scavenged by the antioxidant defense system [14]. However, there are a number of chronic inflammatory conditions, such as aging [15], atherosclerotic heart disease [16], Alzheimer's disease [17], as well as a variety of lung [18] and liver diseases [19, 20] whereby the production of free radicals overwhelms the antioxidant defense system, leading to a condition known as oxidative stress (Fig. 48.1).

Physiological levels of free radicals are essential for cell differentiation, cell growth, cell apoptosis, and immunity against invading microorganisms [21–23]. However, when

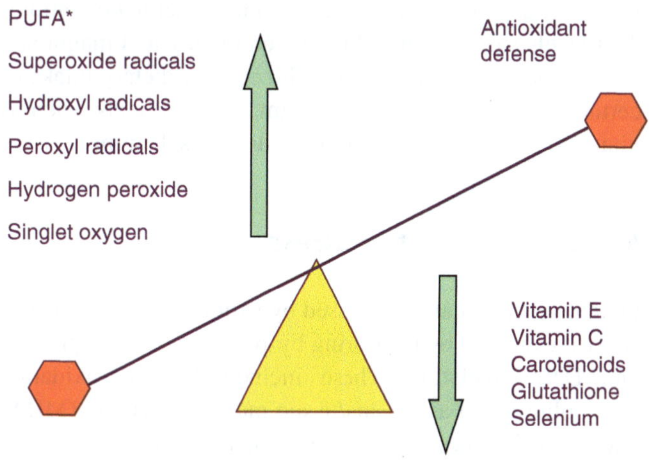

Fig. 48.1 Oxidative stress

E.A. Gabriel, S.A. Gabriel (eds.), *Inflammatory Response in Cardiovascular Surgery*, DOI 10.1007/978-1-4471-4429-8_48, © Springer-Verlag London 2013

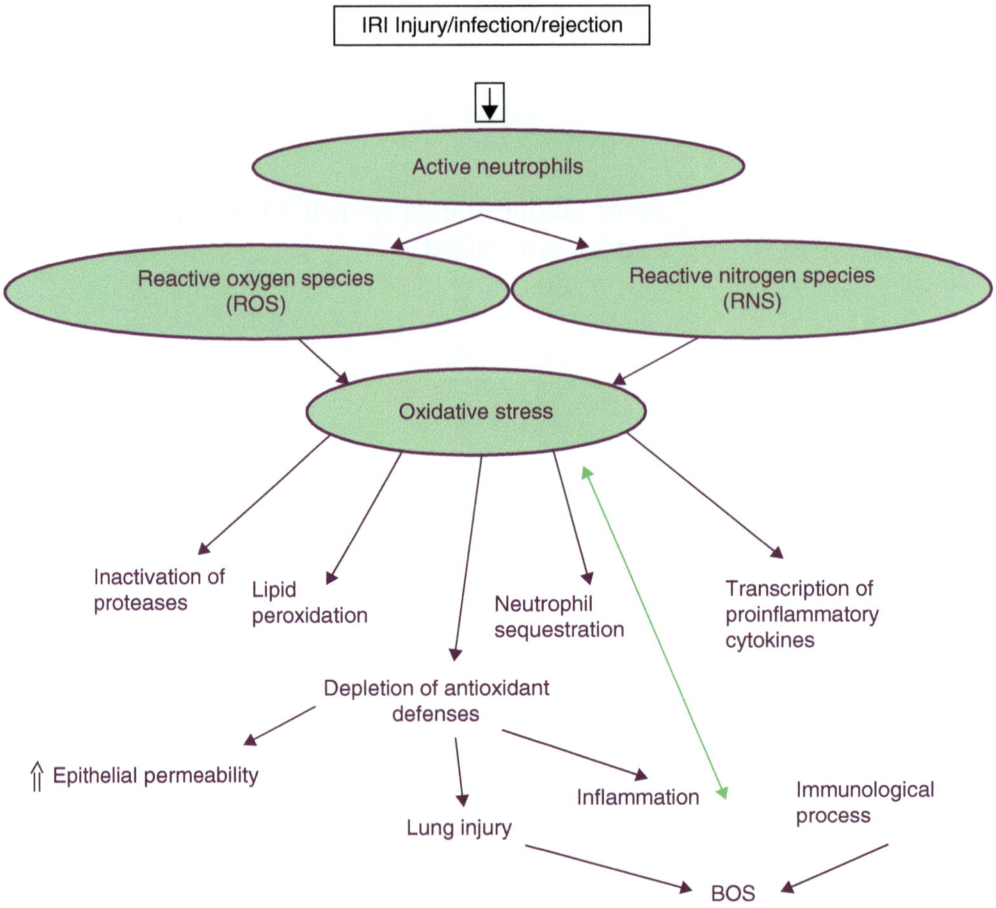

Fig. 48.2 Effects of oxidative stress

these free radicals overwhelm the antioxidant defense system, oxidative stress occurs. ROS/RNS are increased during processes such as immunological reactions, inflammation, infections, and ischemia-reperfusion injury. Excess production of ROS/RNS can cause oxidative damage to DNA as well as modify proteins, carbohydrates, and lipids, resulting in cellular injury (Fig. 48.2). On the other hand, antioxidant levels can be reduced by the chronicity and magnitude of these processes and can be influenced by dietary intake of certain types of fat and antioxidant micronutrients, such as vitamin E, ascorbic acid, carotenoids, and selenium.

Measuring Oxidative Stress

Oxidative stress can be assessed by various laboratory analyses, for example, by measuring by-products of lipid, protein, and DNA oxidation. These include, lipid peroxidation metabolites such as plasma/tissue malondialdehyde (MDA) and 8-isoprostanes [24], protein oxidation parameters, such as protein carbonyls, total thiols, advanced oxidation protein products, and nitrotyrosine [25, 26], and measures of DNA damage, such as DNA strand breaks and guanine oxidation products (8-OHdG) [27, 28].

The antioxidant system can also be assessed by measuring antioxidant enzymes such as glutathione peroxidase (GPx), superoxide dismutase (SOD), and catalase (CAT) or by analysis of micronutrients such as antioxidant vitamin E, C, or carotenoids.

Evidence of Oxidative Stress in Lung Transplantation

Oxidative stress is a condition whereby prooxidants overwhelm the antioxidant defense system, and this may contribute to the pathogenesis of BOS by inducing increased tissue injury and inflammation.

Three studies have reported antioxidants in lung transplant recipients and measured oxidative stress parameters. In a small cross-sectional study, Madill [29] reported that lung recipients with severe stages of BOS were more oxidatively stressed compared to those patients with a milder stages of BOS and non-BOS lung recipients. This was indicated by increased BALF levels of LPO and oxidized glutathione. However, there were no significant differences in nutritional intake of vitamin A, C, or E or plasma antioxidant vitamin levels of retinol, vitamin C, or α- and γ-tocopherol among the three groups.

Williams et al. [30] in a prospective study also reported increased BALF MDA levels in lung recipients 2 weeks and 12 months post-transplant when compared to non-transplant controls ($p<0.05$). The authors reported no significant improvement in antioxidant status (serum or BALF) from 2 weeks to over 1 year post-lung transplant, indicating that lung recipients remain oxidatively stressed.

Another study [31] performed in 15 cystic fibrosis patients taking vitamin supplements, including 8,000 IU (1,200 μg) vitamin A and 300 IU (248 mg) vitamin E, assessed antioxidant vitamin levels. Serum vitamin A and vitamin E levels were determined pre-transplant and again at approximately 15 months post-transplant. Pre-transplant serum vitamin A levels were within the normal range, whereas post-transplant, they significantly increased. Similar results were seen regarding serum vitamin E levels. No measurements were conducted in BALF to assess lung antioxidant status or oxidative stress. Supplementation in these lung transplant patients with both vitamin A and E (8,000 IU, 300 IU, respectively) remained the same pre- and post-transplant to prevent vitamin deficiencies. The increase in vitamin E and A serum vitamin levels post-transplant may have been due to increased compliance or reduced oxidative stress post-transplant due to lower lung infectious rates related to CF.

In summary, only three studies have been conducted examining oxidative stress and lung transplantation. Two studies documented an increase in lipid peroxidation along with a weakened antioxidant status in lung transplants recipients not taking vitamin supplementation. The third study examining CF patients indicated that antioxidant vitamin supplementation helps maintains vitamin levels.

In addition to ischemia-reperfusion injury and inflammation associated with rejection and infection, nutritional factors may contribute to oxidative stress by either creating a prooxidant status or affecting the antioxidant defense system. Prooxidant nutritional factors include obesity and/or malnutrition, as well as intake of dietary fat, particularly polyunsaturated fatty acid (PUFA). Conversely, nutritional factors contributing to the antioxidant defense systems are antioxidant micronutrients such as vitamins E, C, and carotenoids. In addition, antioxidant enzymes and trace elements such as selenium may also play a role.

Nutritional Factors and Oxidative Stress

Obesity

We are currently encountering an obesity epidemic [32]. Recent studies have indicated that decreased energy intake resulted in decreased oxidative stress, measured by decreased plasma MDA levels in non-obese subjects compared to obese participants [33].

Obesity is associated with a heightened state of inflammation [34, 35], resulting in oxidative stress. Increased body weight is positively associated with inflammation, measured by C-reactive protein levels (a biomarker of inflammation) in obese compared to non-obese individuals [36, 37].

Obesity is also prevalent in other solid organ transplant recipients [38–41]. However, in the lung transplant population, there is minimal information on the association of obesity and the development of BOS.

Kanasky et al. [42] examined 85 post-lung transplant recipients (34 % were overweight/obese) and determined that obesity had a negative effect on post-transplant survival. The most powerful predictor of mortality was BMI, with an increased risk of death of 7 % for each 1.0 unit (kg/m^2) increase. These authors also reported that there was no difference in the development of BOS and/or infection in the obese compared to the non-obese group. Another study also reported a negative impact of high pre-transplant BMI [43]. Culver examined 46 lung transplant patients with BMI >30 kg/m^2 and reported a significant increase in 90-day mortality in obese lung transplant patients when compared to non-obese [OR 3.16 (CI: 1.05–9.48)]. Previously, we have reported that high body mass index (BMI) pre-transplantation was shown to increase morbidity and/or mortality within 90 days post-lung transplantation [44]. A retrospective chart review [45] of 826 lung transplant recipients from 12 international transplant centers reported that substantial weight gain occurred within the first year post-transplant. In this study, higher weight gain was associated with better subsequent survival [45].

Taken together, these studies indicate that there is a high prevalence of obesity post-lung transplantation and that this may affect survival, although the results are mixed. Only one small retrospective study looked at the relationship between obesity and BOS and did not find any increased risk of BOS in obese subjects.

Malnutrition

In addition to obesity, malnutrition can also be associated with oxidative stress because of possible micronutrient deficiencies due to inadequate intake and/or malabsorption [46]. In the pre-transplant lung literature, the effect of malnutrition and oxidative stress has been reported mainly in cystic fibrosis (CF) patients [47]. CF patients have malabsorption of fat-soluble vitamins A, E, and carotenoids [48, 49]. In addition, repeated or chronic infections as well as respiratory failure can increase catabolism and anorexia, contributing to malnutrition. Furthermore, chronic inflammation generates more ROS/RNS via neutrophil and macrophage activation and 'respiratory burst' [50, 51]. Therefore, the effect of reduced intake and increased malabsorption of micronutrient antioxidants, combined with greater demand of antioxidants for scavenging free radicals, will enhance oxidative stress in this patient population [50].

Some studies reported on malnutrition, malabsorption, and low micronutrient levels pre-transplantation, particularly the CF population. In general, in the studies reported, oxidative stress was shown to be elevated. However, there is a paucity of studies reporting on nutritional status, dietary intake, and plasma levels of antioxidant micronutrients in post-lung transplant patients. Nutritional intake also influences oxidative stress.

Nutrition Intake

Polyunsaturated Fatty Acid (PUFA)

The type of PUFA ingested in the diet can influence oxidative stress and the demand for antioxidants. It can also influence underlying inflammation. Long-chain PUFAs are more prone to lipid peroxidation (LPO) because they have more double bonds. The greater the number of double bonds in the PUFAs, the more susceptible they are to LPO [52–54].

Hydroxyl radicals produced by activated neutrophils initiate a free radical chain reaction by attacking the double bonds of PUFA within the membrane phospholipids. Omega-6 PUFAs, such as arachidonic acid, and omega-3 PUFAs, such as eicosapentaenoic acid (EPA) and docosahexanoic acid (DHA), are prone to LPO, particularly in an environment deficient in vitamin E. Both PUFA and vitamin E are influenced by diet.

In addition, the type of PUFA influences inflammation. Omega-3 PUFAs, such as α-linolenic acid, eicosapentaenoic acid (EPA), and docosahexaenoic acid (DHA), contained in walnuts, soybeans, flax seed oil, and fish [55], have antiinflammatory effects by decreasing the production of eicosanoids and leukotrienes [56]. However, omega-6 PUFAs, such as linoleic acid found in vegetable oils and arachidonic acid found in animal fat sources, are classified as proinflammatory [57] as they produce two potent inflammatory mediators, eicosanoids and leukotrienes [56]. Therefore, the type of PUFA can influence oxidative stress depending on its predisposition to lipid peroxidation and its effect on inflammation. Both PUFA and vitamin E levels can be influenced by dietary intake.

The University of Toronto Lung Transplant Program conducts about 100 lung transplants/year, and patients with cystic fibrosis (CF) represent 25 % of this population (UHN lung transplant data statistics; December 2011). These patients generally require high-calorie and high-fat nutrition care plans to optimize their nutritional status [58], along with pancreatic enzymes and vitamin supplementation to correct for malabsorption. In addition to the underlying disease, this regimen will influence oxidative stress depending on the proportion and type of fat absorbed and the ratio of PUFA:vitamin E. High fat requirements lead to increased intake of PUFA, which leads to increased oxidative stress.

Because of its antiinflammatory effect, omega-3 PUFA is often given to cystic fibrosis (CF) patients as a supplement. Omega 3 supplements contain vitamin E to prevent LPO. In a Cochrane systematic review [59], results indicated that CF patients supplemented with ω-3 had (1) improved lung function, (2) improved clinical status, (3) reduced volume of sputum, and (4) increased essential fatty acids (efa) in neutrophil membranes. Few minor adverse effects were reported. Another study in CF patients found no change in oxidative stress with fish oil supplementation [60], suggesting that vitamin E from supplementation was sufficient to prevent lipid peroxidation. Studies on the effect of ω-3 PUFA supplementation have not been reported in the lung transplant population. Antioxidant intake and/or supplementation can also influence oxidative stress.

Antioxidants

Observational studies examining a possible protective role of antioxidants in lung diseases have been summarized in several review articles [61–63]. Dietary studies form the bulk of these reports.

Current dietary guidelines from Health Canada *Eating Well with Canada's Food Guide* recommend seven food guide servings of fruit and vegetables per day (HC Pub:4651; Cat: H164-38/1-2007E SSBN:0-662-44467-1). Consuming foods based on this recommendation will provide a diet rich in antioxidants, including vitamins C, E, and β-carotene, among others. Many dietary antioxidants work synergistically [64] to promote their protective effects as they exist in a natural environment and are biochemically balanced [65].

To our knowledge, there are no studies examining fruit and vegetable intake in lung transplant recipients. However, in the patients with lung disease, diets rich in antioxidants have shown beneficial effects on lung function described as high maximal forced expired ventilation in 1 s (FEV_1). Cross-sectional studies have been conducted on 12,000 subjects with various lung etiologies, indicating that intake of fruits and vegetables improves lung function [61–63, 66]. As well, large longitudinal studies have also reported a positive association between overall dietary intake of fruits and vegetables and FEV_1 [67–71]. Furthermore, fruit and vegetable consumption has shown beneficial effects on decreasing respiratory symptoms and disease severity [72]. Even low intake of fruit and vegetables compared to no consumption achieved a positive effect on lung function [61]. Similarly, one longitudinal study [67] reported an inverse association (RR = 0.73) between fruit intake and the incidence of chronic non-specific lung disease.

Studies on the intake of fruits and vegetables and the effect on oxidative stress measurements have been conducted. In a crossover study [73], increased consumption of ten servings of fruits and vegetables resulted in a significant reduction of oxidative stress measured as oxygen radical absorbance capacity (ORAC) from baseline to post-consumption [73].

Dietary studies examining the association between lung function (described as high maximal FEV_1) and intake of individual antioxidants provide conflicting results. Indeed, while some cross-sectional studies found a positive association between vitamin C and lung function [74–77], along with two longitudinal studies [69, 70], others failed to find any such association [67, 78].

The evidence for intake of vitamin E is also conflicting. Cross-sectional studies [74, 75, 78] and one longitudinal study [69] report a positive association between intake of vitamin E and lung function, whereas one cross-sectional [76] and one longitudinal study report no association [79].

Although less well studied, research indicates that intake of β-carotene shows similar trends. Two cross-sectional studies [76, 80] along with a longitudinal study [69] indicate a beneficial association, whereas one cross-sectional study reports no benefit [67].

Studies involving patients with a variety of lung diseases have reported positive associations between plasma vitamin E, vitamin C, and β-carotene antioxidant levels and FEV_1 [79, 81].

Supplementation studies in patients with lung diseases have reported very disappointing results. The Alpha-Tocopherol, Beta-Carotene Cancer Prevention (ATBC) study [82, 83] describes a RCT of 28,000 male smokers who were supplemented with a daily dose of 50 IU of vitamin E, 20 mg β-carotene, both, or placebo for 5–8 years. Unexpected results indicated that vitamin E supplementation, increased the risk of death from hemorrhagic stroke, and β-carotene increased lung cancer mortality and ischemic heart disease.

The CARET study [84] tested effects of combined treatment of β-carotene (30 mg/day) and retinyl palmitate (25,000 IU/day) in 18,000 men and women with a history of smoking. Results from this study found increased risk of both lung cancer and coronary artery disease in treated patients compared to controls.

Therefore, most of these epidemiological studies showed some beneficial effect from antioxidants on various respiratory diseases. However, intervention studies were disappointing. Presently, minimal studies examining antioxidant status in lung transplant patients have been undertaken. One study [85] reported low BALF ascorbic acid and glutathione levels in BOS lung recipients when compared to non-BOS recipients. The second study [30] indicated elevated plasma and BALF MDA levels and low serum and BALF ascorbic acid levels up to 12 months after lung transplantation. No dietary intake assessment was performed, and no intervention studies were conducted.

In the lung disease population, increased oxidative stress has been adequately documented in pre-transplant patients [47, 50, 86–91] as well as early post-lung transplantation in relation to ischemia-reperfusion injury (IRI). However, oxidative stress in long-term lung recipients is not well studied [29, 30].

It is important to keep in mind that, in the broader context, research studies examining antioxidant supplementation in patients with a variety of disease conditions such as atherosclerosis [92] and Alzheimer's disease [93] have also been disappointing, underlying the difficulties regarding decisions for the dosing, timing, type and combination of supplements, duration of the intervention, and outcome measures. Results from primary and secondary intervention trials with 400 IU vitamin E every other day plus 500 mg vitamin C daily have reported increased mortality in both healthy controls and patients with diseases [94–96]. The evidence is even more convincing that antioxidant supplementation with the goal of reducing the risk of cardiovascular disease is not supported by the findings from current randomized controlled studies [97, 98]. Similarly, 400 IU vitamin E every other day along with daily 500 mg vitamin C supplementation, neither alone nor together, reduced the risk of prostate or total cancers [99–101]. However, some of these studies have been criticized for not examining an oxidative stress biomarker, thus making it difficult to identify individuals who may have benefited from supplementation [102]. Therefore, based on these past studies, optimal antioxidant vitamin supplementation studies may be very challenging to design.

Another potential intervention would be a dietary modification [103]. Initiating nutrition strategies to improve the total antioxidant capacity (TAC) of lung recipients' diets represents a possible dietary alteration. Some authors agree that improving the patients' overall nutrition intake may prove more beneficial than antioxidant supplementation [104]. As well, some authors have reported that high TAC foods (consisting of red berries, spinach, coffee, olive oil, among others) can minimize inflammation [105–109]. More recently, Giuseppe reported that subjects consuming higher TAC foods demonstrated a significant improvement in FEV_1 when compared to those with lowered intakes of TAC foods [110]. These types of diets may be more beneficial than consuming additional pills and may have other beneficial compounds that have not yet been identified [111].

However, before recommending antioxidant supplementation in lung transplant recipients, we should assess its benefit and determine what appropriate dose and combination would be most successful, as well as the duration of treatment [112, 113]. We may also want to determine if we could identify the 'more oxidized' lung transplant patient at an earlier stage for supplementation with extra antioxidants [114]. Furthermore, we will need to examine if supplementation leads to minimization of the inflammatory process evident in chronic rejection, a condition that significantly decreases long-term outcomes in lung transplant patients. If so, would this reduce oxidative stress and, as a result, have a clinical impact on FEV_1 and the development of BOS?

Conclusion

Oxidative stress can be generated early post-lung transplantation in relation to ischemia reperfusion injury and longer term with infectious episodes and /or chronic rejection. Nutritional factors as well as nutritional intake may also impact the state of oxidative stress in this patient population. Very little has been published on nutritional factors and oxidative stress in the lung transplant population. However, preliminary research results have been most noticeably encouraging to conduct more extensive clinical studies to determine if oxidative stress post-lung transplantation leads to improved clinical outcomes. Larger and more detailed studies in lung transplantation are needed.

References

1. Hertz MI, Taylor DO, Trulock EP, Boucek MM, Mohacsi PJ, Edwards LB, et al. The registry of the international society for heart and lung transplantation: nineteenth official report—2002. J Heart Lung Transplant. 2002;21(9):950–70.
2. Fiser SM, Tribble CG, Long SM, Kaza AK, Kern JA, Jones DR, et al. Ischemia-reperfusion injury after lung transplantation increases risk of late bronchiolitis obliterans syndrome. Ann Thorac Surg. 2002;73(4):1041–8.
3. Hertz MI. Immunosuppression for prevention of bronchiolitis obliterans. Curr Opin Transpl. 2000;5(4):402–6.
4. Jungraithmayr W, Draenert A, Marquardt K, Weder W. Ultrastructural changes in acute lung allograft rejection: novel insights from an animal study. J Heart Lung Transplant. 2012;31(1):94–100.
5. Bando K, Paradis IL, Similo S, Konishi H, Komatsu K, Zullo TG, et al. Obliterative bronchiolitis after lung and heart-lung transplantation. J Thorac Cardiovasc Surg. 1995;110(1):4–14.
6. El-Gamel A, Sim E, Hasleton P, Hutchinson J, Yonan N, Egan J, et al. Transforming growth factor beta (TGF-β) and obliterative bronchiolitis following pulmonary transplantation. J Heart Lung Transplant. 1999;18(9):828–37.
7. Girgis RE, Tu I, Berry GJ. Risk factors for the development of obliterative bronchiolitis after lung transplantation. J Heart Lung Transplant. 1996;15:1200–8.
8. Jain R, Hachem RR, Morrell MR, Trulock EP, Chakinala MM, Yusen RD, et al. Azithromycin is associated with increased survival in lung transplant recipients with bronchiolitis obliterans syndrome. J Heart Lung Transplant. 2010;29(5):531–7.
9. Vos R, Vanaudenaerde BM, Ottevaere A, Verleden SE, De Vleeschauwer SI, Willems-Widyastuti A, et al. Long-term azithromycin therapy for bronchiolitis obliterans syndrome: divide and conquer? J Heart Lung Transplant. 2010;29(12):1358–68.
10. DiGiovine B, Lynch JP, Matinez FJ, Flint A, Whyte RI, Iannettoni M, et al. Bronchoalveolar lavage neutrophilia is associated with obliterative bronchiolitis after lung transplantation: role of IL-8. J Immunol. 1996;157:4194–202.
11. Snyder L, Ash C, Jackson W, Howel D, Willner DA, Palmer S. Cytomegalovirus pneumonitis is a risk for bronchiolitis obliterans syndrome in lung transplantation. Am J Respir Crit Care Med. 2010;181:1391–6.
12. Madill J, Aghdassi E, Arendt B, Gutierrez C, Chow CW, Hartman-Craven B, et al. Lung transplantation: does oxidative stress contribute to the development of bronchiolitis obliterans syndrome? Transplant Rev. 2009;23(2):103–10.
13. Chabot F, Mitchell JA, Gutteridge JMC, Evans T. Reactive oxygen species in acute lung injury. Eur Respir J. 1998;11:745–57.
14. Sies H. Oxidative stress: introduction. In: Sies H, ed. Oxidative stress: oxidants and antioxidants. San Diego: Academic; 1991. p. xv–xxii.
15. Kregel K, Zhang HJ. An integrated view of oxidative stress in aging: basic mechanisms, functional effects, and pathological consideration. Am J Physiol Regul Integr Comp Physiol. 2007;292:R18–36.
16. Esterbauer H, Wag G, Puhl H. Lipid peroxidation and its role in atherosclerosis. Br Med Bull. 1993;49(566):576.
17. Christen Y. Oxidative stress and Alzheimer disease. Am J Clin Nutr. 2000;71(2):621S–9.
18. Gonzalez-Flecha B. Oxidant mechanisms in response to ambient air particles. Mol Aspects Med. 2004;25:169–82.
19. Houglum K, Bedossa P, Chojkier M. TGF-beta and collagen-alpha 1 (I) gene expression are increased in hepatic acinar zone 1 of rats with iron overload. Am J Physiol. 1994;267(5 Pt 1):G908–13.
20. Houglum K, Filip M, Witztum JL, Chojkier M. Malondialdehyde and 4-hydroxynonenal protein adducts in plasma and liver of rats with iron overload. J Clin Invest. 1990;86(6):1991–8.
21. Heyland D, Dhaliwal R, Suchner U, Berber MM. Antioxidant nutrients: a systematic review or trace elements and vitamins in the critically ill patient. Intensive Care Med. 2005;31:327.
22. Barrera G, Pizzimenti S, Dianzani MU. Lipid peroxidation: control of cell proliferation, cell differentiation and cell death. Mol Aspects Med. 2008;29(1–2):1–8.
23. van der Vliet A. NADPH oxidases in lung biology and pathology: host defense enzymes, and more. Free Radic Biol Med. 2008;44(6):938–55.
24. Halliwell B, Chirico S. Lipid peroxidation: its mechanism, measurement, and significance. Am J Clin Nutr. 1993;57(suppl):715S–25.
25. Tabassum H, Parvez S, Rehman H, Banerjee BD, Raisuddin S. Catechin as an antioxidant in liver mitochondrial toxicity: inhibition of tamoxifen-induced protein oxidation and lipid peroxidation. J Biochem Mol Toxicol. 2007;21(3):110–7.
26. Kayali R, Cakatay U, Tekeli F. Male rats exhibit higher oxidative protein damage than females of the same chronological age. Mech Ageing Dev. 2007;128(5–6):365–9.
27. Collins A, Cadet J, Epe B, Gedik C. Problems in the measurement of 8-oxoguanine in human DNA. Report of a workshop, DNA oxidation, held in Aberdeen, UK, 19–21 January, 1997. Carcinogenesis. 1997;18(9):1833–6.
28. Cooke MS, Evans MD, Dizdaroglu M, Lunec J. Oxidative DNA damage: mechanisms, mutation, and disease. FASEB J. 2003;17(10):1195–214.
29. Madill J, Aghdassi E, Arendt BM, Gutierrez C, Singer L, Chow C, et al. Oxidative stress and nutritional intakes in lung patients with bronchiolitis obliterans syndrome. Transplant Proc. 2009;41(9): 3838–44.
30. Williams A, Riise G, Anderson B, Kjellström C, Scherstén H, Kelly F. Compromised antioxidant status and persistent oxidative stress in lung transplant recipients. Free Radic Res. 1999;30:383–93.
31. Stephenson A, Brotherwood M, Robert R, Durie P, Verjee Z, Chaparro C, et al. Increased vitamin A and E levels in adult cystic fibrosis patients after lung transplantation. Transplantation. 2005;79(5):613–5.
32. Heymsfield SB. How large is the energy gap that accounts for the obesity epidemic? Am J Clin Nutr. 2009;89(6):1717–8.
33. Skalicky J, Muzakova V, Kandar R, Meloun M, Rousar T. Oxidative stress and metabolic syndrome in obese adults with and without controlled diet restriction. Bratisl Lek Listy. 2009;110(3):152–7.
34. Esposito K, Ciotola M, Giugliano D. Mediterranean diet, endothelial function and vascular inflammatory markers. Public Health Nutr. 2006;9(8A):1073–6.
35. Egger G, Dixon J. Non-nutrient causes of low-grade, systemic inflammation: support for a 'canary in the mineshaft' view of obesity in chronic disease. Obes Rev. 2011;12(5):339–45.
36. Dietrich M, Jialal I. The effect of weight loss on stable biomarker of inflammation, C-reactive protein. Nutr Rev. 2005;63(1):22–8.

37. Wu B, Fukuo K, Suzuki K, Yoshino G, Kazumi T. Relationships of systemic oxidative stress to body Fat distribution, adipokines and inflammatory markers in healthy middle-aged women. Endocr J. 2009;56(6):773–82.
38. de Mattos AM, Shibagaki Y, Russo K, Rivinus A, Prather J, Markovich A, et al. Study 2: relationship between pretransplant obesity and posttransplant cardiovascular events, diabetes mellitus, and graft and patient survival in renal transplant recipients. Transplant Rev. 2003;17(4):S38.
39. Thuluvath PJ. Morbid obesity with one or more other serious comorbidities should be a contraindication for liver transplantation. Liver Transpl. 2007;13(12):1627–9.
40. Williams JJ, Lund LH, LaManca J, Kunavarapu C, Cohen DJ, Heshka S, et al. Excessive weight gain in cardiac transplant recipients. J Heart Lung Transplant. 2006;25(1):36–41.
41. Aalten J, Christiaans MH, de Fijter H, Hené R, Homan van der Heijde J, Roodnat J, et al. The influence of obesity on short- and long-term graft and patient survival after renal transplantation. Transpl Int. 2006;19(11):901–7.
42. Kanasky Jr WF, Anton SD, Rodrigue JR, Perri MG, Szwed T, Baz MA. Impact of body weight on long-term survival after lung transplantation. Chest. 2002;121(2):401–6.
43. Culver DA, Mazzone PJ, Khandwala F, Blazey HC, DeCamp MM, Chapman JT. Discordant utility of ideal body weight and body mass index as predictors of mortality in lung transplant recipients. J Heart Lung Transplant. 2005;24(2):137–44.
44. Madill J, Gutierrez C, Grossman J, Allard J, Chan C, Hutcheon M, et al. Nutritional assessment of the lung transplant patient: body mass index as a predictor of 90–day mortality following transplantation. J Heart Lung Transplant. 2001;20(3):288–96.
45. Singer LG, Brazelton TR, Doyle RL, Morris RE, Theodore J. Weight gain after lung transplantation. J Heart Lung Transplant. 2003;22(8):894–902.
46. Halliwell B. Free radicals and antioxidants: a personal view. Nutr Rev. 1994;52(8):253–65.
47. Wood L, Fitzgerald D, Gibson P, Cooper D, Collins C, Garg M. Oxidative stress in cystic fibrosis: dietary and metabolic factors. J Am Coll Nutr. 2001;20(2):157–65.
48. Wood LG, Fitzgerald DA, Gibson PG, Cooper DM, Garg ML. Increased plasma fatty acid concentrations after respiratory exacerbations are associated with elevated oxidative stress in cystic fibrosis patients. Am J Clin Nutr. 2002;75(4):668–75.
49. Wood LG, Fitzgerald DA, Garg ML. Hypothesis: vitamin E complements polyunsaturated fatty acids in essential fatty acid deficiency in cystic fibrosis. J Am Coll Nutr. 2003;22:253–7.
50. Wood LG, Fitzgerald DA, Lee AK, Garg ML. Improved antioxidant and fatty acid status of patients with cystic fibrosis after antioxidant supplementation is linked to improved lung function. Am J Clin Nutr. 2003;77(1):150–9.
51. Papas KA, Sontag MK, Pardee C, Sokol RJ, Sagel SD, Accurso FJ, et al. A pilot study on the safety and efficacy of a novel antioxidant rich formulation in patients with cystic fibrosis. J Cyst Fibros. 2008;7(1):60–7.
52. Shahar E, Folsom AR, Melnick SL, Tockman MS, Comstock GW, Gennaro V, et al. Dietary n-3 polyunsaturated fatty acids and smoking-related chronic obstructive pulmonary disease. N Engl J Med. 1994;331(4):228–34.
53. Schwartz J. Role of polyunsaturated fatty acid in lung disease. Am J Clin Nutr. 2000;71(suppl):397s–406.
54. Halliwell B. Reactive oxygen species in living systems: source, biochemistry, and role in human disease. Am J Med. 1991;91:14S–22.
55. Anderson BM, Ma D. Are all n-3 polyunsaturated fatty acids created equal? Lipids Health Dis. 2009;8(33):1–20.
56. Matsuyama W, Mitsuyama H, Watanabe M, Oonakahara K, Higashimoto I, Osame M, et al. Effects of omega-3 polyunsaturated fatty acids on inflammatory markers in COPD. Chest. 2005;128(6): 3817–27.
57. James MJ, Gibson RA, Cleland LG. Dietary polyunsaturated fatty acids and inflammatory mediator production. Am J Clin Nutr. 2000;71(1(suppl)):343S–8.
58. Clinical Practice Guidelines on Growth and Nutrition Subcommittee, Ad Hoc Working Group, Stallings VA, Stark LJ, Robinson KA, Feranchak AP, et al. Evidence-based practice recommendations for nutrition-related management of children and adults with cystic fibrosis and pancreatic insufficiency: results of a systematic review. J Am Diet Assoc. 2008;108(5):832–9.
59. McKarney C, Everard M, N'Diaye T. Omega-3 fatty acids (from fish oils) for cystic fibrosis. Cochrane Database Syst Rev. 2007;(4):CD002201.
60. Durieu I, Vericel E, Guichardant D, Roth H, Steghens JP, Drai J, et al. Fatty acids platelets and oxidative markers following intravenous n-3 fatty acids administration in cystic fibrosis: an open pilot observational study. J Cyst Fibros. 2007;6(5):320–6.
61. Romieu I, Trenga C. Diet and obstructive lung diseases. Epidemiol Rev. 2001;23:268–71.
62. Romieu I, Meneses F, Ramirez M, Ruiz S, Perez A, Padilla R, et al. Antioxidant supplementation and respiratory functions among workers exposed to high levels of ozone. Am J Respir Crit Care Med. 1998;158:226–32.
63. Kelly F. Vitamins an respiratory disease: antioxidant micronutrients in pulmonary health an disease. Proc Nutr Soc. 2005;64:510–26.
64. Niki E, Noguchi N, Tsuchihashi H, Gotoh N. Interaction among vitamin C, vitamin E, and beta-carotene. Am J Clin Nutr. 1995;62(6):1322S.
65. Herbert V. Prooxidant effects of antioxidant vitamins: introduction. J Nutr. 1996;126:1197S–200.
66. Romieu I. Nutrition and lung health [State of the Art]. Int J Tuberc Lung Dis. 2005;9(4):362–74.
67. Miedema I, Feskens E, Heederik D, Kromhout D. Dietary determinants of long-term incidence of chronic nonspecific lung diseases. The zutphen study. Am J Epidemiol. 1993;138(1):37–45.
68. Carey IM, Strachan DP, Cook DG. Effects of changes in fresh fruit consumption on ventilatory function in healthy British adults. Am J Respir Crit Care Med. 1998;158:728–33.
69. Butland BK, Fehily AM, Elwood PC. Diet, lung function decline in a cohort of 2512 middle aged men. Thorax. 2000;55:102–8.
70. McKeever T, Scrivener S, Broadfield E, Jones Z, Britton J, Lewis S. Prospective study of diet and decline in lung function in a general population. Am J Respir Crit Care Med. 2002;165:1299–303.
71. Varraso R, Fung TT, Barr RG, Hu FB, Willett W, Camargo Jr CA. Prospective study of dietary patterns and chronic obstructive pulmonary disease among US women. Am J Clin Nutr. 2007;86(2):488–95.
72. Schünemann H, Freudenheim J, Grant B. Epidemiologic evidence linking antioxidant vitamins to pulmonary function and airway obstruction. Epidemiol Rev. 2001;23(2):248–67.
73. Cao G, Booth S, Sadowski J, Prior R. Increases in human plasma antioxidant capacity after consumption of controlled diets high in fruits and vegetables. Am J Clin Nutr. 1998;68:1081–7.
74. Britton JR, Pavord ID, Richards KA, Knox AJ, Wisniewski AF, Lewis SA, et al. Dietary antioxidant vitamin intake and lung function in the general population. Am J Respir Crit Care Med. 1995;151:1383–7.
75. Schwartz J, Weiss ST. Relationship between dietary vitamin C intake and pulmonary function in the First National Health and Nutrition Examination Survey (NHANES I). Am J Clin Nutr. 1994;59:110–4.
76. Grievink L, Smit H, Ocké M, Van 't Veer P, Kromhout D. Dietary intake of antioxidant (pro)-vitamins, respiratory symptoms and pulmonary function: the MORGEN study. Thorax. 1998;53:166–71.
77. Tujague J, Bastaki M, Holland N, Balmes JR, Tager IB. Antioxidant intake, GSTM1 polymorphism and pulmonary function in healthy young adults. Eur Respir J. 2006;27(2):282–8.
78. Morabia AA, Soreenson A, Kumanyika SK, Abbey H, Cohen BH, Chee E. Vitamin A, cigarette smoking and airway obstruction. Am Rev Respir Dis. 1989;140:1312–6.

79. McKeever TM, Britton J. Diet and asthma. Am J Respir Crit Care Med. 2004;170:725–9.
80. Chuwers P, Barnhart S, Blanc P, Brodkin CA, Cullen M, Kelly T, et al. The protective effect of beta-carotene and retinol on ventilatory function in an asbestos-exposed cohort. Am J Respir Crit Care Med. 1997;155:1066–71.
81. Hu G, Cassano PA. Antioxidant nutrients and pulmonary function: the third national health and nutrition examination survey (NHANES III). Am J Epidemiol. 2000;151(10):975–81.
82. The ATBC Cancer Prevention Study Group. The alpha-tocopherol, beta-carotene lung cancer prevention study: design, methods, participant characteristics, and compliance. Ann Epidemiol. 1994;4(1):1–10.
83. The Alpha-Tocopherol Beta Carotene Cancer Prevention Study Group. The effect of vitamin E and beta carotene on the incidence of lung cancer and other cancers in male smokers. N Engl J Med. 1994;330:1029–35.
84. Omenn G. Chemoprevention of lung cancers: lessons from CARET, the beta-carotene and retinol efficacy trial, and prospects for the future. Eur J Cancer Prev. 2007;16(3):184–91.
85. Riise GC, Williams A, Kjellstrom C, Schersten H, Andersson BA, Kelly FJ. Bronchiolitis obliterans syndrome in lung transplant recipients is associated with increased neutrophil activity and decreased antioxidant status in the lung. Eur Respir J. 1998;12 (1):82–8.
86. Kelly F, Mudway I, Blomberg A, Frew A, Sandstrom T. Altered lung antioxidant status in patients with mild asthma. Lancet. 1999;354:482–3.
87. Schock B, Young I, Brown V, Fitch P, Shields M. Antioxidants and oxidative stress in BAL fluid of atopic asthmatic children. Pediatr Res. 2002;53(3):375–81.
88. Portal B, Richard M, Faure H, Hadjian A, Favier A. Altered antioxidant status and increased lipid peroxidation in children with cystic fibrosis. Am J Clin Nutr. 1995;61(4):843–7.
89. Back EI, Frindt C, Nohr D, Frank J, Ziebach R, Stern M, et al. Antioxidant deficiency in cystic fibrosis: when is the right time to take action? Am J Clin Nutr. 2004;80:374–84.
90. Renner S, Rath R, Rust P, Lehr S, Frischer T, Elmadfa I, et al. Effects of β-carotene supplementation for six months on clinical and laboratory parameters in patients with cystic fibrosis. Thorax. 2001;56:48–52.
91. Bowler RP, Velsor LW, Duda B, Chan ED, Abraham E, Ware LB, et al. Pulmonary edema fluid antioxidants are depressed in acute lung injury. Crit Care Med. 2003;31(9):2309–15.
92. Thomson MJ, Puntmann V, Kaski JC. Atherosclerosis and oxidant stress: the end of the road for antioxidant vitamin treatment? Cardiovasc Drugs Ther. 2007;21:195–210.
93. Boothby LA, Doering PL. Vitamin C and vitamin E for Alzheimer's disease. Ann Pharmaocother. 2005;39(12):2073–80.
94. Bjelakovic G, Nikolova D, Gluud LL, Simonetti RG, Gluud C. Antioxidant supplements for prevention of mortality in healthy participants and patients with various diseases. Cochrane Database Syst Rev. 2008;(2):CD007176.
95. Bjelakovic G. Mortality in randomized trials of antioxidant supplements for primary and secondary prevention: systematic review and meta-analysis. JAMA. 2007;297(8):842–57.
96. Miller ER, Pastor-Barriuso R, Dalal D, Riemersma RA, Appel LJ, Guallar E. Meta-analysis: high-dosage vitamin E supplementation may increase all-cause mortality. Ann Intern Med. 2005;142(1): 37–46.
97. Sesso HD, Buring JE, Christen WG, Kurth T, Belanger C, MacFadyen J, et al. Vitamins E and C in the prevention of cardiovascular disease in men: the Physicians' health study II randomized controlled trial. JAMA. 2008;300(18):2123–33.
98. Vivekananthan DP, Penn MS, Sapp SK, Hsu A, Topol EJ. Use of antioxidant vitamins for the prevention of cardiovascular disease: meta-analysis of randomized trials. Lancet. 2003;361(9374):2017–23.
99. Hennekens CH, Buring JE, Manson JE, Stampfer M, Rosner B, Cook NR, et al. Lack of effect of long-term supplementation with beta carotene on the incidence of malignant neoplasms and cardiovascular disease. N Engl J Med. 1996;334(18):1145–9.
100. Gaziano JM, Glynn RJ, Christen WG, Kurth T, Belanger C, MacFadyen J, et al. Vitamins E and C in the prevention of prostate and total cancer in men: the Physicians' health study II randomized controlled trial. JAMA. 2009;301(1):52–62.
101. Lippman SM, Klein EA, Goodman PJ, Lucia MS, Thompson IM, Ford LG, et al. Effect of selenium and vitamin E on risk of prostate cancer and other cancers: the selenium and vitamin E cancer prevention trial (SELECT). JAMA. 2009;301(1):39–51.
102. Heinecke JW. Is the emperor wearing clothing? Clinical trials of vitamin E and the LDL oxidation hypothesis. Arterioscler Thromb Vasc Biol. 2001;21:1261–4.
103. Berger MM. Can oxidative damage be treated nutritionally? Clin Nutr. 2005;24(2):172–83.
104. Lampe JW. Health effects of vegetables and fruit: assessing mechanisms of action in human experimental studies. Am J Clin Nutr. 1999;70(3):475S–90.
105. Pellegrini N, Salvatore S, Valtuena S, Bedogni G, Porrini M, Pala V, et al. Development and validation of a food frequency questionnaire for the assessment of dietary total antioxidant capacity. J Nutr. 2007;137(1):93–8.
106. Pellegrini N, Serafini M, Salvatore S, Del Rio D, Bianchi M, Brighenti F. Total antioxidant capacity of spices, dried fruits, nuts, pulses, cereals and sweets consumed in Italy assessed by three different in vitro assays. Mol Nutr Food Res. 2006;50(11):1030–8.
107. Pellegrini N, Serafini M, Colombi B, Del Rio D, Salvatore S, Bianchi M, et al. Total antioxidant capacity of plant foods, beverages and oils consumed in Italy assessed by three different in vitro assays. J Nutr. 2003;133(9):2812–9.
108. Pellegrini N, Riso P, Porrini M. Tomato consumption does not affect the total antioxidant capacity of plasma. Nutrition. 2000;16(4):268–71.
109. Brighenti F, Valtuena S, Pellegrini N. Total antioxidant capacity of the diet is inversely and independently related to plasma concentration of high-sensitivity C-reactive protein in adult Italian subjects. Br J Nutr. 2005;93(5):619–25.
110. di Giuseppe R, Arcari A, Serafini M, Di Castelnuovo A, Zito F, De Curtis A, et al. Total dietary antioxidant capacity and lung function in an Italian population: a favorable role in premenopausal/never smoker women. Eur J Clin Nutr. 2012;66:61–8.
111. Scalbert A, Johnson IT, Saltmarsh M. Polyphenols: antioxidants and beyond. Am J Clin Nutr. 2005;81:215S–7.
112. Meyers DG, Maloley PA, Weeks D. Safety of antioxidant vitamins. Arch Intern Med. 1996;156(9):925–35.
113. Krinsky HI. Human requirements for fat-soluble vitamins, and other things concerning these nutrients. Mol Aspects Med. 2003;24:317.
114. Halliwell B. Establishing the significance and optimal intake of dietary antioxidants: the biomarker concept. Nutr Rev. 1999;57(4): 104–13.

Part XV

Ventricular Assist Device

Mechanical Unloading and Heart Remodeling Features

49

Nikolaos A. Diakos, Omar Wever-Pinzon, Anthony S. Zannas, and Stavros G. Drakos

Introduction

Left ventricular assist devices (LVADs) are increasingly used in the everyday clinical practice to either 'bridge' end-stage heart failure (HF) patients to heart transplantation or as a permanent ('destination') therapy. Myocardial remodeling driven by excess pressure and volume load is believed to be responsible for the vicious cycle of progressive myocardial dysfunction in chronic HF [1]. This mechanistic model led to the hypothesis that LVAD support would disrupt this cycle and, by providing profound volume and pressure unloading, allow for a reversal of stress-related compensatory responses of the overloaded myocardium [2–4]. This in turn would lead to subsequent structural and functional "reverse remodeling" at organ and tissue levels [2–4].

Limited clinical data have suggested that LVAD therapy can occasionally reverse the complex process of chronic myocardial remodeling to the point where a subset of patients can be successfully weaned from the LVAD ("bridge to recovery") [5–8]. Achieving sustained myocardial recovery after LVAD explantation in a patient with chronic HF is one of the most desirable goals in the treatment of heart disease [9]. Consequently, the mechanisms that might facilitate LVAD unloading-induced myocardial reverse remodeling have become the subject of intensive research [2–4], and this has been favored by the fact that the LVAD patient population possesses a series of significant research advantages. However, fundamental questions at the basic science, translational, and clinical level remain unanswered.

N.A. Diakos, MD (✉) • O. Wever-Pinzon, MD
S.G. Drakos, MD
Heart Failure Program (Division of Cardiology) and Molecular Medicine Program (Eccles Institute of Human Genetics), University of Utah, Salt Lake City, UT, USA
e-mail: ndiakos@u2m2.utah.edu

A.S. Zannas, MD, MSc
Department of Psychiatry, Duke University Medical Center, Durham, NC 27710, USA

Effects of LVAD-Induced Unloading on Myocardial Structure

Key changes that have been described in the failing myocardium after LVAD unloading include alterations in cardiomyocyte hypertrophy, extracellular matrix, microvasculature, and adrenergic pathways-sympathetic innervation, among others. These effects are summarized in Table 49.1 and will be described in this section.

Cardiac Hypertrophy – Atrophy

Hypertrophic growth of cardiomyocytes is the common mechanism by which the heart reduces stress on the failing ventricular wall. Pulsatile LVAD unloading has been repeatedly shown to induce regression of cardiac myocyte hypertrophy – cell length, width, and thickness [10]. This is in agreement with data showing that pulsatile LVAD unloading reverses the altered cardiac production of natriuretic peptides along with parallel reductions in myocardial mass and myocyte size [4]. Regarding the exact mechanisms governing hypertrophy regression during pulsatile LVAD support, reviewed in detail elsewhere, ongoing investigations examining the complex role of Akt kinase/cyclooxygenase-2, mitogen-activated protein kinases (MAPK)/extracellular signal-related kinases (Erks),

Table 49.1 Cardiac remodeling parameters favorably altered with LVAD unloading

Hypertrophy
Contractile dysfunction
Calcium cycling
Cytoskeletal proteins (sarcomeric, non-sarcomeric, membrane)
Beta-adrenergic signaling
Metabolism and bioenergetics
Myocyte death (apoptosis, autophagy, stress)
Endothelium and microvasculature
Sympathetic innervation
Circulating neurohormones, cytokines

E.A. Gabriel, S.A. Gabriel (eds.), *Inflammatory Response in Cardiovascular Surgery*, DOI 10.1007/978-1-4471-4429-8_49, © Springer-Verlag London 2013

and Akt kinase/glycogen synthase kinase 3β (GSK3β) underscore their importance in the pathogenesis and regulation of cardiac hypertrophy. Whether the primary stimulus for the regression of hypertrophy is directly related to mechanical unloading/stretch or to circulating systemic factors needs to be further investigated. Interestingly, a study from the Harefield group examining myocytes from pulsatile LVAD patients with and without myocardial functional recovery demonstrated that myocytes from both groups had similar reductions in cell size, suggesting that hypertrophy regression might not be specifically related to the structural signature of LVAD-induced myocardial recovery [11].

Animal models of prolonged unloading in nonfailing, nonhypertrophic myocardium by means of heterotopic transplantation or LVAD or severing the chordae tendinae of the mitral papillary muscle suggested that mechanical unloading could lead to cardiac myocyte atrophy. Whether this phenomenon applies only to nonfailing and nonhypertrophic or also to hypertrophic and failing myocardium unloaded by LVAD is controversial. One animal study of hypertrophic failing hearts indicated that unloading by means of heterotopic transplantation resulted in a decrease of cardiac myocyte size beyond normal values [12]. However, in two human HF studies, unloading by means of pulsatile LVAD support also revealed a decrease of cardiac myocyte size, but not beyond the size of normal donor cardiac myocytes [13, 14]. In a later study from our group in which light microscopy findings were complemented by ultrastructural and metabolic data, we did not identify any evidence suggesting cardiac myocyte atrophy or degeneration during pulsatile LVAD support [14]. More research needs to be performed to clarify whether prolonged mechanical unloading with the currently utilized continuous flow LVADs affects basic protein degradation pathways (calcium-dependent calpain system, ubiquitin proteasome system, and lysosomal proteolysis) and/or fetal gene program overexpression, which have been implicated in cardiac hypertrophy and atrophic remodeling .

Finally, a recent study examined cardiomyocyte DNA content, nuclear morphology, and the number of nuclei per cell before and after LVAD support [15]. After unloading, the number of polyploid cardiomyocytes and cardiomyocyte DNA content declined, whereas an increase in binucleated cardiomyocytes was observed. The authors hypothesized that the vast polyploidy of cardiomyocytes in the failing human heart was a result of hypertrophic growth associated with repeated rounds of DNA synthesis that despite completion of DNA replication did not result in cell division. The increase in binucleated cardiomyocytes could suggest that reduction of noxious hypertrophic stimuli through LVAD unloading might have led to beneficial cardiomyocyte duplication and regeneration. These findings suggest that there is a dynamic and plastic regulation of cardiomyocyte content in HF, which strengthens the notion that at least a proportion of cardiomyocytes are not terminally differentiated and could reenter the cell cycle during regenerative processes. Of course, this hypothesis requires further confirmation.

Extracellular Matrix

Remodeling of extracellular matrix, specifically an increase in fibrosis, is a hallmark feature of myocardial remodeling in chronic HF. Altered collagen metabolism is responsible for ventricular dilatation and for changes in systolic and diastolic function. Investigations of the effect of mechanical unloading on extracellular matrix have shown conflicting results: one group of investigators has reported decreased fibrosis, while others found an increase in fibrosis associated with an increase in cross-linked collagen and myocardial stiffness [2, 3, 10]. The explanation for the contradictory observations is not clear, with some attributing the inconsistent results to differences in the methodology employed [2, 3]. Applying recent advances in whole-field digital microscopy, we addressed this issue using digital histopathology and advanced image analysis techniques, an approach that reduces observer bias, increases the amount of myocardial tissue analyzed, and permits comprehensive endocardium-to-epicardium evaluation [14]. This eliminates the confounding effect of endocardial or epicardial sampling known to be associated with different degrees of fibrosis. In failing hearts, interstitial and total fibrosis was higher compared with normal myocardium, and the collagen content increased further after LVAD unloading [14].

Changes in the neurohormonal milieu seen after LVAD implant support the above findings. While older studies indicated that circulating levels of many neurohormones (plasma epinephrine, norepinephrine, arginine, vasopressin, renin, and angiotensin II) decrease after LVAD implant, the effects of LVAD unloading on the *myocardial tissue* renin-angiotensin-aldosterone system (RAAS) components (including the profibrotic and prohypertrophic angiotensin II) seem to be more complicated. Klotz et al. recently published results of the first study that systematically analyzed the different components of RAAS in paired myocardial tissue samples obtained before and after LVAD implantation [16]. Renin levels in the pre-LVAD myocardium were the highest ever reported in human cardiac tissue (100× normal), and the myocardial aldosterone level was also elevated (250× normal). After LVAD support, myocardial renin and aldosterone levels markedly decreased, but, in contrast with this finding, myocardial angiotensin I and II levels increased five to ten fold [16]. The increase in the myocardial level of angiotensin II during LVAD support was accompanied by a seven fold rise in myocardial norepinephrine content [16]. Increased norepinephrine levels are also known to lead to cardiac fibrosis. The same group of investigators reported an increase in the ratio of matrix metalloproteinases (MMPs) to tissue inhibitors of metalloproteinases (TIMP-1) in end-stage HF, which normalized after LVAD unloading, favoring decreased collagen degradation and hence increased fibrosis [17]. Collectively, these post-LVAD myocardial biomarker alterations are compatible with the structural findings, suggesting increased post-LVAD fibrosis. Whether the observed increase in fibrosis is a manifestation of further progression of cardiac remodeling that LVAD unloading failed to reverse or a direct result of LVAD actively inducing an increase in fibrosis warrants further investigation.

Endothelium and Microvasculature

Myocardial microvascular density is reduced in patients with HF. LVAD unloading has been shown to lead to changes in the expression of genes involved in the regulation of vascular organization and migration. In agreement with these findings, our group demonstrated that pulsatile LVAD unloading resulted in increased microvascular density in failing human hearts [14]. We also found strong evidence of endothelial cell activation by both immunohistochemistry (the endothelial activation marker major histocompatibility complex class-II, MHC-II) and by electron microscopy (ultrastructure analysis) [14]. The findings of a post-LVAD increase in microvascular density and endothelial cell activation were also accompanied by increased interstitial and total myocardial fibrosis [14]. This suggests that the recently described mechanistic link between the endothelium and cardiac fibrosis during the cardiac remodeling process – "endothelial to mesenchymal transition" via pathways directly implicated in cardiomyocyte hypertrophy [18, 19] – might also apply to human myocardium. Obviously, direct proof for such a mechanism requires lineage tracing possible only in genetically manipulated animal models [18, 19]. Of note, work done in our laboratory has shown that endothelial proliferation and migration, hallmarks of angiogenesis, must be balanced by mechanisms that stabilize the endothelium so that a functional vascular network may be established and maintained [20–22]. An imbalance in these competing signals after LVAD implantation may contribute to the increase in microvascular density, endothelial activation, and cardiac fibrosis.

Beta-Adrenergic Signal Transduction

The changes in the β-adrenergic receptor (AR) system in the failing heart are well known. Typically, the β1-AR density is selectively reduced, and the remaining β1- and β2-AR are desensitized. The response of cardiomyocytes to β-adrenergic stimulation with isoproterenol after long-term LVAD support was characterized by an increase in the magnitude of contraction and shortening of the time to peak contraction and time to 50 % relaxation [23]. In isolated trabecular muscles of failing human hearts with and without LVAD support, Ogletree-Hughes et al. found that unloading restores the density of β-AR in cardiomyocytes [24]. They also found that muscle from hearts that had been supported with LVAD produced an inotropic response to isoproterenol similar to nonfailing hearts, significantly stronger than that observed with muscles from failing hearts that had not been mechanically supported. However, the receptor density alone did not predict the magnitude of the inotropic response [24]. Similarly, in another study, an increase in β-adrenergic density and a prominent normalization in the location of the receptors in the myocardium were observed following ventricular unloading [25]. The potentially important role of β-AR signaling in the reverse remodeling process that occurs in mechanically assisted failing hearts is also supported by experimental observations showing that β2-AR stimulation results in inotropic support of the heart and decreases apoptosis, while β1-AR causes progressive cardiomyopathy and HF.

Altogether, these observations suggest that it might be beneficial to combine ventricular unloading with an augmentation of β2-AR signaling to enhance reverse remodeling. In this direction, in order to maximize the efficiency of LVAD as a bridge to recovery, M.H. Yacoub combined mechanical unloading with the selective β2 agonist clenbuterol to take advantage of the therapeutic effects of β2-AR signaling on the heart as well as of the antiatrophic effects of clenbuterol on the mechanically unloaded myocardium and on skeletal muscles [26]. According to the Harefield protocol, clenbuterol is added to standard medical treatment for HF, including β1-blockade, angiotensin-converting enzyme, or angiotensin-II inhibition, spironolactone and digoxin, when maximal regression of the LV end-diastolic and end-systolic diameters has been reached, usually after approximately 2 months of LVAD support, and when they have remained stable for at least 2 weeks. Using this strategy, Yacoub's group was able to remove LVAD successfully from 11 out of 15 patients suffering from non-ischemic cardiomyopathy, and excellent cardiac function was preserved during long-term follow-up [7].

Whether stimulation of β2-AR with clenbuterol best takes advantage of the beneficial effects of β2-AR signaling described earlier in order to enhance the effectiveness of chronic mechanical unloading, with myocardial recovery as a target, certainly needs further investigation.

Effects of LVAD-Induced Unloading on Myocardial Function

Ventricular remodeling is associated with a rightward shift of the pressure-volume loop toward larger volumes, while pulsatile LVAD unloading results in a leftward shift in the direction of a normal physiological relationship. Both continuous flow

Table 49.2 LVAD bridge to recovery studies

	Study design	*N*	Adjuvant drug therapy protocol	Unloading duration (m)	Recovery[a] *N*, (%)
US LVAD Working group 2007 [5]	P	67	Not standardized	4.5	6 (9)
Berlin group 2008 [6]	R	188	Not standardized	4	35 (19)
Harefield group 2006 [7]	P	15	Yes	11	11 (73)
Harefield group 2011 [8]	P	20	Yes	9	12 (60)
University of Athens-Harefield group 2007 [4]	P	8	Yes	7	4 (50)
Vancouver group 2011 [28]	P	17	Not standardized	7	4 (23)
Gothenburg group 2007 [29]	P	18	Not standardized	7	3 (17)
Osaka group 2005 [30]	R	11	Not standardized	15	5 (45)
Pittsburgh group 2010 [31]	R	18	Not standardized	8	6 (33)
Multicenter 2002 [32]	R	271	N/A	2	22 (8)
Columbia group 1998 [33]	R	111	N/A	6	5 (4.5)

HF heart failure, *LVAD* left ventricular assist device, *m* months, *N* number of patients, *N/A* not applicable, *P* prospective studies, *R* retrospective studies

[a]Defined as LVAD explantation due to functional myocardial recovery

and pulsatile flow LVADs are associated with significant volume unloading and subsequent decrease in LV end-diastolic diameter. However, pulsatile LVADs seem to have a more pronounced volume unloading effect compared with continuous flow LVADs [10]. Continuous flow LVADs, in addition to LV unloading, have also been associated with significant left atrial volume unloading and improved left atrial function at 3–6 months after LVAD implantation [10].

LVAD unloading results in increased cardiac output and near normalization of pulmonary artery pressures and LV systolic and diastolic pressures. These changes are comparable regardless of the etiology of HF and are similar in magnitude in pulsatile and continuous flow LVADs. Etz et al. reported that continuous flow LVADs implanted in patients with medically refractory pulmonary hypertension resulted in a significant reduction in mean pulmonary artery pressures and pulmonary vascular resistance, and these patients were subsequently successfully transplanted [27].

Left ventricular unloading by LVAD also has significant effects on the right ventricle (RV). LVAD unloading will typically result in a decrease in RV afterload and improved RV geometry and systolic function [4]. However, higher than optimal continuous flow LVAD unloading can result in a leftward shift of the interventricular septum with a resulting compromise in RV systolic function and RV failure [4].

Exercise intolerance in patients with chronic HF is associated with respiratory muscle weakness and poor outcomes [10]. In a study where cardiopulmonary exercise testing was done before and after continuous flow LVAD placement, we observed that all patients had a restrictive ventilatory pattern before LVAD implantation. This improved during LVAD support and was associated with a significant increase in the anaerobic threshold, peak work rate, and exercise duration, findings consistent with other investigations [10].

Experience from "Bridge to Recovery Studies"

The main results of key clinical outcome studies investigating LVAD used as a bridge to recovery are summarized in Table 49.2 [4–8, 28–33]. Most of the clinical outcome studies that addressed myocardial recovery during LVAD support were retrospective, and the results, as far as the success of LVAD weaning and of achieving sustained myocardial recovery, varied significantly (Table 49.2). These inconsistencies can be explained by numerous limitations in the study design, such as (1) absence of a pre-specified protocol to monitor functional myocardial recovery, (2) absence of a pre-specified protocol for the use of adjuvant pharmacotherapy with potential anti-remodeling effects, (3) variable duration of LVAD support, (4) lack of standardized LVAD explantation criteria, and (5) diversity of the populations studied in their propensity for recovery. With the exception of three recent studies from Berlin, Harefield, and Vancouver [8, 28, 34], the majority of the devices utilized in the bridge to recovery studies have so far included first generation, pulsatile LVADs. The most effective approach aimed at recovery of myocardial function reported so far is that of the Harefield protocol, which tested mechanical unloading combined with aggressive anti-remodeling drug therapy, including the beta-2 agonist clenbuterol, in advanced non-ischemic cardiomyopathy patients [4, 7, 8]. Reproducibility of these results in larger patient cohorts and in a randomized fashion would be of great importance.

Future Directions

The impact of the etiology of HF on the potential for myocardial recovery is not well understood (Table 49.3, target 2). Direct comparisons between ischemic and non-ischemic

Table 49.3 LVAD unloading and myocardial recovery: unsolved issues – future directions

Unsolved issues-ongoing research targets
Target 1: Correlate structural and functional findings
Target 2: Impact of HF etiology on the potential of myocardial recovery
Target 3: Role of HF duration on prospect of cardiac reverse remodeling
Target 4: Extent of pre LVAD remodeling
Target 5: Type of unloading: pulsatile vs. continuous vs. counterpulsation
Target 6: Targeted adjuvant therapies
Target 7: Functional and structural evaluation protocols
Target 8: Optimal duration of mechanical unloading
Target 9: Determinants of myocardial recovery

patients were performed in only a few studies. The likely candidates for reverse remodeling induced by LVAD unloading usually include patients with non-ischemic cardiomyopathy of different etiologies: idiopathic, hypertensive, peripartum, familial, alcoholic, etc. However, ischemic cardiomyopathy patients who have suffered myocardial infarction and have large areas of non-infarcted myocardium that 'remodeled' over the years could also be considered candidates [4]. This latter concept deserves further investigation and could combine the excision of scarred myocardium, using LV reconstruction techniques (e.g., Dor operation) with LVAD unloading. It can be argued that with this approach the index event that triggered the cascade of cardiac remodeling progression – the post-myocardial infarction scar– has been eliminated [4]. In contrast, in most non-ischemic cardiomyopathy cases, the index event that caused progressive ventricular remodeling and HF often remains undetermined, most likely persists despite an initially successful reversal of the process by mechanical unloading, and might recur and cause further progression of HF after the termination of LVAD support. This might explain why long-term freedom from recurrent HF in the largest bridge to recovery series in non-ischemic cardiomyopathy patients was 74 and 66 % at 3–5 years, respectively [6].

The importance of the duration of HF on the prospect for cardiac reverse remodeling also needs further study. Data from two series of patients that were successfully bridged to sustained recovery have identified 'duration of HF history' (i.e., time from HF symptoms onset) as an important predictor of favorable response [6, 8]. In terms of the cardiac remodeling trajectory, the time from the index event that triggered the HF syndrome, rather than the time from symptom onset, would be an even more meaningful target (Table 49.3, target 3). However, we need to acknowledge that in the clinical research arena this may be a target too hard to achieve. The index event can often be determined in ischemic cardiomyopathy patients, but it may be hard to identify in non-ischemic patients. Even in ischemic cardiomyopathy, other factors such as ischemia induced by non-culprit lesions, repetitive stunning, etc., add to the complexity. Insofar as the 'HF history duration' can be viewed as a surrogate of potential irreversibility of chronic remodeling, it may be argued that a more direct research target would be the identification of the degree of pre-LVAD structural or molecular remodeling beyond which there is 'no return.' Indeed, Bruckner et al. have reported that patients with worse hypertrophy and higher degrees of fibrosis at baseline (the time of LVAD implantation) were by far less likely to show recovery of LV systolic function during LVAD unloading [35]. More research needs to be done to determine what degree of pre-LVAD myocardial remodeling changes preclude unloading-induced reversibility and thus provide useful guidance for patient selection (Table 49.3, target 4).

Another important issue in need of further investigation is the definition of the specific type of mechanical unloading that best promotes reverse remodeling (Table 49.3, target 5). Various LVAD types have been tested in the experimental and clinical arenas during the last half century: pulsatile, non pulsatile/continuous flow, and counterpulsatile. Mainly for engineering reasons, the clinical field has recently shifted from pulsatile to continuous flow LVADs. Whether these devices also have different effects on the biological outcomes needs to be further investigated. Consequently, whether the prospects of LVAD-induced reverse remodeling are better served by pulsatile, non-pulsatile, or counterpulsation devices, and by full or partial unloading, is unknown. Future studies must be designed targeting the identification of specific ventricular-assist device properties that would best promote reverse remodeling.

The potential impact of the following important issues also needs to be clarified: the concept of targeted adjuvant drug therapies (introduced by Sir Magdi H. Yacoub) [26], the optimal duration of mechanical unloading, and the development of advanced protocols to monitor the unloaded myocardium during LVAD support (Table 49.3, targets 6, 7, 8). These latter imaging protocols could include either conventional imaging techniques (echocardiography, nuclear imaging, computed tomography) or molecular imaging techniques. They will need to address the challenging issue of reliable testing of the heart's performance under both decreased and increased loading conditions – the so-called 'off-pump' or 'turn-down' studies. These monitoring protocols should also evaluate the short- and long-term impact of LVAD support on the right ventricle (RV). The published studies gave conflicting results on this issue. Some investigations have shown evidence of improved RV structure and function after LVAD support, suggesting that the normalization of both the hemodynamic status and the neurohormonal milieu also has favorable effects on the RV. On the contrary, Klotz et al. found that biventricular assist device support resulted in significant reverse structural and functional remodeling of both the RV and the LV, while RV reverse remodeling was not seen during LVAD support alone [36]. The authors concluded that a lesser degree of volume unloading provided to the RV during LVAD support may not be sufficient to result in significant reverse structural and functional remodeling of the RV. In fact, it is not uncommon after LVAD implant to find the net effect on the RV to be the one of overloading, rather than unloading, a result of the higher cardiac output offsetting the benefit derived from the LVAD-induced decrease of pulmonary pressures.

References

1. Katz AM. Maladaptive growth in the failing heart: the cardiomyopathy of overload. Cardiovasc Drugs Ther. 2002;16:245–9.
2. Soppa GK, Barton PJ, Terracciano CM, et al. Left ventricular assist device-induced molecular changes in the failing myocardium. Curr Opin Cardiol. 2008;23:206–18.
3. Klotz S, Jan Danser AH, Burkhoff D. Impact of left ventricular assist device (LVAD) support on the cardiac reverse remodeling process. Prog Biophys Mol Biol. 2008;97:479–96.
4. Drakos SG, Terrovitis JV, Anastasiou-Nana MI, Nanas JN. Reverse remodeling during long-term mechanical unloading of the left ventricle. J Mol Cell Cardiol. 2007;43:231–42.
5. Maybaum S, Mancini D, Xydas S, et al. Cardiac improvement during mechanical circulatory support: a prospective multicenter study of the LVAD Working Group. Circulation. 2007;115:2497–505.
6. Dandel M, Weng Y, Siniawski H, et al. Prediction of cardiac stability after weaning from left ventricular assist devices in patients with idiopathic dilated cardiomyopathy. Circulation. 2008;118:S94–105.
7. Birks EJ, Tansley PD, Hardy J, et al. Left ventricular assist device and drug therapy for the reversal of heart failure. N Engl J Med. 2006;355:1873–84.
8. Birks EJ, George RS, Hedger M, et al. Reversal of severe heart failure with a continuous-flow left ventricular assist device and pharmacological therapy: a prospective study. Circulation. 2011;123(4):381–90.
9. Drakos SG, Charitos EI, Nanas SN, et al. Ventricular-assist devices for the treatment of chronic heart failure. Expert Rev Cardiovasc Ther. 2007;5:571–84.
10. Drakos SG, Kfoury AG, Selzman CH, et al. Left ventricular assist device unloading effects on myocardial structure and function: current status of the field and call for action. Curr Opin Cardiol. 2011;26:245–55.
11. Terracciano CM, Hardy J, Birks EJ, et al. Clinical recovery from end-stage heart failure using left – ventricular assist device and pharmacological therapy correlates with increased sarcoplasmic reticulum calcium content but not with regression of cellular hypertrophy. Circulation. 2004;109:2263–5.
12. Oriyanhan W, Tsuneyoshi H, Nishina T, et al. Determination of optimal duration of mechanical unloading for failing hearts to achieve bridge to recovery in a rat heterotopic heart transplantation model. J Heart Lung Transplant. 2007;26:16–23.
13. Jacquet L, Zerbe T, Stein KL, et al. Evolution of human cardiac myocyte dimension during prolonged mechanical support. J Thorac Cardiovasc Surg. 1991;101:256–9.
14. Drakos SG, Kfoury AG, Hammond EH, et al. Impact of mechanical unloading on microvasculature and associated central remodeling features of the failing human heart. J Am Coll Cardiol. 2010;56:382–91.
15. Wohlschlaeger J, Levkau B, Brockhoff G, et al. Hemodynamic support by left ventricular assist devices reduces cardiomyocyte DNA content in the failing human heart. Circulation. 2010;121:989–96.
16. Klotz S, Burkhoff D, Garrelds IM, et al. The impact of left ventricular assist device-induced left ventricular unloading on the myocardial renin-angiotensin-aldosterone system: therapeutic consequences? Eur Heart J. 2009;30:805–12.
17. Klotz S, Foronjy RF, Dickstein ML, et al. Mechanical unloading during left ventricular assist device support increases left ventricular collagen cross-linking and myocardial stiffness. Circulation. 2005;112:364–74.
18. Zeisberg EM, Tarnavski O, Zeisberg M, et al. Endothelial-to-mesenchymal transition contributes to cardiac fibrosis. Nat Med. 2007;13:952–61.
19. Towbin JA. Scarring in the heart – a reversible phenomenon? N Engl J Med. 2007;357:1767–8.
20. Whitehead KJ, Chan AC, Navankasattusas S, et al. The cerebral cavernous malformation signaling pathway promotes vascular integrity via Rho GTPases. Nat Med. 2009;15:177–84.
21. Jones CA, London NR, Chen H, et al. Robo4 stabilizes the vascular network by inhibiting pathologic angiogenesis and endothelial hyperpermeability. Nat Med. 2008;14:448–53.
22. Wilson BD, Ii M, Park KW, et al. Netrins promote developmental and therapeutic angiogenesis. Science. 2006;313:640–4.
23. Dipla K, Mattiello JA, Jeevanandam V, et al. Myocyte recovery after mechanical circulatory support in humans with end-stage heart failure. Circulation. 1998;97:2316–22.
24. Ogletree-Hughes ML, Stull LB, Sweet WE, et al. Mechanical unloading restores beta-adrenergic responsiveness and reverses receptor downregulation in the failing human heart. Circulation. 2001;104:881–6.
25. Bick RJ, Grigore AM, Poindexter BJ, et al. Left ventricular unloading with an assist device results in receptor relocalization as well as increased beta-adrenergic receptor numbers: are these changes indications for outcome? J Card Surg. 2005;20:332–6.
26. Yacoub MH. A novel strategy to maximize the efficacy of left ventricular assist devices as a bridge to recovery. Eur Heart J. 2001;22:534–40.
27. Etz CD, Welp HA, Tjan TD, et al. Medically refractory pulmonary hypertension: treatment with nonpulsatile left ventricular assist devices. Ann Thorac Surg. 2007;83:1697–705.
28. Lamarche Y, Kearns M, Josan K, et al. Successful weaning and explantation of the Heartmate II left ventricular assist device. Can J Cardiol. 2011;27(3):358–62.
29. Liden H, Karason K, Bergh CH, et al. The feasibility of left ventricular mechanical support as a bridge to cardiac recovery. Eur J Heart Fail. 2007;9:525–30.
30. Matsumiya G, Monta O, Fukushima N, et al. Who would be a candidate for bridge to recovery during prolonged mechanical left ventricular support in idiopathic dilated cardiomyopathy? J Thorac Cardiovasc Surg. 2005;130:699–704.
31. Simon MA, Primack BA, Teuteberg J, et al. Left ventricular remodeling and myocardial recovery on mechanical circulatory support. J Card Fail. 2010;16:99–105.
32. Farrar DJ, Holman WR, McBride LR, et al. Long-term follow-up of Thoratec ventricular assist device bridge-to-recovery patients successfully removed from support after recovery of ventricular function. J Heart Lung Transplant. 2002;21:516–21.
33. Mancini DM, Beniaminovitz A, Levin H, et al. Low incidence of myocardial recovery after left ventricular assist device implantation in patients with chronic heart failure. Circulation. 1998;98:2383–9.
34. Krabatsch T, Schweiger M, Dandel M, et al. Is bridge to recovery more likely with pulsatile left ventricular assist devices than with nonpulsatile-flow systems? Ann Thorac Surg. 2011;91:1335–40.
35. Bruckner BA, Razeghi P, Stetson S, et al. Degree of cardiac fibrosis and hypertrophy at time of implantation predicts myocardial improvement during left ventricular assist device support. J Heart Lung Transplant. 2004;23:36–42.
36. Klotz S, Naka Y, Oz MC, Burkhoff D. Biventricular assist device-induced right ventricular reverse structural and functional remodeling. J Heart Lung Transplant. 2005;24:1195–201.

Part XVI

Stem Cells in Cardiovascular Surgery

50 Cytokine Profiles in Cardiac Diseases and Marrow Stromal Cells Therapy

Nasser Alkhamees, Alice Le Huu, and Dominique Shum-Tim

Introduction

Worldwide, it has been estimated that cardiac surgeons perform over 800,000 coronary artery bypass graft (CABG) procedures per year [1]. With the advent of percutaneous coronary intervention (PCI), the number of patients undergoing CABG has declined in recent years. PCI presents a rapid, non-invasive technique for revascularization, but has also created several daunting tasks for cardiac surgeons. Surgeons are increasingly faced with patients suffering from acute myocardial infarction (MI) who have failed PCI and are suffering from advanced heart failure. These patients are often hemodynamically unstable, and the challenge is further confounded by a full-fledged inflammatory response from an evolving MI. As surgeons, the tendency is to focus on the clinical and technical aspects of patient care. However, on a biochemical level, the inflammatory process encompasses every facet of a cardiac surgeon's practice. Understanding the biochemical basis of the inflammatory response allows for a greater appreciation of physiopathological mechanisms responsible for heart disease.

In addition, the basis of the inflammatory process is an intricate interaction between cytokines. Acting as mediators for intercellular communication, these molecules are responsible for propagating damage sustained during an MI, eventually culminating in the development of congestive heart failure (CHF) [2–4]. Paradoxically, recent studies demonstrate that cytokines are paramount to stem cell therapy [5, 6]. Research is increasingly focused on cytokines in the hope of developing new therapeutic modalities aimed at the treatment and prevention of ischemic heart disease. Consequently, comprehension of the inflammatory cascade is increasingly indispensable.

Myocardial Infarction and the Inflammatory Reaction

The sudden rupture of an atherosclerotic plaque leads to the formation of a thrombus within a coronary artery. As the thrombus occludes the vessel and blood flow is interrupted, cardiomyocyte death quickly ensues [7]. Rapid revascularization can decrease the proportion of cell death and thus preserve heart function. However, cardiomyocytes damaged by the initial insult will release chemotactic factors and cytokines that will provoke an intense inflammatory response. Rapid recruitment of leucocytes to the affected area is essential for healing and subsequent scar formation after an MI. Unfortunately, the inflammatory response is non-specific and continued propagation of this process damages healthy, viable myocardium untouched by the initial insult [8].

The inflammatory response is controlled by cytokines, which are soluble proteins produced by damaged cells. Following an MI, cytokines may be classified into two distinct categories: pro- and antiinflammatory cytokines. Proinflammatory cytokines frequently found in ischemic heart disease consist of TNF-α, interlukin-1β, IL-6, and IL-8 [9, 10]. They are primarily responsible for the stimulation and enhancement of inflammation. In contrast, antiinflammatory cytokines are responsible for tempering the inflammatory response, the most important being IL-10, which is a powerful

N. Alkhamees, MD • A. Le Huu, MD, MSc
Divisions of Cardiac Surgery and Surgical Research, Department of Surgery, McGill University Health Center, Montreal, QC, Canada

D. Shum-Tim, MD, CM, MSc, FRCSC, FACS, FAHA (✉)
Divisions of Cardiac Surgery and Surgical Research, Department of Surgery, McGill University Health Center, Montreal, H3G 1A4 QC, Canada

The Montreal Children's Hospital, The Montreal General Hospital, Montreal, QC, Canada

Department of Surgery, McGill University, Montreal, QC, Canada
e-mail: dshumtim@yahoo.ca

E.A. Gabriel, S.A. Gabriel (eds.), *Inflammatory Response in Cardiovascular Surgery*,
DOI 10.1007/978-1-4471-4429-8_50, © Springer-Verlag London 2013

inhibitor of proinflammatory cytokines IL- α, IL-1β, TNF-α, and IL-8 [11]. An important caveat when classifying cytokines into distinct categories is that the molecules often have multiple functions and may exert pro- and antiinflammatory roles depending on their milieu.

The Cytokines Cascade

Proinflammatory cytokines TNF-α, IL-1β, IL-6, and IL-8 upregulate the inflammatory cascade and induce myocardial damage. Clinically, increased levels of these cytokines are directly proportional to the risk of future ischemic events [12]. TNF-α, released early after an MI, stimulates the expression of other proinflammatory cytokines. It is also responsible for upregulation of chemokines, stimulating the degradation of the extracellular matrix by reducing collagen synthesis and enhancing matrix metalloproteinase (MMP) activity in cardiac fibroblasts [12]. Concurrently, TNF- α enhances cardiomyocyte apoptosis. TNF- α also promotes end organ dysfunction by suppressing cardiac contractility though inhibition of intracellular calcium during systole, leading to decreased contractility [3, 4]. A potent proinflammatory cytokine, TNF- α may also have antiinflammatory properties. Specifically, studies suggest that TNF-α may exert a cytoprotective function by preventing or delaying myocyte apoptosis following MI [13, 14].

IL- 1β and IL-6 are proinflammatory cytokines that function as acute phase reactants. Both of these cytokines demonstrate elevated levels early after an MI and remain elevated after the initial insult [8, 11, 15]. They are found to cause myocyte hypertrophy in vitro [16, 17]. IL-8 is released upon myocardial injury [18]. It appears to function as a chemoattractant, acting on neutrophils and T-lymphocytes, leading to increased myocardial destruction [19].

The most prominent antiinflammatory cytokine is IL-10, produced by Th_2 lymphocytes. It appears to inhibit the production of proinflammatory cytokines IL-1 α, IL-1β, TNF-α, and IL-8 by monocytes [11]. Consequently, increasing the production of IL-10 may reduce the damage inflicted on the myocardium by a pronounced proinflammatory reaction.

In patients suffering from an MI or in CHF, studies show that lower ratios of pro-/antiinflammatory cytokines were associated with improved ventricular function. Chen et al. demonstrated that the pro-/antiinflammatory ratio might be crucial to ventricular remodeling. Following induction of acute myocardial infarction in 88 Lewis rats, the animals were subsequently injected with culture medium or mesenchymal stem cells. PCR analysis was used to determine the ratio of IL-1β/IL-10, IL-6/IL-10, and IL-8/10 produced at 24 h, 1 week, and 2 weeks. A baseline echocardiography was performed before the study and at intervals after stem cell injection. Upon termination of the study, the heart tissue was harvested, and histopathological analysis was completed.

Rats injected with mesenchymal stem cells had significantly lower ratios of pro-/antiinflammatory cytokines compared with control groups. Although levels of both pro- and antiinflammatory cytokines were upregulated, the actual ratios were lower than the control groups because of significantly higher levels of IL-10 (antiinflammatory) cytokine. In addition, rats injected with mesenchymal cells had a decreased ratio of MMP-2/tissue inhibitor of metalloproteinases-1 (TIMP-1).

Functionally, the results were equally impressive. After 12 h, rats injected with mesenchymal stem cells demonstrated improved ejection fractions compared to control groups. This improvement was sustained up to 2 weeks after the MI. Histological examination showed significantly lower levels of extracellular matrix deposition, reduced tissue injury, and decreased inflammatory cell infiltration. Consequently, at a cellular level, decreased ratios of pro-/antiinflammatory cytokines led to significantly less cellular destruction following an MI. The cellular improvements culminated in clinically improved ventricular function [20].

This experiment couples mesenchymal cell implantation with the production of inflammatory cytokines and suggests that the paracrine function of cells is crucial to the regenerative process. Another study by Guo et al. found that implantation of mesenchymal cells resulted in lower levels of proinflammatory cytokines TNF-α, IL-1β, and IL-6. These results were correlated with clinical parameters that demonstrated decreased ventricular dilatation and thickening [21]. Following the acute event, IL-1 and IL-6 continue to contribute to organ dysfunction by inducing myocyte hypertrophy [16, 17]. This cellular change is a crucial contributor to the pathophysiological changes culminating in the development of heart failure.

Proinflammatory cytokines may also be useful prognostic indicators, by providing measures of clinical outcome. Upregulation of IL-8 has been associated with increased myocardial damage measured through higher levels of troponin release [19]. Similarly, in patients with chronic heart failure, increased plasma levels of proinflammatory cytokines correlate with increased severity and poor clinical outcome [22–24]. In addition, patients in end-stage heart failure produce abundant levels of proinflammatory cytokines [25]. Torre-Amione et al. demonstrated that implanting a left ventricular assist device in patients with heart failure resulted in a significant reduction of TNF-α levels [26]. This suggests that high ventricular pressures and hemodynamic volume may play a role in TNF-α activation. It is thought that TNF-α induces myocardial dysfunction by inhibiting the increase of intracellular calcium during systole and by induction of nitric oxide [3].

Cellular Cardiomyoplasty

Heart failure is the end result of histopathological and structural changes to the myocardium resulting in left ventricular (LV) remodeling. The core component of this process is cardiomyocyte death and the resultant loss of myocardial cell mass. Conventional management of ischemic heart disease has focused on palliation of symptoms without addressing the inadequate regenerative capabilities possessed by the myocardium. However, in the last two decades, research has been increasingly focused on cell-based therapy to recruit, regenerate, and prevent further cell loss while promoting angiogenesis.

Cellular cardiomyoplasty consists of transplanting stem cells to sites of cardiac injury, restoring blood flow and contractility to areas previously infarcted or scarred myocardium [27]. Studies have shown that stem cell transplantation can limit scar expansion, ventricular dilation, and improve ventricular function after myocardial injury [28–31]. The process by which stem cell therapy repairs damaged myocardium, leading to significant recovery of cardiac function, is unknown. To date, the following mechanisms have been proposed:

- *Trans-differentiation*: Studies have shown that injection of MSCs into infarcted myocardium resulted in mesenchymal stem cells (MSC) undergoing trans-differentiation into cardiomyocytes [32]. Injected MSCs expressed cardiomyocyte markers and aligned with host cardiomyocytes, forming intercalated discs [33–35]. However, the quantity of stem cells presented at the site of injury was disproportionately lower than the functional recovery obtained solely on the basis of neo-myocardial regeneration. Consequently, MSC trans-differentiation into cardiomyocytes remains controversial [36–39].
- *Angiogenesis*: Many studies have demonstrated that stem cells promote angiogenesis. In vivo, endothelial progenitor cells have been successfully used for neovascularization of ischemic myocardium [40]. Similar results were achieved in humans using endothelial progenitor cells (EPC) and bone marrow mononuclear cells [41, 42]. It remains unclear if angiogenesis alone can result in the significant functional improvement.
- *Cell fusion*: This mechanism is a derivative of stem cell plasticity. Orlic et al. demonstrated that bone marrow-derived cells (BMDCs) transplanted into acute myocardial infarction models were integrated into damaged myocardium and expressed connexin-43. This implies the formation of gap junctions with the host myocardium [32]. In contrast, Nygren et al. suggest that BMDCs fusion with cardiomyocytes is a transient and hematopoietic phenomenon, with no BMDCs observed within damaged myocardium 28 days post-implantation [43].
- *Paracrine effect*: Proponents of this hypothesis believe that stem cells release active endogenous factors that influence the local milieu rather than exerting a regenerative mechanism. Urbanek et al. found that growth factors (HGF, IGF-1) attract cardiac stem cells to infarcted myocardium and stimulate them to proliferate [44]. In addition, MSCs exposed to hypoxic conditions express vascular endothelial growth factor (VEGF) [45–47]. Secretion of VEGF enhances cell survival, and upregulation of VEGF results in angiogenesis within ischemic myocardium [48–50]. In a similar manner, Rehman et al. demonstrated that the secretion of another molecule, HGF, also resulted in angiogenesis and a significant reduction in endothelial cell apoptosis [51]. Currently, this hypothesis is the most widely accepted mechanism of action for cardiomyoplasty.

Conclusion

Proinflammatory cytokines play a central role in the propagation of an MI and subsequent development of heart failure. However, because of the pleiotropic and redundant nature of cytokines, further studies are required to fully elucidate the cellular and molecular events associated with the inflammatory cytokine cascade. It is evident that cytokines, through network modulation, may alter the outcome of the disease, and influence patient prognosis. Therefore, extensive comprehension of the inflammatory cascade is essential to the development of therapeutic modalities aimed at ischemic heart disease.

Despite incomplete knowledge about the inflammatory cytokine cascade, clinical trials involving cardiomyoplasty already have debuted. Early data published from the Stem Cell Infusion in Patients with Ischemic Cardiomyopathy (SCIPIO) phase 1 trial are encouraging [52]. Patients who received autologous cardiac stem cells by intracoronary infusion 4 months post-coronary bypass grafting demonstrated a 24 % reduction in infarct size and 8.2 % improvement in ejection fraction. These clinical gains are indisputable and demonstrate that further research focused on understanding the mechanisms of stem cell therapy, proper selection of cell type, optimization of cell delivery, and survival will bring cellular cardiomyoplasty to the forefront of treatments aimed at eradicating congestive heart failure.

References

1. Selnes OA et al. Neurobehavioural sequelae of cardiopulmonary bypass. Lancet. 1999;353(9164):1601–6.
2. Jacobs M et al. Tumor necrosis factor-alpha at acute myocardial infarction in rats and effects on cardiac fibroblasts. J Mol Cell Cardiol. 1999;31(11):1949–59.
3. Yokoyama T et al. Cellular basis for the negative inotropic effects of tumor necrosis factor-alpha in the adult mammalian heart. J Clin Invest. 1993;92(5):2303–12.
4. Engel D et al. Cardiac myocyte apoptosis provokes adverse cardiac remodeling in transgenic mice with targeted TNF overexpression. Am J Physiol Heart Circ Physiol. 2004;287(3):H1303–11.

5. Kinnaird T et al. Marrow-derived stromal cells express genes encoding a broad spectrum of arteriogenic cytokines and promote in vitro and in vivo arteriogenesis through paracrine mechanisms. Circ Res. 2004;94(5):678–85.
6. Kamihata H et al. Implantation of bone marrow mononuclear cells into ischemic myocardium enhances collateral perfusion and regional function via side supply of angioblasts, angiogenic ligands, and cytokines. Circulation. 2001;104(9):1046–52.
7. Lilly LS. Heart disease. Lippincott Williams & Wilkins: Boston; 2003.
8. Frangogiannis NG, Smith CW, Entman ML. The inflammatory response in myocardial infarction. Cardiovasc Res. 2002;53(1):31–47.
9. Amado LC et al. Cardiac repair with intramyocardial injection of allogeneic mesenchymal stem cells after myocardial infarction. Proc Natl Acad Sci USA. 2005;102(32):11474–9.
10. Frangogiannis NG et al. IL-10 is induced in the reperfused myocardium and may modulate the reaction to injury. J Immunol. 2000;165(5):2798–808.
11. Yang Z, Zingarelli B, Szabo C. Crucial role of endogenous interleukin-10 production in myocardial ischemia/reperfusion injury. Circulation. 2000;101(9):1019–26.
12. Kilic T et al. Relation between proinflammatory to anti-inflammatory cytokine ratios and long-term prognosis in patients with non-ST elevation acute coronary syndrome. Heart. 2006;92(8):1041–6.
13. Monden Y et al. Soluble TNF receptors prevent apoptosis in infiltrating cells and promote ventricular rupture and remodeling after myocardial infarction. Cardiovasc Res. 2007;73(4):794–805.
14. Kurrelmeyer KM et al. Endogenous tumor necrosis factor protects the adult cardiac myocyte against ischemic-induced apoptosis in a murine model of acute myocardial infarction. Proc Natl Acad Sci USA. 2000;97(10):5456–61.
15. Wollert KC, Drexler H. The role of interleukin-6 in the failing heart. Heart Fail Rev. 2001;6(2):95–103.
16. Yokoyama T et al. Tumor necrosis factor-alpha provokes a hypertrophic growth response in adult cardiac myocytes. Circulation. 1997;95(5):1247–52.
17. Fuchs M et al. Role of interleukin-6 for LV remodeling and survival after experimental myocardial infarction. FASEB J. 2003;17(14): 2118–20.
18. Kukielka GL et al. Interleukin-8 gene induction in the myocardium after ischemia and reperfusion in vivo. J Clin Invest. 1995;95(1): 89–103.
19. Ivey CL et al. Neutrophil chemoattractants generated in two phases during reperfusion of ischemic myocardium in the rabbit. Evidence for a role for C5a and interleukin-8. J Clin Invest. 1995;95(6): 2720–8.
20. Chen G et al. Marrow stromal cells for cell-based therapy: the role of antiinflammatory cytokines in cellular cardiomyoplasty. Ann Thorac Surg. 2010;90(1):190–7.
21. Guo J et al. Anti-inflammation role for mesenchymal stem cells transplantation in myocardial infarction. Inflammation. 2007; 30(3–4):97–104.
22. Levine B et al. Elevated circulating levels of tumor necrosis factor in severe chronic heart failure. N Engl J Med. 1990;323(4): 236–41.
23. MacGowan GA et al. Circulating interleukin-6 in severe heart failure. Am J Cardiol. 1997;79(8):1128–31.
24. Tsutamoto T et al. Interleukin-6 spillover in the peripheral circulation increases with the severity of heart failure, and the high plasma level of interleukin-6 is an important prognostic predictor in patients with congestive heart failure. J Am Coll Cardiol. 1998;31(2): 391–8.
25. Torre-Amione G et al. Tumor necrosis factor-alpha and tumor necrosis factor receptors in the failing human heart. Circulation. 1996;93(4):704–11.
26. Torre-Amione G et al. Proinflammatory cytokine levels in patients with depressed left ventricular ejection fraction: a report from the Studies of Left Ventricular Dysfunction (SOLVD). J Am Coll Cardiol. 1996;27(5):1201–6.
27. Taylor DA. Cell-based myocardial repair: how should we proceed? Int J Cardiol. 2004;95 Suppl 1:S8–12.
28. Sakai T et al. Autologous heart cell transplantation improves cardiac function after myocardial injury. Ann Thorac Surg. 1999;68(6):2074–80; discussion 2080–1.
29. Strauer BE et al. Repair of infarcted myocardium by autologous intracoronary mononuclear bone marrow cell transplantation in humans. Circulation. 2002;106(15):1913–8.
30. Yousef M et al. The BALANCE Study: clinical benefit and long-term outcome after intracoronary autologous bone marrow cell transplantation in patients with acute myocardial infarction. J Am Coll Cardiol. 2009;53(24):2262–9.
31. Jain M et al. Cell therapy attenuates deleterious ventricular remodeling and improves cardiac performance after myocardial infarction. Circulation. 2001;103(14):1920–7.
32. Orlic D et al. Bone marrow cells regenerate infarcted myocardium. Nature. 2001;410(6829):701–5.
33. Pittenger MF, Martin BJ. Mesenchymal stem cells and their potential as cardiac therapeutics. Circ Res. 2004;95(1):9–20.
34. Toma C et al. Human mesenchymal stem cells differentiate to a cardiomyocyte phenotype in the adult murine heart. Circulation. 2002;105(1):93–8.
35. Wang T et al. Cell-to-cell contact induces mesenchymal stem cell to differentiate into cardiomyocyte and smooth muscle cell. Int J Cardiol. 2006;109(1):74–81.
36. Kawada H, Ogawa M. Bone marrow origin of hematopoietic progenitors and stem cells in murine muscle. Blood. 2001;98(7):2008–13.
37. Wagers AJ et al. Little evidence for developmental plasticity of adult hematopoietic stem cells. Science. 2002;297(5590):2256–9.
38. Castro RF et al. Failure of bone marrow cells to transdifferentiate into neural cells in vivo. Science. 2002;297(5585):1299.
39. Murry CE et al. Haematopoietic stem cells do not transdifferentiate into cardiac myocytes in myocardial infarcts. Nature. 2004; 428(6983):664–8.
40. Orlic D et al. Mobilized bone marrow cells repair the infarcted heart, improving function and survival. Proc Natl Acad Sci USA. 2001;98(18):10344–9.
41. Assmus B et al. Transplantation of progenitor cells and regeneration enhancement in acute myocardial infarction (TOPCARE-AMI). Circulation. 2002;106(24):3009–17.
42. Losordo DW, Dimmeler S. Therapeutic angiogenesis and vasculogenesis for ischemic disease: part II: cell-based therapies. Circulation. 2004;109(22):2692–7.
43. Nygren JM et al. Bone marrow-derived hematopoietic cells generate cardiomyocytes at a low frequency through cell fusion, but not transdifferentiation. Nat Med. 2004;10(5):494–501.
44. Urbanek K et al. Cardiac stem cells possess growth factor-receptor systems that after activation regenerate the infarcted myocardium, improving ventricular function and long-term survival. Circ Res. 2005;97(7):663–73.
45. Xu M et al. In vitro and in vivo effects of bone marrow stem cells on cardiac structure and function. J Mol Cell Cardiol. 2007; 42(2):441–8.
46. Li W et al. Bcl-2 engineered MSCs inhibited apoptosis and improved heart function. Stem Cells. 2007;25(8):2118–27.
47. Gnecchi M et al. Evidence supporting paracrine hypothesis for Akt-modified mesenchymal stem cell-mediated cardiac protection and functional improvement. FASEB J. 2006;20(6):661–9.
48. Tse HF et al. Paracrine effects of direct intramyocardial implantation of bone marrow derived cells to enhance neovascularization in chronic ischaemic myocardium. Eur J Heart Fail. 2007;9(8):747–53.

49. Tang YL et al. Autologous mesenchymal stem cell transplantation induce VEGF and neovascularization in ischemic myocardium. Regul Pept. 2004;117(1):3–10.
50. Cheng AS, Yau TM. Paracrine effects of cell transplantation: strategies to augment the efficacy of cell therapies. Semin Thorac Cardiovasc Surg. 2008;20(2):94–101.
51. Rehman J et al. Secretion of angiogenic and antiapoptotic factors by human adipose stromal cells. Circulation. 2004;109(10):1292–8.
52. Bolli R et al. Cardiac stem cells in patients with ischaemic cardiomyopathy (SCIPIO): initial results of a randomised phase 1 trial. Lancet. 2011;378(9806):1847–57.

Hypoxic Preconditioning of Cardiac Progenitor Cells for Ischemic Heart

51

Shiyue Xu and Gangjian Qin

Introduction

Ischemic heart disease is the leading cause of morbidity and mortality in western countries. According to the data from the American Heart Association, coronary artery disease causes about one of every six deaths in the United States. Each year, an estimated 785,000 Americans will have a new coronary attack, about 470,000 will have a recurrent attack, and an additional 195,000 will have a silent first myocardial infarction. Thus, approximately every 25 s, an American will have a coronary event; approximately every minute, someone will die of one [1].

The pathophysiological process underlying most ischemic heart disease is atherosclerosis of coronary arteries. Atheroma formation, with or without thrombus, can lead to stenosis in coronary arteries, resulting in a reduction in coronary blood flow and oxygen supply. A sudden and significant reduction in coronary blood flow, most commonly from rupture of plaques in the coronary arteries, can cause myocardial infarction. A large number of cardiomyocytes die, and cardiac muscles in the infarcted area lose their striations. The death of cardiomyocytes invokes the recruitment of inflammatory cells at the infarct border, which remove the necrotic cell debris by phagocytosis [2]. As a result, the infarct area becomes thin and non-contractile and may lead to infarct rupture, which accounts for 15–30 % of deaths in the first week after infarction [3, 4].

The acute phase of infarction is always followed by a chronic phase of remodeling related to fibroblast proliferation and collagen deposition. In the chronic phase, collagen deposition is the primary determinant of structural and mechanical changes. A rapid increase of the collagen amount in the infarcted zones strengthens the necrotic cardiac muscle and makes it stiff and resistant to distension. However, collagen deposition also occurs in the uninfarcted remote myocardial region, particularly in the interstitium. These changes, collectively, result in adverse remodeling of ischemic heart, which contributes to ventricular stiffness and dysfunction [5]. Furthermore, due to the loss of cardiomyocytes and adverse remodeling, ischemic heart often shows both systolic (decreased contraction) and diastolic (decreased relaxation) dysfunction and ultimately fails; a large portion of patients who suffer from myocardial infarction die from heart failure [1, 6].

In the past decade, a tremendous amount of scientific knowledge about the pathophysiology and molecular mechanisms of myocardial infarction and heart failure has been learned; nevertheless, therapeutic options for these devastating diseases remain limited. Traditional therapies, such as angioplasty and thrombolytic agents, can relieve only the cause of infarction; no existing medication or procedure can effectively replace cardiac scarring (i.e., fibrotic tissue) with functional contractile tissue. Newer therapies that incorporate recently identified populations of stem/progenitor cells may regenerate cardiac tissue directly by inducing neovasculogenesis and cardiogenesis [7–15]. Resident cardiac stem/progenitor cells (CSPCs) may be particularly suitable for resurrecting dead myocardium because they are endogenous components of the adult heart and appear to be responsible for the physiologic and pathologic turnover of cardiac myocytes and other cardiac cells [16]. In this chapter, we will introduce different types of CSPCs identified and various strategies to enhance the effectiveness of these cells for cardiac regeneration, with a particular focus on the treatment of cells with hypoxic preconditioning.

Cardiac Stem/Progenitor Cells

For a long time, the human heart has been considered a terminally differentiated, postmitotic organ. The number of cardiomyocytes was determined on the day of birth, and there

S. Xu, MD • G. Qin, MD (✉)
Department of Medicine, Cardiology,
Feinberg Cardiovascular Research Institute,
Northwestern University Feinberg School of Medicine,
303 E Chicago Ave, Tarry 14-721, 60611 Chicago, IL, USA
e-mail: g-qin@northwestern.edu

E.A. Gabriel, S.A. Gabriel (eds.), *Inflammatory Response in Cardiovascular Surgery*,
DOI 10.1007/978-1-4471-4429-8_51, © Springer-Verlag London 2013

was not regeneration of these cells throughout life. However, in the past decade, a population of multipotent undifferentiated cells termed "cardiac stem/progenitor cells (CSPCs)" was found in adult human hearts as well as other mammalian animals [17]. Evidence suggests that CSPCs can give rise to cardiomyocytes, vascular endothelial cells, and smooth muscle cells and contribute to cardiomyocyte turnover and myocardial recovery following injury [16]. Studies focusing on the biology and therapeutic potential of CSPCs are growing exponentially. Like any other types of stem/progenitor cells, the true identity of CSPCs remains debated.

$Lin^-c\text{-}kit^+$ Cells

The $Lin^-c\text{-}kit^+$ CSPCs were first reported by Beltrami et al. in 2003 [7]. They found that this population of cells in the adult rat hearts are self-renewing, clonogenic, and multipotent, giving rise to at least three differentiated cell types including cardiomyocytes, vascular endothelial and smooth muscle cells. When injected into ischemic heart of animals, these cells regenerated well-differentiated myocardium and encompassed a significant portion of the ventricle [7]. Subsequently, $Lin^-c\text{-}kit^+$ CSPCs were extensively characterized by many laboratories across different species of animals including mice and humans [17]. In a recent clinical trial conducted by Bolli et al., one million autologous CSPCs were administered via coronary artery in patients with post-infarction left ventricular dysfunction at a mean of 113 days after coronary artery bypass grafting (CABG). After a 4-month follow-up in 23 patients (16 cardiac stem cell-treated patients, 7 control-treated patients), the investigators found that the left ventricular ejection fraction (LVEF) and the quality of life in the CSPCs-treated patients were significantly better than those in control-treated patients [18].

$Isl1^+$ Cells

The LIM-homeodomain transcription factor islet-1 (isl1)-positive cells were initially identified as a population of embryonic progenitors that contribute to the embryonic heart formation, comprising most of the cells in the right ventricle, both atria, the outflow tract, and specific regions of the left ventricle [19]. By using genetic fate-mapping techniques, Moretti et al. identified a subset of primordial $isl1^+$ cardiovascular progenitors with the transcriptional signature of $isl1^+/Nkx2.5^+/flk1^+$, which are multipotent and play a critical role in embryo heart development [20]. They found that those $isl1^+$ cells isolated from the second heart field of the embryonic heart can give rise to cardiomyocytes, endothelial and smooth muscle cells in vitro and are essential for cardiogenesis. Subsequently, $isl1^+$ cardiac progenitors were identified also in postnatal myocardia of rats, mice, and humans [12]. These cells were capable of renewal and fully differentiation into cardiomyocytes.

$Sca\text{-}1^+$ Cells

Stem cell antigen-1 (Sca-1) is a member of the Ly-6 family and was initially suggested as a surface marker of hematopoietic stem cells [21]. Oh et al. identified a group of cells in the adult heart that express Sca-1 and possess cardiac progenitor cell properties [8]. Using a magnetic cell sorting system, Katsuhisa Matsuura et al. isolated $Sca\text{-}1^+$ cells from adult murine hearts and induced these cells to express cardiac transcription factors and contractile proteins, form sarcomeric structure, and beat spontaneously in vitro following oxytocin treatment [10]. Recently, several subpopulations of $Sca\text{-}1^+$ cardiac progenitor cells have been further characterized [22, 23]. Like other CSPCs, $Sca\text{-}1^+$ cells are able to home to the infarcted myocardium, differentiate into cardiomyocytes, and integrate with host cells in the infarcted myocardium of animals [8, 10, 22, 23].

Side Population (SP) Cells

SP cells were first described by Margaret et al. when they stained murine bone marrow cells with the Hoechst 33342 [24]. They found that these cells resisted Hoechst staining, had phenotypic markers of multipotent hematopoietic stem cells, and contributed to the bone marrow reconstitution in lethally irradiated mice. Recently the concept of SP cells has been introduced to identify stem/progenitor cells in the adult heart. In a study from Hierlihy et al., a resident side population was found in the post-natal mouse heart [25]. They showed that the cardiac SP cells were capable of forming cardiomyocytes when co-cultured with primary cardiomyocytes. Pfister et al. further demonstrated that only $CD31^-$ $Sca1^+$ cardiac SP cells exhibit the potential of cardiomyogenic differentiation [26]. These investigators also reported that Abcg2, one of the ATP-binding cassette (ABC) transporter superfamily members, plays an important role in regulating the proliferation, differentiation, and survival of cardiac SP cells [27]. Furthermore, cardiac SP cells have been shown to be involved in both early heart development and the repair of adult hearts [9].

Cardiosphere Cells

Cardiosphere is a cluster of self-adhering undifferentiated cells grown from subcultures of postnatal atrial or ventricular biopsy specimens [11]. In vitro study showed that cardiosphere cells express stem and endothelial progenitor cell antigens; they are clonogenic and capable of self-renewal and diverse differentiation including myocytes and vascular cells [11]. Smith et al. demonstrated that cardiosphere-derived cells developed from cardiospheres exhibited biophysical features of cardiomyocytes when co-cultured with neonatal rat ventricular myocytes and that engraftment of human cardiosphere-derived cells in immunodeficient mice can increase the percentage of viable myocardium in the infarct zone and improve left ventricular ejection fraction [15]. In a recent clinical trial conducted by Makkar et al., autologous cardiosphere-derived cells were administrated at escalating doses (12.5–25 million cells) by intracoronary infusion in 17 patients at 1.5–3 months after myocardial infarction. After a 6-month follow-up in 25 patients (17 patients receiving cardiosphere-derived cells, 8 patients receiving standard treatment), these investigators reported that patients treated with cardiosphere-derived cells showed a reduction in scar mass and increase in viable heart mass, regional contractility, and regional systolic wall thickening as compared with control patients. However, there were no significant changes in end-diastolic volume, end-systolic volume, and LVEF between groups by 6 months [28]. Toward enhancing the therapeutic index of these cells, we further purified CSPCs from the cardiosphere-derived cells by depleting the cells that express hematopoietic lineage markers (Lin^-) and enriching c-kit^+ cells; these cardiosphere-derived, Lin^-c-kit^+ cells (CLK cells) demonstrate an enhanced regenerative capacity [29].

In summary, although many different types of CSPCs have been identified, their regenerative capacity, long-term engraftment in the ischemic heart tissue, and benefit to cardiac function have been modest in various pre-clinical animal models and, more recently, in clinical studies [30]. Methods to maximize their therapeutic potential are becoming the focus of research in the field.

Enhancement of the Cardiac Stem/Progenitor-Cell Function

Cardiac regeneration by CSPCs involves a series of integrated steps, including homing, proliferation, differentiation, and survival. Thus, enhancing CSPC function through these steps would aid in the design of better strategies for cardiac cell therapy.

Expansion and Differentiation

CSPC expansion and differentiation are the foundation of cardiac regeneration. Several laboratories have reported that Wnt/β-catenin signaling plays a key role in promoting expansion and self-renewal of CSPCs, including isl^+ cells [31–33] (Fig. 51.1). Limana et al. reported that administration of high-mobility group box 1 protein (HMGB1) to the ischemic heart after permanent coronary artery ligation resulted in the formation of new myocytes in the infarcted zone through activating the proliferation and differentiation of endogenous cardiac c-kit^+ progenitor cells [34]. Smart et al. used a small protein called thymosin b4 to re-activate the expression of a key embryonic epicardial gene, Wilm's tumor 1 (Wt1), in the endogenous CSPCs in the ischemic heart and induced *de novo* cardiogenesis [35]. Boni et al. demonstrated that Notch1 can regulate the differentiation ability of cardiac progenitor cells through Notch1 intracellular domain (N1ICD), and RBP-J; inhibition of Notch1 in infarcted mice impaired the differentiation of resident CSPCs into the myocyte lineage [36] (Fig. 51.1). In addition, a number of growth factors and signaling molecules involved in cell growth and survival, including Akt, c-kit, and insulin-like growth factor-1 (IGF-1), have been shown to play important roles in the differentiation and expansion of CSPCs [37–39].

Survival

Survival of stem cells is one of the main barriers to effective cell therapy. The hostile myocardium environment, such as persistent ischemia and inflammation, challenge the survival of all types of cells. It has been observed that within a day of myocardial infarction, 40 % of resident cardiac progenitor cells are depleted [13], emphasizing the importance of enhancing the survival of CSPCs. Lu et al. demonstrated that pretreatment of Sca-1^+ cells with IGF-1 can promote cell survival both in vitro and in vivo [40]. The survival rate of the pre-conditioned Sca-1^+ cells was 5.5 fold higher than that of the non-preconditioned cells. In addition, Konstantinos et al. reported that transplantation of bone marrow-derived mesenchymal stem cells (MSCs) can stimulate the survival of the host endogenous c-kit^+ CSPCs after infarction, and the improvements of CSPC survival lead to amelioration of cardiac function [41].

Homing and Recruitment

When administered intravenously or through coronary artery, the CSPCs need to home to the damaged cardiac tissue, whereas at local tissue, the densely packed cardiac cells, extracellular matrix, and replacement fibrotic tissues impose a significant physical barrier to the cell recruitment. Compelling evidence now suggests that enhancement of CSPC migration can enhance the repair of ischemic heart. Goichberg et al. demonstrated that Ephrin A1, through interacting with EphA2 receptor, promotes the motility of cardiac stem cells in vitro and their migration to the area of damage in vivo [42]. Liang et al. found that upregulation of SDF-1 in the infarcted myocardium induces migration

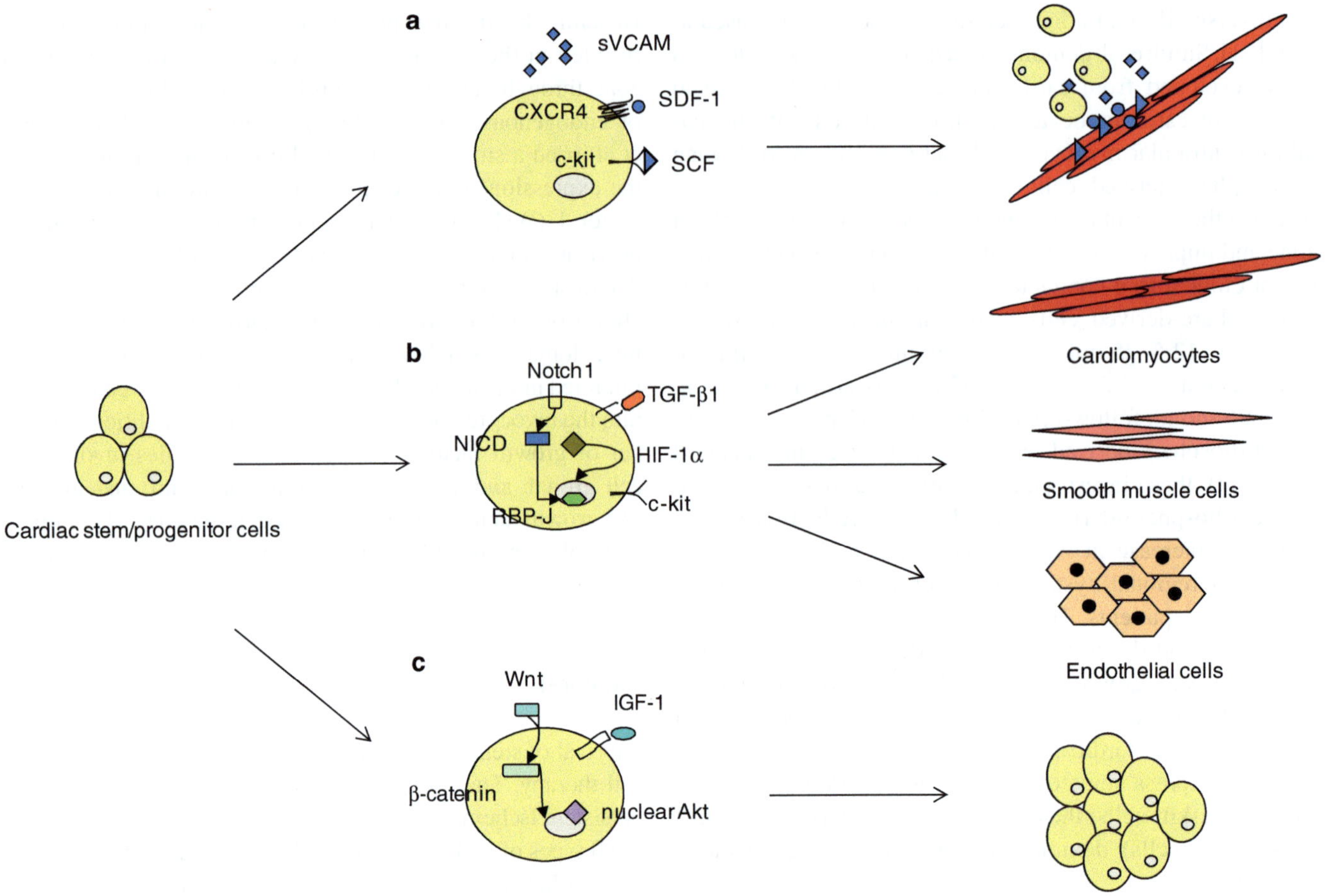

Fig. 51.1 Mechanisms that regulate CSPC migration (**a**), differentiation (**b**), and proliferation (**c**). *CXCR4* C-X-C chemokine receptor type 4, *SDF-1* stromal cell-derived factor-1, *sVCAM* soluble vascular cell adhesion molecules, *SCF* stem cell factor, *NICD* Notch1 intracellular domain, *RBP-J* J kappa-recombining binding protein, *TGF-β1* transforming growth factor beta 1, *HIF-1α* hypoxia-inducible factor 1α, *IGF-1* insulin-like growth factor 1 (see text for detailed discussions)

of $Sca1^{+}CD31^{-}$ cardiac SP cells [43]. In addition, the soluble VCAM-1 (sVCAM-1) has also been shown to exert a positive effect on the migration of cardiac stem cells [44]. Short exposure to hypoxia has also been shown to increase the migration of CSPCs [45]. All of these studies suggest the importance of homing and recruitment of the CSPCs in cardiac repair and may provide a therapeutic strategy in the treatment of ischemic heart diseases.

Hypoxic Preconditioning of Cardiac Stem/Progenitor Cells

Hypoxia is the most common pathological state of ischemic diseases including ischemic heart disease, and severe hypoxia causes cardiac cell death. However, accumulating evidence now suggests that hypoxia has a variety of effects on embryonic and adult stem cells, from proliferation and pluripotency maintenance to adaptive stress response, which are largely dependent on the O_2 level, time of exposure, and specific tissue microenvironment [46]. Hypoxic preconditioning of stem cells can induce a series of protective responses that adapt these cells to the hostile environment of damaged tissues; therefore, it can be employed as a strategy to enhance the effectiveness of cell therapy.

General Mechanisms of Hypoxic Preconditioning in the Regulation of Stem/Progenitor-Cell Function

It is well established that preconditioning of hearts with mild ischemia/hypoxia stimuli can significantly limit the damage from a subsequent serious cardiac ischemia such as myocardial infarction. However, how hypoxic pre-treatment of stem/progenitor cells affects their functional capacity is incompletely understood, and a number of molecules and signaling pathways have been reported to be involved in the process.

Hypoxia-Inducible Factor-1 (HIF-1)

The HIF-1 transcription factor is known as a master regulator for cells to sense O_2 levels in the tissue microenvironment and mount an appropriate cellular response to hypoxia [47]. Its pivotal role in the hypoxic preconditioning is well supported by a large body of literature [48]. Hypoxia results in a reduced degradation of HIF-1a via the proteasome pathway; the accumulated protein induces the expression of a diverse range of target genes, including erythropoietin, vascular endothelial growth factor, and Bcl-2 family members, which augment stem cell function [49, 50] and markedly enhance stem cell survival under severe hypoxia, oxidative stress, or in the inflammatory environment [51–53].

Akt

Akt is a hub of several important survival pathways in many types of cells. Recently, it has been shown to participate in hypoxic preconditioning of stem cells. Phosphorylation (activation) of Akt is significantly increased in adipose-derived stem cells during hypoxic preconditioning, and inhibition of Akt abolishes the protective effect of the hypoxic preconditioning [54]. Similarly, hypoxic treatment of mesenchymal stem cells (MSCs) results in an upregulation of several pro-survival and angiogenic factors, including HIF-1a, VEGF, and the phosphorylated Akt [55, 56]. These data suggest that Akt is critical for the protective effect of hypoxic preconditioning [57].

Mitogen-Activated Protein (MAP) Kinases

It has been shown that the intermittent hypoxia-induced delayed cardioprotection is mediated by p38 MAPK and ERK 1/2 and blocked by p38 MAPK inhibitor [58]. This indicates that the protective effect of hypoxic preconditioning may be, at least partially, dependent on MAPK pathways. In addition, JNK and ERK have been reported to exert an anti-apoptotic effect of ischemic/hypoxic preconditioning on stem cells and regulate cell function by interacting with additional molecular pathways [59]. Furthermore, inhibition of ERK attenuates the beneficial effect of ischemic preconditioning on the pig myocardium [60]. In addition to Akt and MAPKs, protein kinase C (PKC) has also been shown to play a role in ischemic preconditioning in the rat heart [61].

Endothelial Nitric Oxide Synthase (eNOS)

eNOS is an important regulator of stem/progenitor cell biology as well as vascular function. Uemura et al. found that hypoxic treatment significantly increases the level of eNOS in bone marrow stem cells. When injected into the infarcted myocardium in mice, the hypoxic pretreated bone marrow cells exhibit better survival than control non-treated cells [62]. Interestingly, Ii et al. demonstrated that endothelial progenitor cells (EPCs) are recruited to the ischemic pre-conditioned myocardium and exert a protective effect through NOS expression [63].

Iron Channels

Hu et al. demonstrated that hypoxic preconditioning can increase the migratory capacity of bone marrow mesenchymal stem cells via upregulation of Kv2.1 expression and FAK activity [64]. The importance of calcium was also noted by another study in which Yu et al. found that calcium/calmodulin-dependent protein kinase II is critical for the beneficial effect of intermittent hypoxic preconditioning in the ischemic-reperfusion-induced cardiac dysfunction [65]. Thus, iron channels may participate in the hypoxic preconditioning in ischemic heart diseases.

Taken together, these experimental findings provide a general understanding of the mechanisms involved in hypoxic preconditioning of stem/progenitor cells. However, more in-depth investigations are warranted to unravel the molecular details.

Hypoxic Preconditioning of Cardiac Stem/Progenitor Cells (CSPCs)

Compared with other types of stem/progenitor cells, CSPCs seem to be the obvious choice for cell-based cardiac repair. However, the success of this approach is determined in part by the same factors that cause the endogenous cardiac repair system to fail. Within a day of myocardial infarction, 40 % of resident CSPCs are depleted [13], and the barriers imposed by cardiac damage may limit the proliferation and self-renewal of the remaining resident cells, thereby preventing restoration of the progenitor-cell pool. At present, these limitations are often addressed by using ex vivo expansion protocols to generate a sufficient number of cells for transplantation into the ischemic heart. However, only a very small number of transplanted stem/progenitor cells are retained in the ischemic myocardium [66], and poor cell retention is one of the primary barriers to the effectiveness of cell therapy [67]. Thus, techniques that enhance the recruitment and retention of transplanted stem/progenitor cells are crucial to adequately replenish the resident progenitor cell pool and to maximize its regenerative potential. Toward this goal, we have initiated a series of studies investigating the effect of hypoxic preconditioning on the recruitment of intravenously administered cells to ischemic heart tissue and the preservation of heart function in murine models of myocardial infarction.

To enrich potent CPSCs, we selected the hematopoietic-lineage-negative (Lin^-) and c-kit-positive ($c\text{-}kit^+$) cells (CLK cells) from cardiospheres grown from explants of adult mouse hearts [29]. Because CXCR4 plays a critical role during SDF-1-mediated recruitment of circulating stem/progenitor cells to ischemic myocardium [68, 69], we evaluated the expression of CXCR4 in CLK cells. When cultured under normoxic conditions, CXCR4 expression was rather modest; however, both the number of cells expressing CXCR4 and the amount of CXCR4 protein expressed increased rapidly after just 4 h in hypoxic culture [29]. The elevation in CXCR4 expression was preceded by an increase in the expression of HIF-1α, and transfection of CLK cells with a HIF-1α small-interference RNA (siRNA) diminished hypoxia-induced CXCR4 expression. Furthermore, the hypoxia-induced CXCR4 expression is associated with a markedly increased CLK-cell migration toward SDF-1, and when CXCR4 expression was knocked down by infecting CLK cells with a lentiviral vector encoding CXCR4 shRNA, the hypoxia-induced enhancement of CLK-cell migration was abolished. Collectively, these observations indicate that the migratory activity of CLK cells is increased by hypoxia and that the mechanism of enhancement is dependent on an HIF-1α-mediated increase in CXCR4 expression.

To determine whether hypoxia-induced CLK-cell migration was accompanied by enhanced CLK-cell recruitment to ischemic myocardium, and to assess the differentiation of the recruited CLK cells, CLK cells were transduced with retroviral vector pCL-MFG-LacZ (CLK-LacZ cells). Hypoxic preconditioning was associated with a ~2.5-fold increase in CLK-cell recruitment to ischemic myocardium as assessed 24 h after CLK cell injection. Importantly, pretreatment of CSPCs with CXCR4 antagonist AMD3100 during the course of hypoxic preconditioning diminished the increase in CLK-cell recruitment, suggesting that the SDF-1/CXCR4 axis plays a pivotal role (Fig. 51.2). Our observation is supported by studies reported by van Oorschot et al., which also demonstrated that short-term hypoxia increased the migratory and invasive capacities of CSPCs [45]. In addition, we assessed CLK cell differentiation at 4 weeks after injection of lacZ-transgenic CLK cells; histological analyses revealed that the lacZ$^+$ cells in the ischemic myocardium co-expressed cardiac troponin I, von Willebrand factor, and smooth muscle actin, indicating that the transplanted CLK cells had differentiated into cardiomyocytes, endothelial cells, and vascular smooth muscle cells, respectively. Therefore, hypoxic preconditioning enhances CLK cell migration, recruitment, and differentiation.

After observing the dramatic hypoxia-induced increase in CLK-cell recruitment to ischemic myocardium, we investigated whether hypoxic preconditioning enhanced the therapeutic benefit of CLK cells. At week 4, functional analyses indicated that both left ventricular fractional shortening and the ejection fraction were better preserved in mice administered hypoxic-preconditioned CLK cells than in mice treated with normoxia-cultured CLK cells. Histological analyses indicated that peri-infarct capillary density and infarct wall thickness in the left ventricle were significantly greater, and infarct size was significantly smaller, in hearts from mice administered hypoxic-preconditioned cells than from mice treated with normoxia-cultured cells, and hypoxic-preconditioned cells were also associated with lower heart weights and a lower heart-weight:body-weight ratio. Collectively, these results indicate that the therapeutic benefits of CLK-cell administration after myocardial infarction are enhanced by hypoxic preconditioning.

The ischemic myocardium is known to produce an abundance of chemo-active, -attractive, or -repulsive, agents [70, 71], and these chemotactic signals, along with specific cell-matrix and cell-cell interactions, modulate the regenerative capacity of progenitor cells [67]. Accordingly, we performed protein array experiments to compare the levels of more than 300 mouse cytokines released from hypoxia- and normoxia-treated CLK cells into the culture medium. Hypoxic treatment was associated with higher levels of numerous factors, including chemokines (e.g., TCA-3, SDF-1, 6Ckine), vascular growth factors (e.g., VEGF, Osteopontin, bFGF, EPO, SCF), and factors involved in cardiac differentiation (e.g., Activin A, TGF-β, and Dkk-1), which also contribute to the cardiac repair (Fig. 51.2). The increase in SDF-1 secretion by CLK cells is particularly interesting. Recent studies have shown that SDF-1 is cardioprotective and that pretreatment of BM-derived mesenchymal stem cells (MSCs) with SDF-1 enhances cell survival, proliferation, and engraftment, and improves cardiac function after myocardial infarction in animals [72–74]. Our results indicate that SDF-1 is one of the chemokines and growth factors secreted by hypoxia-preconditioned CLK cells, which suggests that the apparent benefit associated with systemically administered hypoxia-preconditioned CLK-cells evolves, at least in part, through paracrine mechanisms.

Outlook

Ischemic heart disease and consequent heart failure remain the leading cause of morbidity and mortality worldwide; traditional therapies can only relieve symptoms and slow the disease progress. In the past decade, stem/progenitor cells have emerged as an optimal strategy of treatment, and CSPCs, in particular, can directly regenerate cardiac tissue by inducing neovasculogenesis and cardiogenesis. At present, the regenerative capacity of CSPCs is rather limited, and their clinical uses are still at infancy. One of the major barriers to the successful CSPC therapy is the hostile environment of the infarcted cardiac tissue, which quickly depletes endogenous CSPCs and limits the expansion and differentiation of the exogenously administered cells.

Recently, hypoxic preconditioning has emerged as a promising strategy to improve CSPC therapy. Studies from our laboratory and others have shown that hypoxic

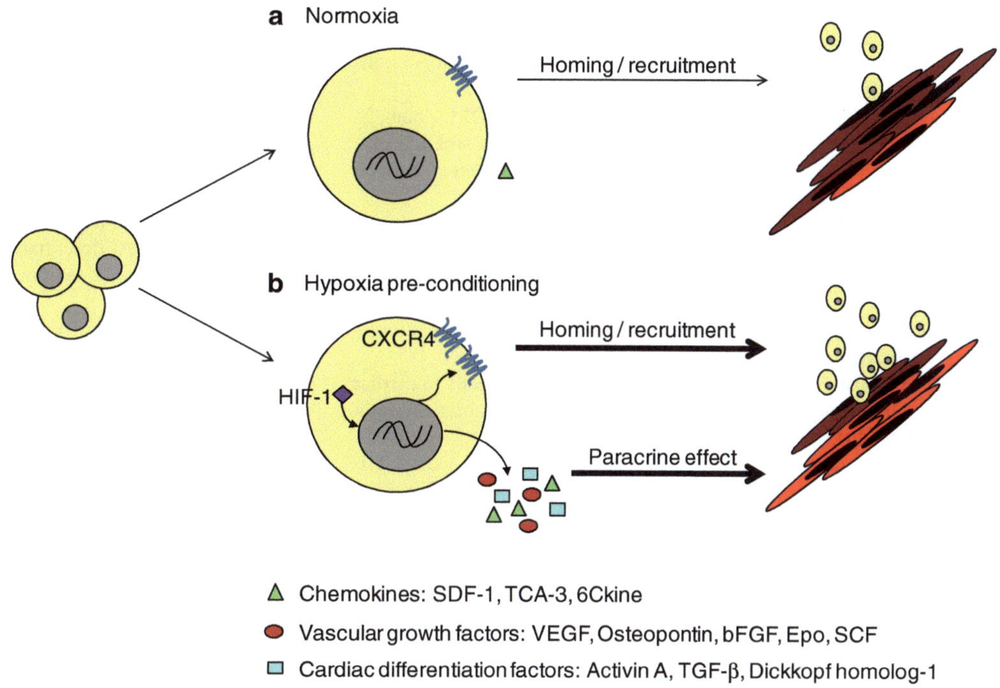

Fig. 51.2 Hypoxic preconditioning of CLK cardiac stem cells enhances repair of the infarcted myocardium. (**a**) Hypoxic pretreatment of CLK cardiac stem cells upregulates the expression of CXCR4 and SDF-1 through HIF-1 and augments the recruitment of CLK cells to the ischemic myocardium. (**b**) Hypoxic pretreatment also increases the secretion of paracrine factors that promote chemotaxis, vascular growth, and cardiac differentiation. TCA-3, also named chemokine (C-C motif) ligand 1, CCL1, or I-309; 6Ckine, also named chemokine (C-C motif) ligand 21A, CCL21A, secondary lymphoid-tissue chemokine (SLC), or Exodus-2; Epo, erythropoietin

pretreatment of CSPCs significantly increases their migratory capability and survival, and when administered systemically, the hypoxia-preconditioned CSPCs homed to the infarcted myocardium more efficiently than normoxia-cultured cells, which lead to significantly improved cardiac function and reduced infarct size. Hypoxia activates CSPCs through multiple mechanisms in which HIF-1α-mediated SDF-1/CXCR4 upregulation appears to play a critical role.

It is well known that during ischemia, hypoxia stimulates a series of adaptive cellular responses that favor the survival of cardiomyocytes, and transient episodes of ischemia have been shown to protect the ischemic heart. Thus, patients experiencing a cardiovascular event could benefit, at least theoretically, from ischemic preconditioning, but this cardioprotective strategy has yet to be effectively employed clinically. One of the primary barriers limiting the effectiveness of ischemic preconditioning is the need to apply this strategy before the ischemic event occurs rather than after the unanticipated onset of myocardial ischemia experienced by patients who present with acute myocardial infarction or who survive cardiac arrest. Hypoxic preconditioning may be a more viable therapeutic approach, because the cellular components could be obtained and preconditioned with hypoxia in advance for administration after a subsequent ischemic event.

Acknowledgements This work was supported by NIH grants R01 HL093439 and R01 HL113541 and American Heart Association grant 0430135N (to G.Q.) and the State Scholarship Fund of China (to S.X.).

References

1. Writing Group M, Roger VL, Go AS, Lloyd-Jones DM, Benjamin EJ, Berry JD, et al. Heart disease and stroke statistics – 2012 update: a report from the American Heart Association. Circulation. 2012;125(1):e2–220.
2. van den Borne SW, Diez J, Blankesteijn WM, Verjans J, Hofstra L, Narula J. Myocardial remodeling after infarction: the role of myofibroblasts. Nat Rev Cardiol. 2010;7(1):30–7.
3. Birnbaum Y, Chamoun AJ, Anzuini A, Lick SD, Ahmad M, Uretsky BF. Ventricular free wall rupture following acute myocardial infarction. Coron Artery Dis. 2003;14(6):463–70.
4. Wehrens XH, Doevendans PA. Cardiac rupture complicating myocardial infarction. Int J Cardiol. 2004;95(2–3):285–92.
5. Opie LH, Commerford PJ, Gersh BJ, Pfeffer MA. Controversies in ventricular remodelling. Lancet. 2006;367(9507):356–67.
6. Katz AM. The cardiomyopathy of overload: an unnatural growth response. Eur Heart J. 1995;16(Suppl O):110–4.
7. Beltrami AP, Barlucchi L, Torella D, Baker M, Limana F, Chimenti S, et al. Adult cardiac stem cells are multipotent and support myocardial regeneration. Cell. 2003;114(6):763–76.
8. Oh H, Bradfute SB, Gallardo TD, Nakamura T, Gaussin V, Mishina Y, et al. Cardiac progenitor cells from adult myocardium: homing, differentiation, and fusion after infarction. Proc Natl Acad Sci USA. 2003;100(21):12313–8.
9. Martin CM, Meeson AP, Robertson SM, Hawke TJ, Richardson JA, Bates S, et al. Persistent expression of the ATP-binding cassette transporter, Abcg2, identifies cardiac SP cells in the developing and adult heart. Dev Biol. 2004;265(1):262–75.
10. Matsuura K, Nagai T, Nishigaki N, Oyama T, Nishi J, Wada H, et al. Adult cardiac Sca-1-positive cells differentiate into beating cardiomyocytes. J Biol Chem. 2004;279(12):11384–91.
11. Messina E, De Angelis L, Frati G, Morrone S, Chimenti S, Fiordaliso F, et al. Isolation and expansion of adult cardiac stem cells from human and murine heart. Circ Res. 2004;95(9):911–21.
12. Laugwitz KL, Moretti A, Lam J, Gruber P, Chen Y, Woodard S, et al. Postnatal isl1^{+} cardioblasts enter fully differentiated cardiomyocyte lineages. Nature. 2005;433(7026):647–53.

13. Mouquet F, Pfister O, Jain M, Oikonomopoulos A, Ngoy S, Summer R, et al. Restoration of cardiac progenitor cells after myocardial infarction by self-proliferation and selective homing of bone marrow-derived stem cells. Circ Res. 2005;97(11):1090–2.
14. Chen X, Wilson RM, Kubo H, Berretta RM, Harris DM, Zhang X, et al. Adolescent feline heart contains a population of small, proliferative ventricular myocytes with immature physiological properties. Circ Res. 2007;100(4):536–44.
15. Smith RR, Barile L, Cho HC, Leppo MK, Hare JM, Messina E, et al. Regenerative potential of cardiosphere-derived cells expanded from percutaneous endomyocardial biopsy specimens. Circulation. 2007;115(7):896–908.
16. Dawn B, Bolli R. Cardiac progenitor cells: the revolution continues. Circ Res. 2005;97(11):1080–2.
17. Leri A, Kajstura J, Anversa P. Role of cardiac stem cells in cardiac pathophysiology: a paradigm shift in human myocardial biology. Circ Res. 2011;109(8):941–61.
18. Bolli R, Chugh AR, D'Amario D, Loughran JH, Stoddard MF, Ikram S, et al. Cardiac stem cells in patients with ischaemic cardiomyopathy (SCIPIO): initial results of a randomised phase 1 trial. Lancet. 2011;378(9806):1847–57.
19. Cai CL, Liang X, Shi Y, Chu PH, Pfaff SL, Chen J, et al. Isl1 identifies a cardiac progenitor population that proliferates prior to differentiation and contributes a majority of cells to the heart. Dev Cell. 2003;5(6):877–89.
20. Moretti A, Caron L, Nakano A, Lam JT, Bernshausen A, Chen Y, et al. Multipotent embryonic isl1+ progenitor cells lead to cardiac, smooth muscle, and endothelial cell diversification. Cell. 2006;127(6):1151–65.
21. van de Rijn M, Heimfeld S, Spangrude GJ, Weissman IL. Mouse hematopoietic stem-cell antigen Sca-1 is a member of the Ly-6 antigen family. Proc Natl Acad Sci USA. 1989;86(12):4634–8.
22. Wang X, Hu Q, Nakamura Y, Lee J, Zhang G, From AH, et al. The role of the sca-1+/CD31 – cardiac progenitor cell population in postinfarction left ventricular remodeling. Stem Cells. 2006;24(7):1779–88.
23. Takamiya M, Haider KH, Ashraf M. Identification and characterization of a novel multipotent sub-population of Sca-1 cardiac progenitor cells for myocardial regeneration. PLoS One. 2011;6(9):e25265.
24. Goodell MA, Brose K, Paradis G, Conner AS, Mulligan RC. Isolation and functional properties of murine hematopoietic stem cells that are replicating in vivo. J Exp Med. 1996;183(4):1797–806.
25. Hierlihy AM, Seale P, Lobe CG, Rudnicki MA, Megeney LA. The post-natal heart contains a myocardial stem cell population. FEBS Lett. 2002;530(1–3):239–43.
26. Pfister O, Mouquet F, Jain M, Summer R, Helmes M, Fine A, et al. CD31 – But Not CD31+ cardiac side population cells exhibit functional cardiomyogenic differentiation. Circ Res. 2005;97(1):52–61.
27. Pfister O, Oikonomopoulos A, Sereti KI, Sohn RL, Cullen D, Fine GC, et al. Role of the ATP-binding cassette transporter Abcg2 in the phenotype and function of cardiac side population cells. Circ Res. 2008;103(8):825–35.
28. Makkar RR, Smith RR, Cheng K, Malliaras K, Thomson LE, Berman D, et al. Intracoronary cardiosphere-derived cells for heart regeneration after myocardial infarction (CADUCEUS): a prospective, randomised phase 1 trial. Lancet. 2012;379(9819):895–904.
29. Tang YL, Zhu W, Cheng M, Chen L, Zhang J, Sun T, et al. Hypoxic preconditioning enhances the benefit of cardiac progenitor cell therapy for treatment of myocardial infarction by inducing CXCR4 expression. Circ Res. 2009;104(10):1209–16.
30. Li Z, Lee A, Huang M, Chun H, Chung J, Chu P, et al. Imaging survival and function of transplanted cardiac resident stem cells. J Am Coll Cardiol. 2009;53(14):1229–40.
31. Cohen ED, Wang Z, Lepore JJ, Lu MM, Taketo MM, Epstein DJ, et al. Wnt/beta-catenin signaling promotes expansion of Isl-1-positive cardiac progenitor cells through regulation of FGF signaling. J Clin Invest. 2007;117(7):1794–804.
32. Kwon C, Arnold J, Hsiao EC, Taketo MM, Conklin BR, Srivastava D. Canonical Wnt signaling is a positive regulator of mammalian cardiac progenitors. Proc Natl Acad Sci USA. 2007;104(26):10894–9.
33. Qyang Y, Martin-Puig S, Chiravuri M, Chen S, Xu H, Bu L, et al. The renewal and differentiation of Isl1+ cardiovascular progenitors are controlled by a Wnt/beta-catenin pathway. Cell Stem Cell. 2007;1(2):165–79.
34. Limana F, Germani A, Zacheo A, Kajstura J, Di Carlo A, Borsellino G, et al. Exogenous high-mobility group box 1 protein induces myocardial regeneration after infarction via enhanced cardiac C-kit+ cell proliferation and differentiation. Circ Res. 2005;97(8):e73–83.
35. Smart N, Bollini S, Dube KN, Vieira JM, Zhou B, Davidson S, et al. De novo cardiomyocytes from within the activated adult heart after injury. Nature. 2011;474(7353):640–4.
36. Boni A, Urbanek K, Nascimbene A, Hosoda T, Zheng H, Delucchi F, et al. Notch1 regulates the fate of cardiac progenitor cells. Proc Natl Acad Sci USA. 2008;105(40):15529–34.
37. Gude N, Muraski J, Rubio M, Kajstura J, Schaefer E, Anversa P, et al. Akt promotes increased cardiomyocyte cycling and expansion of the cardiac progenitor cell population. Circ Res. 2006;99(4):381–8.
38. Li M, Naqvi N, Yahiro E, Liu K, Powell PC, Bradley WE, et al. c-kit is required for cardiomyocyte terminal differentiation. Circ Res. 2008;102(6):677–85.
39. Ellison GM, Torella D, Dellegrottaglie S, Perez-Martinez C, Perezde Prado A, Vicinanza C, et al. Endogenous cardiac stem cell activation by insulin-like growth factor-1/hepatocyte growth factor intracoronary injection fosters survival and regeneration of the infarcted pig heart. J Am Coll Cardiol. 2011;58(9):977–86.
40. Lu G, Haider HK, Jiang S, Ashraf M. Sca-1+ stem cell survival and engraftment in the infarcted heart: dual role for preconditioning-induced connexin-43. Circulation. 2009;119(19):2587–96.
41. Hatzistergos KE, Quevedo H, Oskouei BN, Hu Q, Feigenbaum GS, Margitich IS, et al. Bone marrow mesenchymal stem cells stimulate cardiac stem cell proliferation and differentiation. Circ Res. 2010;107(7):913–22.
42. Goichberg P, Bai Y, D'Amario D, Ferreira-Martins J, Fiorini C, Zheng H, et al. The ephrin A1-EphA2 system promotes cardiac stem cell migration after infarction. Circ Res. 2011;108(9):1071–83.
43. Liang SX, Tan TY, Gaudry L, Chong B. Differentiation and migration of Sca1+/CD31 – cardiac side population cells in a murine myocardial ischemic model. Int J Cardiol. 2010;138(1):40–9.
44. Matsuura K, Honda A, Nagai T, Fukushima N, Iwanaga K, Tokunaga M, et al. Transplantation of cardiac progenitor cells ameliorates cardiac dysfunction after myocardial infarction in mice. J Clin Invest. 2009;119(8):2204–17.
45. van Oorschot AA, Smits AM, Pardali E, Doevendans PA, Goumans MJ. Low oxygen tension positively influences cardiomyocyte progenitor cell function. J Cell Mol Med. 2011;15(12):2723–34.
46. Abdollahi H, Harris LJ, Zhang P, McIlhenny S, Srinivas V, Tulenko T, et al. The role of hypoxia in stem cell differentiation and therapeutics. J Surg Res. 2011;165(1):112–7.
47. Semenza GL. Hypoxia – inducible factors in physiology and medicine. Cell. 2012;148(3):399–408.
48. Ytrehus K. Hypoxia-inducible factor 1 alpha: a new piece in the preconditioning puzzle. Cardiovasc Res. 2008;77(3):443–4.
49. Cameron CM, Harding F, Hu WS, Kaufman DS. Activation of hypoxic response in human embryonic stem cell-derived embryoid bodies. Exp Biol Med (Maywood). 2008;233(8):1044–57.

50. Francis KR, Wei L. Human embryonic stem cell neural differentiation and enhanced cell survival promoted by hypoxic preconditioning. Cell Death Dis. 2010;1:e22.
51. Hu X, Yu SP, Fraser JL, Lu Z, Ogle ME, Wang JA, et al. Transplantation of hypoxia-preconditioned mesenchymal stem cells improves infarcted heart function via enhanced survival of implanted cells and angiogenesis. J Thorac Cardiovasc Surg. 2008;135(4):799–808.
52. Zhao T, Zhang CP, Liu ZH, Wu LY, Huang X, Wu HT, et al. Hypoxia-driven proliferation of embryonic neural stem/progenitor cells–role of hypoxia-inducible transcription factor-1alpha. FEBS J. 2008;275(8):1824–34.
53. Han Y, Kuang SZ, Gomer A, Ramirez-Bergeron DL. Hypoxia influences the vascular expansion and differentiation of embryonic stem cell cultures through the temporal expression of vascular endothelial growth factor receptors in an ARNT-dependent manner. Stem Cells. 2010;28(4):799–809.
54. Stubbs SL, Hsiao ST, Peshavariya HM, Lim SY, Dusting GJ, Dilley RJ. Hypoxic preconditioning enhances survival of human adipose-derived stem cells and conditions endothelial cells in vitro. Stem Cells Dev. 2012;21(11):1887–96.
55. Chacko SM, Ahmed S, Selvendiran K, Kuppusamy ML, Khan M, Kuppusamy P. Hypoxic preconditioning induces the expression of prosurvival and proangiogenic markers in mesenchymal stem cells. Am J Physiol Cell Physiol. 2010;299(6):C1562–70.
56. Liu H, Xue W, Ge G, Luo X, Li Y, Xiang H, et al. Hypoxic preconditioning advances CXCR4 and CXCR7 expression by activating HIF-1alpha in MSCs. Biochem Biophys Res Commun. 2010;401(4):509–15.
57. Hausenloy DJ, Tsang A, Yellon DM. The reperfusion injury salvage kinase pathway: a common target for both ischemic preconditioning and postconditioning. Trends Cardiovasc Med. 2005;15(2):69–75.
58. Beguin PC, Belaidi E, Godin-Ribuot D, Levy P, Ribuot C. Intermittent hypoxia-induced delayed cardioprotection is mediated by PKC and triggered by p38 MAP kinase and Erk1/2. J Mol Cell Cardiol. 2007;42(2):343–51.
59. Hausenloy DJ, Yellon DM. Survival kinases in ischemic preconditioning and postconditioning. Cardiovasc Res. 2006;70(2):240–53.
60. Strohm C, Barancik T, Bruhl ML, Kilian SA, Schaper W. Inhibition of the ER-kinase cascade by PD98059 and UO126 counteracts ischemic preconditioning in pig myocardium. J Cardiovasc Pharmacol. 2000;36(2):218–29.
61. Speechly-Dick ME, Mocanu MM, Yellon DM. Protein kinase C. Its role in ischemic preconditioning in the rat. Circ Res. 1994;75(3):586–90.
62. Uemura R, Xu M, Ahmad N, Ashraf M. Bone marrow stem cells prevent left ventricular remodeling of ischemic heart through paracrine signaling. Circ Res. 2006;98(11):1414–21.
63. Ii M, Nishimura H, Iwakura A, Wecker A, Eaton E, Asahara T, et al. Endothelial progenitor cells are rapidly recruited to myocardium and mediate protective effect of ischemic preconditioning via "imported" nitric oxide synthase activity. Circulation. 2005;111(9):1114–20.
64. Hu X, Wei L, Taylor TM, Wei J, Zhou X, Wang JA, et al. Hypoxic preconditioning enhances bone marrow mesenchymal stem cell migration via Kv2.1 channel and FAK activation. Am J Physiol Cell Physiol. 2011;301(2):C362–72.
65. Yu Z, Wang ZH, Yang HT. Calcium/calmodulin-dependent protein kinase II mediates cardioprotection of intermittent hypoxia against ischemic-reperfusion-induced cardiac dysfunction. Am J Physiol Heart Circ Physiol. 2009;297(2):H735–42.
66. Hofmann M, Wollert KC, Meyer GP, Menke A, Arseniev L, Hertenstein B, et al. Monitoring of bone marrow cell homing into the infarcted human myocardium. Circulation. 2005;111(17):2198–202.
67. Dimmeler S, Zeiher AM, Schneider MD. Unchain my heart: the scientific foundations of cardiac repair. J Clin Invest. 2005;115(3):572–83.
68. Askari AT, Unzek S, Popovic ZB, Goldman CK, Forudi F, Kiedrowski M, et al. Effect of stromal-cell-derived factor 1 on stem-cell homing and tissue regeneration in ischaemic cardiomyopathy. Lancet. 2003;362(9385):697–703.
69. Abbott JD, Huang Y, Liu D, Hickey R, Krause DS, Giordano FJ. Stromal cell-derived factor-1alpha plays a critical role in stem cell recruitment to the heart after myocardial infarction but is not sufficient to induce homing in the absence of injury. Circulation. 2004;110(21):3300–5.
70. Zhang XF, Wang JF, Matczak E, Proper JA, Groopman JE. Janus kinase 2 is involved in stromal cell-derived factor-1alpha-induced tyrosine phosphorylation of focal adhesion proteins and migration of hematopoietic progenitor cells. Blood. 2001;97(11):3342–8.
71. Vandervelde S, van Luyn MJ, Tio RA, Harmsen MC. Signaling factors in stem cell-mediated repair of infarcted myocardium. J Mol Cell Cardiol. 2005;39(2):363–76.
72. Elmadbouh I, Haider H, Jiang S, Idris NM, Lu G, Ashraf M. Ex vivo delivered stromal cell-derived factor-1alpha promotes stem cell homing and induces angiomyogenesis in the infarcted myocardium. J Mol Cell Cardiol. 2007;42(4):792–803.
73. Zhang M, Mal N, Kiedrowski M, Chacko M, Askari AT, Popovic ZB, et al. SDF-1 expression by mesenchymal stem cells results in trophic support of cardiac myocytes after myocardial infarction. FASEB J. 2007;21(12):3197–207.
74. Pasha Z, Wang Y, Sheikh R, Zhang D, Zhao T, Ashraf M. Preconditioning enhances cell survival and differentiation of stem cells during transplantation in infarcted myocardium. Cardiovasc Res. 2008;77(1):134–42.

Index

E.A. Gabriel, S.A. Gabriel (eds.), *Inflammatory Response in Cardiovascular Surgery*,
DOI 10.1007/978-1-4471-4429-8, © Springer-Verlag London 2013

R

S

T

MIX
Papier aus verantwortungsvollen Quellen
Paper from responsible sources
FSC® C105338

If you have any concerns about our products,
you can contact us on
ProductSafety@springernature.com

In case Publisher is established outside the EU,
the EU authorized representative is:
Springer Nature Customer Service Center GmbH
Europaplatz 3, 69115 Heidelberg, Germany

Printed by Libri Plureos GmbH
in Hamburg, Germany